Robotic Hernia Surgery

Omar Yusef Kudsi
Editor

# Robotic Hernia Surgery

## A Comprehensive Illustrated Guide

Springer

*Editor*
Omar Yusef Kudsi
Department of Surgery
Good Samaritan Medical Center, Tufts University School of Medicine
Boston, MA
USA

ISBN 978-3-030-46666-4    ISBN 978-3-030-46667-1 (eBook)
https://doi.org/10.1007/978-3-030-46667-1



This Springer imprint is published by the registered company Springer Nature Switzerland AG
The registered company address is: Gewerbestrasse 11, 6330 Cham, Switzerland

*To my family, I share this publishing achievement with you with love and gratitude.*

# Preface

Technology is evolving at high speed, and just in the past decade surgeons started exploring the use of robotic technology in the field of hernia repair. Surgeons were able to take minimal invasive surgery further by exploring the layers of the abdominal wall and entertained the idea of placing the mesh outside the peritoneal cavity.

The main focus of this atlas is to demonstrate to surgeons how to perform extraperitoneal hernia repair, taking them through a wide variety of abdominal wall hernias. In the past few years, especially through videos and live case observations, surgeons were able to adopt more complex approaches in minimal invasive hernia repair.

This is the first dedicated atlas exploring each available extraperitoneal hernia repair. This is possible via a set of high-quality annotated images showing step-by-step guidance on how to perform the surgery.

Robotic extraperitoneal hernia procedures are considered great teaching procedures especially with a dual teaching console. Teachers and learners are faced with a new dilemma on how to teach and learn with robotic technology. This dilemma will be solved through curriculums, dry and wet laboratories, and wide-open access to robotic technology across institutions.

Surgeons are subject to a cognitive bias called "naïve realism" that gives them the status of "knowing" what's going on. As a result, they often fail to wonder what others are doing and they become less curious, saying "I have done this for many years and it has worked very well." Fortunately, that bubble of perception and isolation is being penetrated by digital media as well as high-speed internet and portable devices. I have to say, an exciting digital surgical era is ahead.

Boston, MA, USA — Omar Yusef Kudsi

# Contents

# Contributors


**Azure Adkins, MD, DABS** Alta Bates Summit Medical Center, Epic Care, Oakland, CA, USA

**Agustin Alvarez, MD** Division of Endocrine Surgery, DeWitt Daughtry Family Department of Surgery, Leonard M. Miller School of Medicine, University of Miami, Miami, FL, USA

**Jeffrey A. Blatnik, MD** Department of Surgery, Section of Minimally Invasive Surgery, Washington University School of Medicine, St. Louis, MO, USA

**Naseem Bou-Ayash, MD** Department of Surgery, Good Samaritan Medical Center, Brockton, MA, USA

**Alfredo M. Carbonell, DO** Department of Surgery, Prisma Health-Upstate, University of South Carolina School of Medicine, Greenville, Greenville, SC, USA

**Leandro Totti Cavazzola, MD, MSc, PhD** Department of Surgery, Universidade Federal do Rio Grande do Sul, Porto Alegre, Rio Grande do Sul, Brazil

General Surgery Section – Hospital de Clínicas de Porto Alegre, Porto Alegre, Rio Grande do Sul, Brazil

**Sora Ely, MD** Department of General Surgery, University of California San Francisco East Bay, Highland Hospital, Oakland, CA, USA

**Fahri Gokcal, MD** Department of Surgery, Good Samaritan Medical Center, Brockton, MA, USA

**Engin Hatipoglu, MD** Department of General Surgery, Cerrahpasa Faculty of Medicine, Istanbul University–Cerrahpasa/Kocamustafapasa, Istanbul, Turkey

**Omar Yusef Kudsi, MD, MBA, FACS** Department of Surgery, Good Samaritan Medical Center, Tufts University School of Medicine, Boston, MA, USA

**Rockson Liu, MD, FACS** Alta Bates Summit Medical Center, Epic Care, Oakland, CA, USA

**Flavio Malcher, MD, MSc** Montefiore Medical Center, Albert Einstein College of Medicine, Bronx, NY, USA

**David J. Morrell, MD** Department of Surgery, Penn State Health Milton S. Hershey Medical Center, Hershey, PA, USA

**Eduardo Parra-Davila, MD, FACS, FASCRS** Good Samaritan Medical Center, West Palm Beach, FL, USA

**Eric M. Pauli, MD, FACS, FASGE** Department of Surgery, Division of Minimally Invasive and Bariatric Surgery, Penn State Health Milton S. Hershey Medical Center, Hershey, PA, USA

**Ibnalwalid Saad, MD** Department of Surgery, Prisma Health-Upstate, University of South Carolina School of Medicine, Greenville, Greenville, SC, USA

**Hakan Seyit, MD** Department of Surgery, University of Health Sciences, Bakirkoy Dr. Sadi Konuk Training and Research Hospital, Bakirkoy, Istanbul, Turkey

**Hany Takla, MD, FACS** Department of General Surgery, Beth Israel Lahey Health, Winchester Hospital, Winchester, MA, USA

# Robotic Subxiphoid Hernia Repair: Transabdominal Preperitoneal (TAPP)

1

Engin Hatipoglu and Omar Yusef Kudsi

## Introduction

Subxiphoid hernias (SHs), are classified as M1 by the European Hernia Society [1]. They usually arise within 3 cm caudal to the ciphoid and are most often encountered as incisional hernias, after sternotomy incisions for cardiac surgery or subcostal incisions for hepatobiliary or foregut procedures [2]. Robotic transabdominal preperitoneal (TAPP) repair for SHs is analogous to the TAPP repair of centrally located hernias, which involves developing a large peritoneal pocket, reducing the hernia sac, closing the hernia defect, placing mesh with wide overlap, and closing the pocket [3]. These hernias' proximity to the costal margin and the diaphragm makes defect closure, adequate mesh overlap, and fixation difficult. Therefore, placing the mesh in the preperitoneal or retrorectus space helps to overcome these technical difficulties. Ensuring a large mesh overlap, even in the absence of mesh fixation, is key to successful robotic TAPP.

## Procedure: Illustrated Steps

Figures 1.1, 1.2, 1.3, 1.4, 1.5, 1.6, 1.7, 1.8, 1.9, 1.10, 1.11, 1.12, 1.13, 1.14, 1.15, 1.16, 1.17, 1.18, 1.19, 1.20, 1.21, 1.22, 1.23, and 1.24 illustrate the technical aspects of robotic TAPP repair of subxiphoid hernia (M1) repair.

E. Hatipoglu
Department of General Surgery, Cerrahpasa Faculty of Medicine, Istanbul University–Cerrahpasa/Kocamustafapasa, Istanbul, Turkey

O. Y. Kudsi (✉)
Department of Surgery, Good Samaritan Medical Center, Tufts University School of Medicine, Boston, MA, USA


O. Y. Kudsi (ed.), *Robotic Hernia Surgery*, https://doi.org/10.1007/978-3-030-46667-1_1

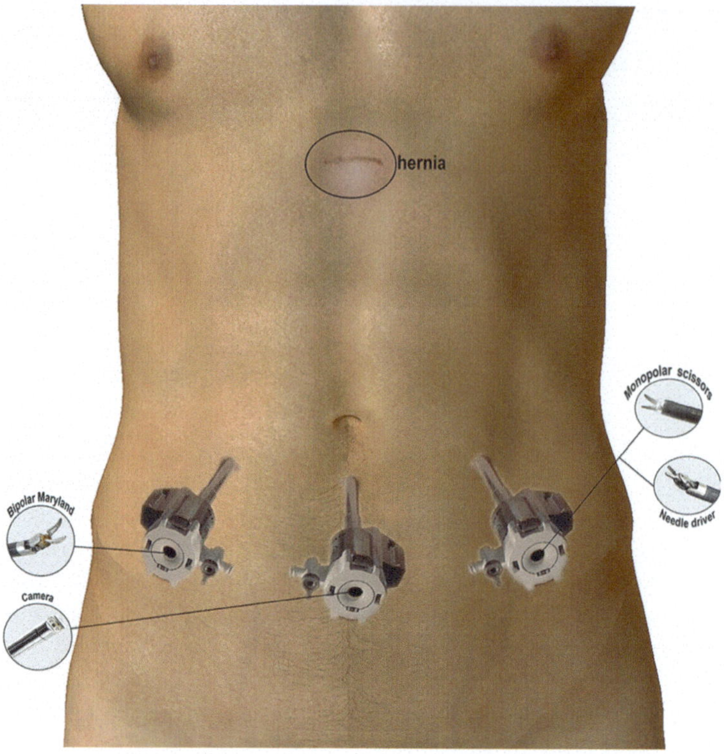


**Fig. 1.1** Trocar position in the robotic transabdominal preperitoneal (TAPP) repair for subxiphoid hernia (SH). Three trocars, one for the camera and the others for instruments, are usually sufficient. After docking of the patient-side cart, the EndoWrist® instruments (Intuitive Surgical Inc., Sunnyvale, CA, USA) are introduced to the abdominal cavity: a bipolar fenestrated Maryland (left arm), and a monopolar scissors (right arm), which is later switched with a needle-driver

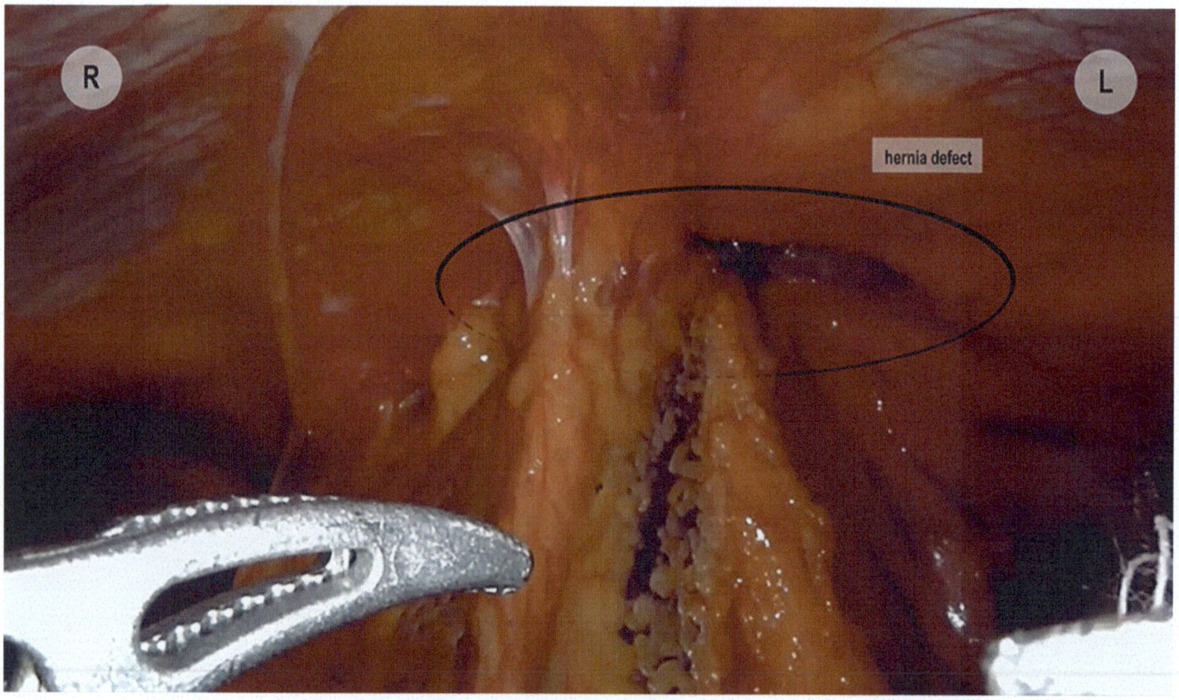


**Fig. 1.2** Initial exploration and adhesions between hernia and omentum

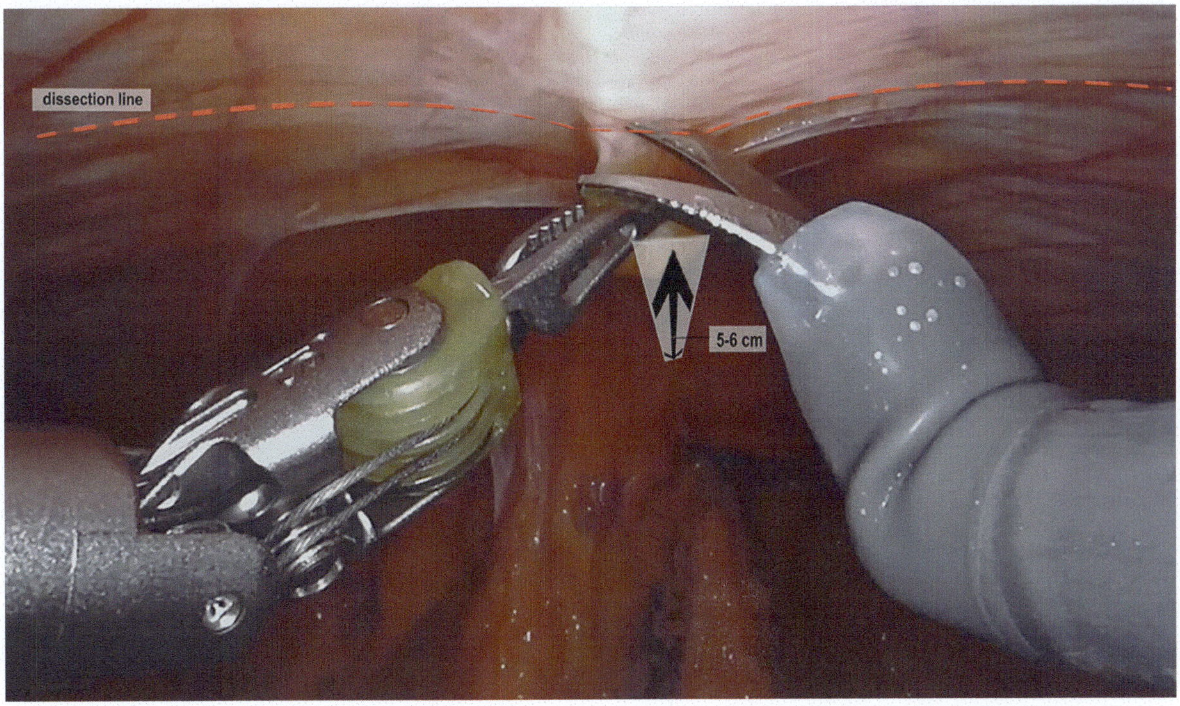


Fig. 1.3 With the use of monopolar scissors and a bipolar Maryland, the peritoneum is grasped and cut at least 5 cm from the defect on the side ipsilateral to the trocars

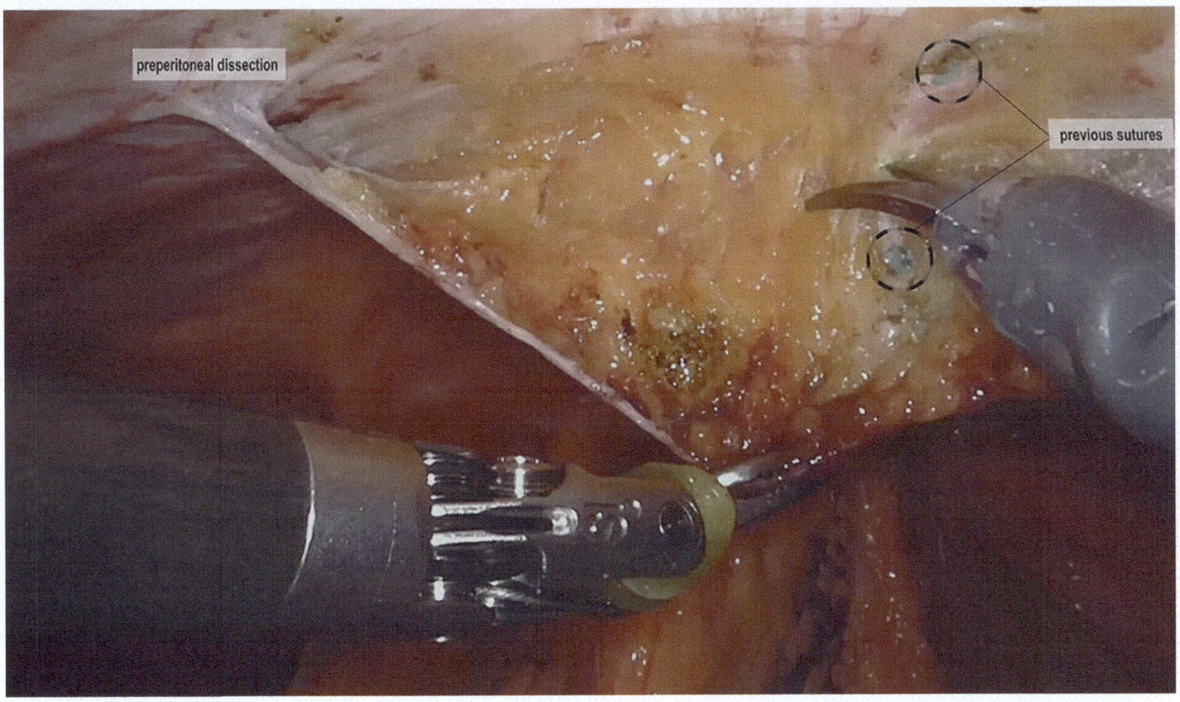


Fig. 1.4 Preperitoneal dissection is started by performing a peritoneal incision. The preperitoneal fat underlying the rectus fascia is revealed

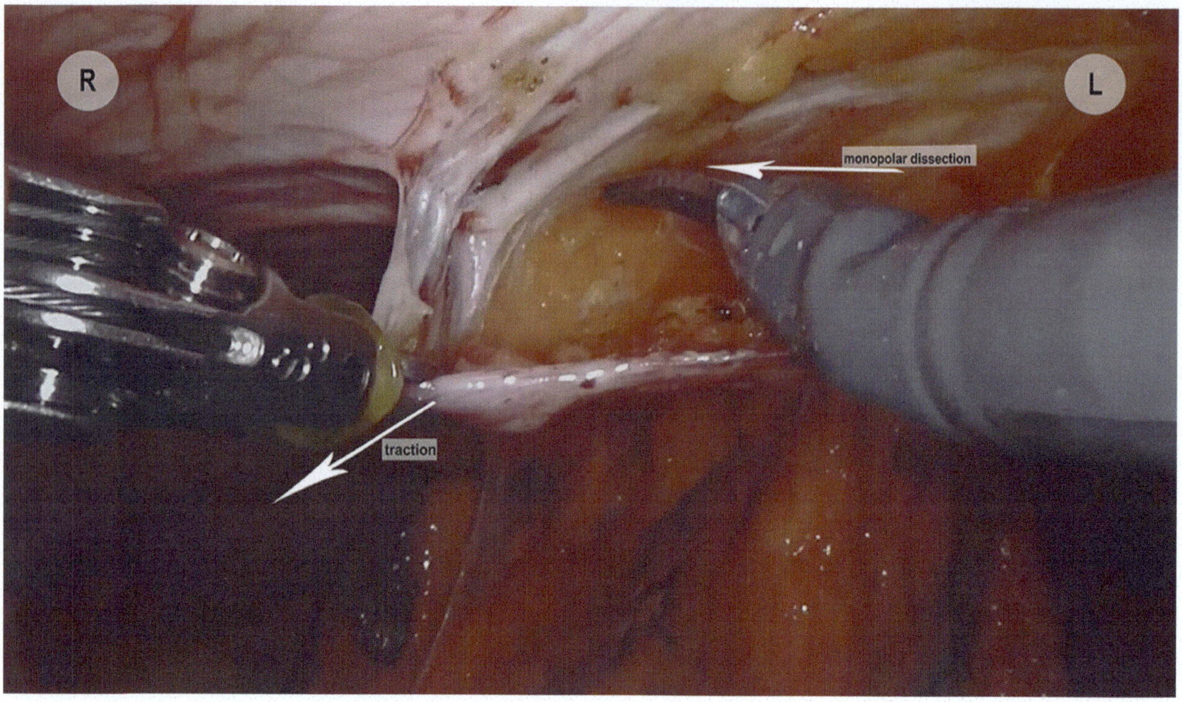


**Fig. 1.5** Throughout dissection of the peritoneal flap, gentle traction should be applied to avoid tearing of the peritoneum

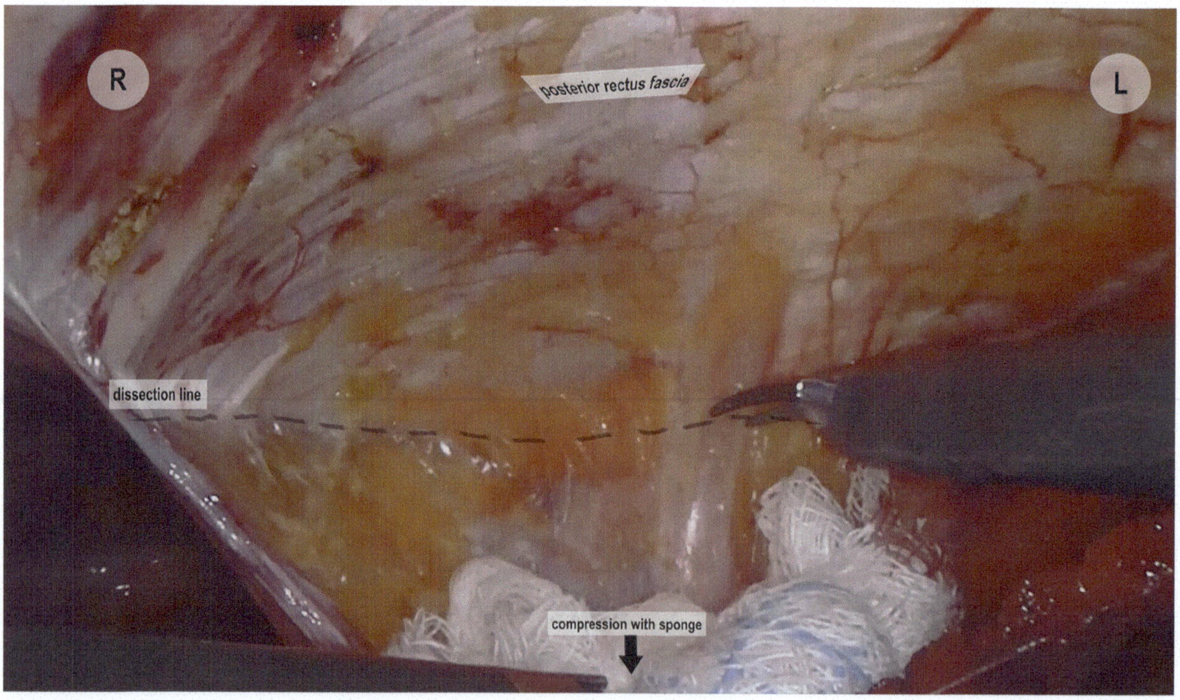


**Fig. 1.6** Gentle traction with a sponge (gauze) against the peritoneal flap helps in recognizing the correct dissection line, conrolling minimal bleeding, and minimizing the risk of peritoneal tears

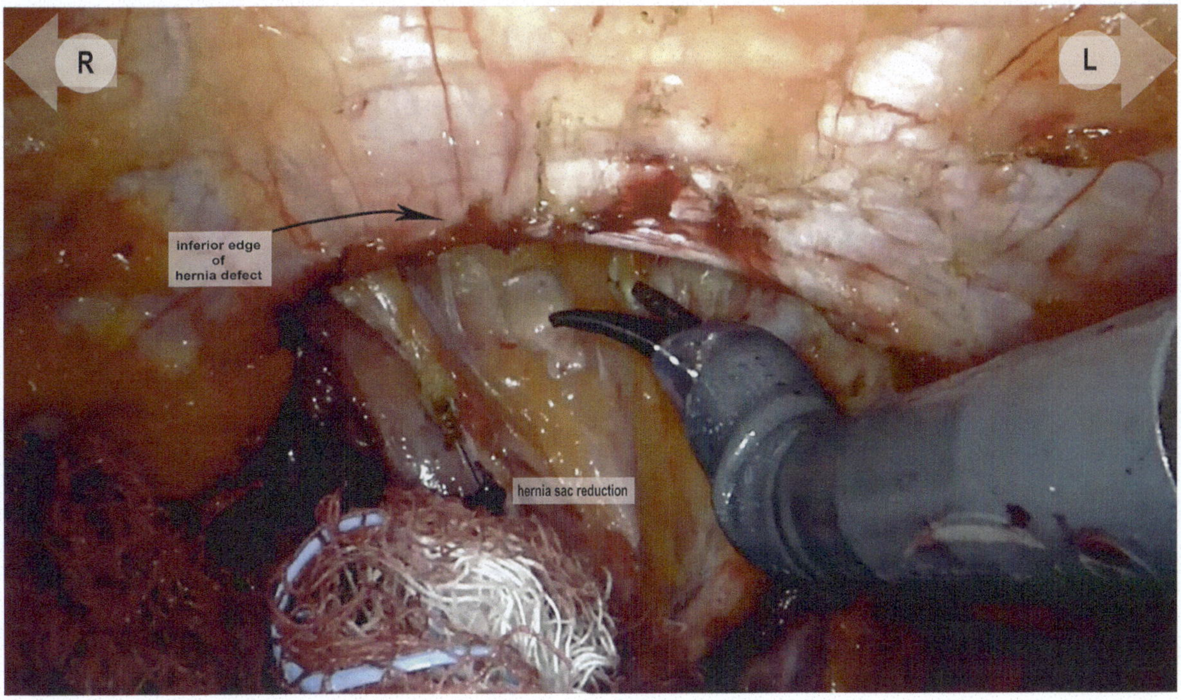


**Fig. 1.7** The peritoneum forms the inner most layer of the hernia sac, and may be difficult to separate without creating peritoneal tears. Any inadvertent tears should be repaired later using absorbable sutures

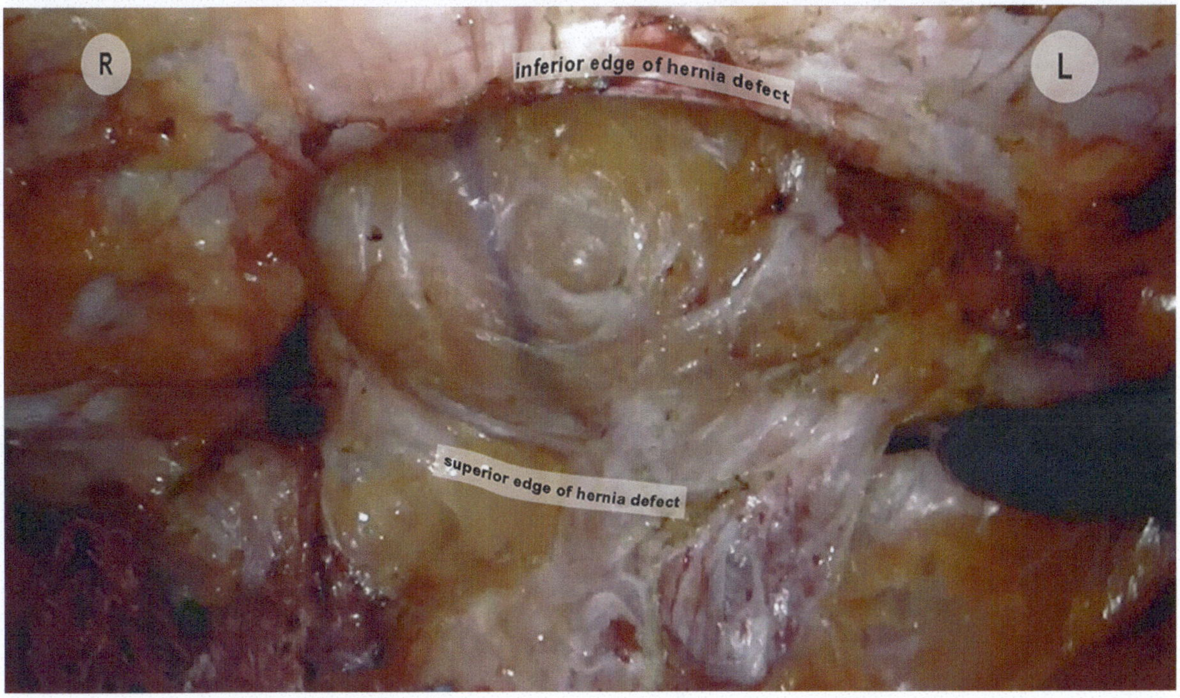


**Fig. 1.8** The hernia sac is reduced and dissection is continued superior to the defect, allowing for placement of an adequately sized mesh

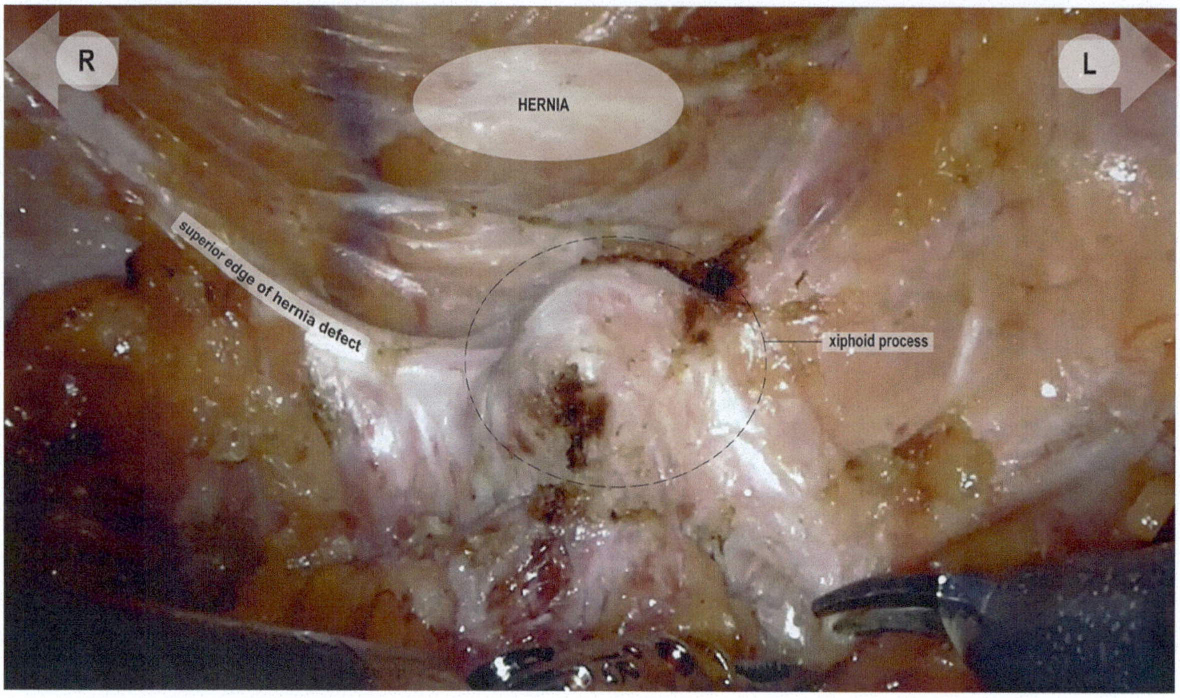


**Fig. 1.9** Retroxiphoid dissection is continued

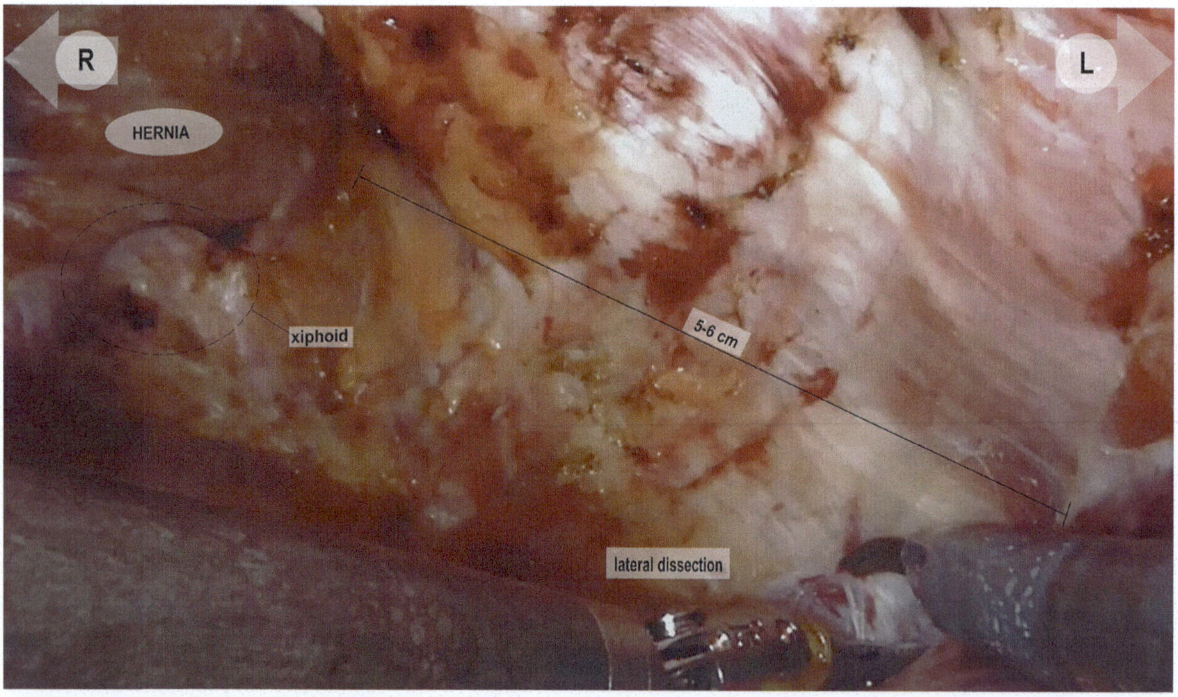


**Fig. 1.10** Left-sided lateral dissection. Preperitoneal dissection should extend 5 cm in all directions from the defect, at least, to provide adequate mesh placement

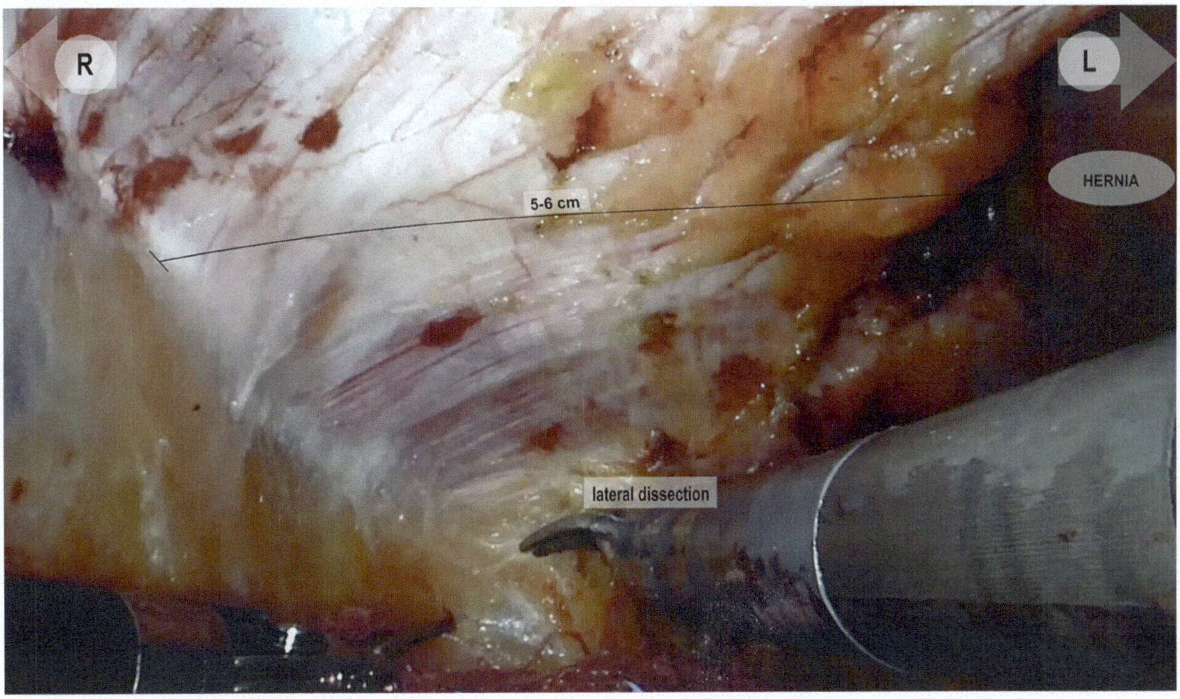


Fig. 1.11 Right-sided lateral dissection

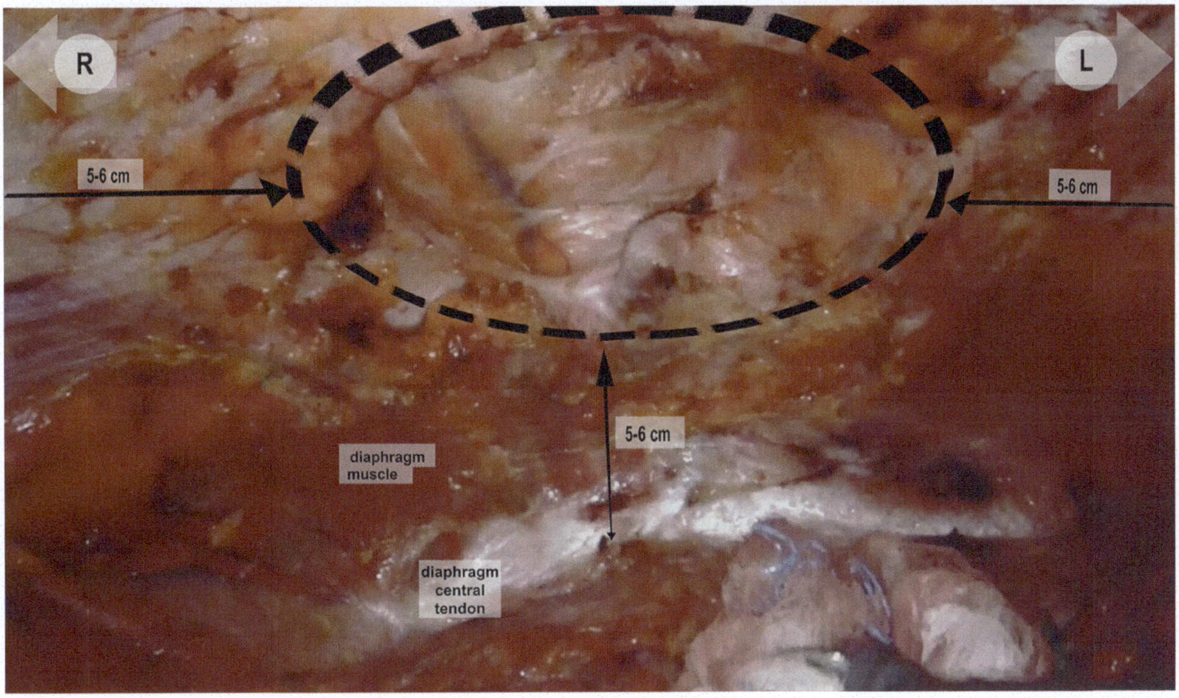


Fig. 1.12 The central tendon of the diaphragm is exposed during cephalic dissection

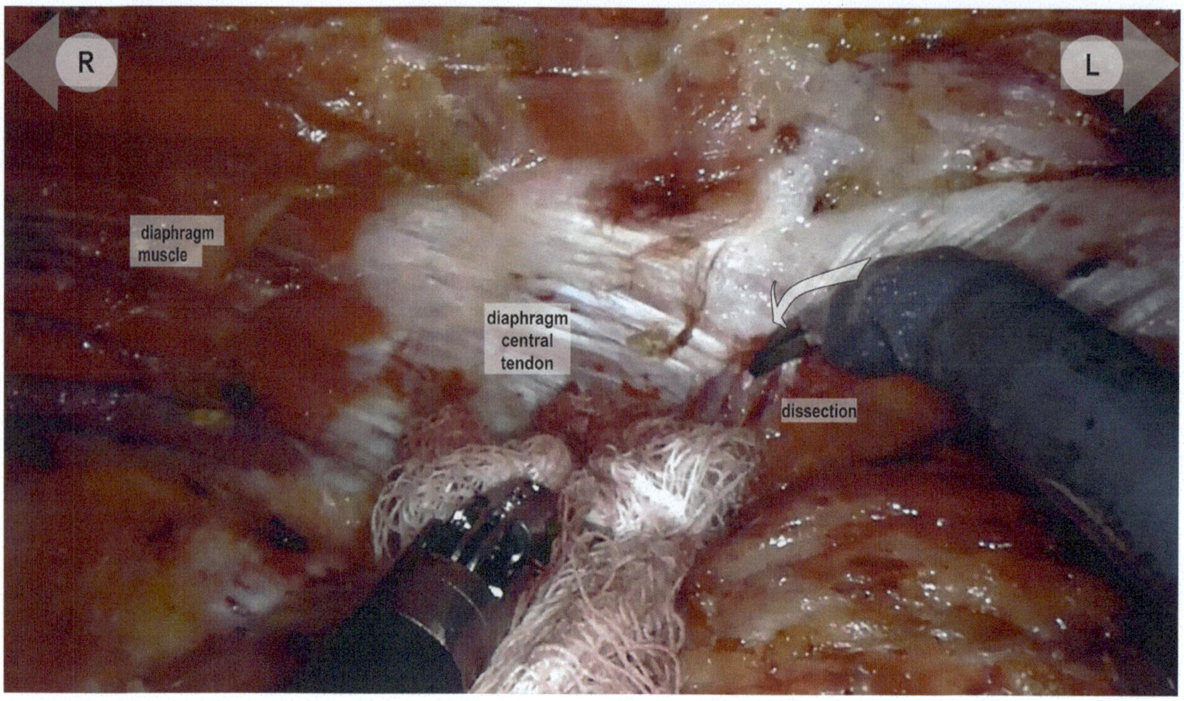


Fig. 1.13 The dissection is carried superiorly to allow for proper mesh overlap over the diaphragm, but care must be taken to avoid violation of the thoracic cavity, central tendon, or pericardium

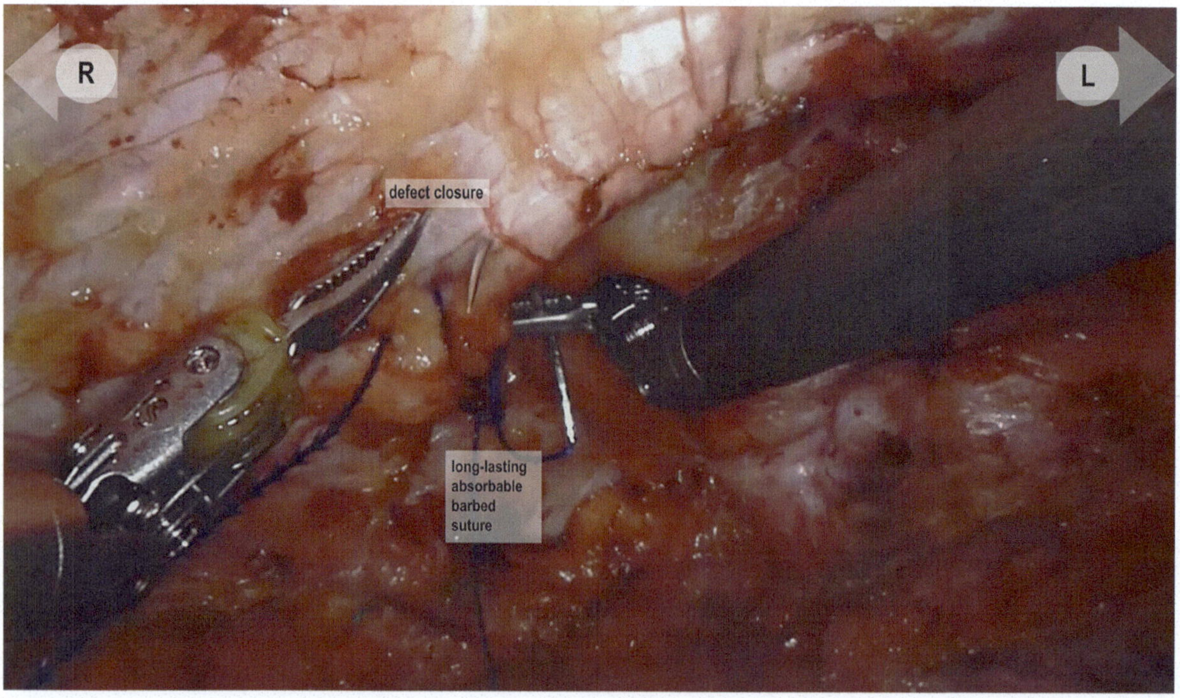


Fig. 1.14 Hernia defect closure is intended to restore abdominal wall anatomy and function, as well as prevent postoperative bulging. The choice of suture material may vary; we perform primary closure of the hernia defect by running a long-lasting, absorbable barbed suture

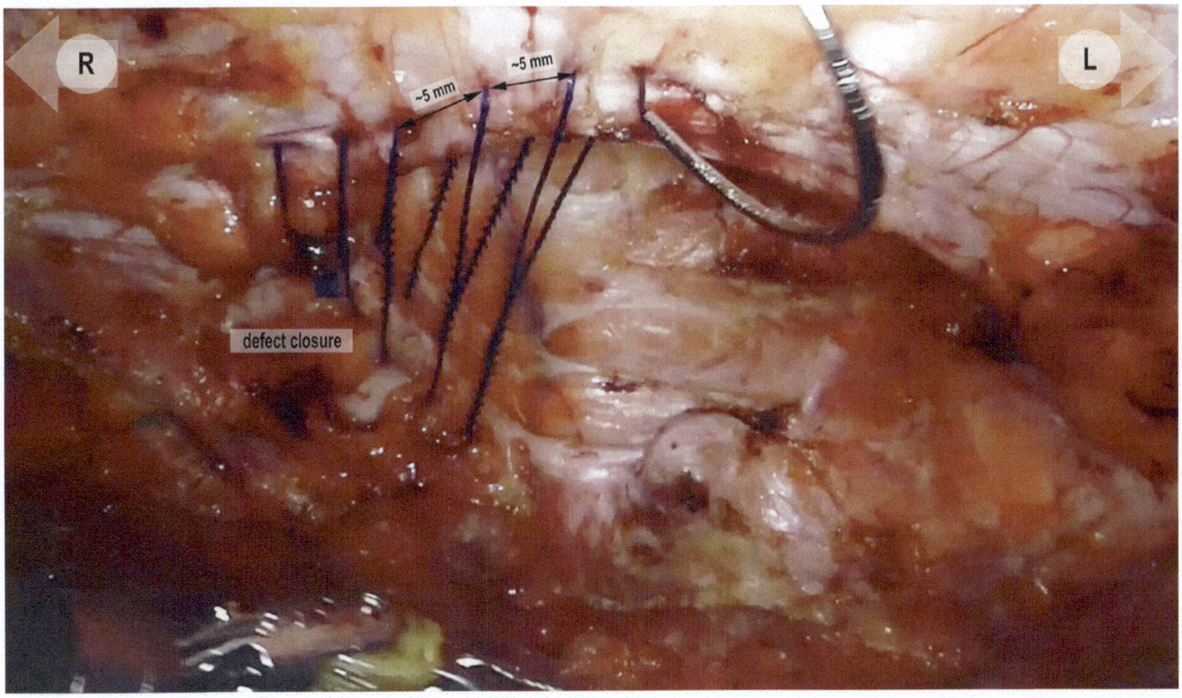


Fig. 1.15 While closing the hernia defect, we prefer to follow the same method used for laparotomy closure: the small-bite technique, taking 5–8 mm bites of fascia and placing stitches every 5 mm in a running fashion

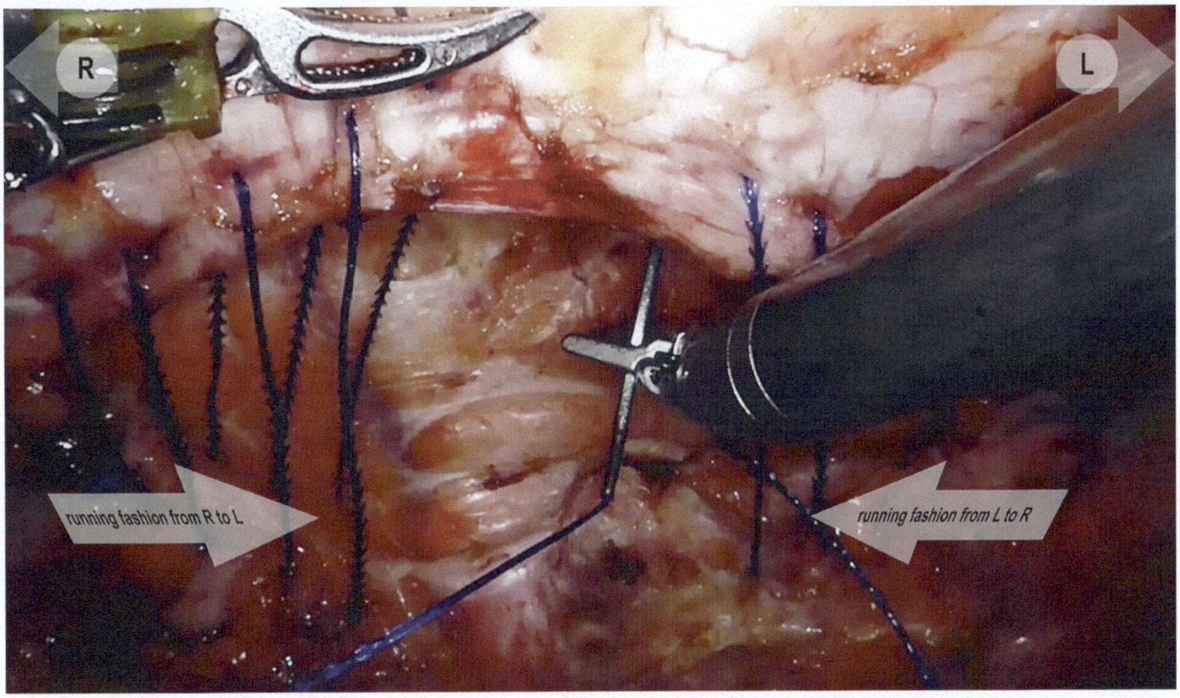


Fig. 1.16 Two separate sutures, starting from either end of the defect, meet in the middle of the defect

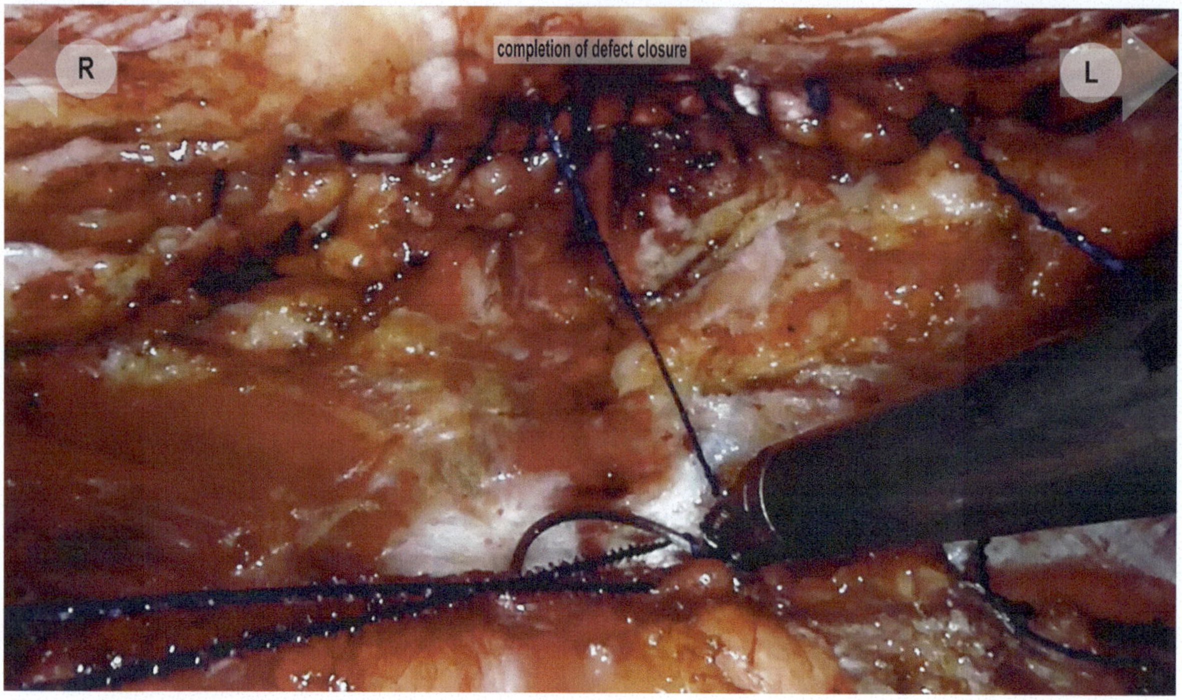


**Fig. 1.17** Before tightening the sutures to complete the defect closure, pneumoperitoneum is reduced to 6–8 mmHg and the anesthesiologist is asked to relax the patient's muscles

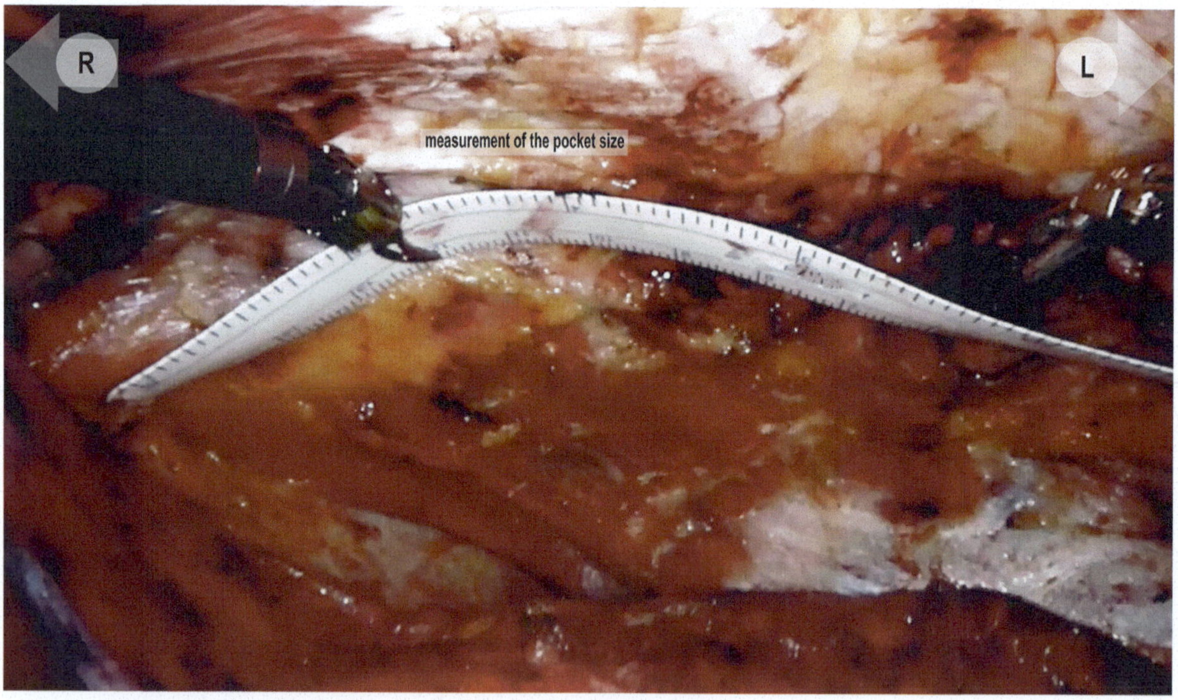


**Fig. 1.18** Pocket size is directly measured by a ruler, which is placed intraperitoneally

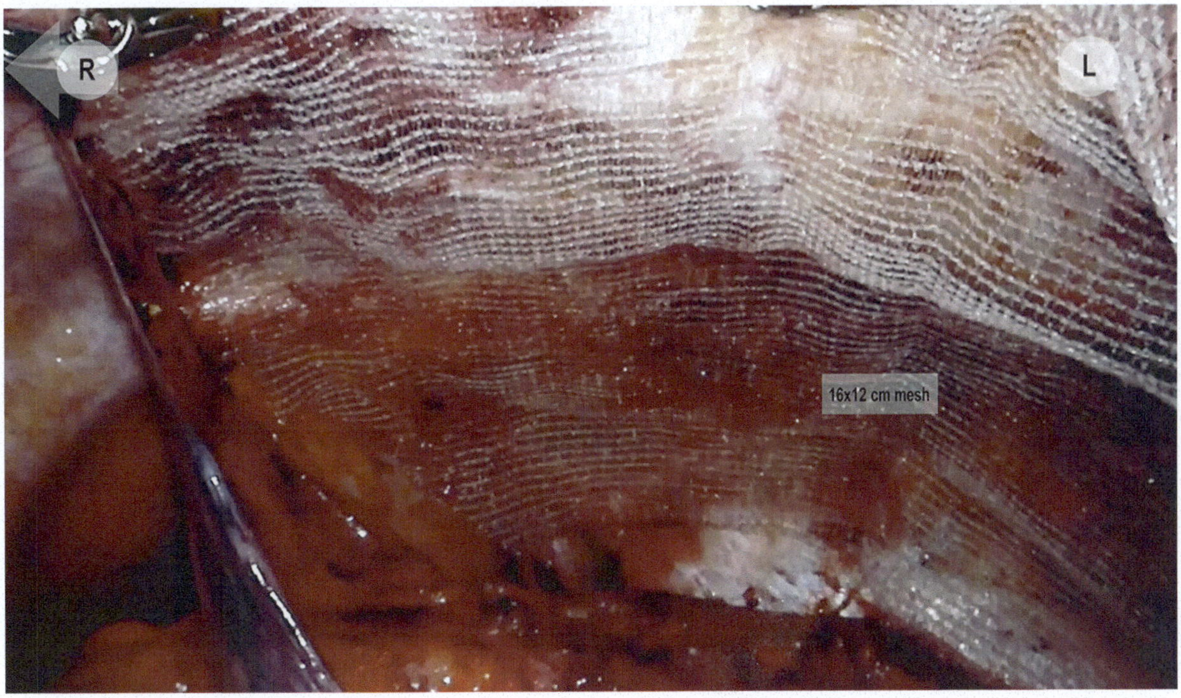


**Fig. 1.19** Adequate mesh coverage is paramount for successful repair and can be achieved with maintaining 5 cm of overalp in all directctions from the defect

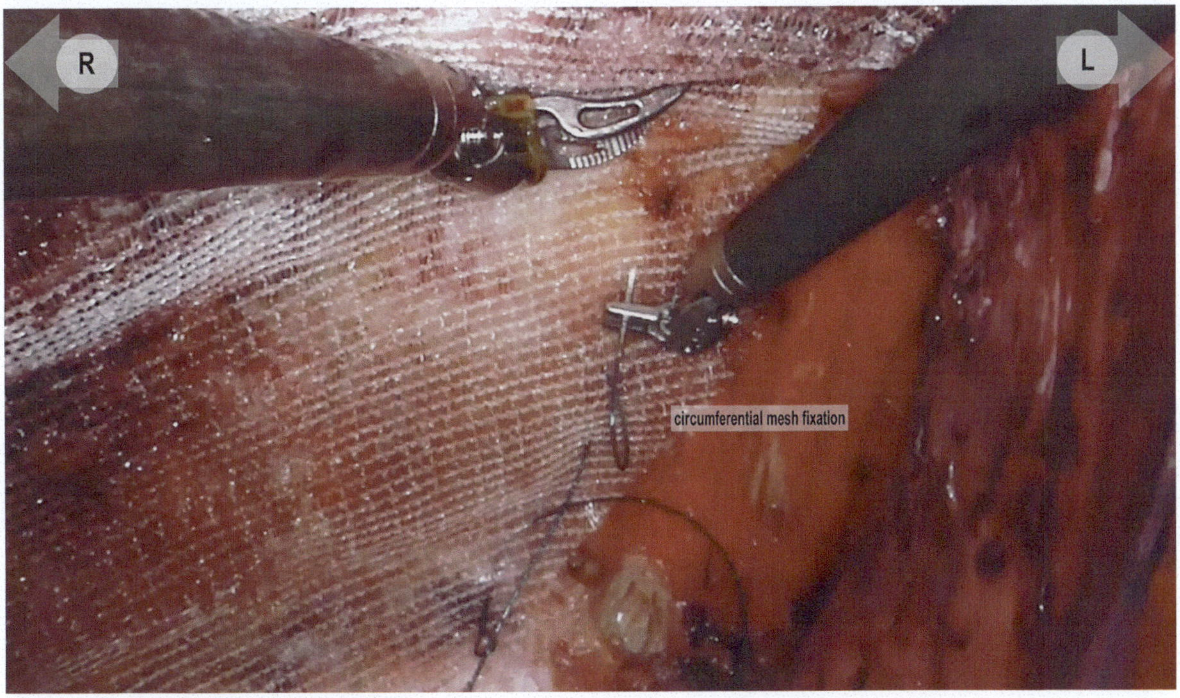


**Fig. 1.20** The mesh must be secured to prevent migration. A circumferential fascial suture technique with barbed absorbable sutures is used to secure the mesh to the posterior fascia

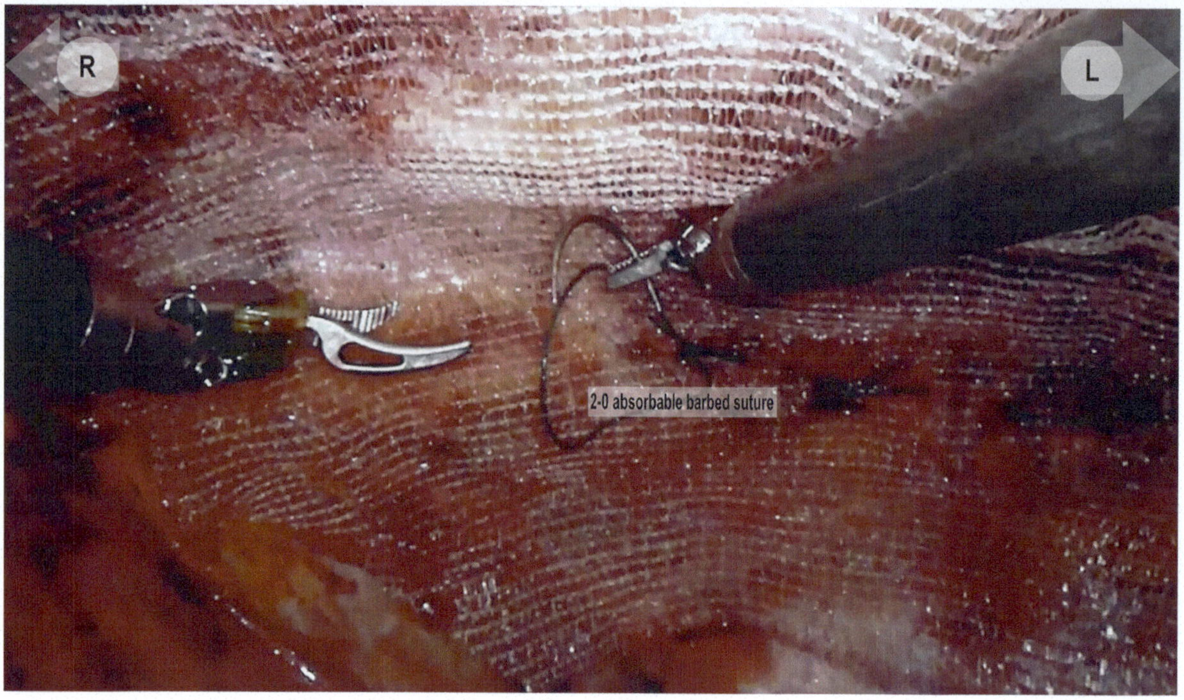


**Fig. 1.21** Fixating the mesh with deep sutures around the central tendon of the diaphragm can cause devastating cardiopulmonary injury. A superficial suture fixation method is preferred, away from the central tendon. The use of self-gripping mesh or glue fixation may also be helpful

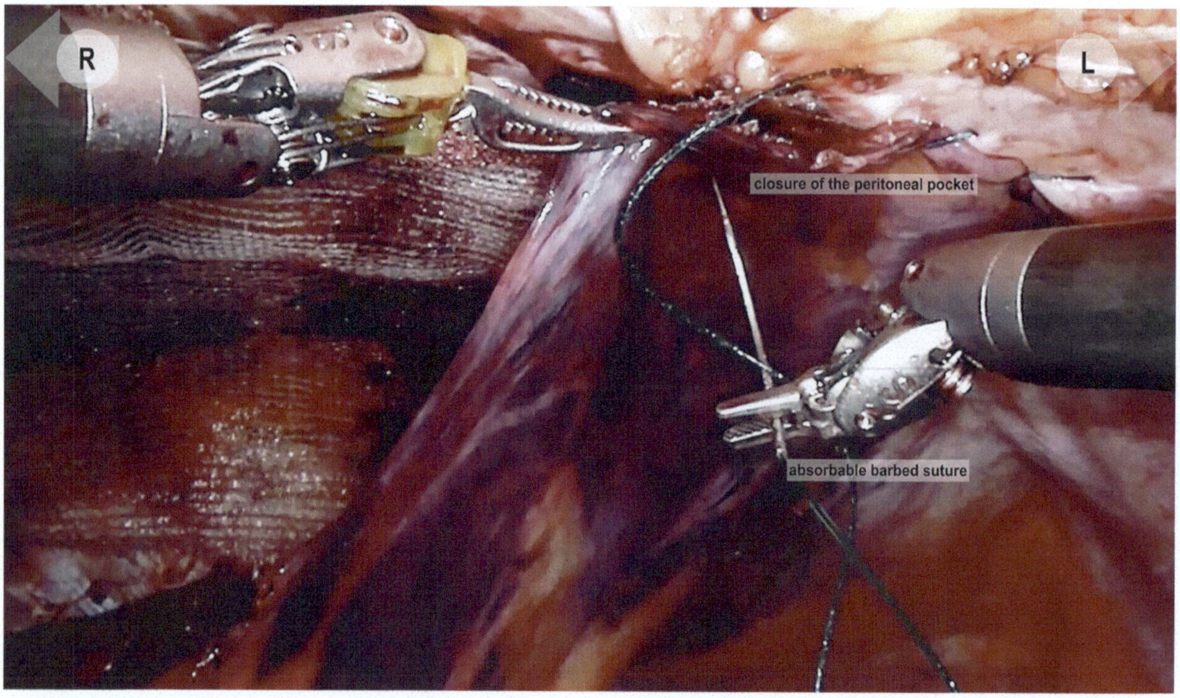


**Fig. 1.22** After mesh fixation and control of bleeding, the next step is closing the peritoneal flap with a rapidly absorbable barbed sture, using a bottom-to-top apprach

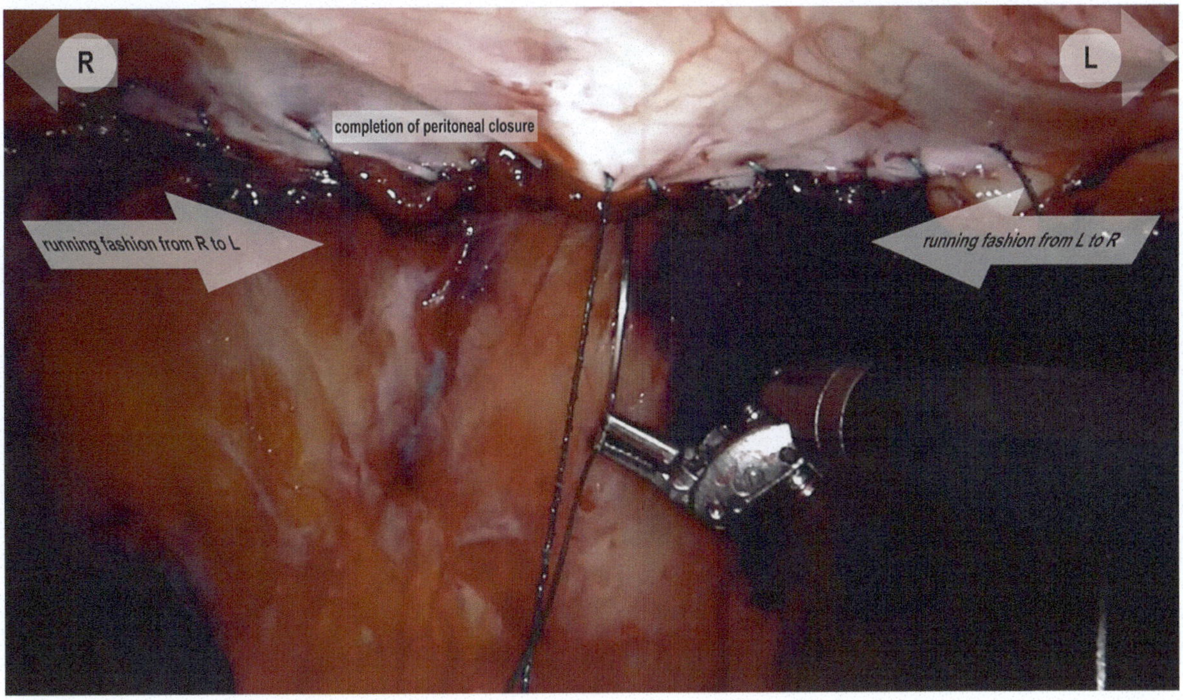


**Fig. 1.23** The risk of intraparietal hernia formation is minimized by using a running short stitch. At the end of the procedure, the peritoneal flap should be examined to ensure that intra-abdominal structures do not come in contact with exposed mesh

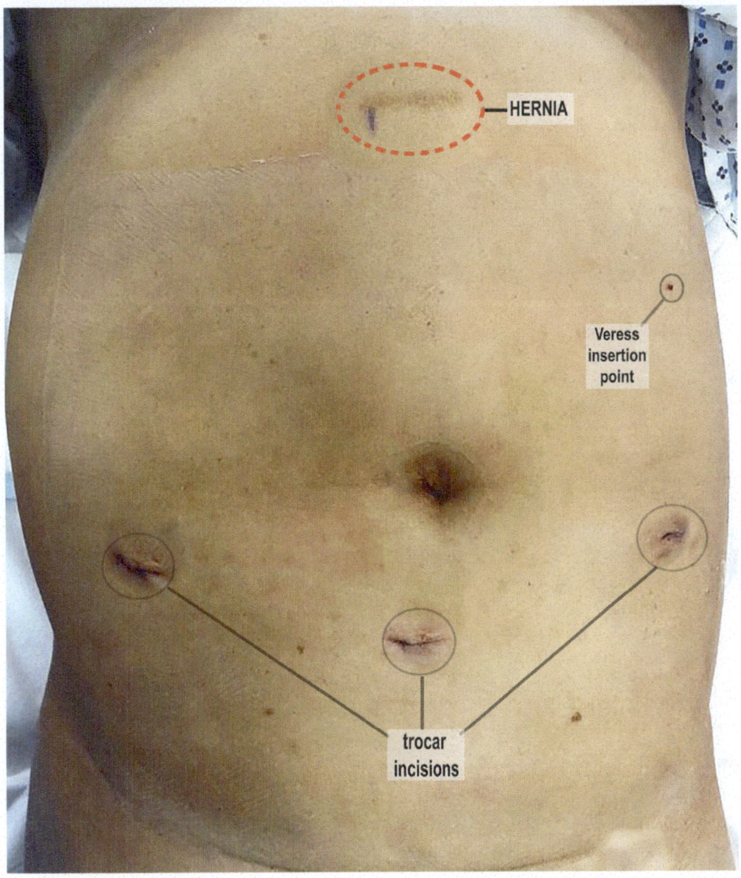


**Fig. 1.24** The trocars are removed and the pneumoperitoneum is released. Long-acting local anesthetic agent is injected at the trocar sites for management of postoperative pain. Skin incisions are sutured

## References

1. Muysoms FE, Miserez M, Berrevoet F, Campanelli G, Champault GG, Chelala E, et al. Classification of primary and incisional abdominal wall hernias. Hernia. 2009;13:407–14.
2. Hope WW, Hooks WB 3rd. Atypical hernias: suprapubic, subxiphoid, and flank. Surg Clin North Am. 2013;93:1135–62.
3. Ballecer C, Parra-Davila E. Robotic ventral hernia repair. In: Novitsky YW, editor. Hernia surgery: current principles. Cham: Springer; 2016. p. 273–86.

# Robotic Epigastric Hernia Repair: Totally Extraperitoneal (TEP)

2

Hany Takla

## Introduction

According to the European Hernia Society, an M2 (primary epigastric hernia) is an abdominal wall hernia located in the area between 3 cm below the xiphoid and 3 cm above the umbilicus. More commonly, however, epigastric hernias coexist with other midline hernias, including umbilical hernias. Moreover, epigastric hernias are usually seen in the context of rectus muscle diastasis, a condition that commonly affects the abdominal wall in middle-aged women after multiple pregnancies, as well as patients who are overweight or obese.

Robotic-assisted enhanced-view totally extraperitoneal (eTEP) epigastric hernia repair should be one of the tools in the surgeon's armamentarium. It has several potential advantages:

- It adequately exposes the retromuscular space, including the midline, which can commonly harbor multiple small defects containing herniated pre-peritoneal fat.
- It allows repair of multiple midline defects as well as rectus muscle diastasis, in theory restoring the functionality of the abdominal wall.
- It allows mesh placement outside of the peritoneal cavity, which allows better mesh incorporation over time and decreases the likelihood of intraperitoneal adhesions.

For these reasons, the overall interest in the eTEP approach and its adoption for repair of various ventral and incisional hernias has been increasing. In addition, it gives access to the fibers of the transversus abdominus muscle, allowing a transversus abdominis release, which is sometimes needed for larger hernias (typically for defects more than 8 cm in width). Also, separating the posterior sheath from the rectus muscle complex theoretically allows closure of both the posterior sheath and the linea alba without undue tension.

## Procedure: Illustrated Steps

Figures 2.1, 2.2, 2.3, 2.4, 2.5, 2.6, 2.7, 2.8, 2.9, 2.10, 2.11, 2.12, 2.13, 2.14, 2.15, 2.16, 2.17, 2.18, 2.19, 2.20, 2.21, 2.22, 2.23, 2.24, 2.25, 2.26, 2.27, 2.28, 2.29, 2.30, 2.31, and 2.32 illustrate our approach for eTEP epigastric hernia repair, including access, exposure, and tips for efficient repair.

H. Takla (✉)
Department of General Surgery, Beth Israel Lahey Health, Winchester Hospital, Winchester, MA, USA


O. Y. Kudsi (ed.), *Robotic Hernia Surgery*, https://doi.org/10.1007/978-3-030-46667-1_2

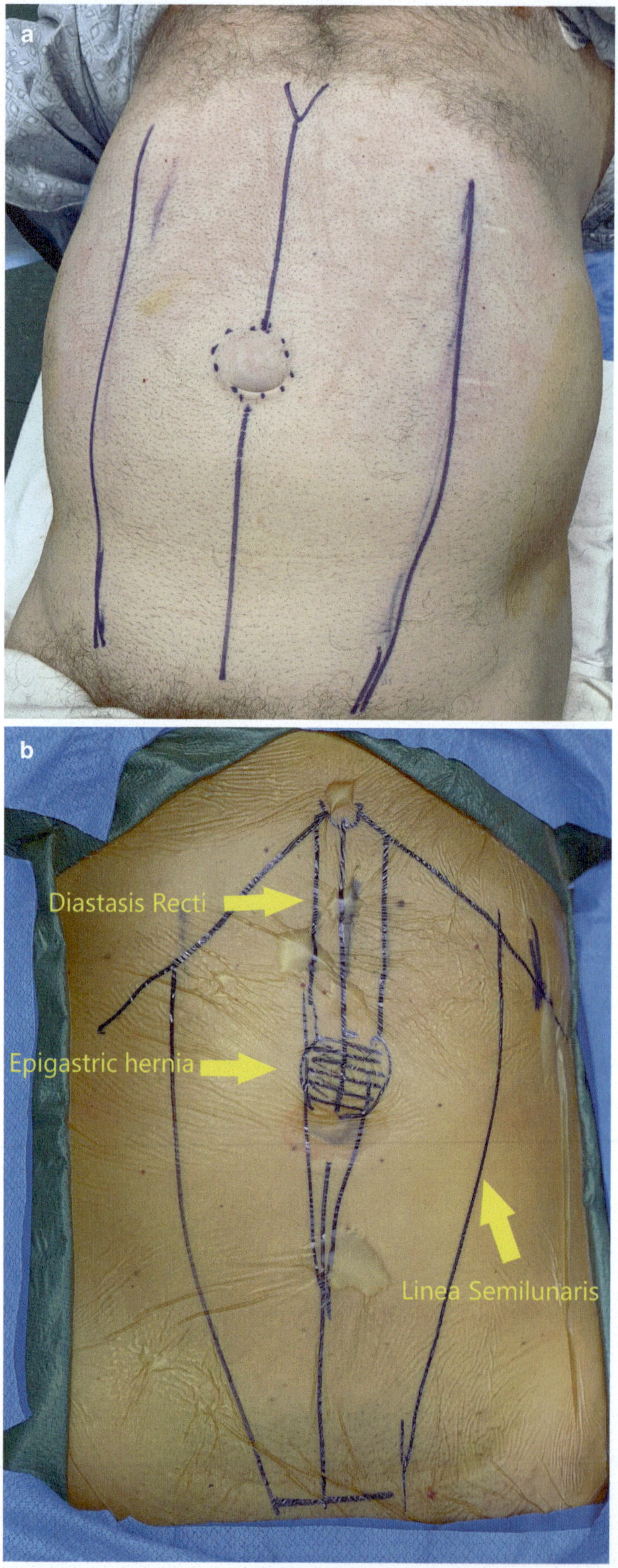


**Fig. 2.1** (**a**) Landmarks marked using ultrasound (US) after a transverse abdominis plane (TAP) block is done by Anesthesia. (**b**) Bilateral linea semilunaris are marked and the span of the rectus muscle bilaterally is measured to ensure adequate space for eTEP. (Typically 8 cm or more is considered adequate.) Midline and diastasis are also visible and can be measured by US

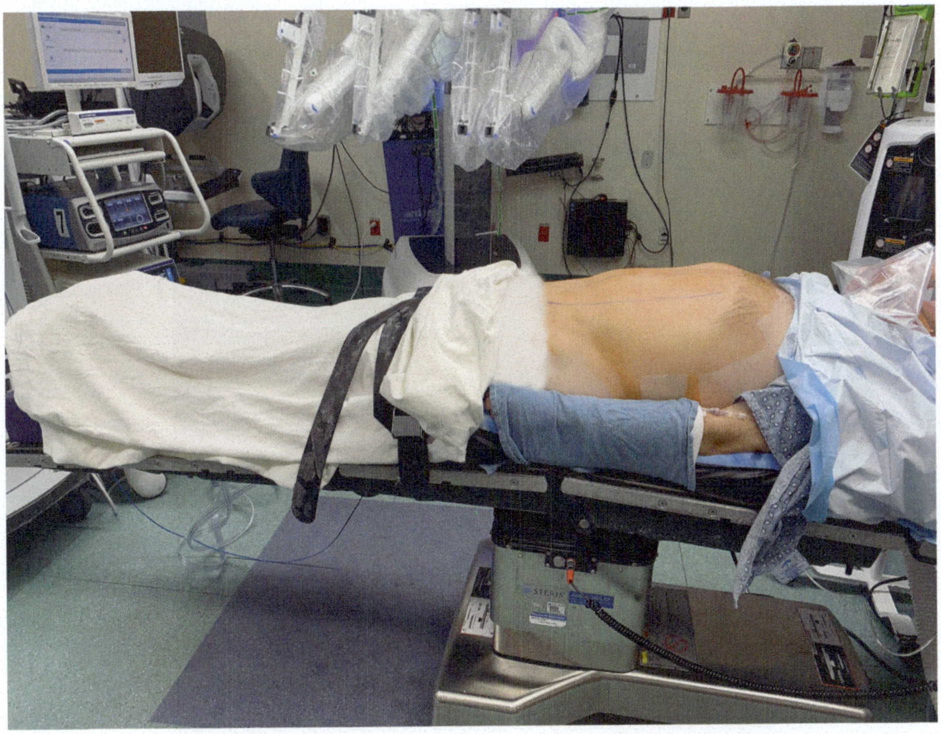

**Fig. 2.2** Patient positioning, with at least the left arm tucked (or trocar side) to allow more mobility for the arms, especially the camera. The bed is slightly flexed, and the patient's face is protected

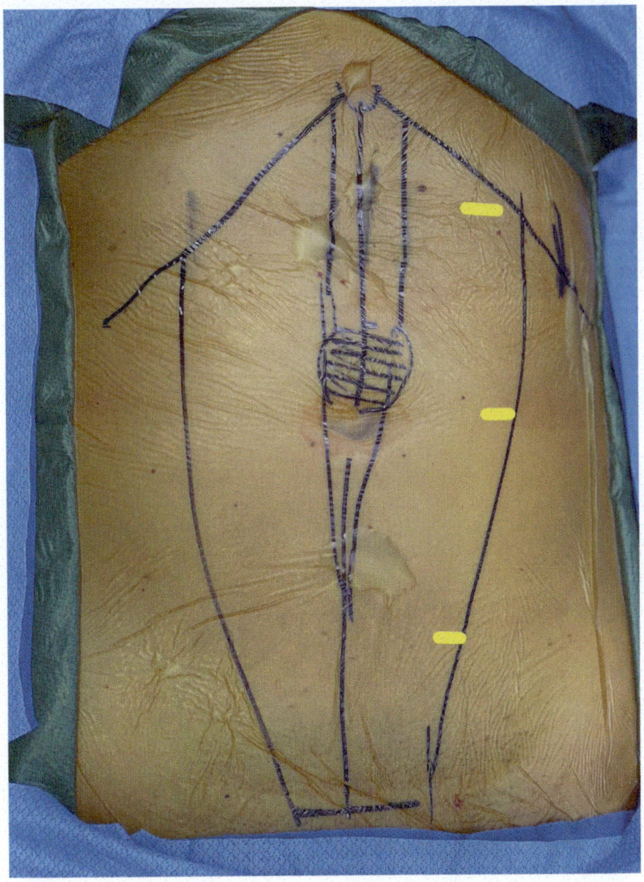

**Fig. 2.3** After draping, the anatomical landmarks are re-marked on the surface

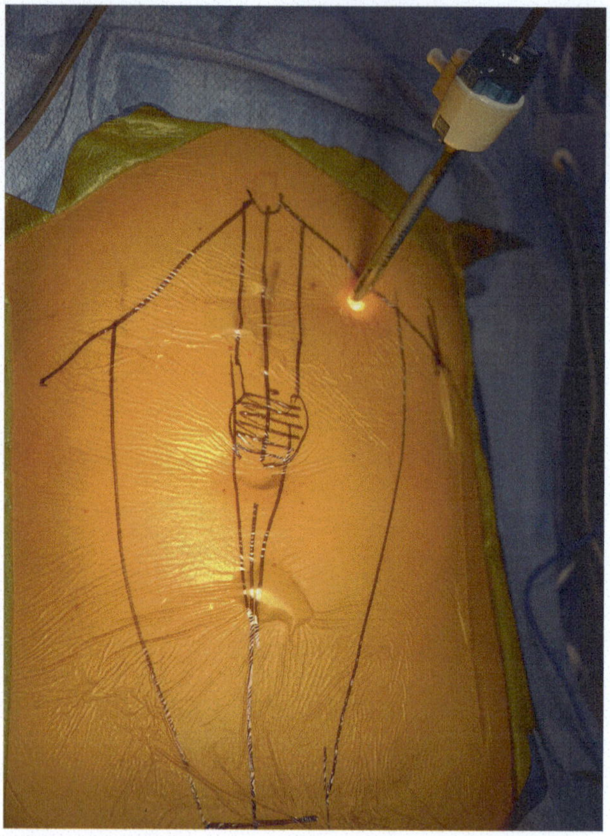

Fig. 2.4 Initial entry in the left upper quadrant is achieved using an Optiview technique, with insufflation

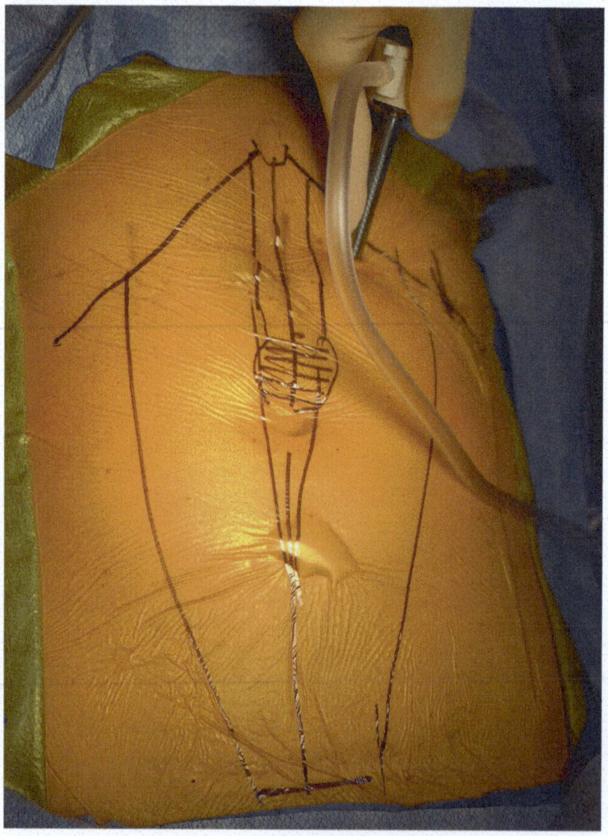

Fig. 2.5 Continue perpendicular until the view seen in Fig. 2.6 is achieved

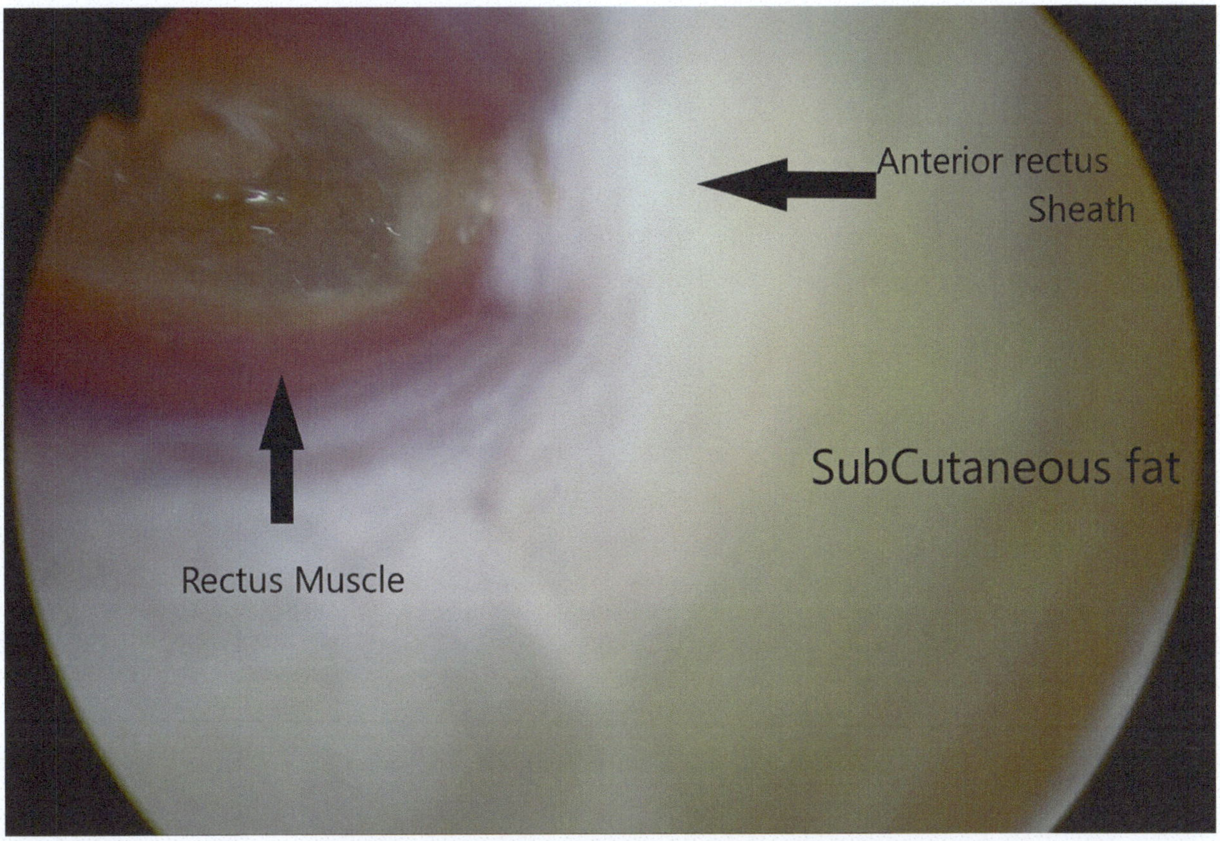


**Fig. 2.6** View after rectus muscle is traversed; the posterior rectus sheath is seen in the background

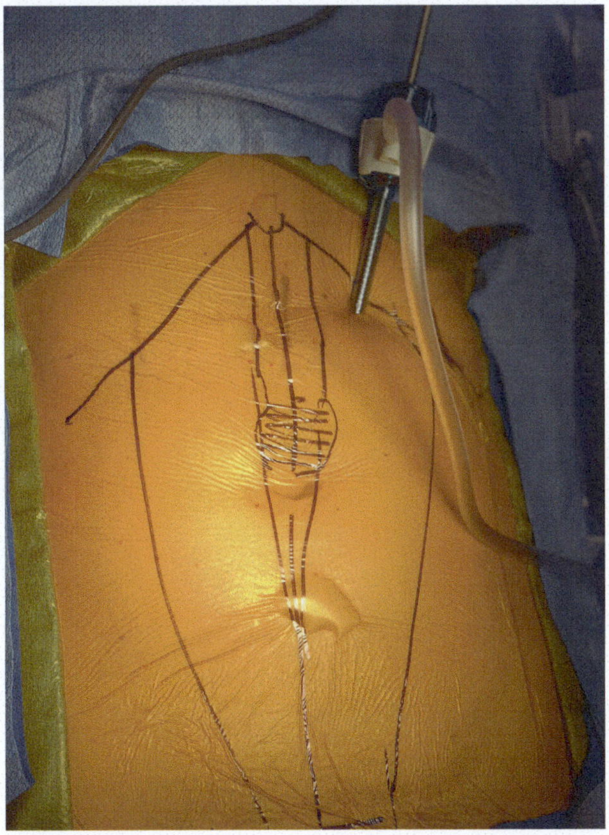

**Fig. 2.7** The trajectory of the port is changed to be parallel to the abdominal wall, and it is advanced in the retromuscular space. A chance is given for $CO_2$ to do some of the dissection

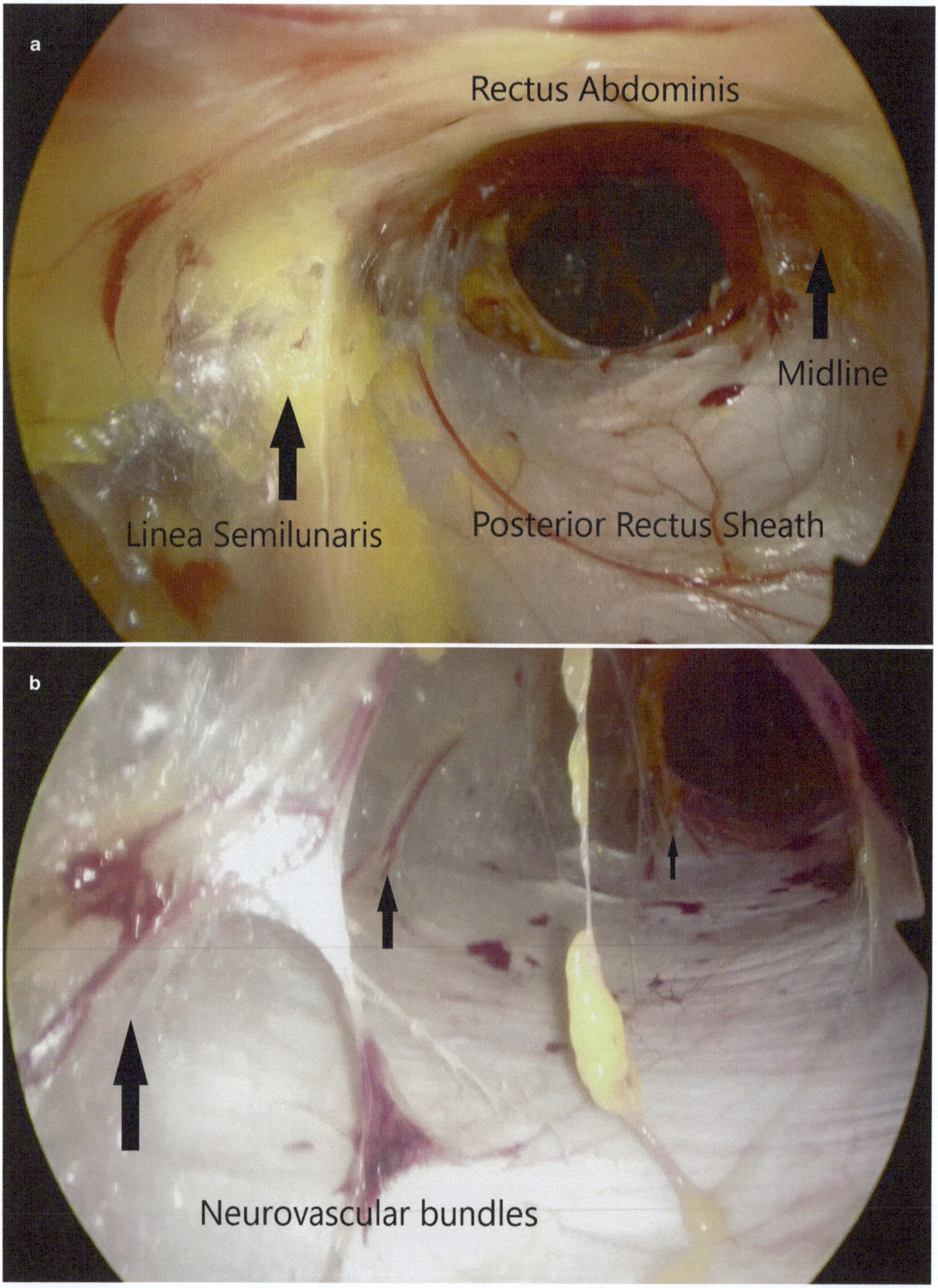


**Fig. 2.8** (**a**) Using blunt dissection with the camera tip, the retromuscular space can be developed to allow for additional port placement. The limits of the space are seen in this picture. (**b**) Neurovascular bundles are preserved

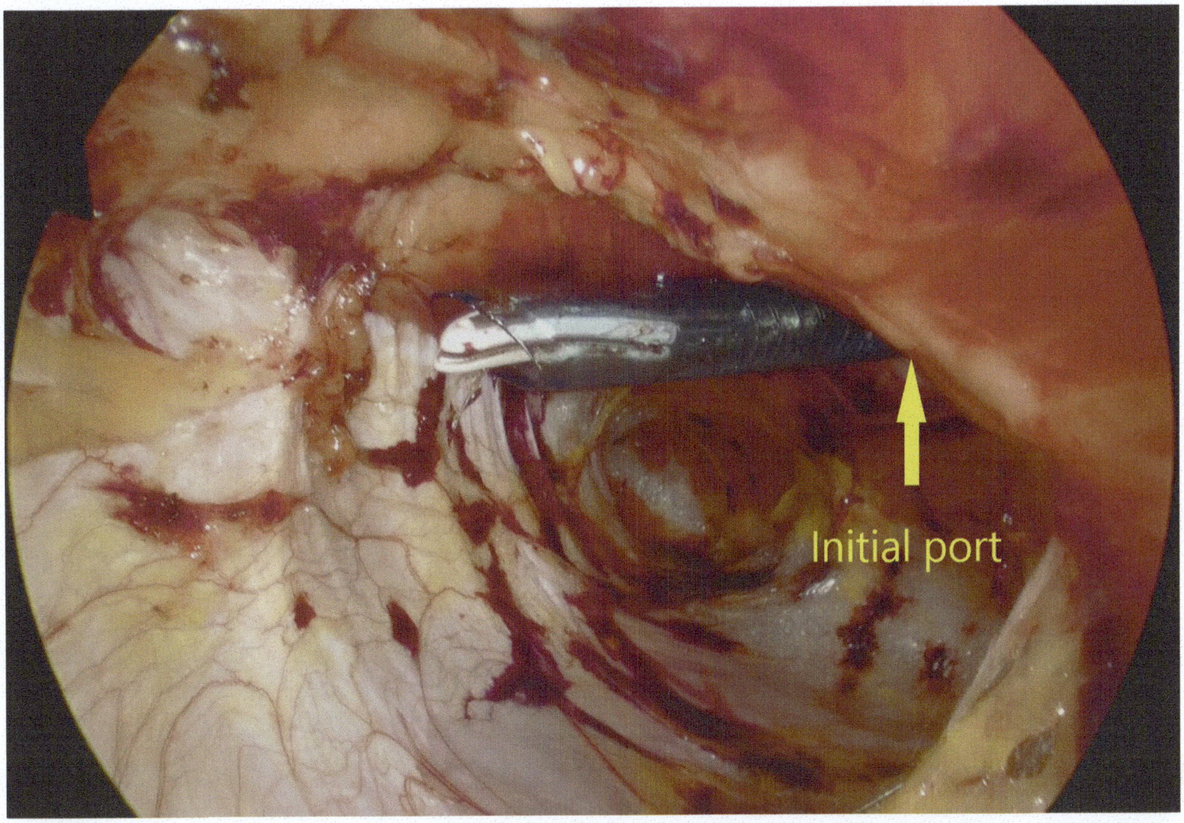


**Fig. 2.9** Additional ports are placed sequentially as the retromuscular space is developed. Laparoscopic instruments can be used in the early learning curve

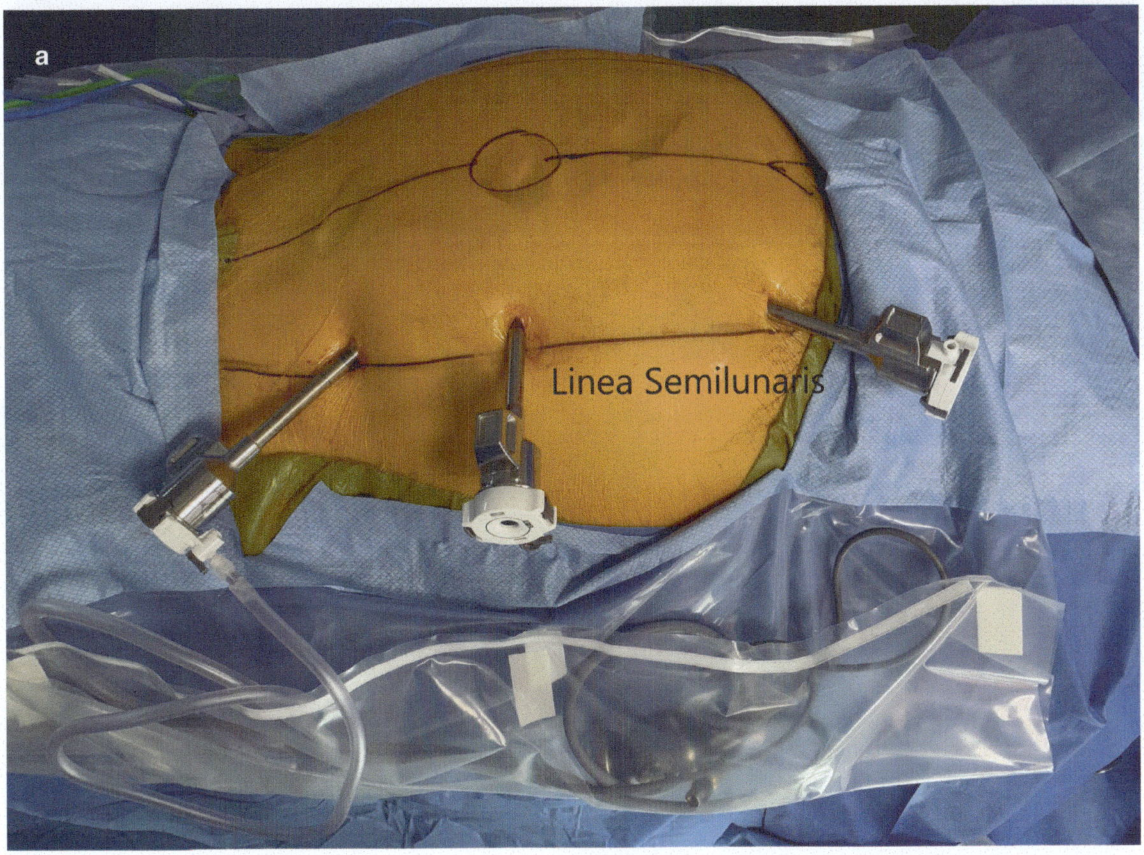


**Fig. 2.10** (**a**) Port placement shown in relation to the linea semilunaris. (**b**) We prefer to use a bariatric-length trocar in the lower quadrant to give more mobility and avoid collisions with the patient's hip or thigh. (**c**) Another view for port placement prior to robot docking

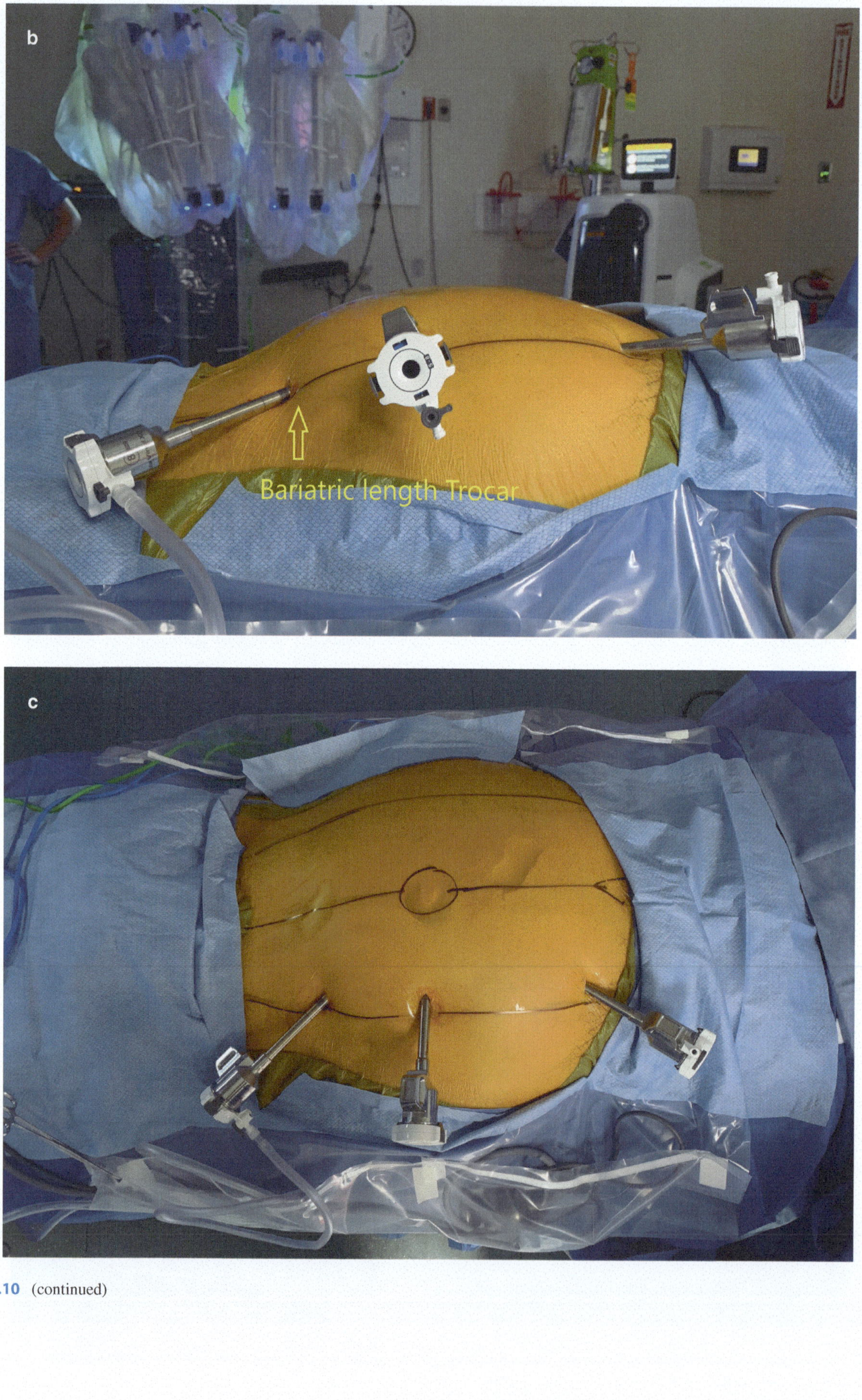


**Fig. 2.10** (continued)

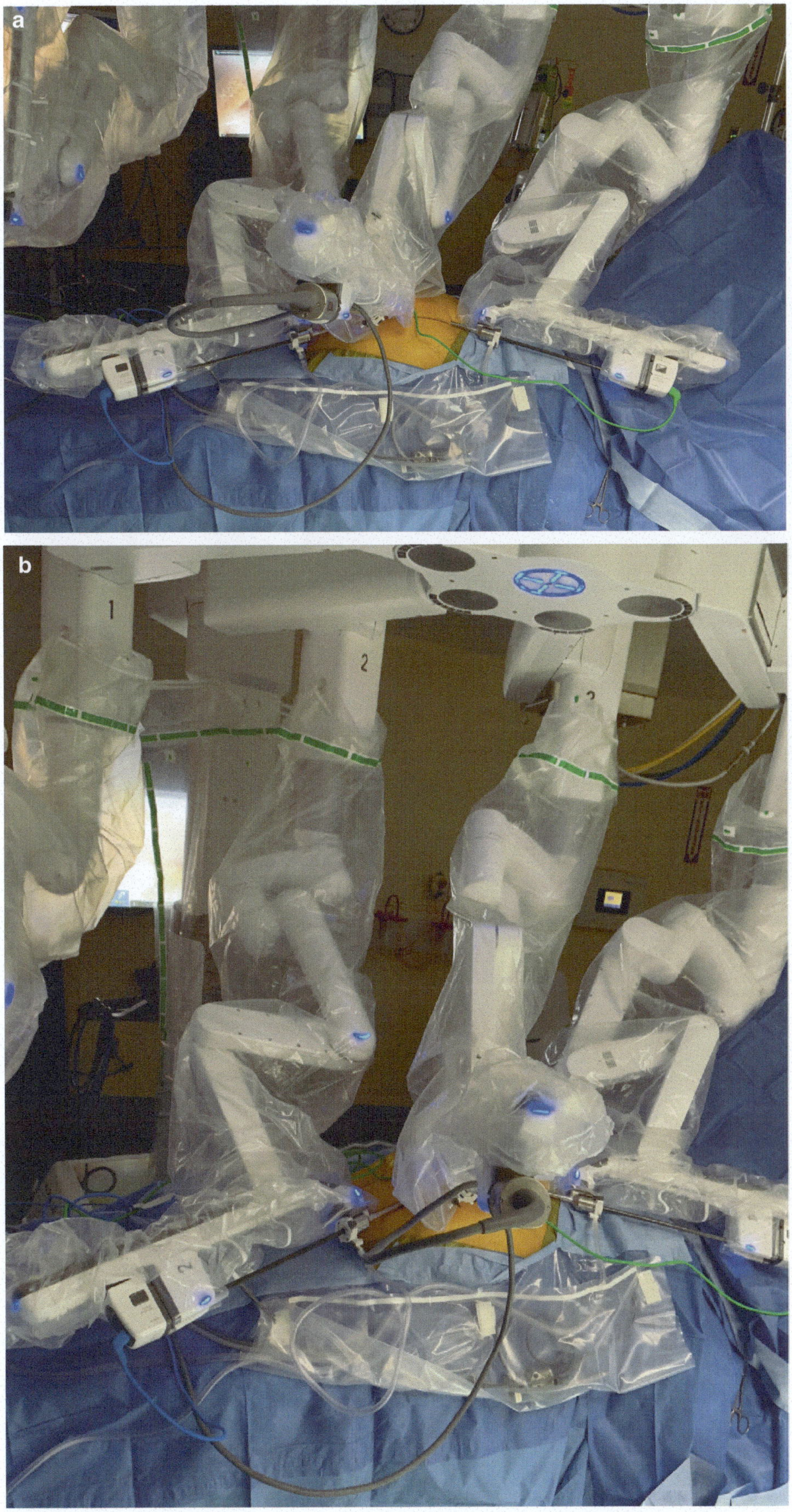

**Fig. 2.11** (**a**) Robot docking. (**b**) and (**c**) When introducing the instruments and due to limited space in an ipsilateral retrorectus space, the instruments must be advanced parallel to the midline rather than perpendicular

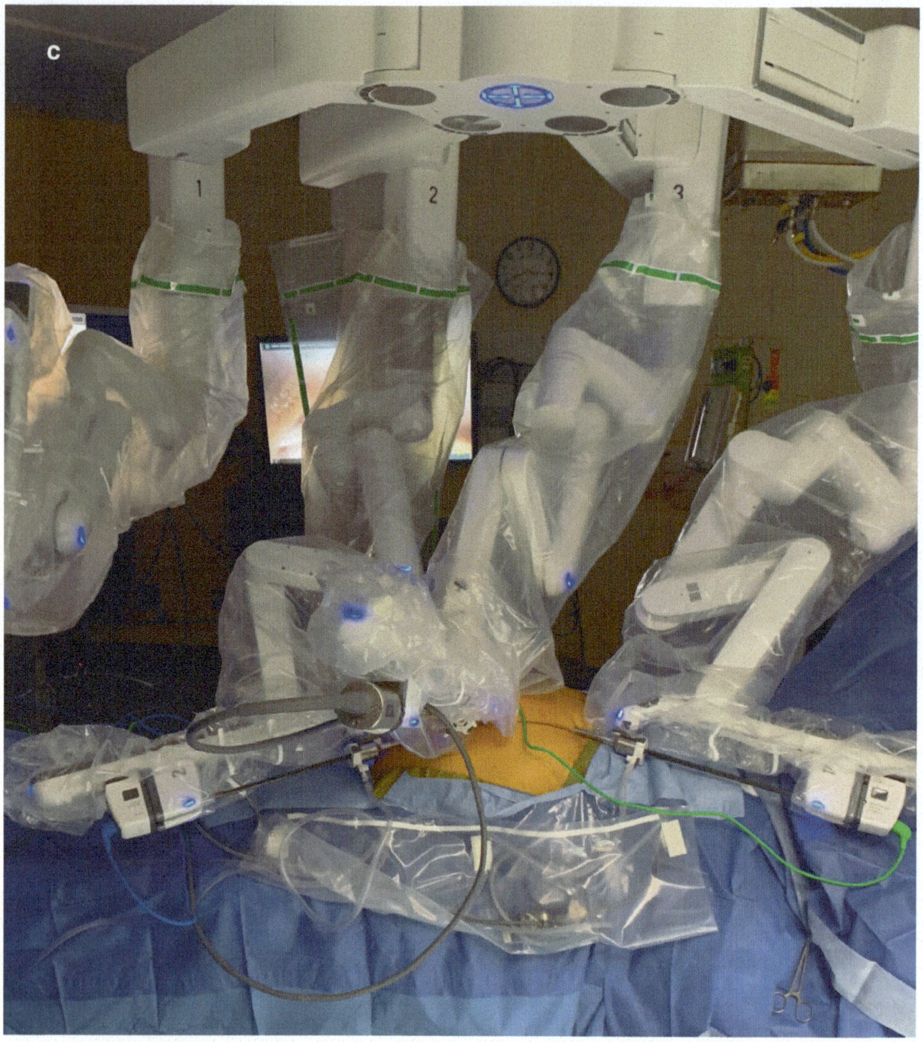


Fig. 2.11 (continued)

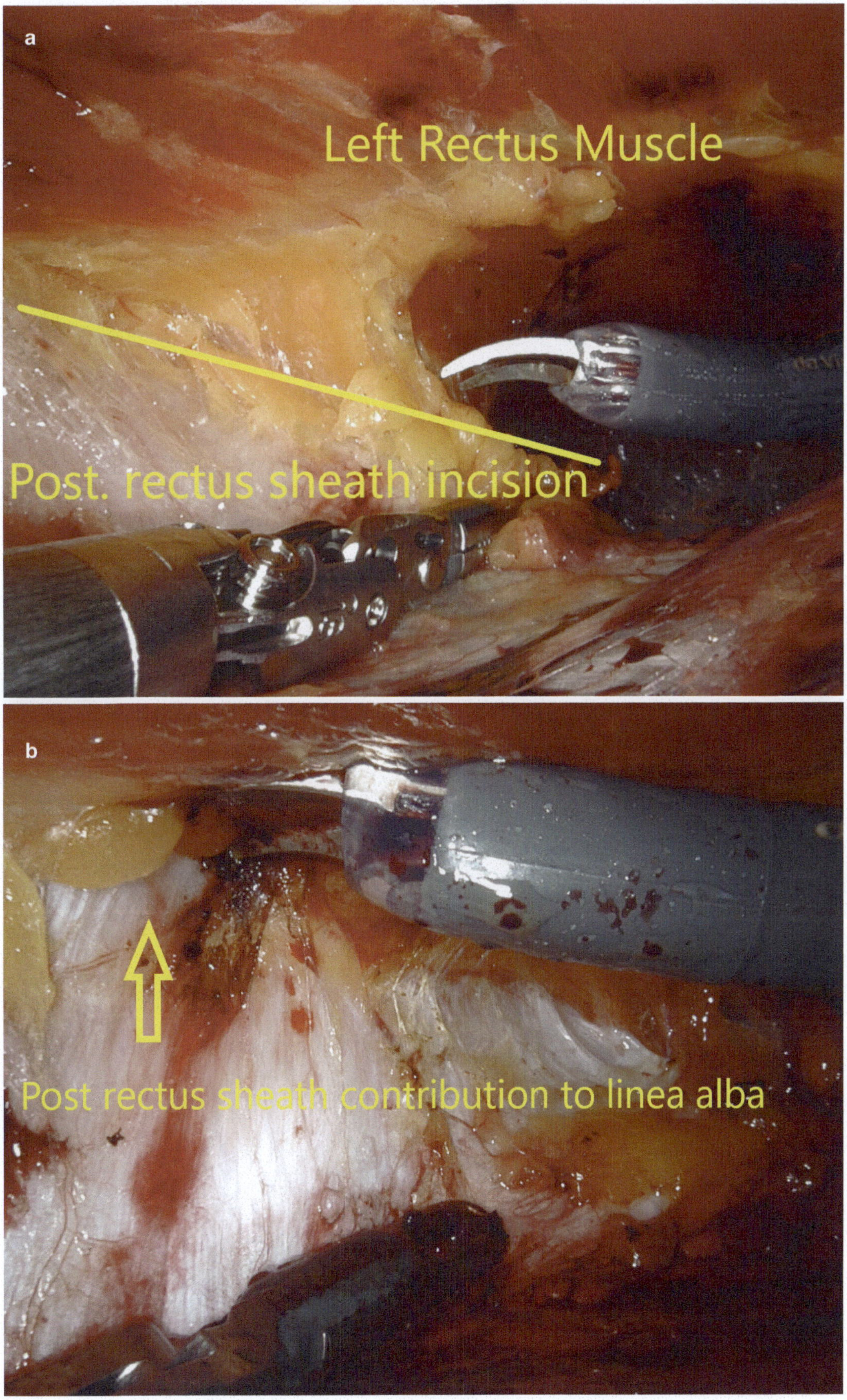


**Fig. 2.12** (**a**) Initial step is posterior rectus sheath incision on the ipsilateral side. (**b**) The posterior rectus sheath contribution to the linea alba should be visualized before incising the ipsilateral posterior rectus sheath

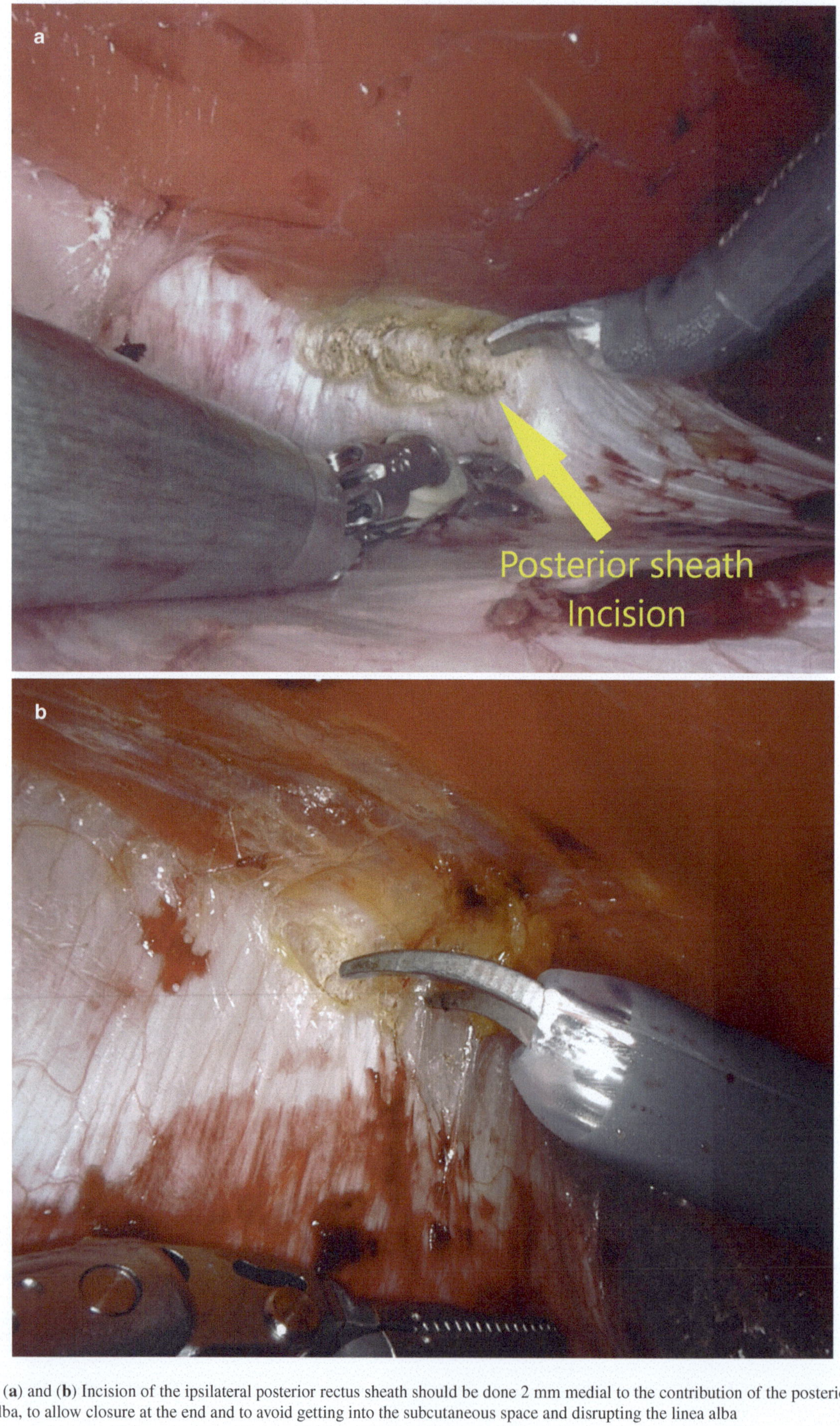


**Fig. 2.13** (**a**) and (**b**) Incision of the ipsilateral posterior rectus sheath should be done 2 mm medial to the contribution of the posterior sheath to the linea alba, to allow closure at the end and to avoid getting into the subcutaneous space and disrupting the linea alba

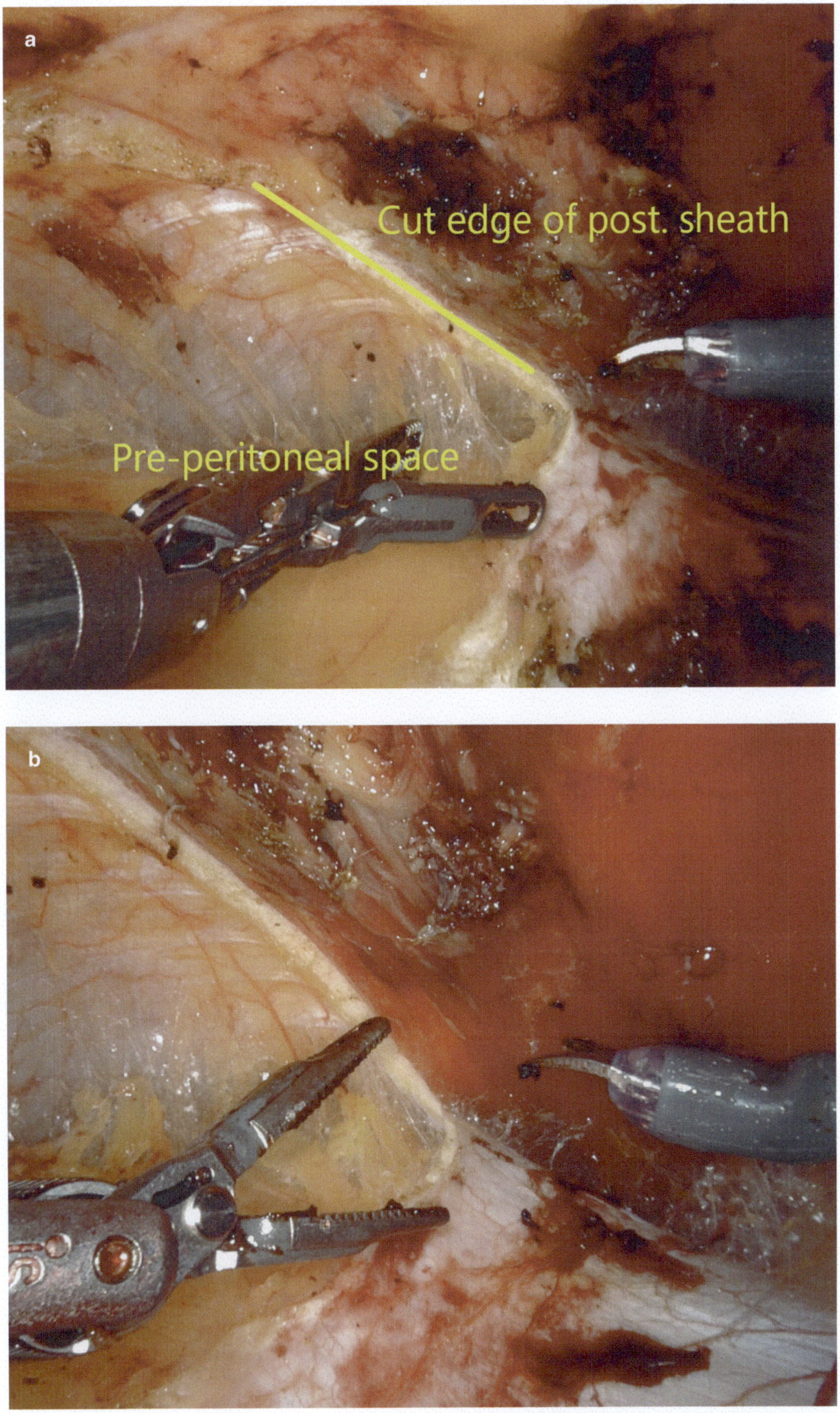


**Fig. 2.14** (**a**) Ipsilateral posterior rectus sheath incision is initiated, exposing the preperitoneal space in the upper abdomen. (**b**) This incision is carried up and down to create more space gradually. (**c**) Crossover in the subxiphoid area for defects just above the umbilicus (M2 hernias)

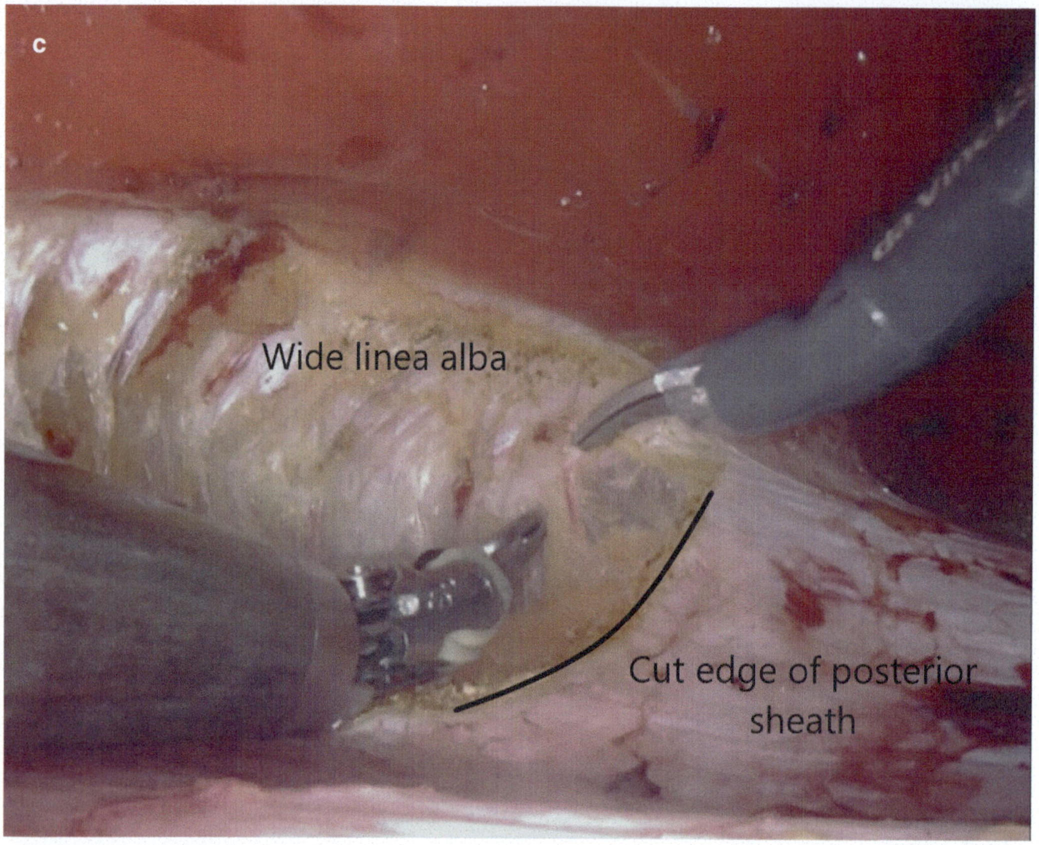


Fig. 2.14 (continued)

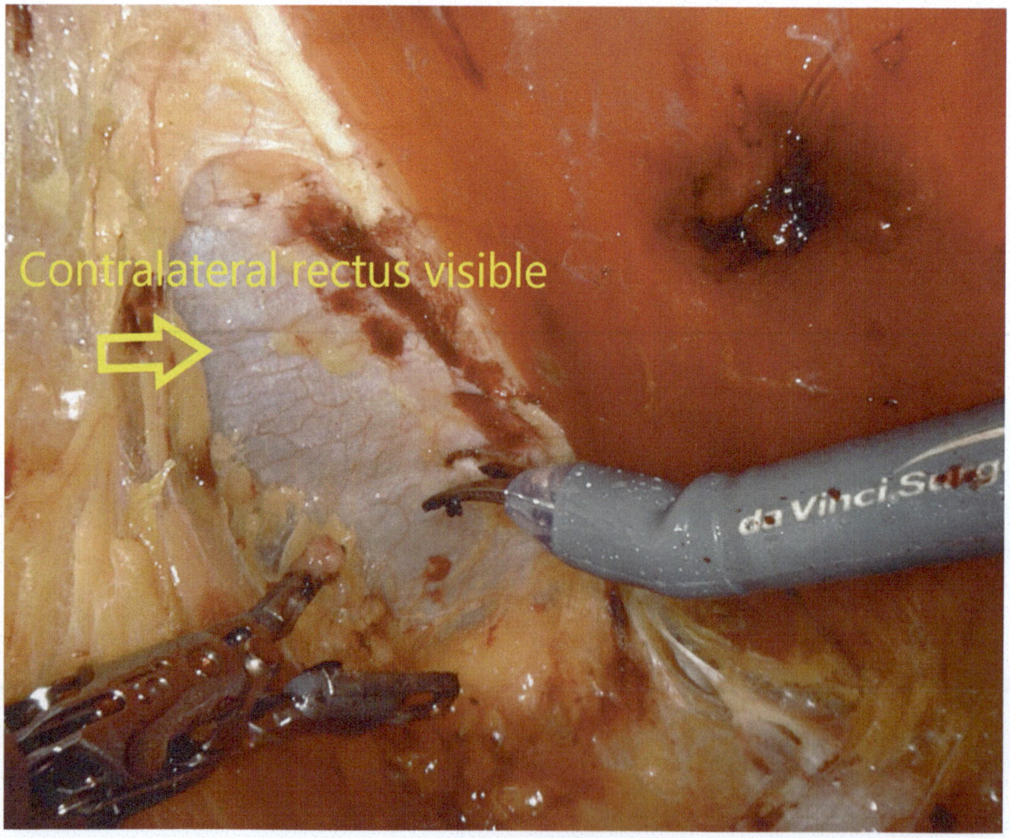


Fig. 2.15 The contralateral rectus muscle is visible through the contralateral posterior rectus sheath after the crossover in the preperitoneal space

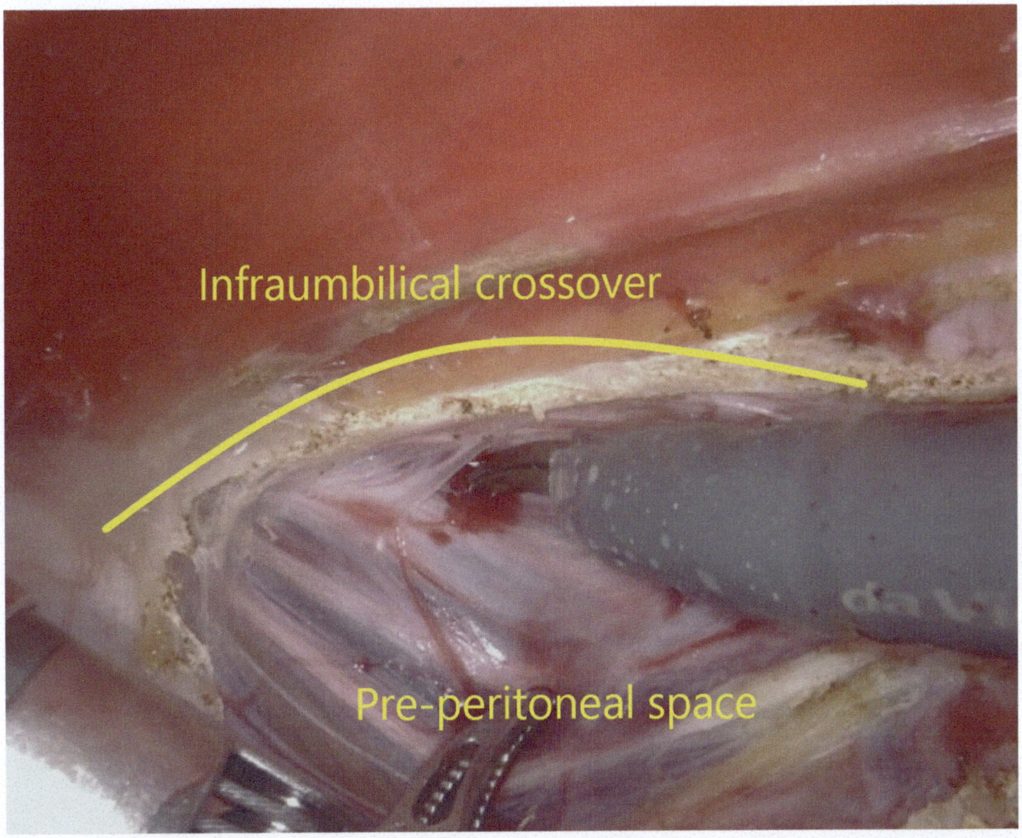


**Fig. 2.16** Crossover in suprapubic area for subxiphoid epigastric hernias (M1 hernias)

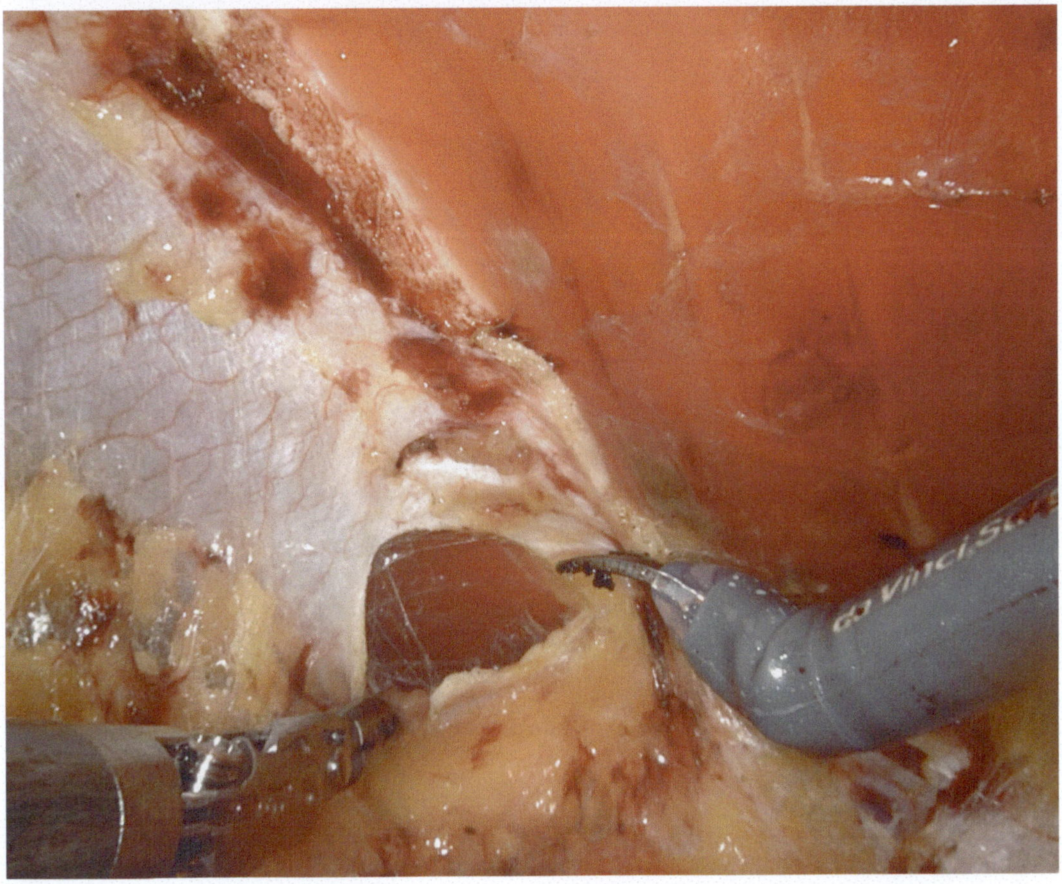

**Fig. 2.17** Incision of contralateral posterior rectus sheath

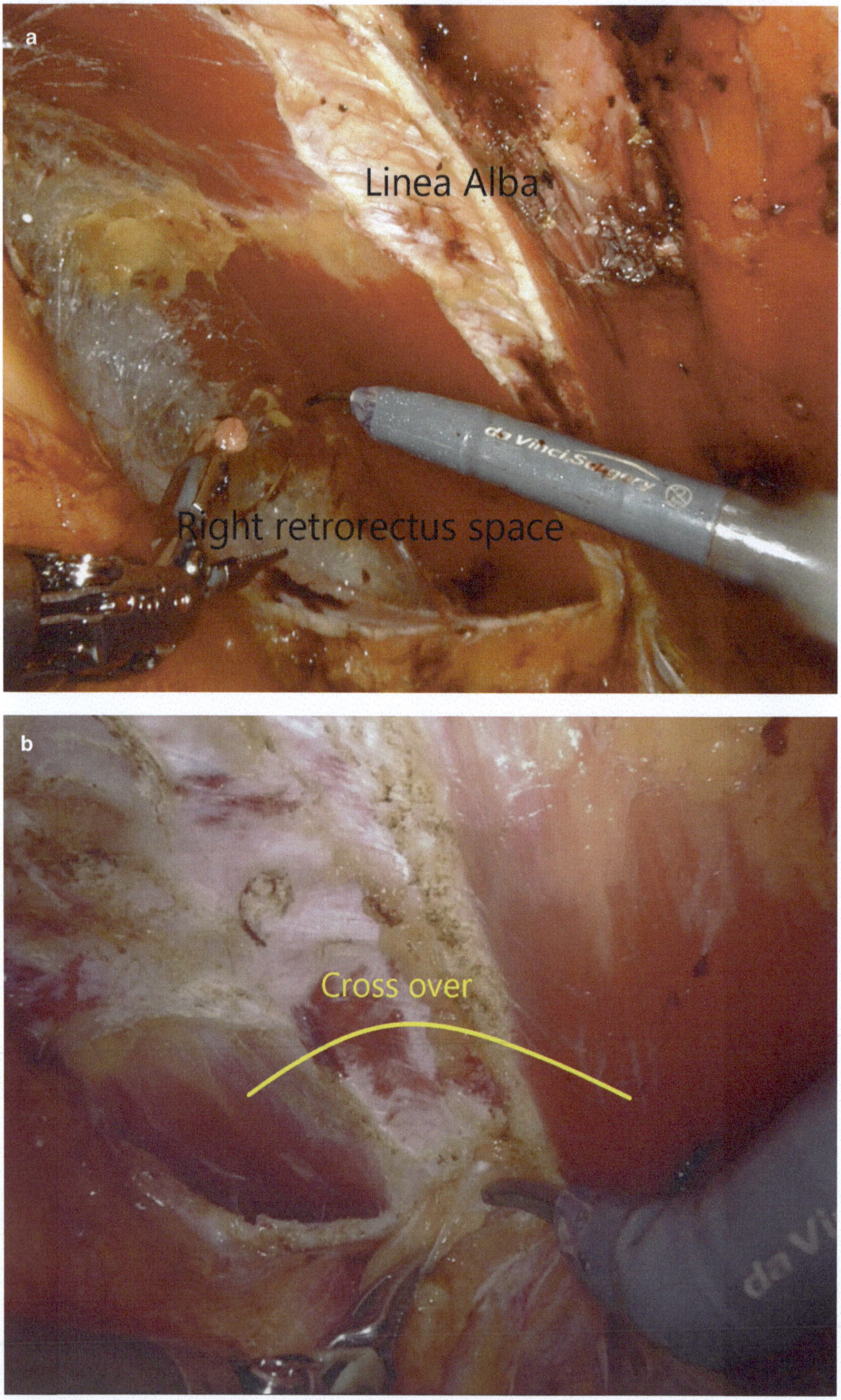


**Fig. 2.18** (**a–c**) Crossover completed in upper abdomen

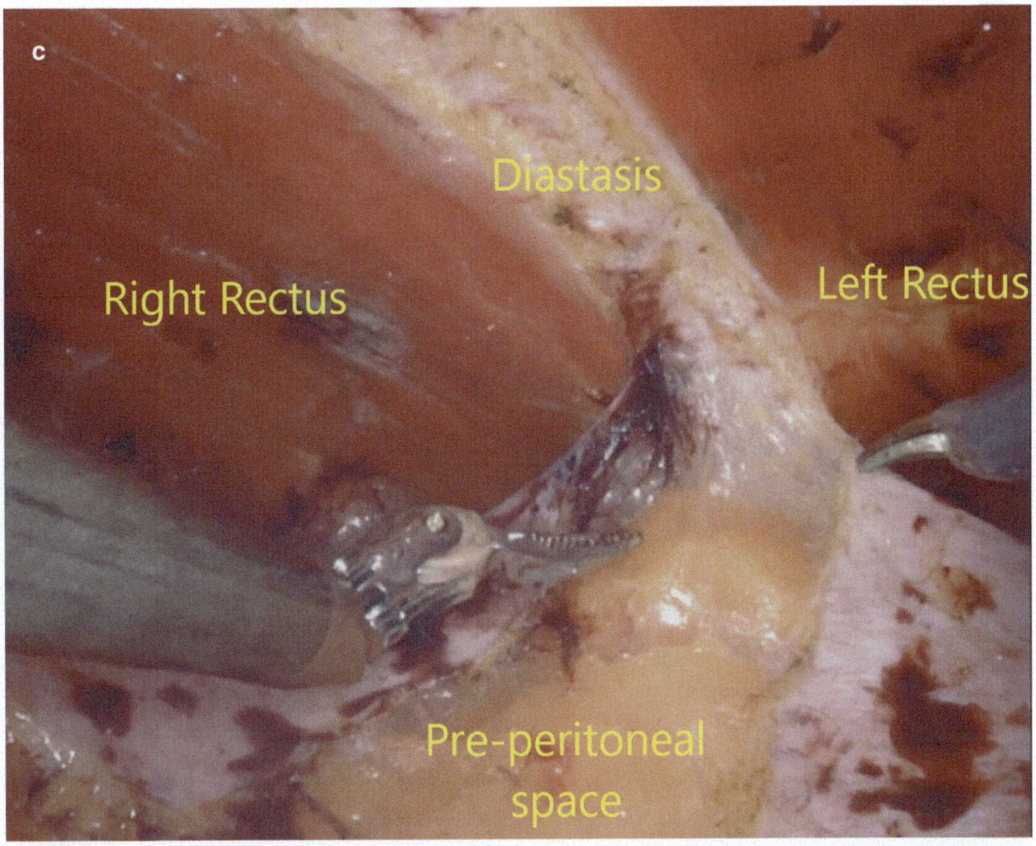


**Fig. 2.18** (continued)

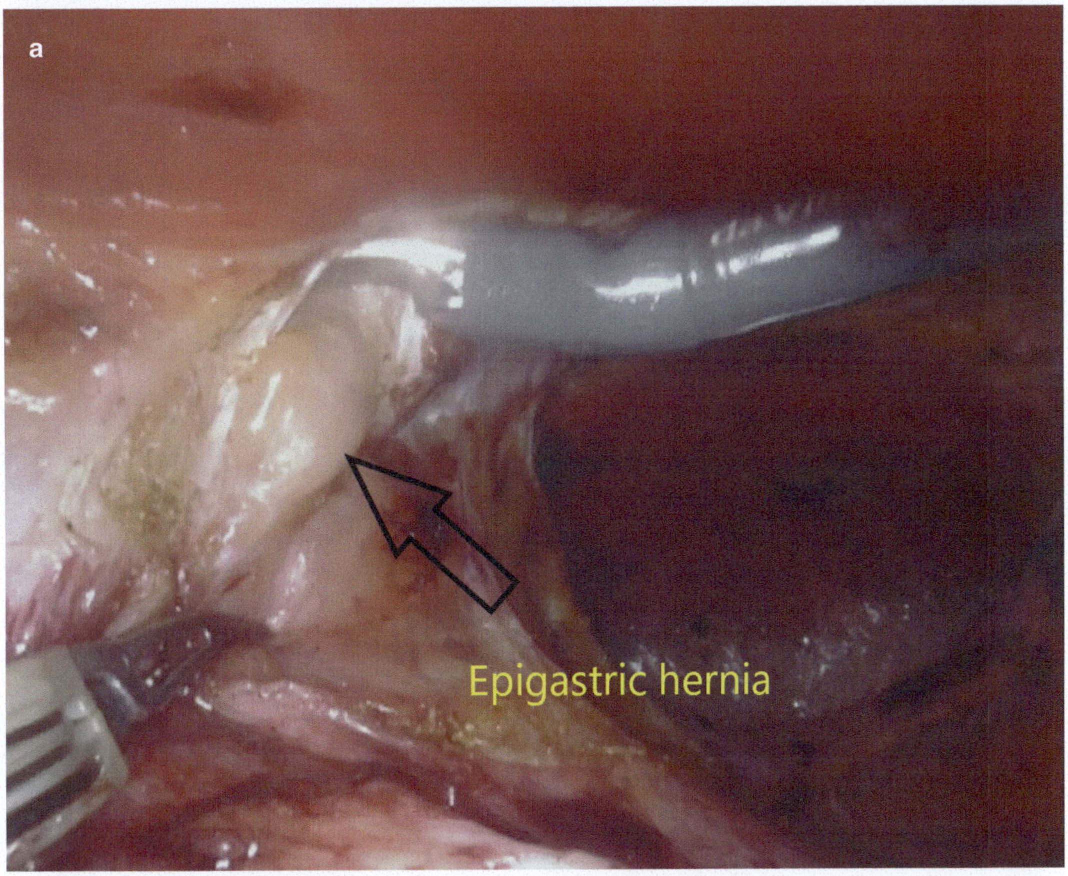


**Fig. 2.19** (**a**) and (**b**) Reduction of epigastric hernia, which usually contains preperitoneal fat

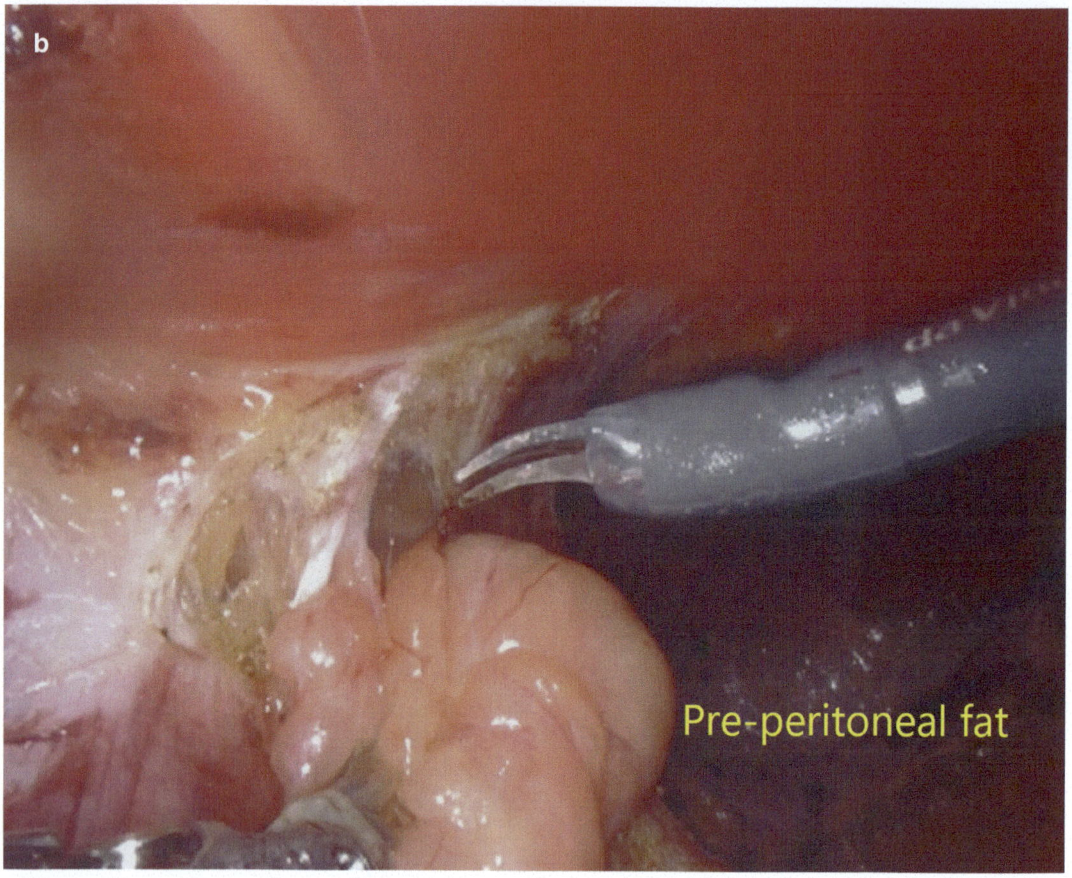


Fig. 2.19 (continued)

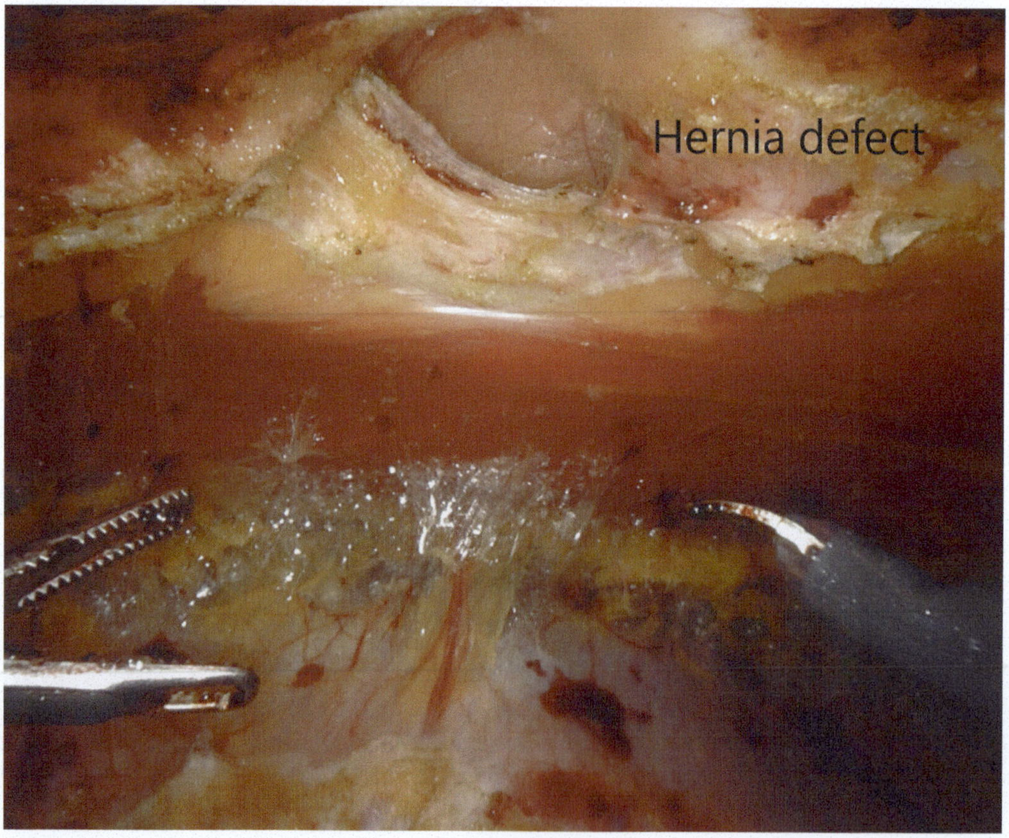


Fig. 2.20 View of hernia defect after reduction of contents

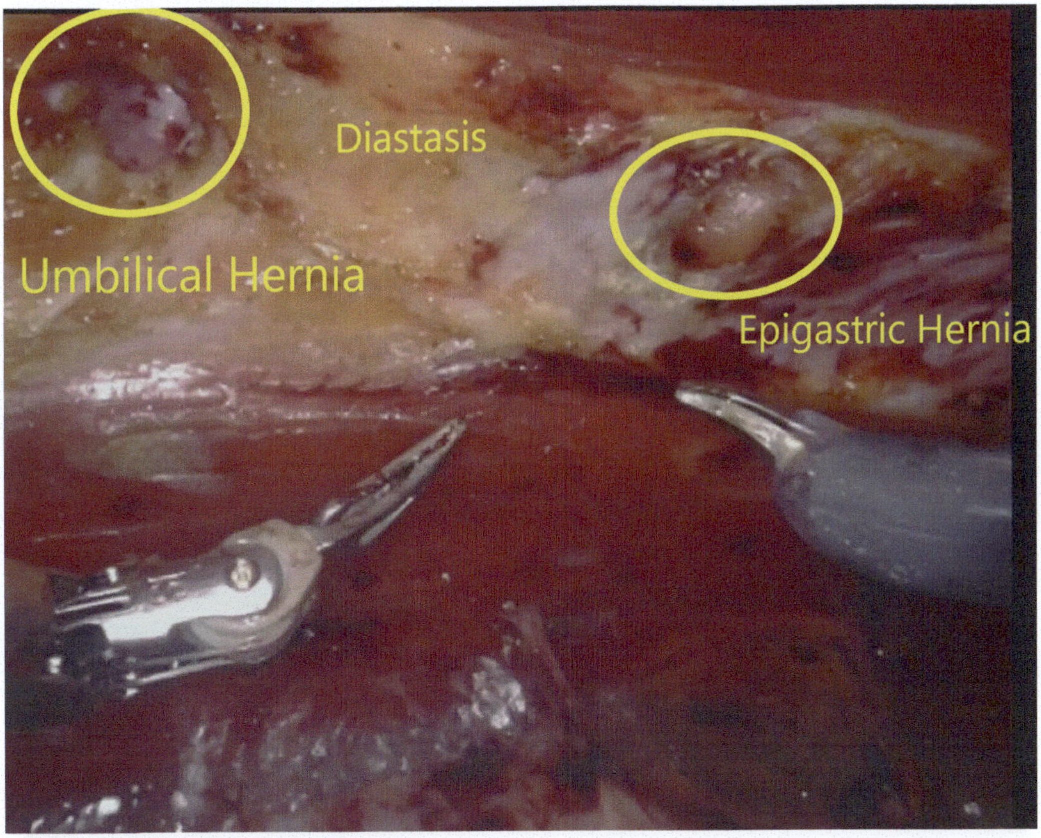


**Fig. 2.21** Midline defects (including diastasis) completely exposed

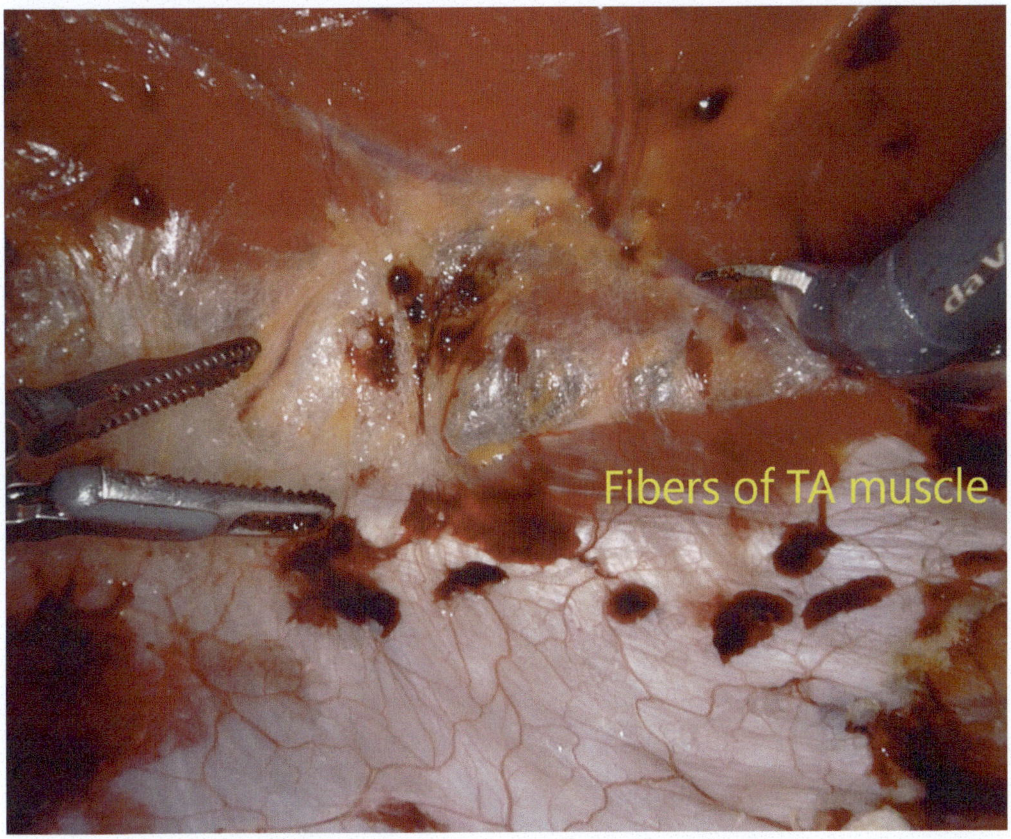


**Fig. 2.22** Fibers of the transversus abdominis (TA) muscles are seen. This is where a TA release could be started. Also, this (in addition to the semilunar lines) marks the extent of the lateral dissection

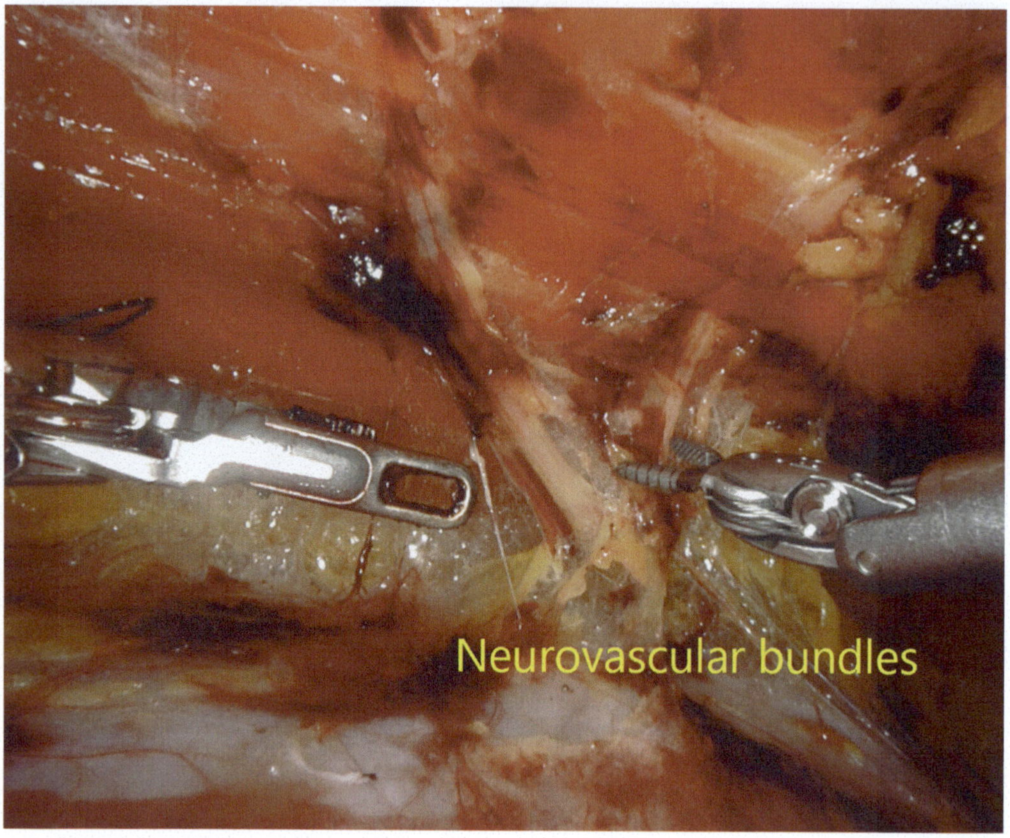


**Fig. 2.23** Neurovascular bundles are also a landmark for the extent of lateral dissection

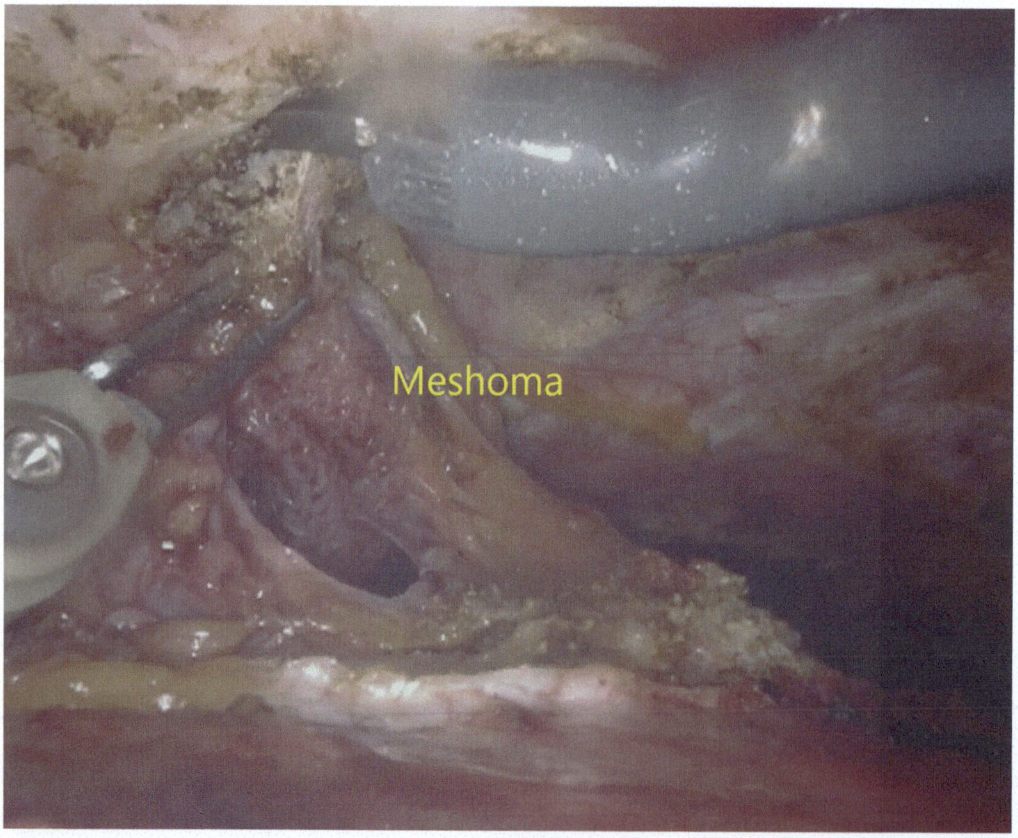


**Fig. 2.24** Excision of a "meshoma" in a recurrent epigastric hernia

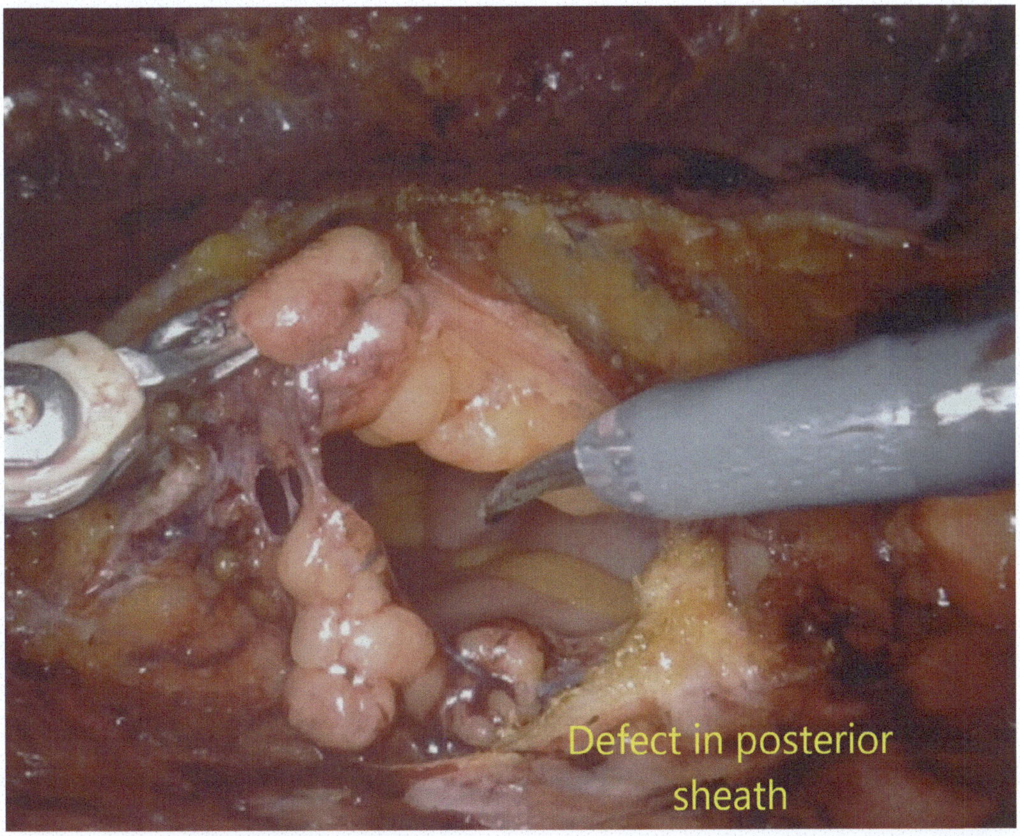


**Fig. 2.25** It is very important in eTEP repairs to identify and close any defects in the posterior sheath, to avoid postoperative interparietal hernia

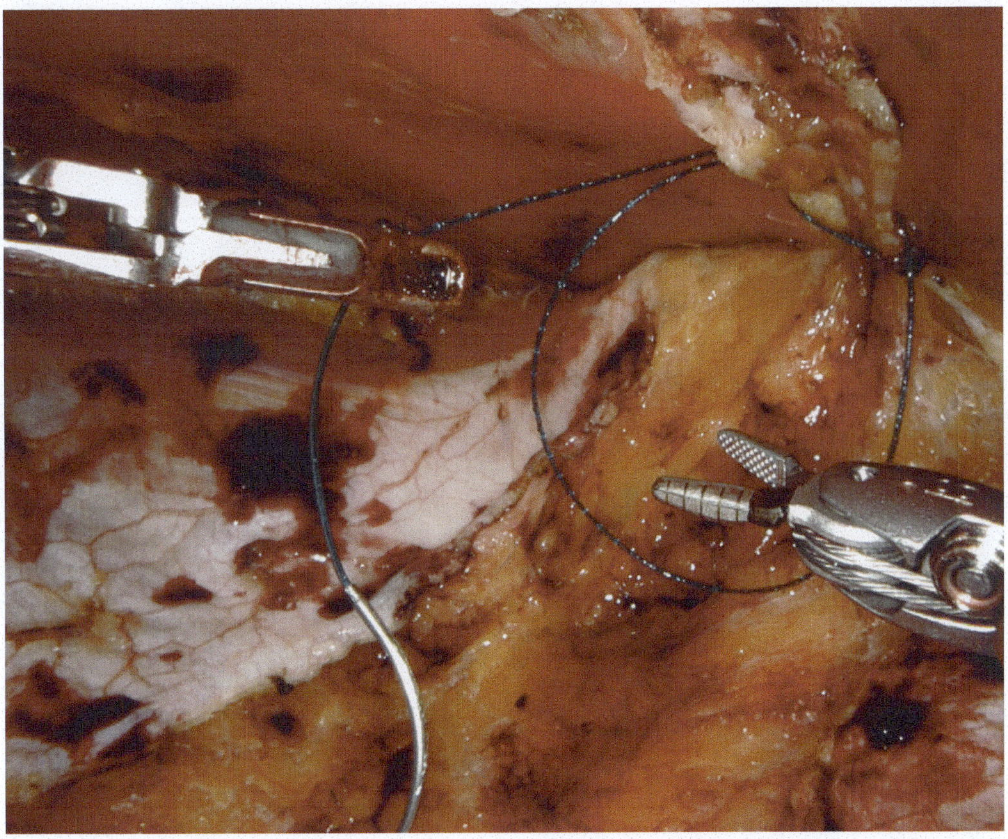

**Fig. 2.26** If repair of diastasis is planned along with hernia defect closure, the closure is started in the subxiphoid area

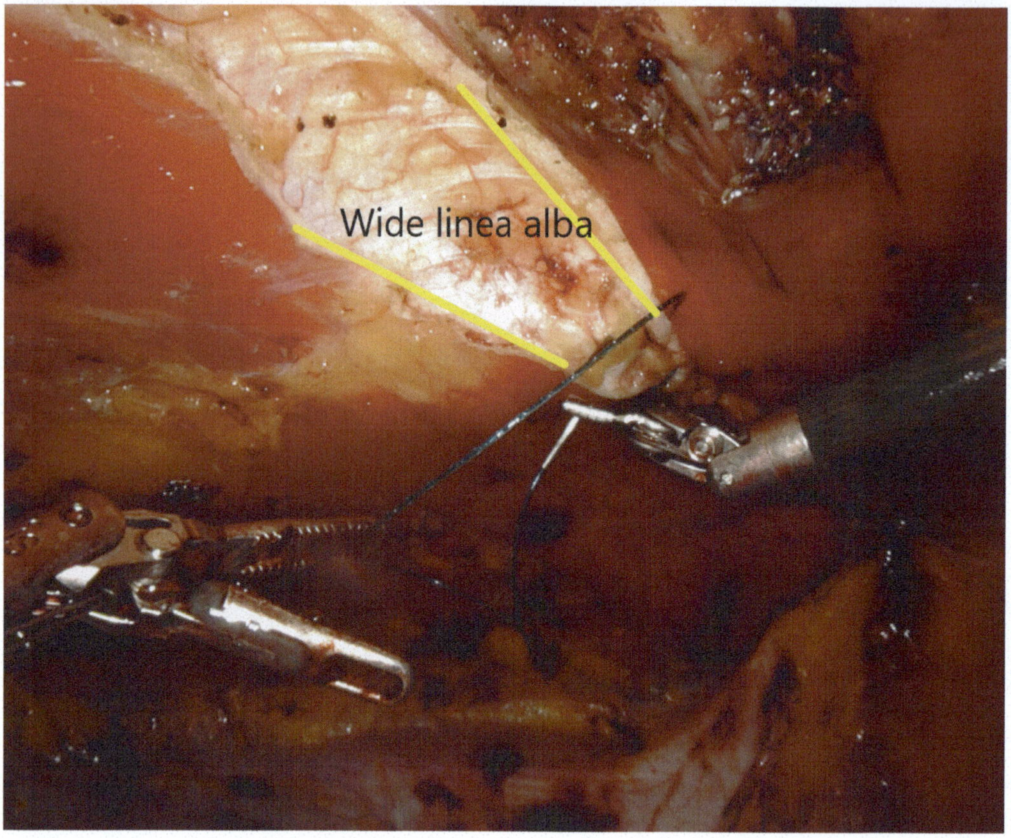


**Fig. 2.27** To reconstitute the midline, it is important to include in the closure bites the cut edge of the posterior rectus sheath on both sides, as well as the linea alba

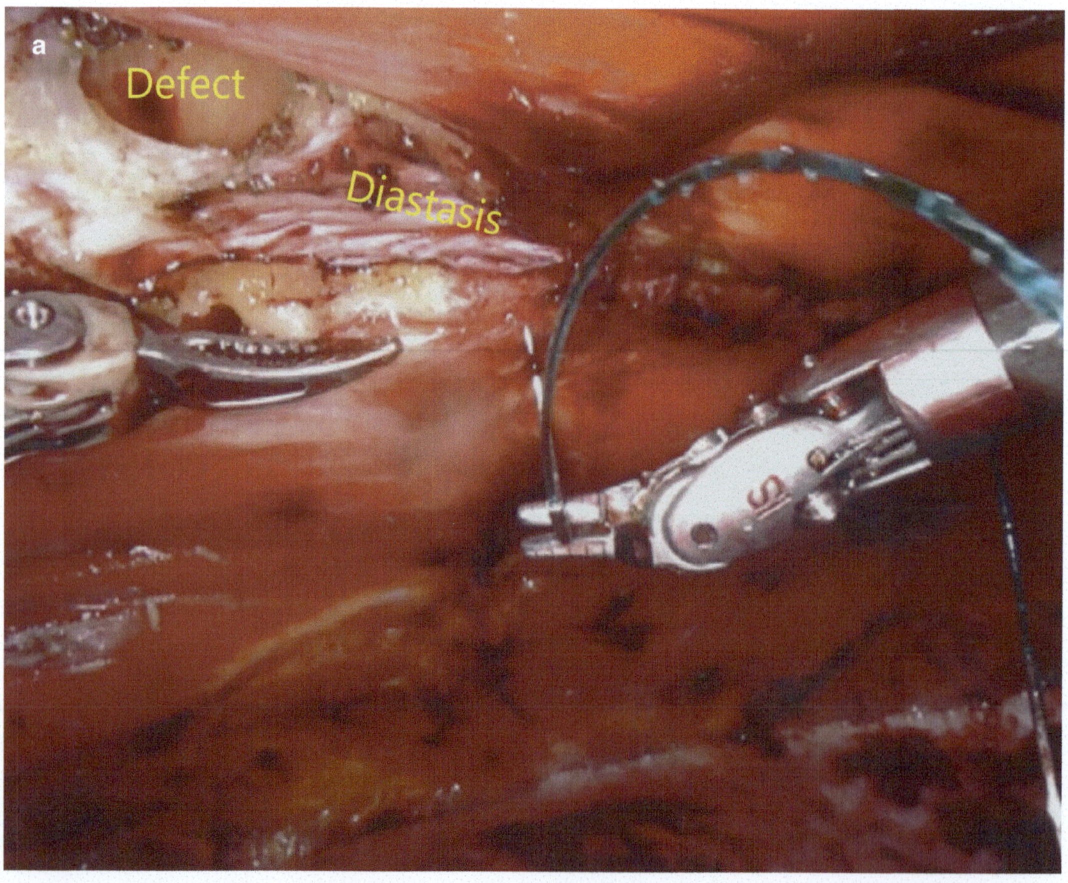


**Fig. 2.28** (**a**) Closure of defect included in midline closure. (**b**) Hernia defect closed and recti muscles reapproximated in the midline

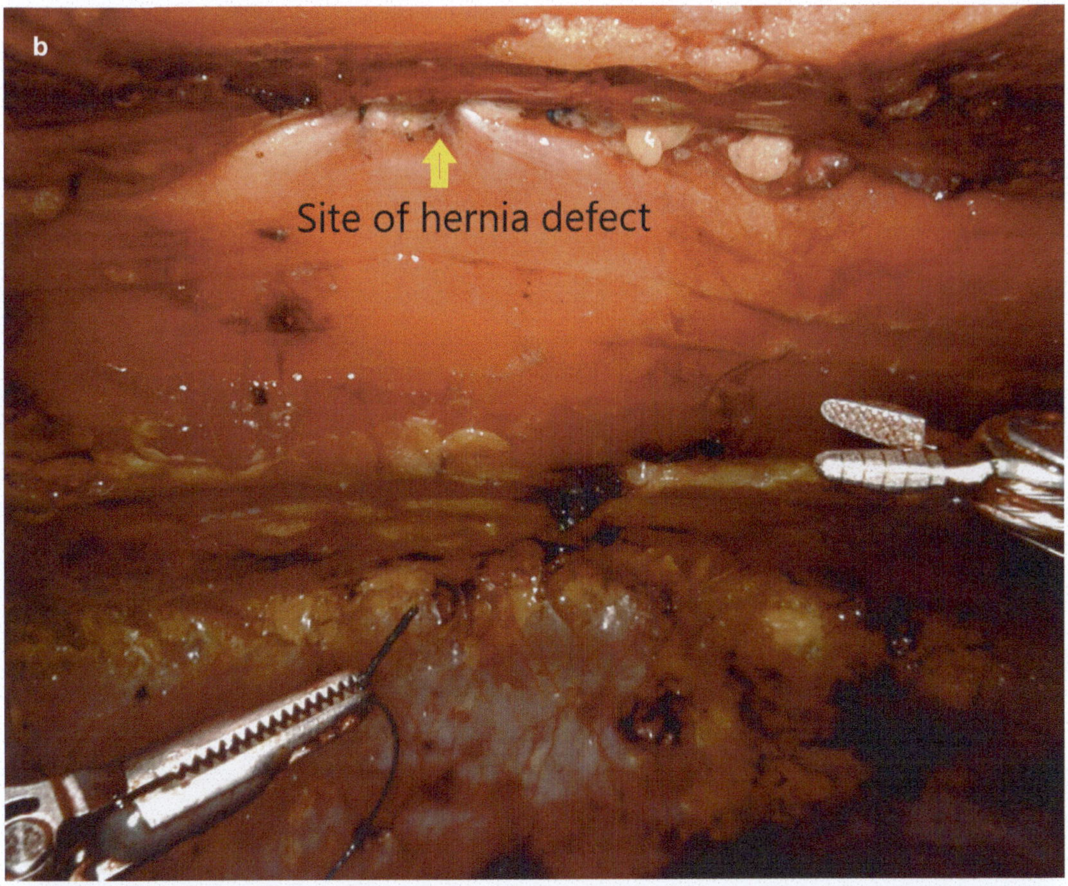


Fig. 2.28 (continued)

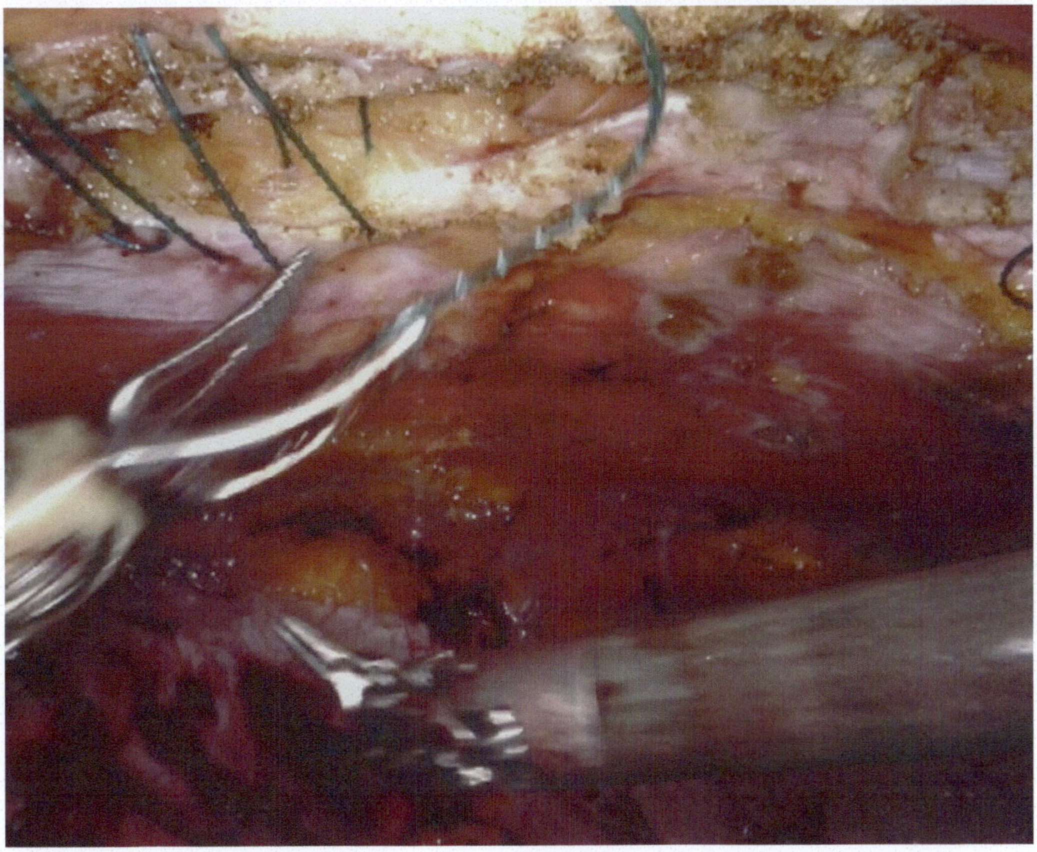

Fig. 2.29 Sequential tightening of closure at an intraabdominal pressure of 8 mmHg

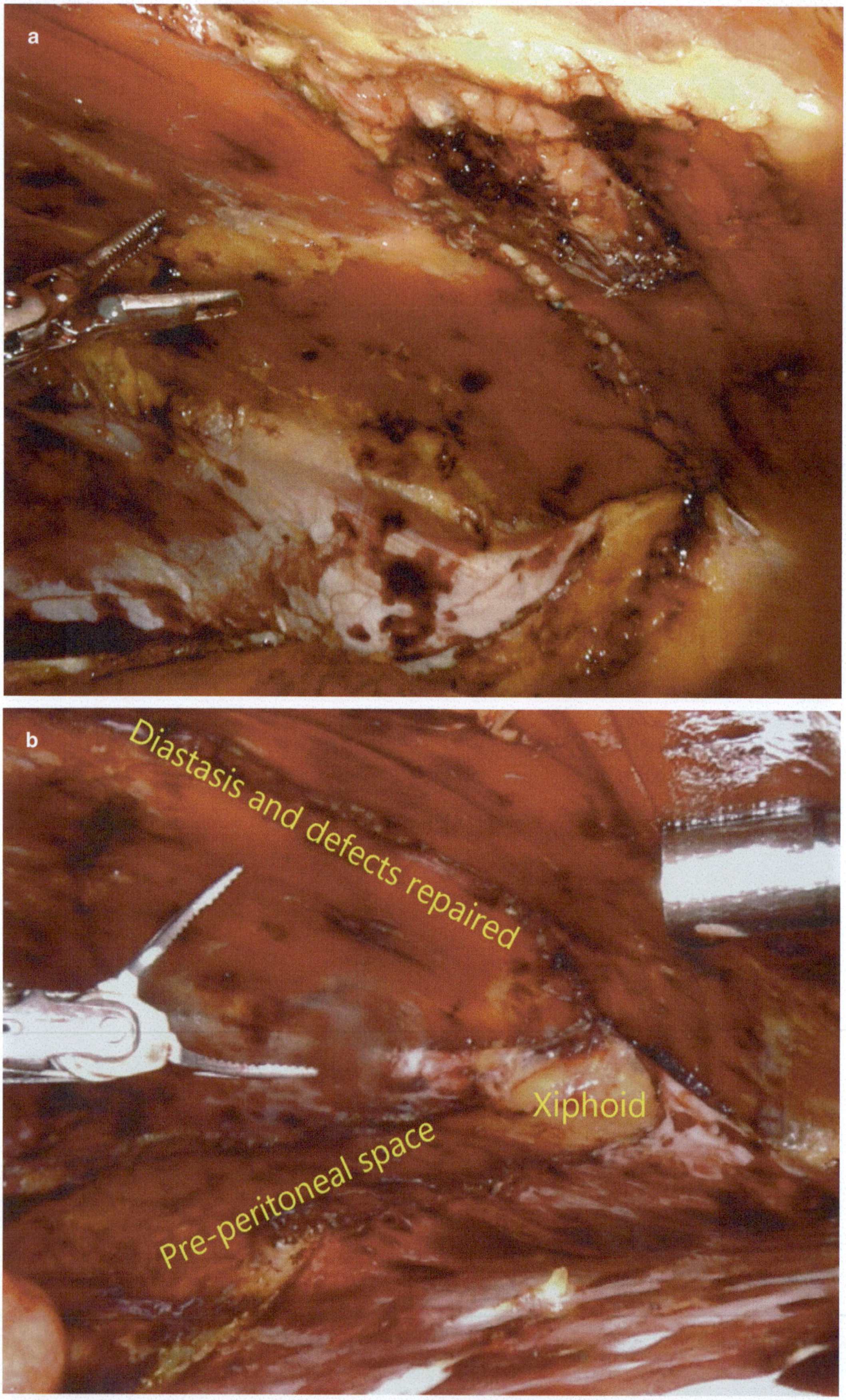


**Fig. 2.30** (**a**) and (**b**) View after completed midline closure to repair diastasis and close all midline hernia defects

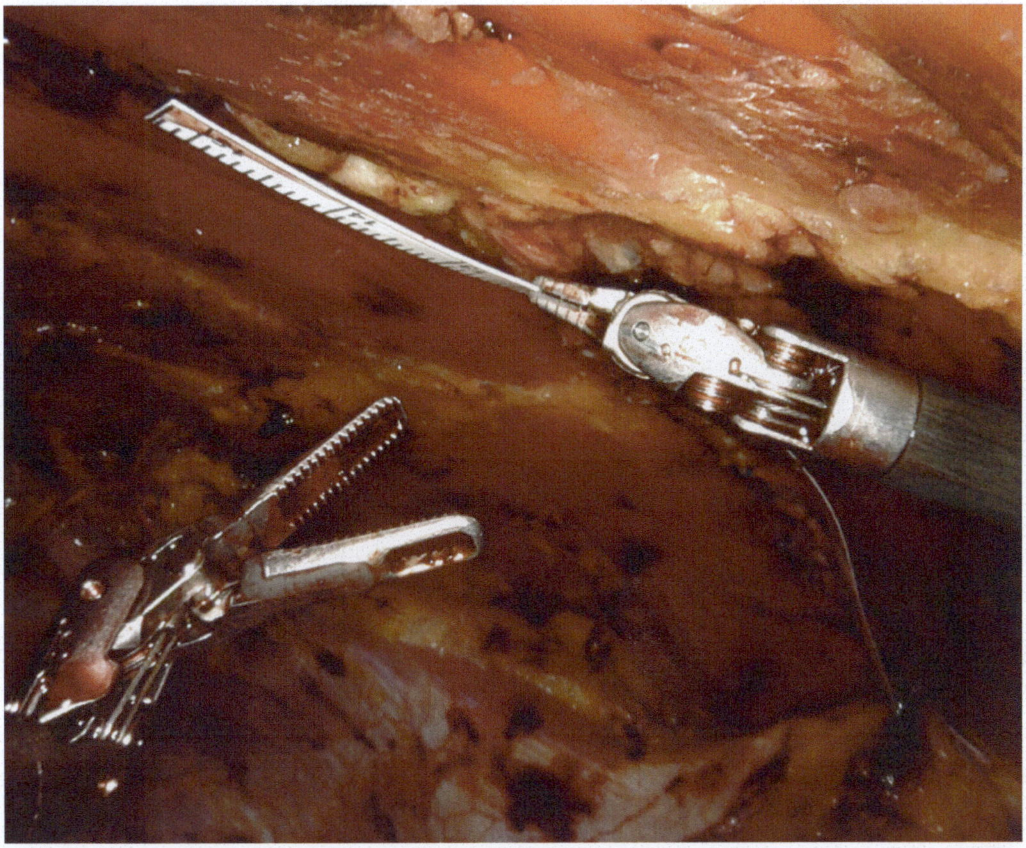

Fig. 2.31 Retromuscular space is measured, in order to fashion a mesh. We typically use a macroporus lightweight or mediumweight polypropylene mesh to reinforce the whole retromuscular space

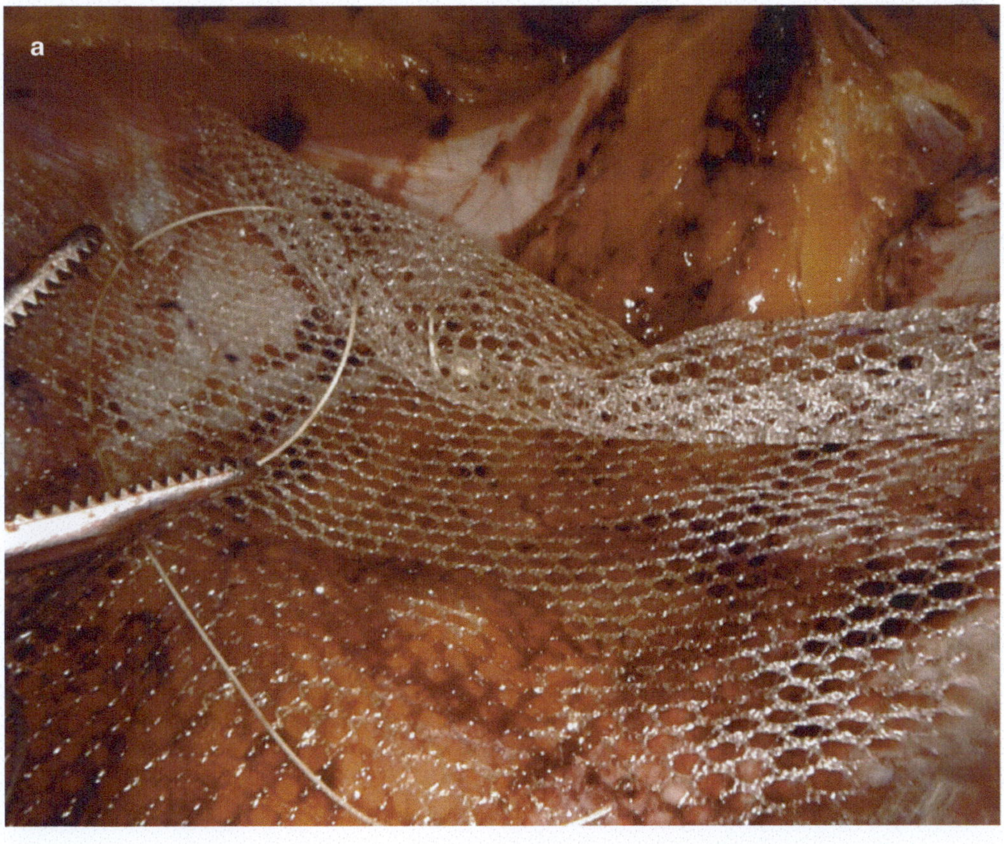


Fig. 2.32 (a) and (b) Mesh placement. We prefer to use a suture tied at the edge of the mesh to help unroll it

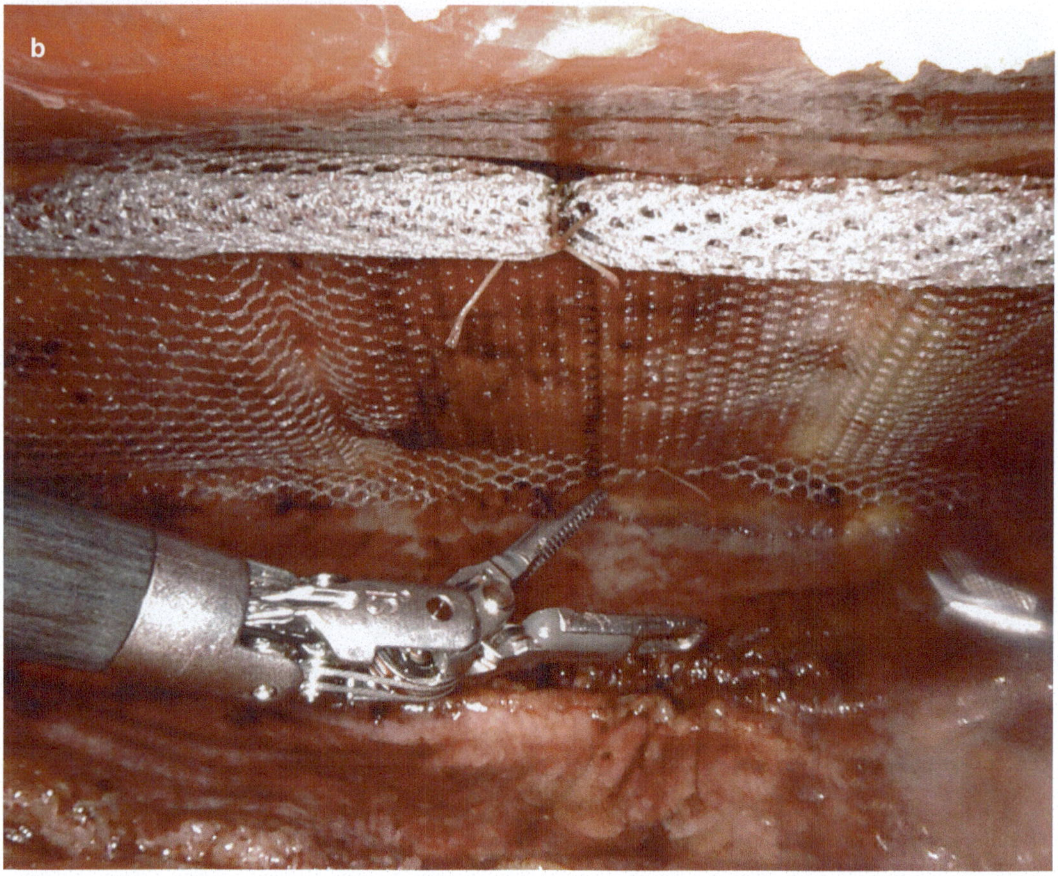


Fig. 2.32 (continued)

## Suggested Reading

Abdalla R, Costa TN, editors. Robotic surgery for abdominal wall hernia repair: a manual of best practices. Cham: Springer International Publishing; 2018.

Belyansky I, Reza Zahiri H, Sanford Z, Weltz AS, Park A. Early operative outcomes of endoscopic (eTEP access) robotic-assisted retromuscular abdominal wall hernia repair. Hernia. 2018;22(5):837–47.

Kudsi OY, Carbonell AM, Yiengpruksawan A, et al., editors. Atlas of robotic surgery. Woodbury: Cine-Med Inc.; 2018.

# 3 Robotic Umbilical Hernia Repair: Totally Extraperitoneal (TEP)

Fahri Gokcal and Omar Yusef Kudsi

## Introduction

In current practice, umbilical hernias can be repaired by several mesh repair techniques, including the retrorectus (Rives-Stoppa) repair. In the Rives-Stoppa technique, the mesh is excluded from the visceral contents and thus does not pose a problem for future abdominal surgery. Furthermore, this technique is increasingly becoming the preferred approach for ventral hernia owing to its durability and long-term outcomes [1].

Minimally invasive ventral hernia repair with totally extraperitoneal (TEP) access, as popularized by Belyansky et al. [2], offers use of the retromuscular space. TEP-access robotic retromuscular ventral hernia repair has several advantages. It may eliminate the need for closure of posterior fascia, which is usually required with standard transabdominal access. Furthermore, placing mesh between the anterior and posterior layers of the abdominal wall can eliminate the need for transfascial fixation, which often causes chronic postoperative pain. Shifting from traditional transabdominal access to TEP access also may lead to a subsequent decrease in trocar-site hernia formation, as all trocar sites are covered with mesh or posterior fascia at the completion of the procedure.

## Procedure: Illustrated Steps

Figures 3.1, 3.2, 3.3, 3.4, 3.5, 3.6, 3.7, 3.8, 3.9, 3.10, 3.11, 3.12, 3.13, 3.14, 3.15, 3.16, 3.17, 3.18, 3.19, 3.20, 3.21, 3.22, 3.23, 3.24, 3.25, 3.26, 3.27, 3.28, 3.29, 3.30, 3.31, 3.32, 3.33, and 3.34 illustrate the technical aspects of robotic TEP-access Rives-Stoppa umbilical hernia repair.

F. Gokcal
Department of Surgery, Good Samaritan Medical Center, Brockton, MA, USA

O. Y. Kudsi (✉)
Department of Surgery, Good Samaritan Medical Center, Tufts University School of Medicine, Boston, MA, USA


O. Y. Kudsi (ed.), *Robotic Hernia Surgery*, https://doi.org/10.1007/978-3-030-46667-1_3

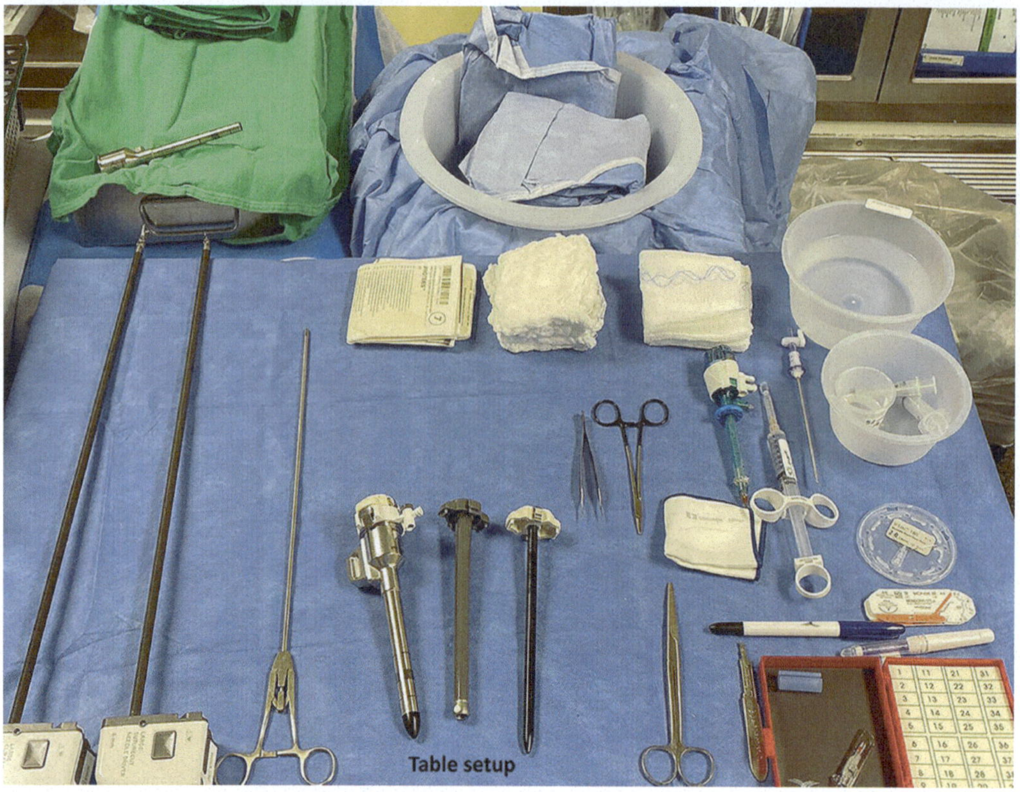


Fig. 3.1 Table setup

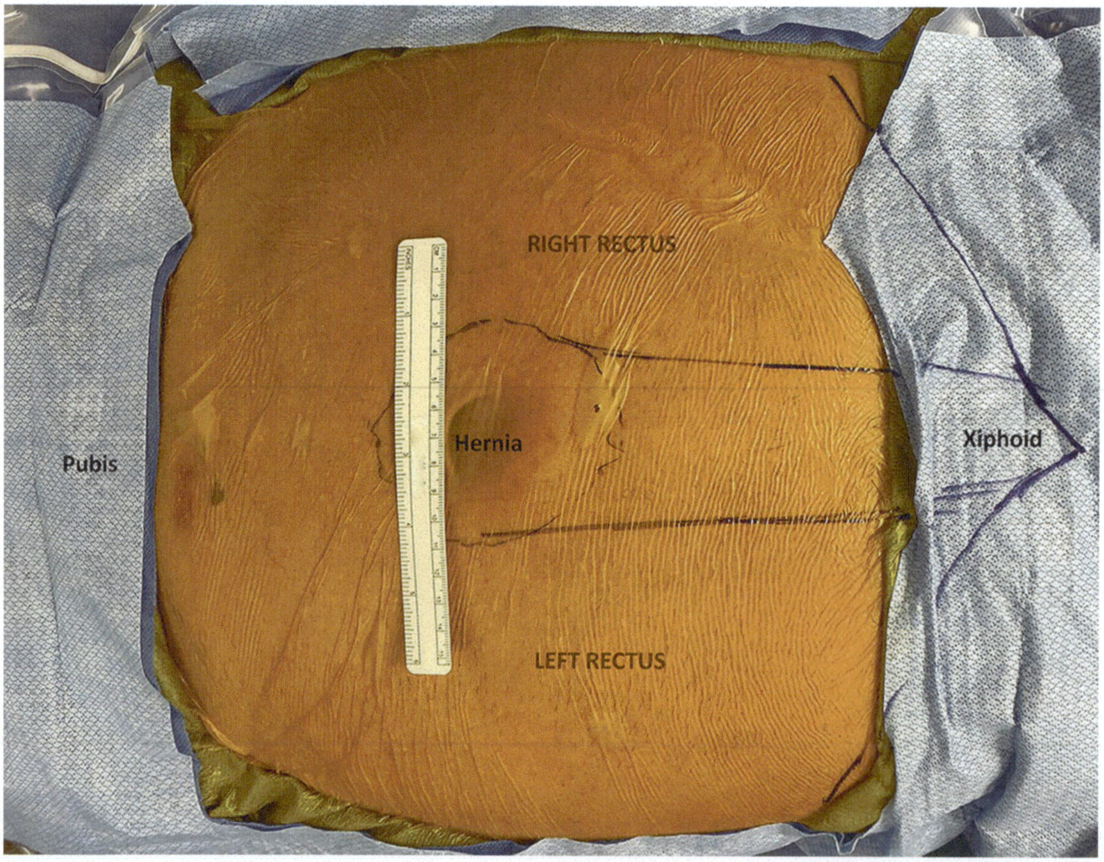


Fig. 3.2 The patient is positioned supine with arms abducted. After draping the surgical site, relevant anatomy is marked, including the xiphoid process, bilateral subcostal margins, symphysis pubis, and linea alba

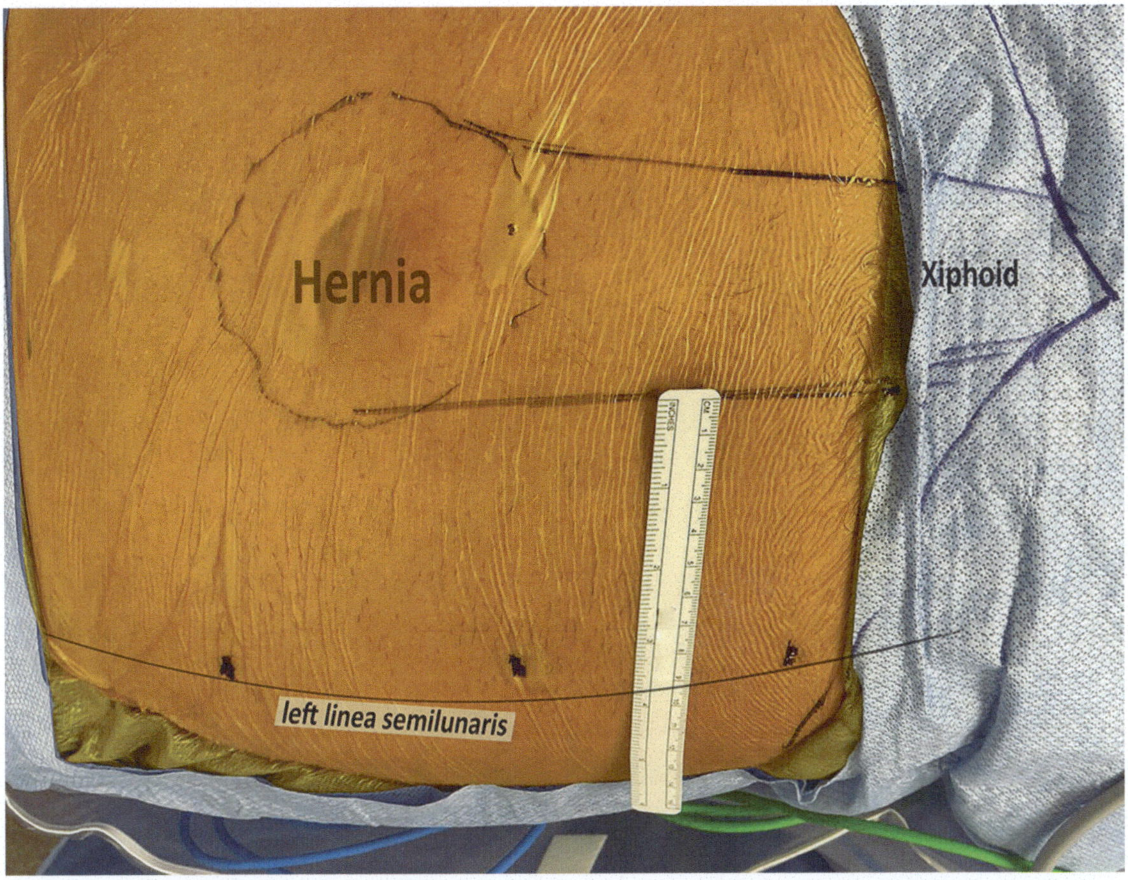


**Fig. 3.3** Trocar sites are marked at least 8–10 cm away from target anatomy

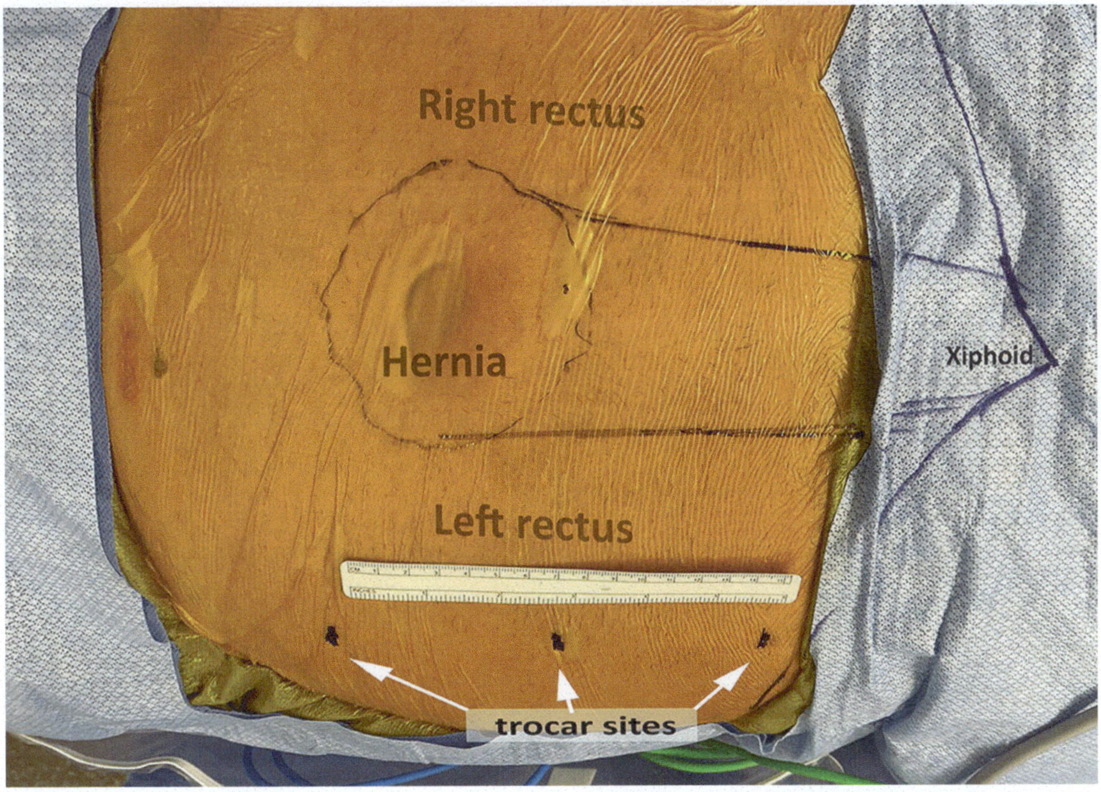


**Fig. 3.4** A distance of 6–8 cm is recommended between trocars to prevent the robotic arms from colliding

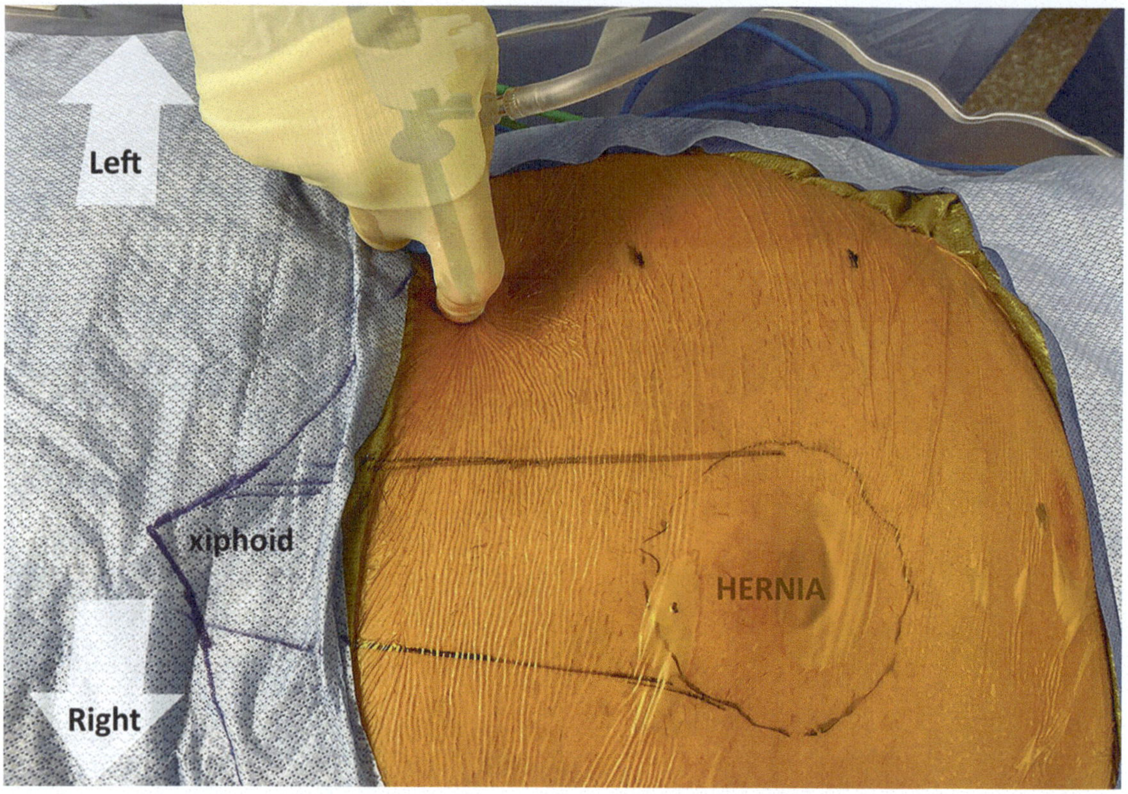


Fig. 3.5 After a skin incision, a 5-mm optical trocar connected to carbon dioxide ($CO_2$) insufflation on high flow and a 5-mm laparoscopic camera are inserted

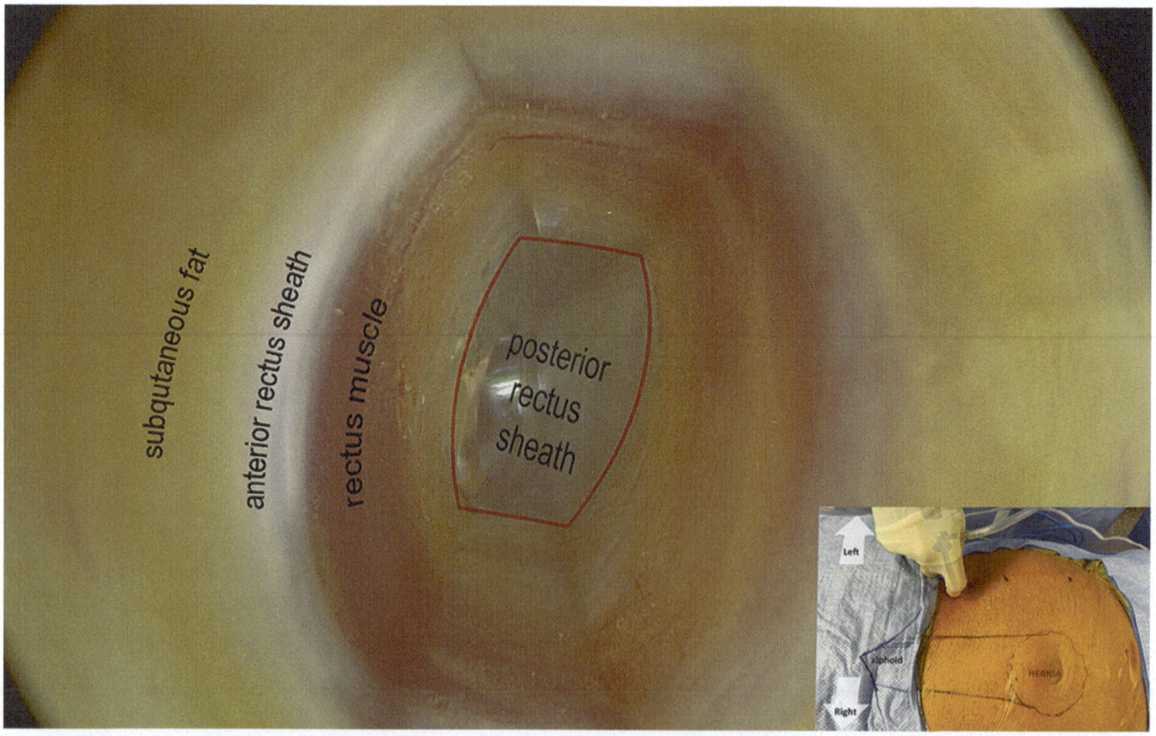


Fig. 3.6 By slowly advancing the trocar perpendicular to the surface, the anterior rectus sheath is visualized, followed by the rectus abdominis muscle

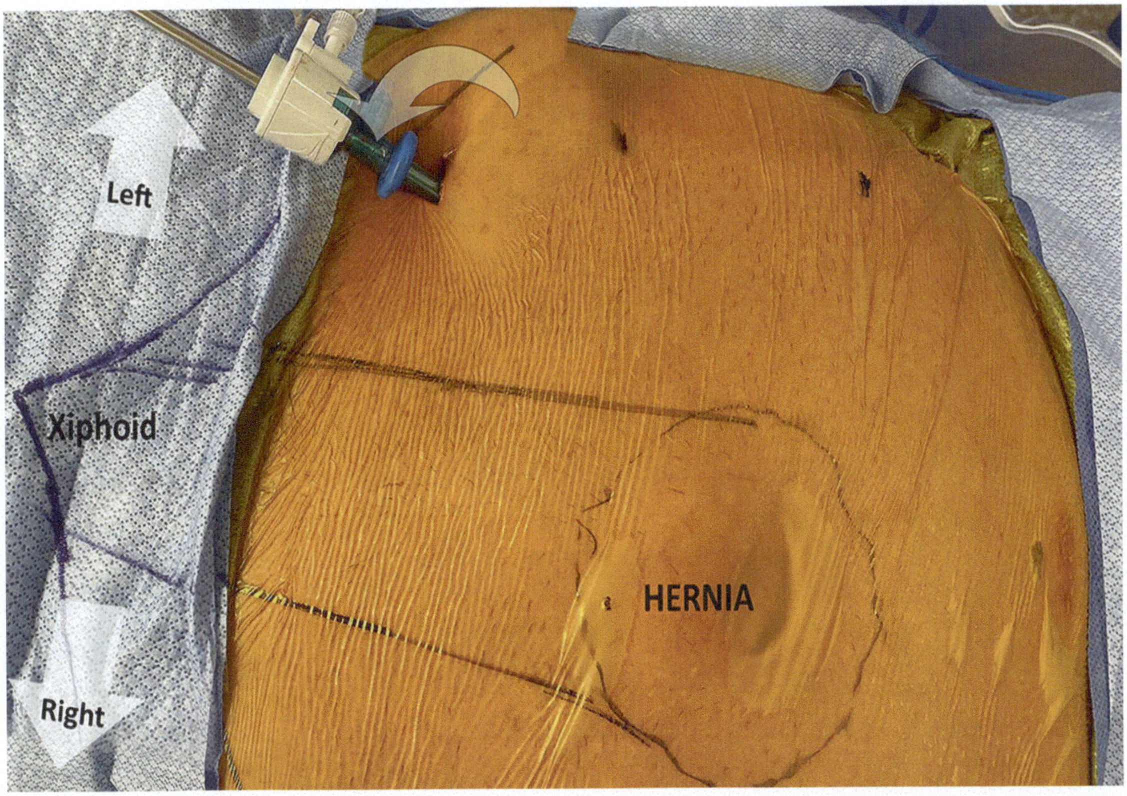


Fig. 3.7 Once the muscle fibers are visualized, the direction of trocar advancement is angled inferiorly, in order to avoid penetrating the posterior rectus sheath

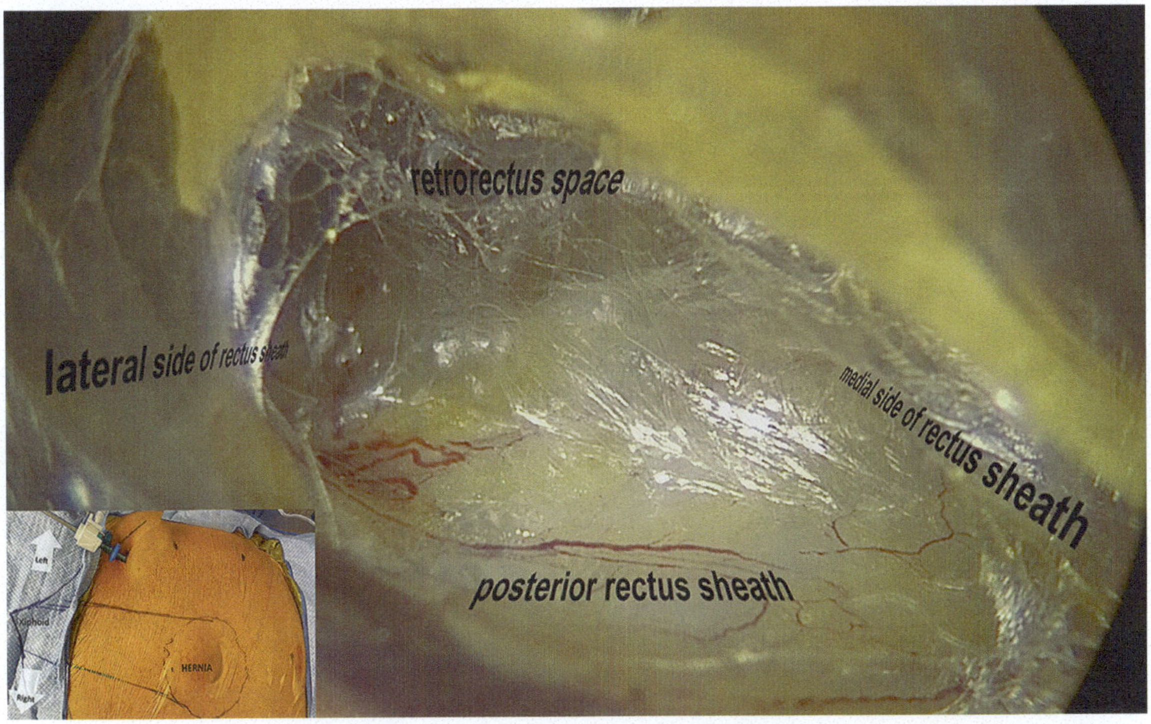


Fig. 3.8 Blunt dissection is performed using the laparoscope and high-pressure $CO_2$ insufflation to obtain a reasonable amount of space in order to insert the other trocars

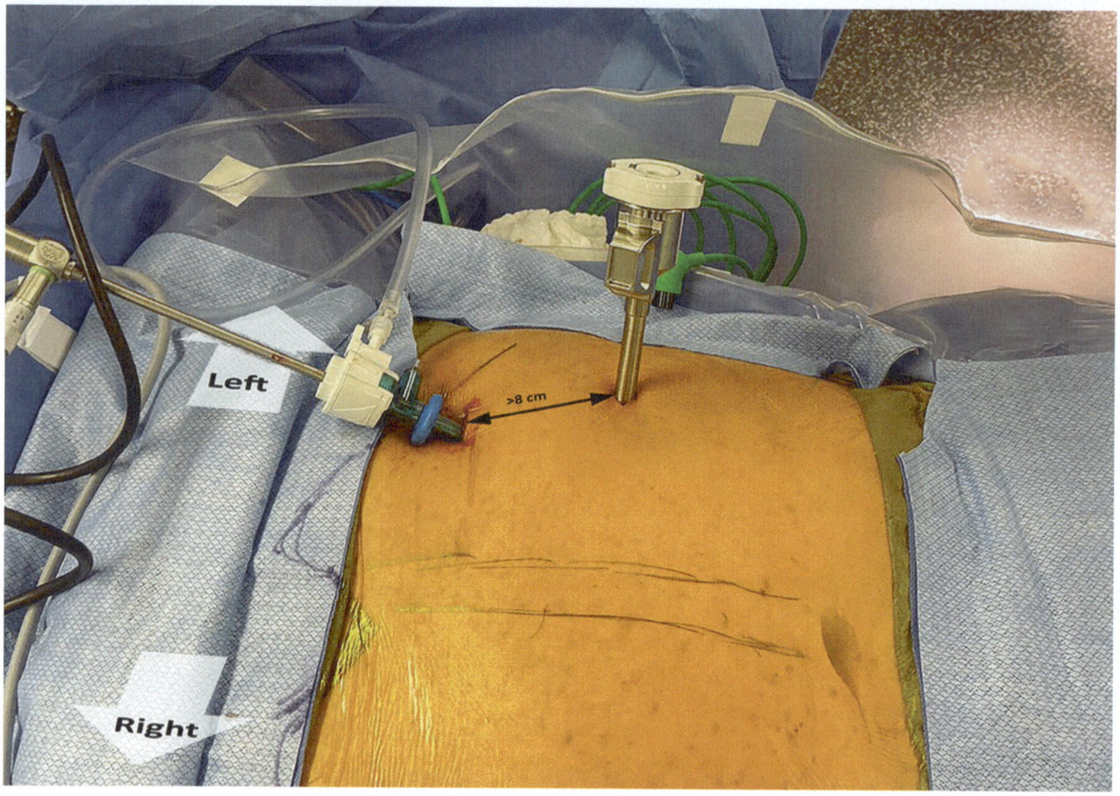


Fig. 3.9 A lateromedial and angled advancement is recommended to insert the trocars, providing a distance of at least 8 cm from the first trocar in order to minimize mechanical interference between the robotic arms

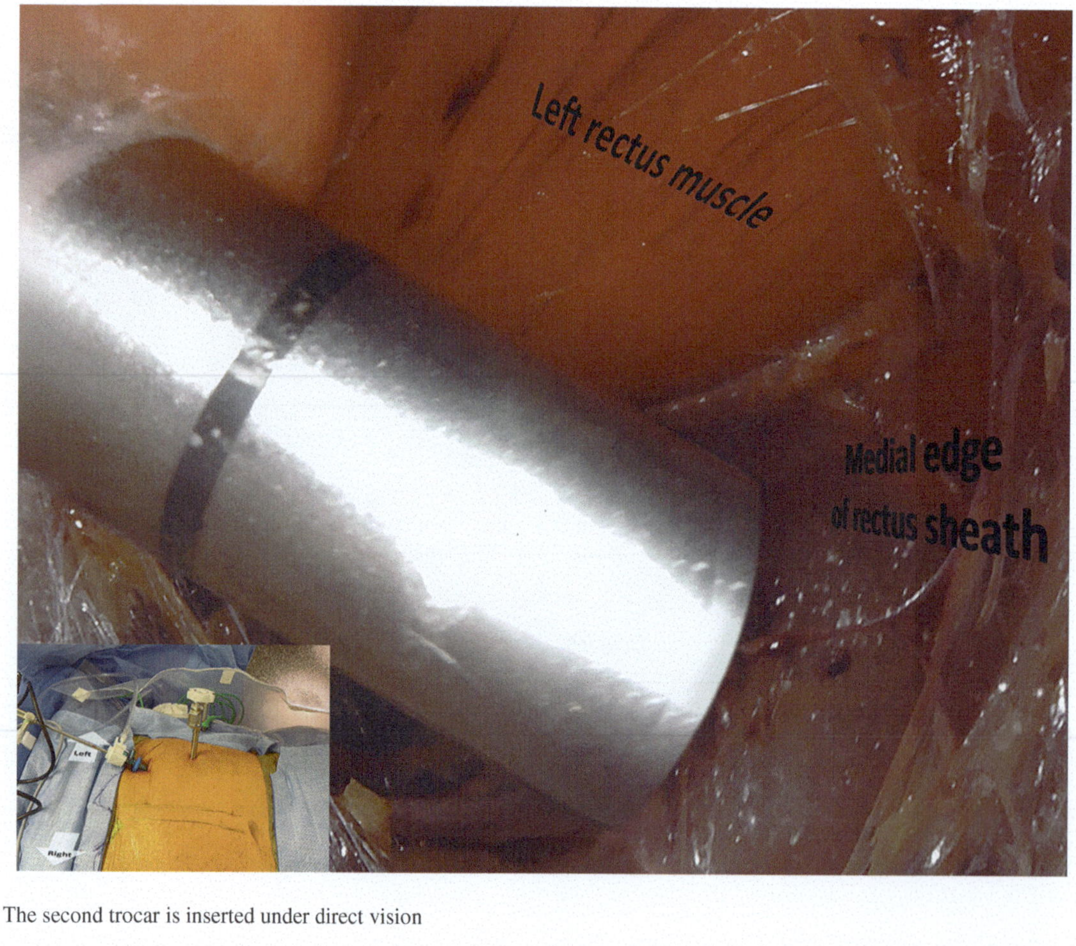


Fig. 3.10 The second trocar is inserted under direct vision

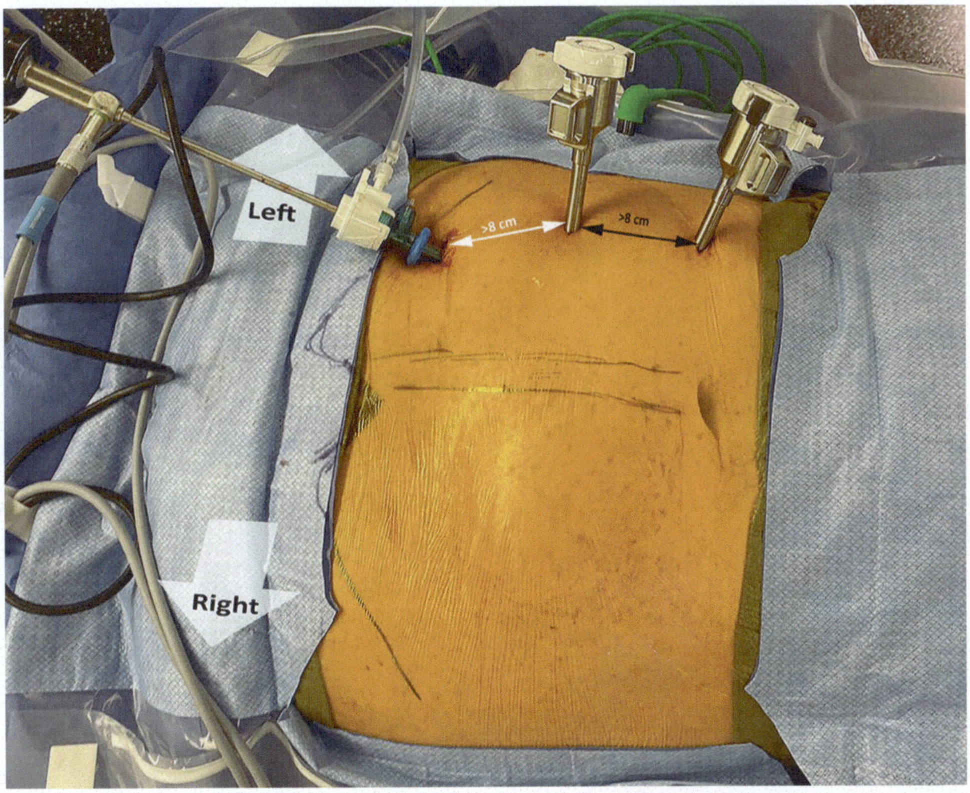


**Fig. 3.11** The third trocar is inserted at least 8 cm from the second trocar, in order to minimize mechanical interference between the robotic arms

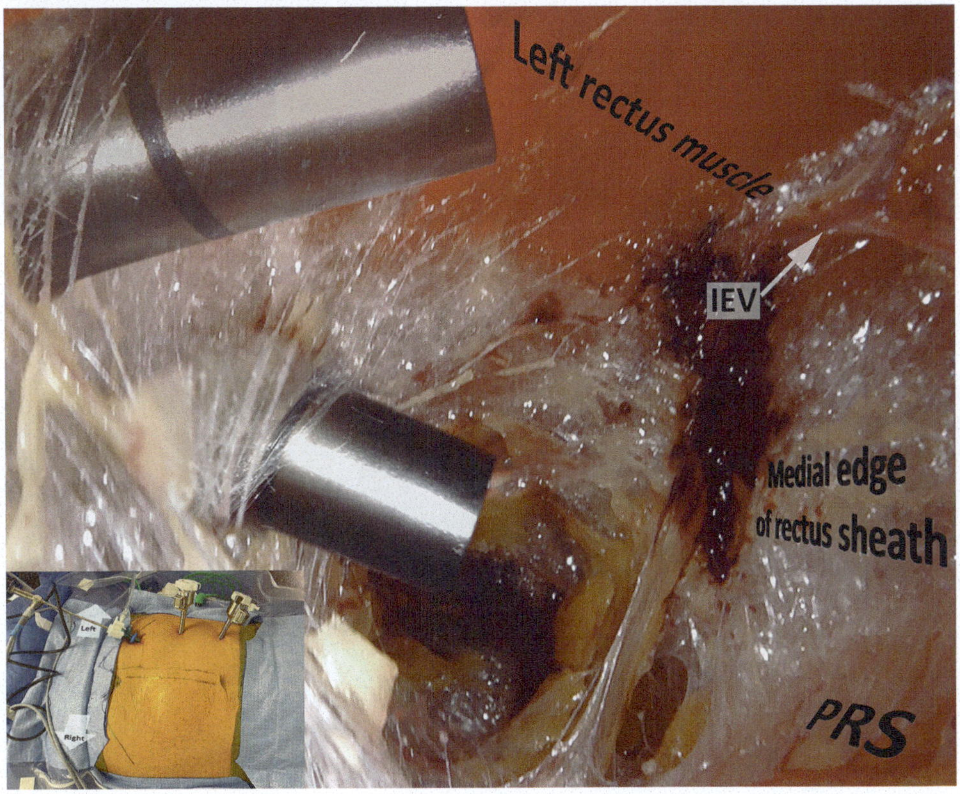


**Fig. 3.12** The third trocar is inserted under direct vision. IEV inferior epigastric vessel; PRS posterior rectus sheath

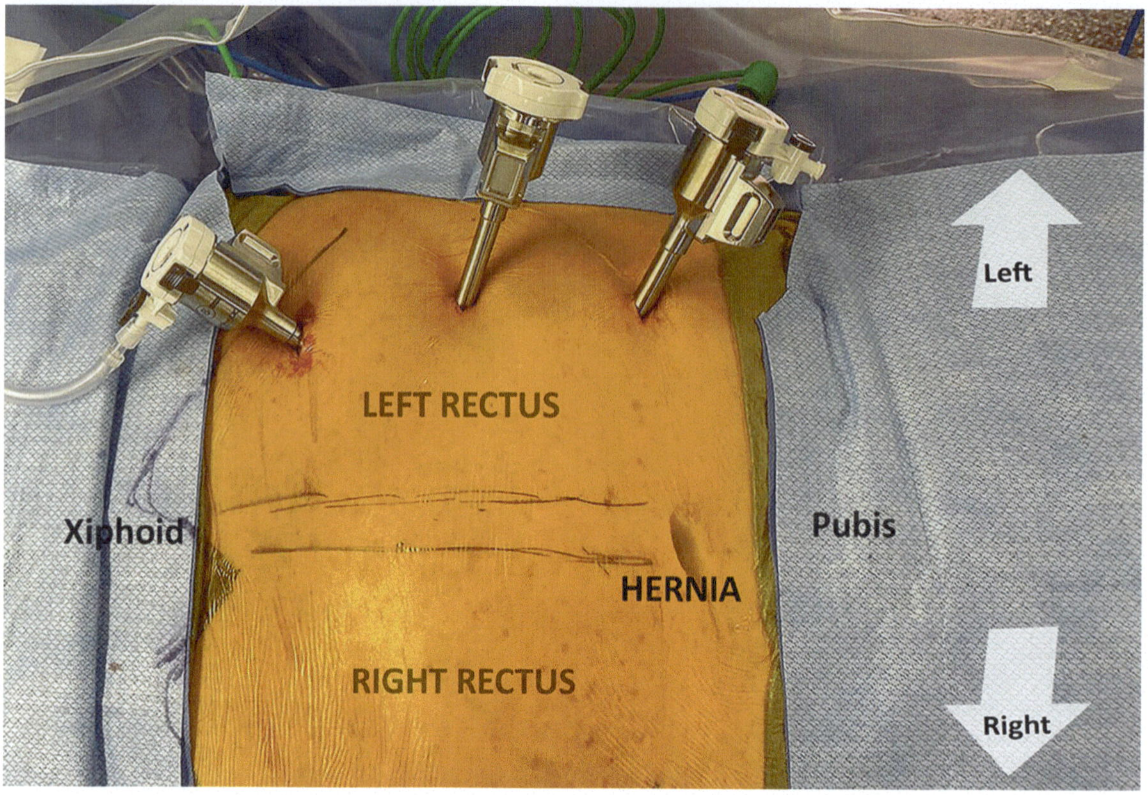


**Fig. 3.13** The initially placed 5-mm trocar is then switched to an 8.5-mm da Vinci trocar (Intuitive Surgical Inc., Sunnyvale, CA, USA)

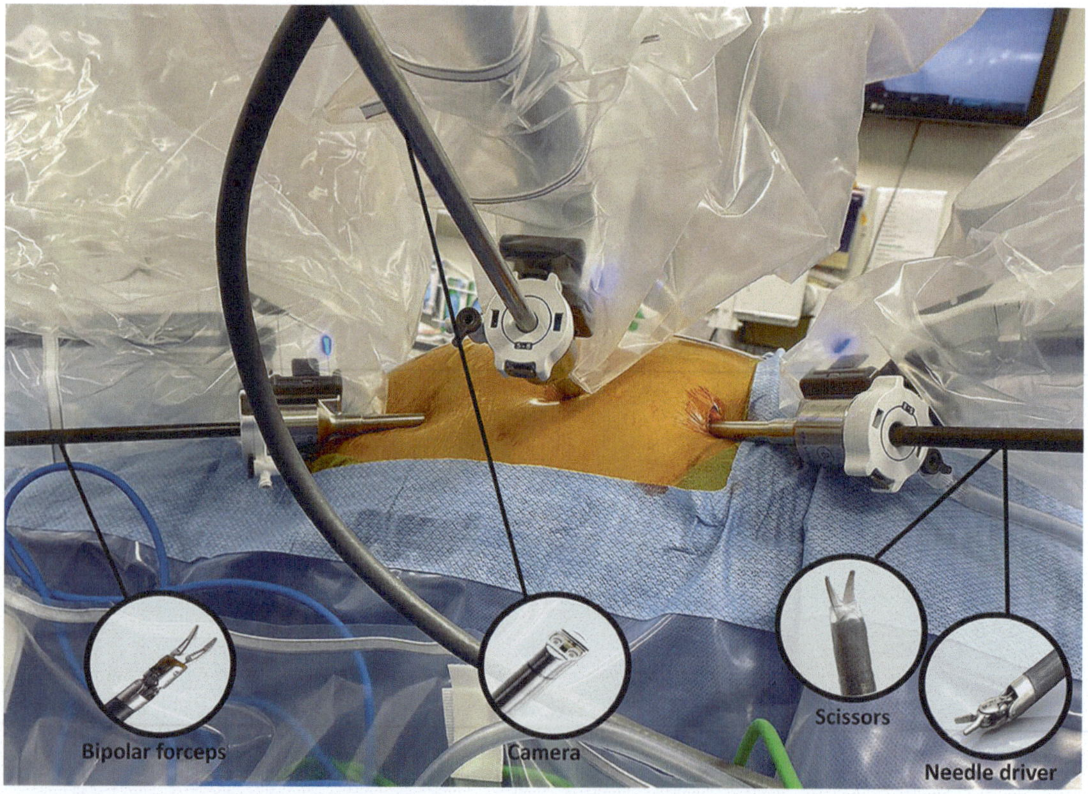


**Fig. 3.14** Once proper trocar placement is achieved, the patient-side cart of the da Vinci surgical system (Model Xi, Intuitive Surgical Inc., Sunnyvale, CA, USA) is docked at the patient's right side. The EndoWrist® instruments (Intuitive Surgical Inc., Sunnyvale, CA, USA) are used as follows: First, a bipolar fenestrated forceps and monopolar curved scissors; later, the scissors are switched to a large suture cut needle driver. The 30°camera is pointed to the target anatomy, and the system will automatically position the boom to ensure an optimal arm configuration for the procedure

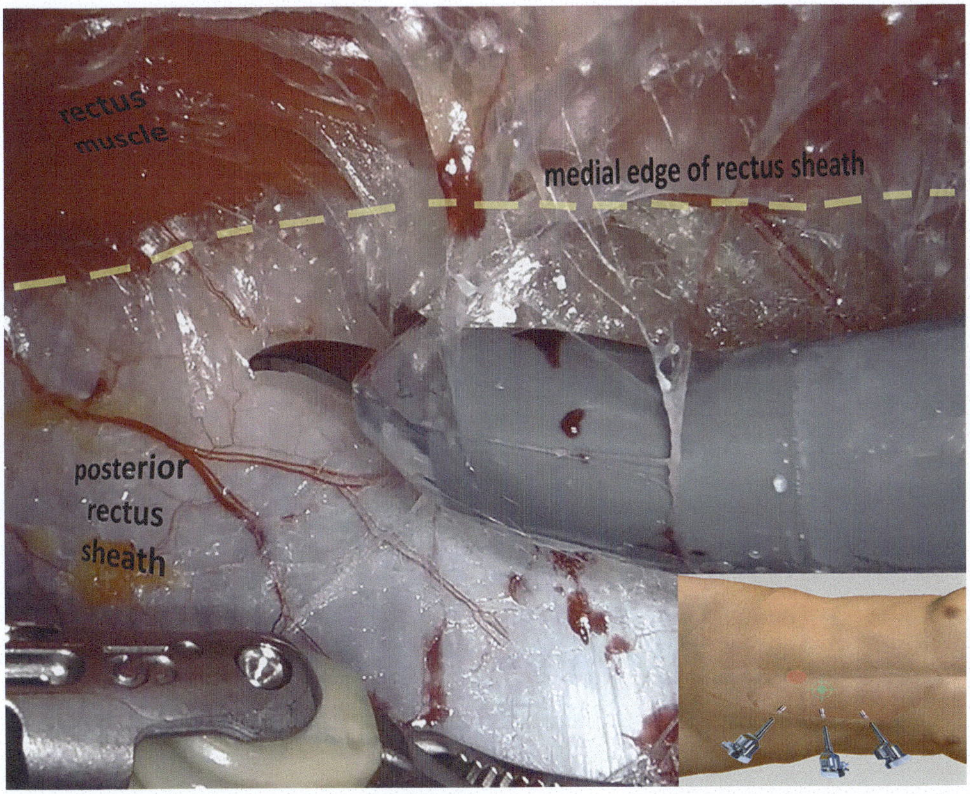


Fig. 3.15 Loose connective tissue between the rectus muscle and rectus sheath is dissected to reach the medial edge of the ipsilateral rectus sheath

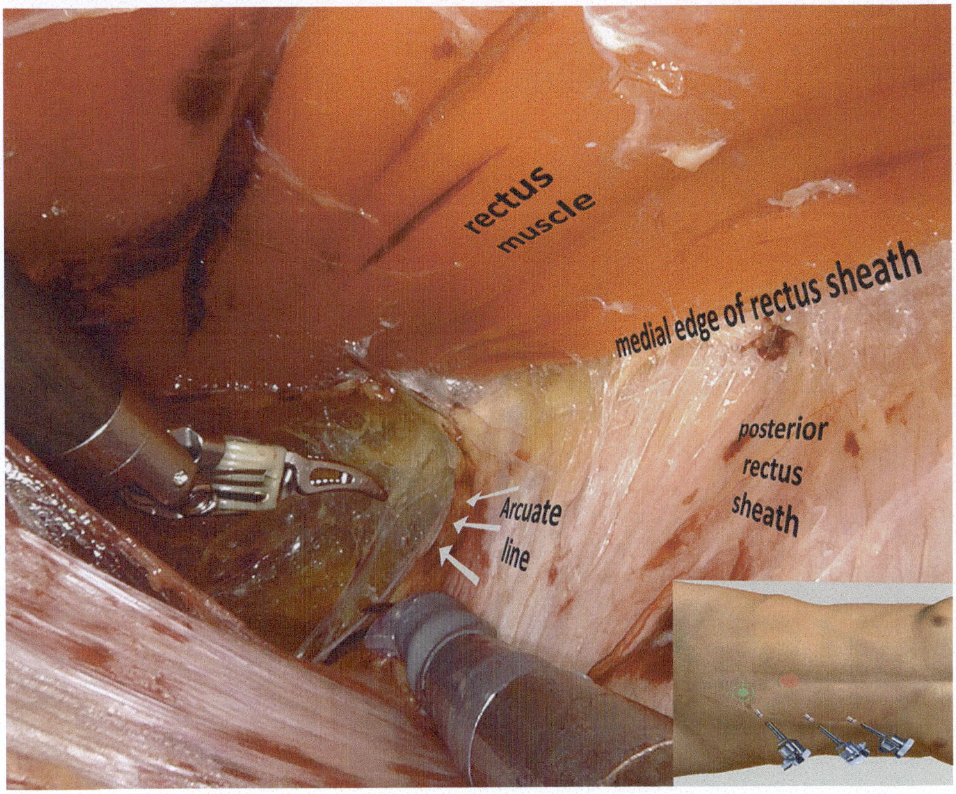


Fig. 3.16 Ipsilateral retrorectus dissection is completed, and the medial edge of the ipsilateral rectus sheath is revealed from the supraumbilical to infraumbilical aspects

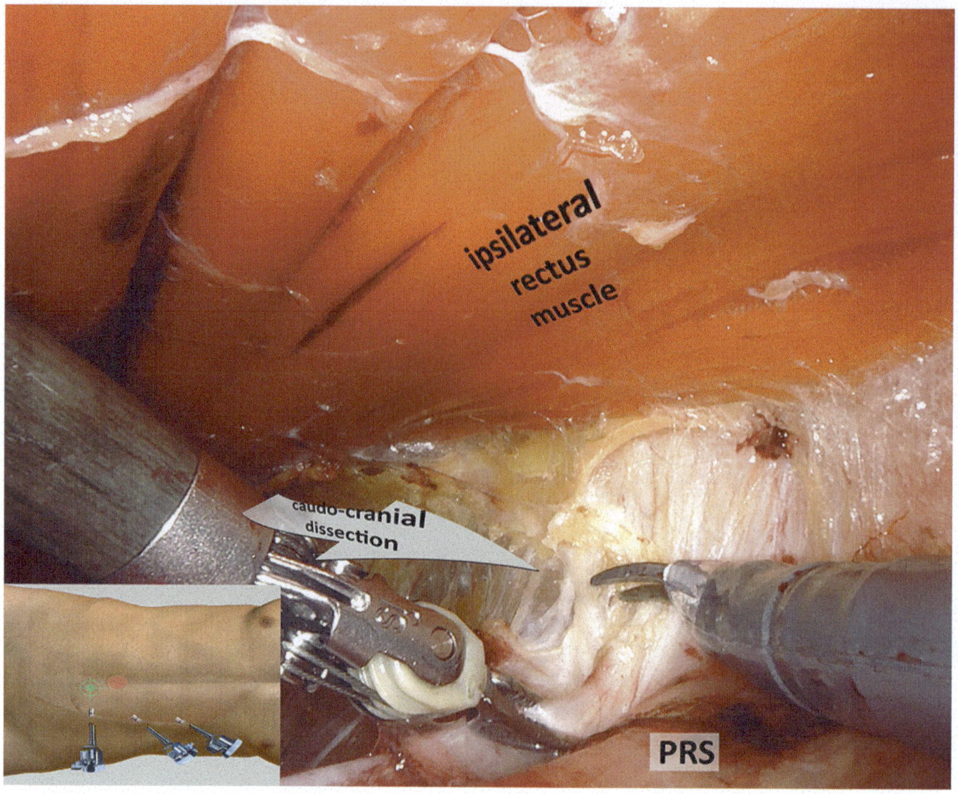


Fig. 3.17 The medial edge of the rectus sheath is incised in the caudocranial direction. PRS posterior rectus sheath

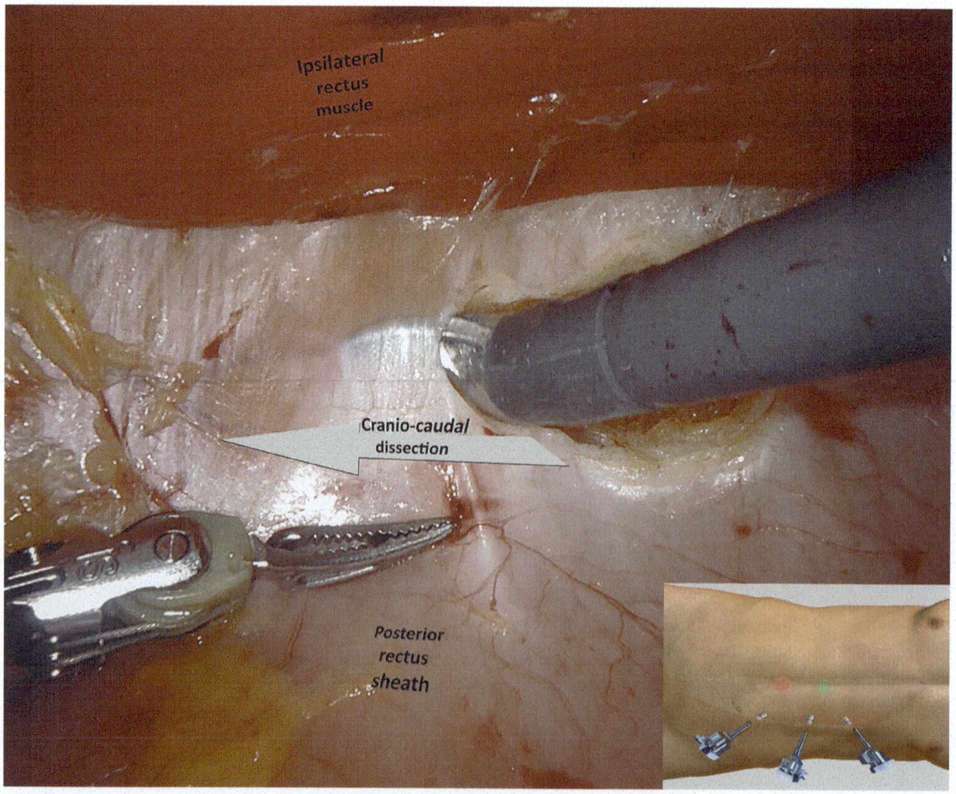


Fig. 3.18 A similar step is repeated for the supraumbilical portion, starting approximately 5–8 cm away from the hernia defect and proceeding in the craniocaudal direction

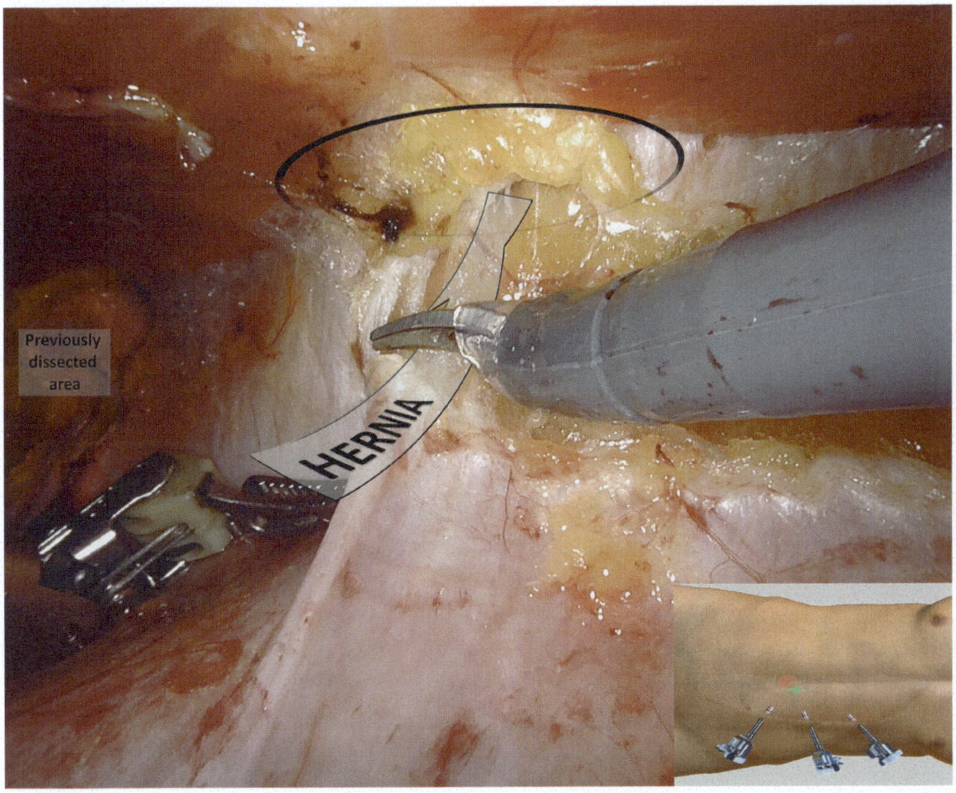


**Fig. 3.19** Caution should be exercised when dividing the posterior rectus sheath in order to prevent inadvertent intraabdominal organ injury, especially in the case of an incarcerated hernia

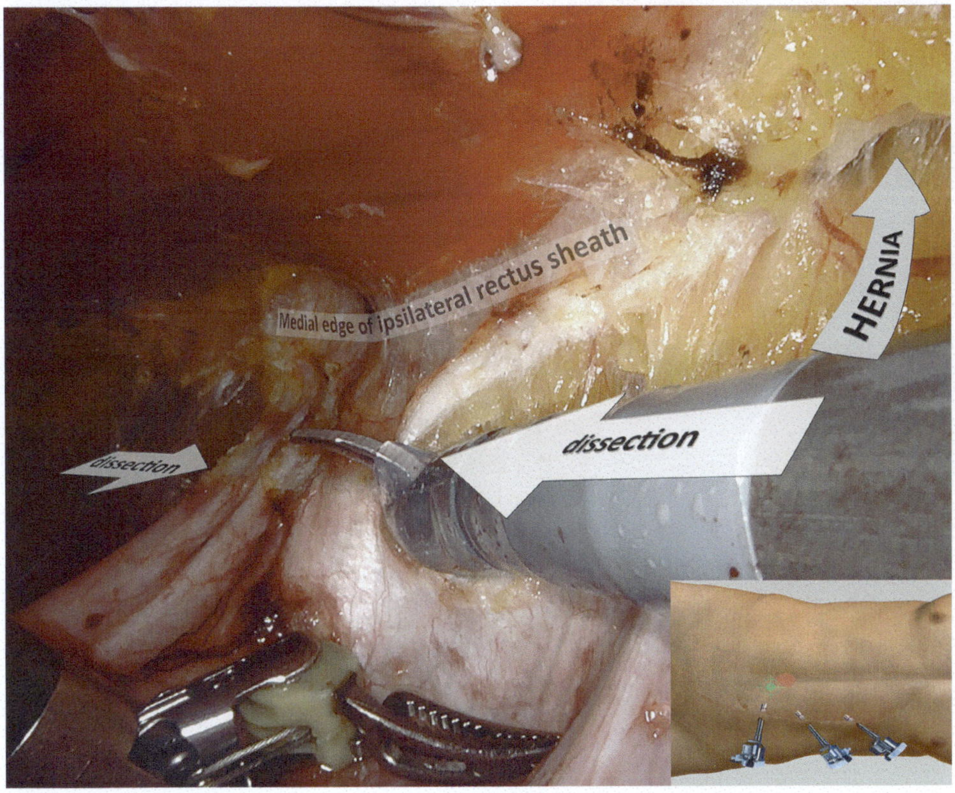


**Fig. 3.20** The division of the medial edge of the posterior rectus sheath is completed by joining the two dissection lines

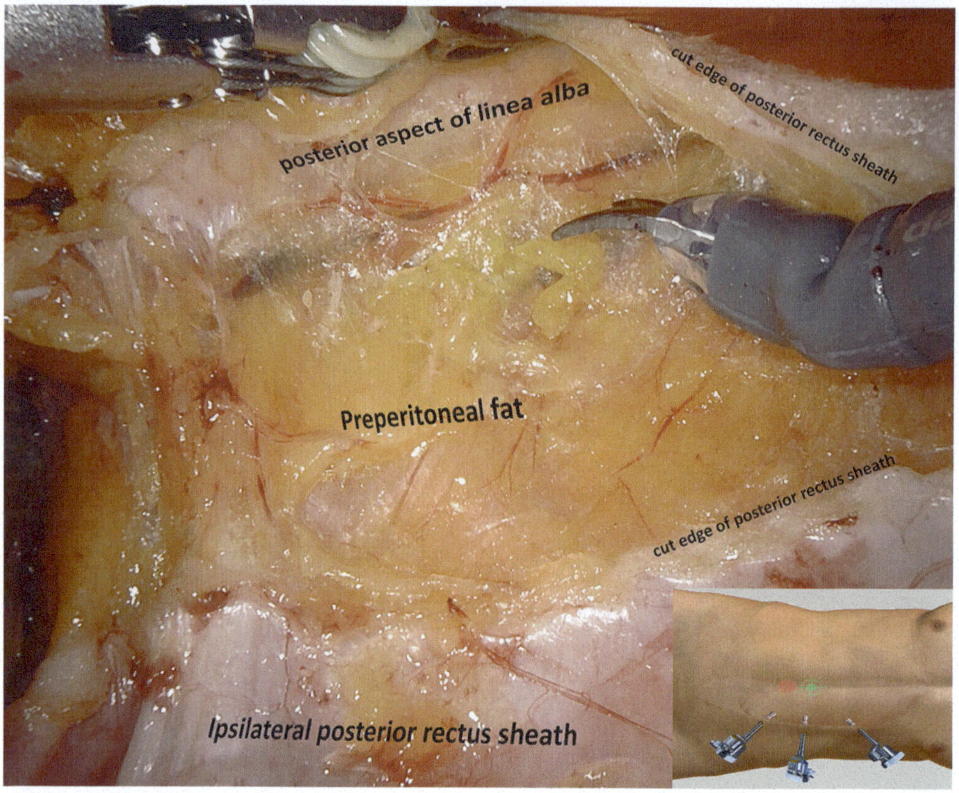


**Fig. 3.21** To enter the contralateral rectus sheath, it is recommended to initiate crossover in a previously unviolated area. The supraumbilical part of the posterior aspect of the linea alba may be a more suitable entry point for this purpose. At this location, the preperitoneal fat is relatively dense because of the contribution of the falciform ligament (superiorly) and umbilical ligaments (inferiorly)

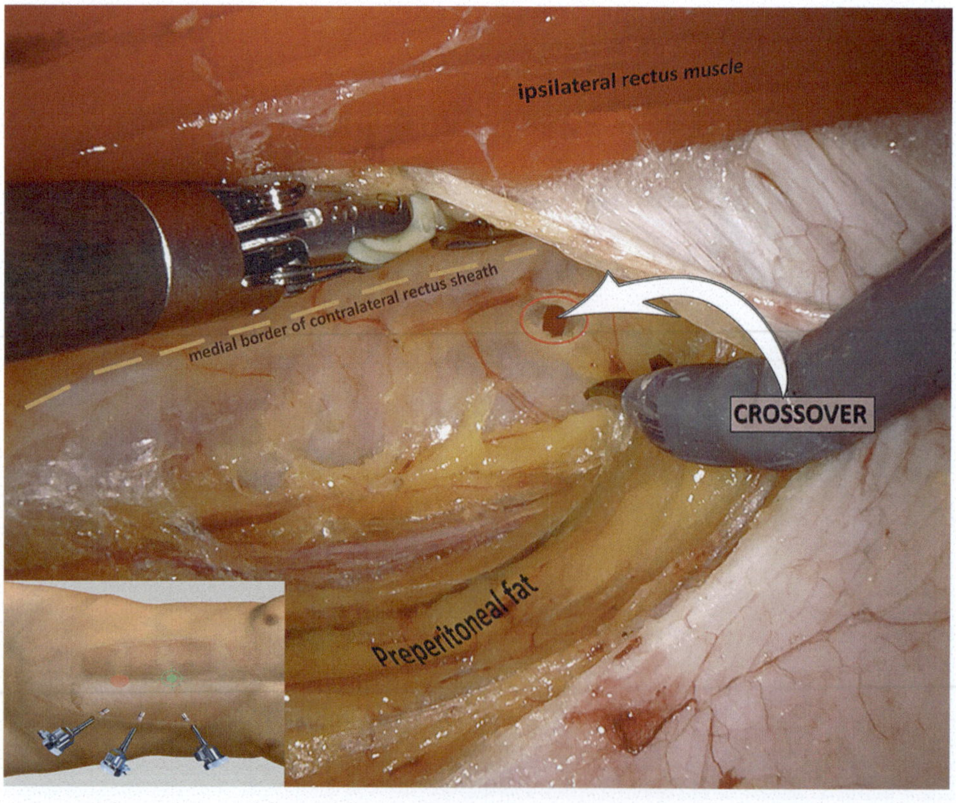


**Fig. 3.22** Once preperitoneal dissection is completed, the contralateral rectus sheath is incised just below the linea alba

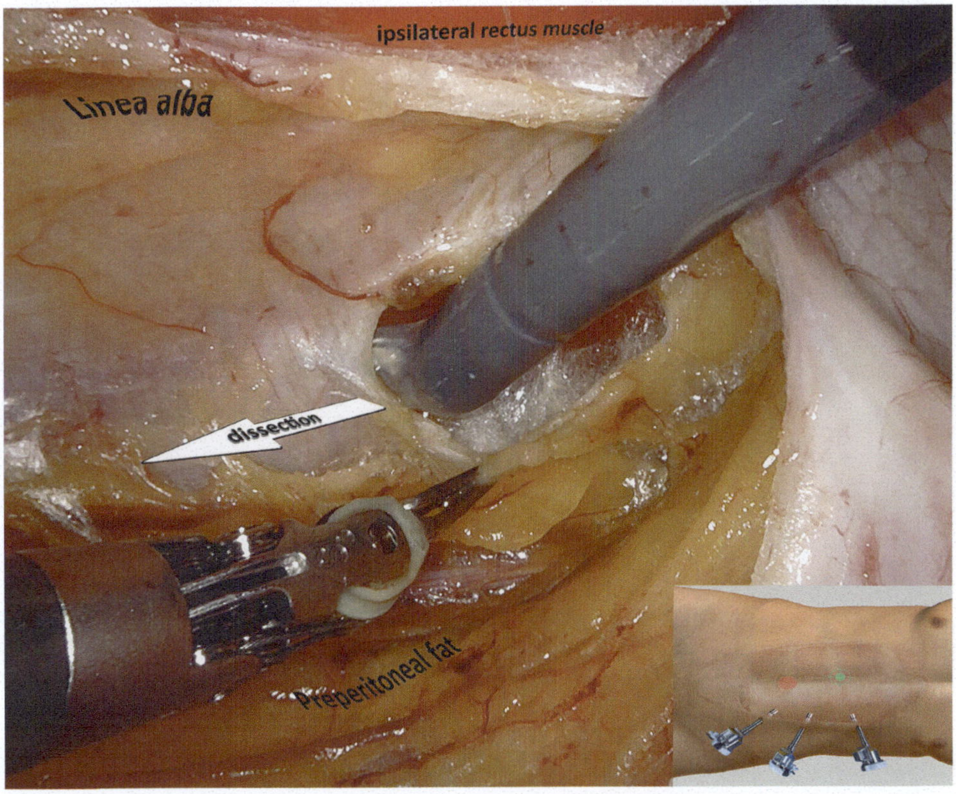


Fig. 3.23 The dissection of the contralateral rectus sheath is carried out toward the hernia defect

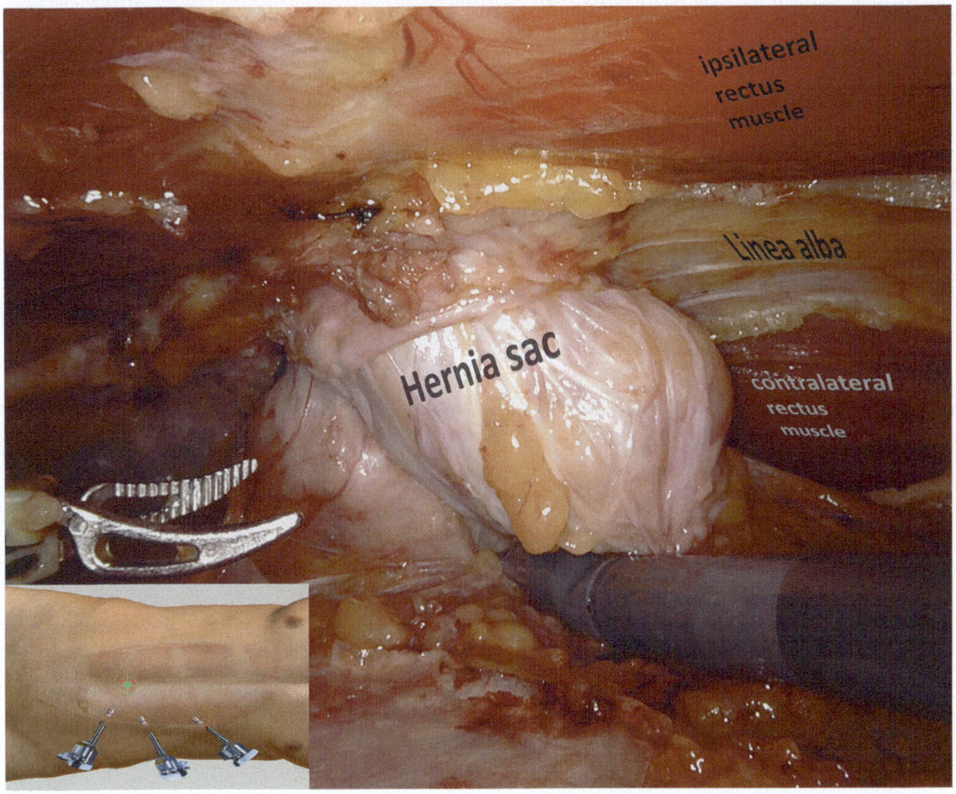


Fig. 3.24 Visceral content of the hernia sac is reduced into the abdominal cavity. Circumferential dissection around the hernia defect and external compression by the bedside assistant or scrub nurse may facilitate this step

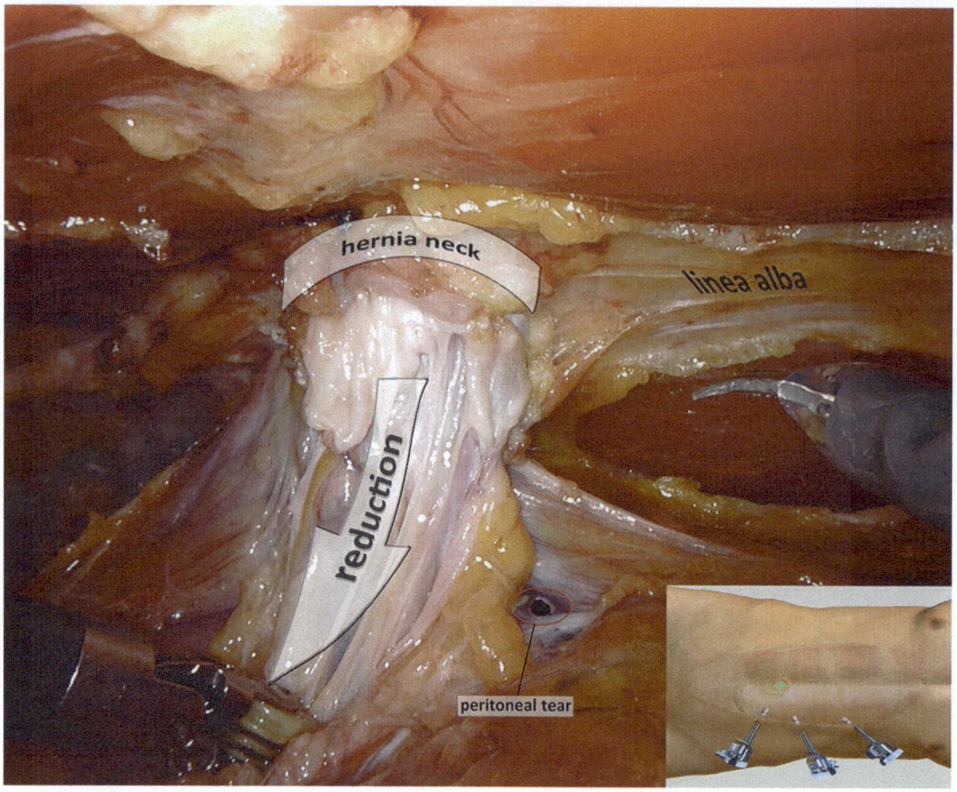


Fig. 3.25 The hernia sac is separated from its distal attachments. Any peritoneal tear should be closed later with an absorbable suture

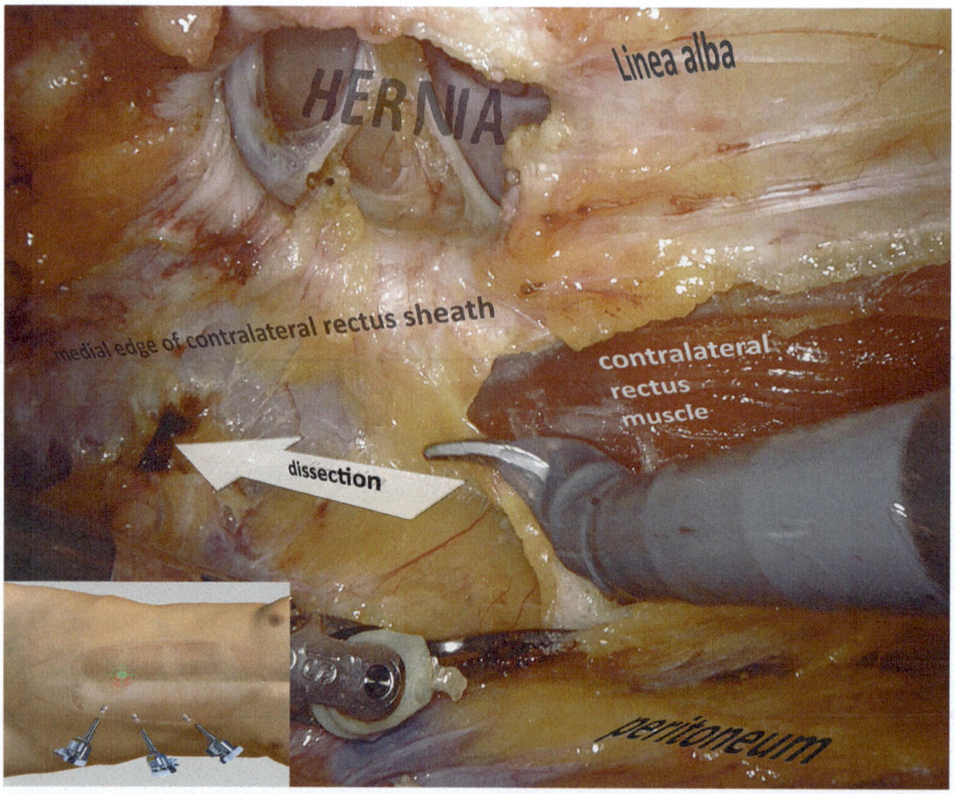


Fig. 3.26 Contralateral medial edge dissection is continued caudally

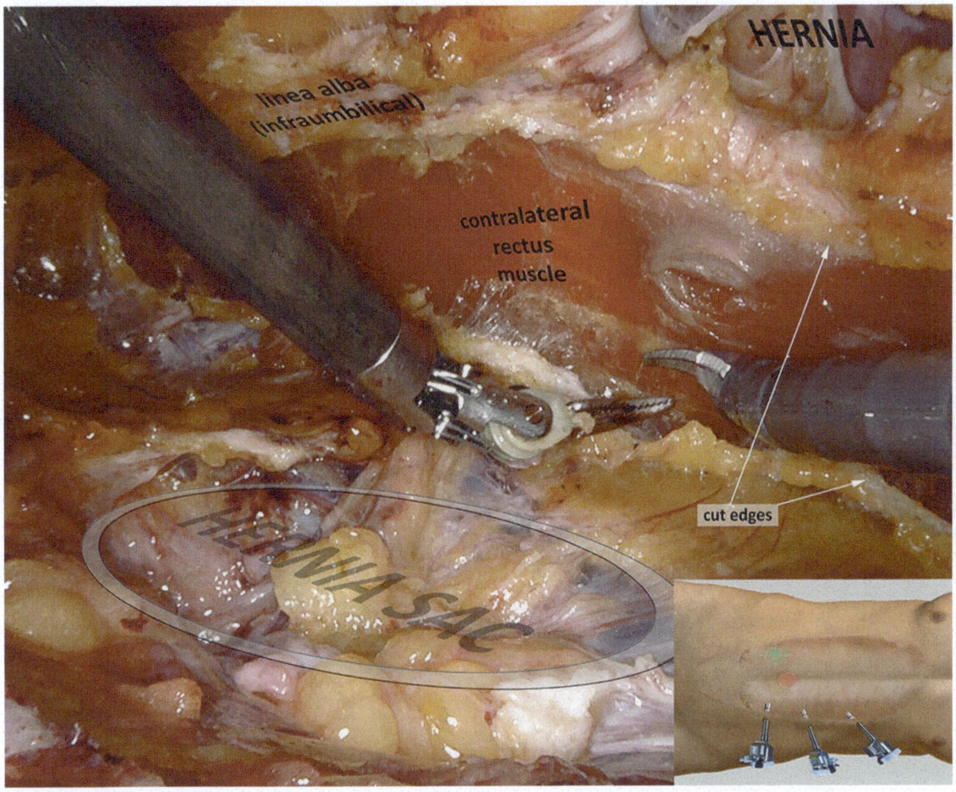


Fig. 3.27 Contralateral retrorectus dissection is performed to reach the lateral edge of the contralateral rectus sheath

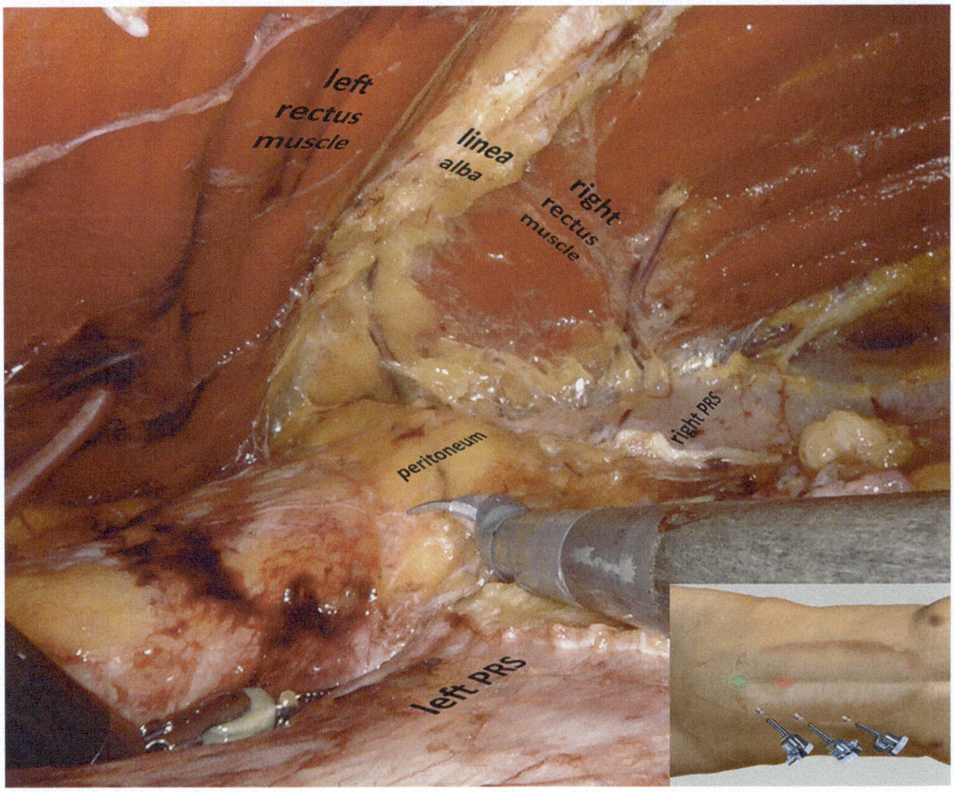


Fig. 3.28 The retrorectus area should be cleared from any adhesions between the rectus muscle and posterior flap in order to deploy the mesh without any wrinkling. PRS posterior rectus sheath

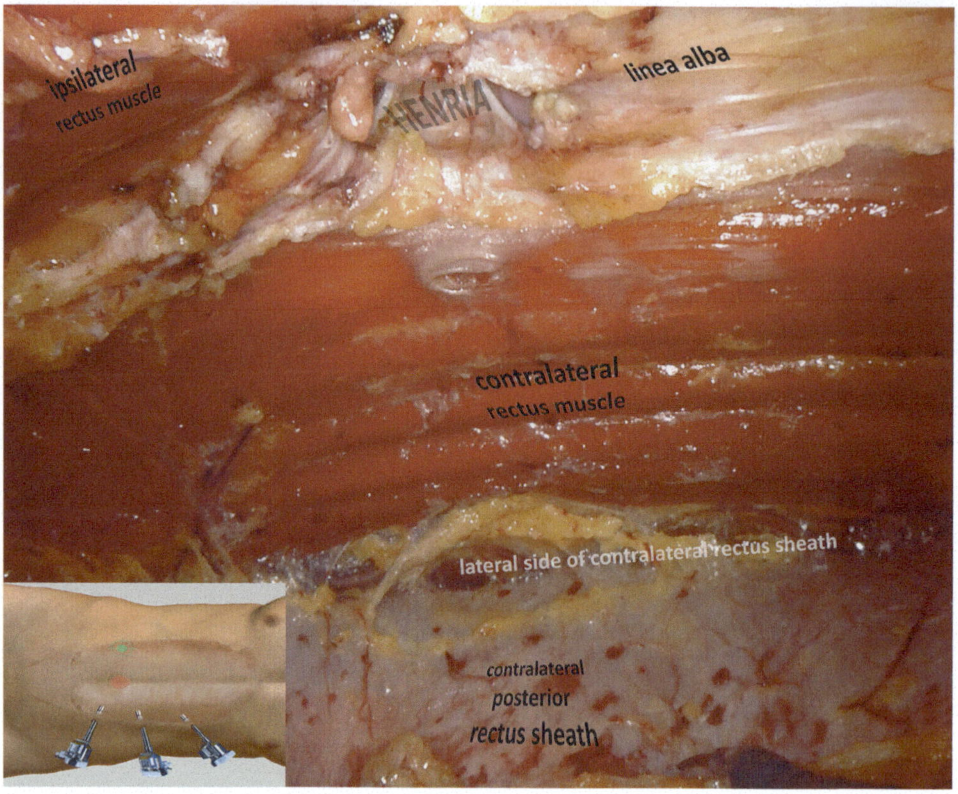


**Fig. 3.29** The border of the Rives-Stoppa repair is formed by the lateral side of the contralateral rectus sheath

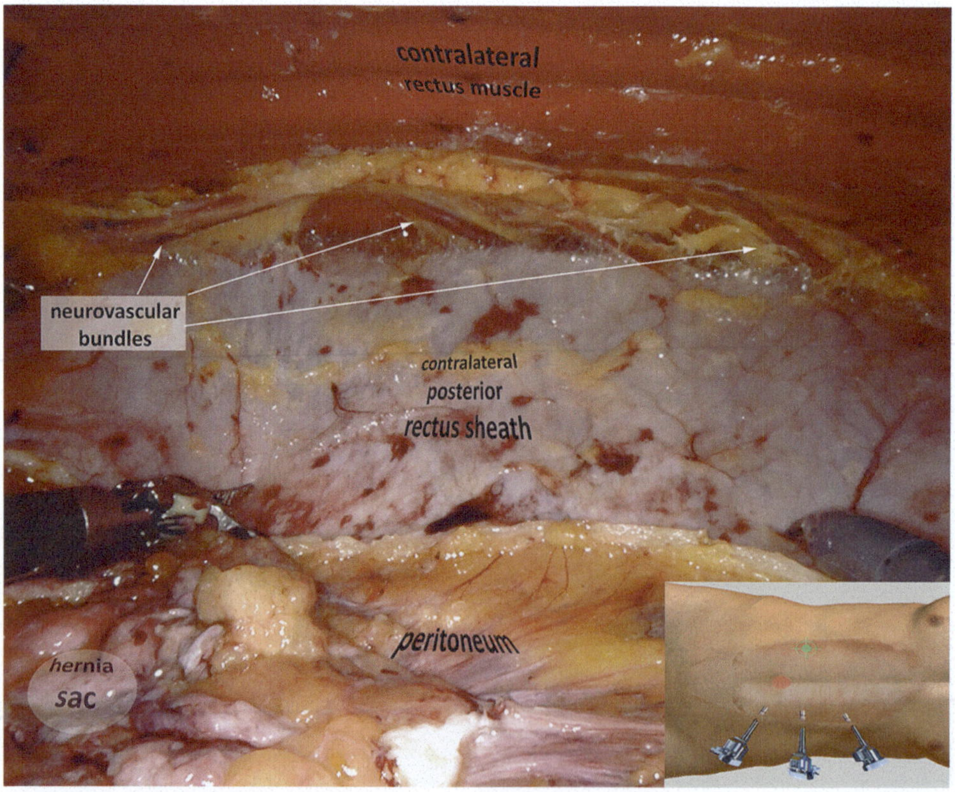


**Fig. 3.30** Neurovascular bundles are spared in the case of a transversus abdominis release

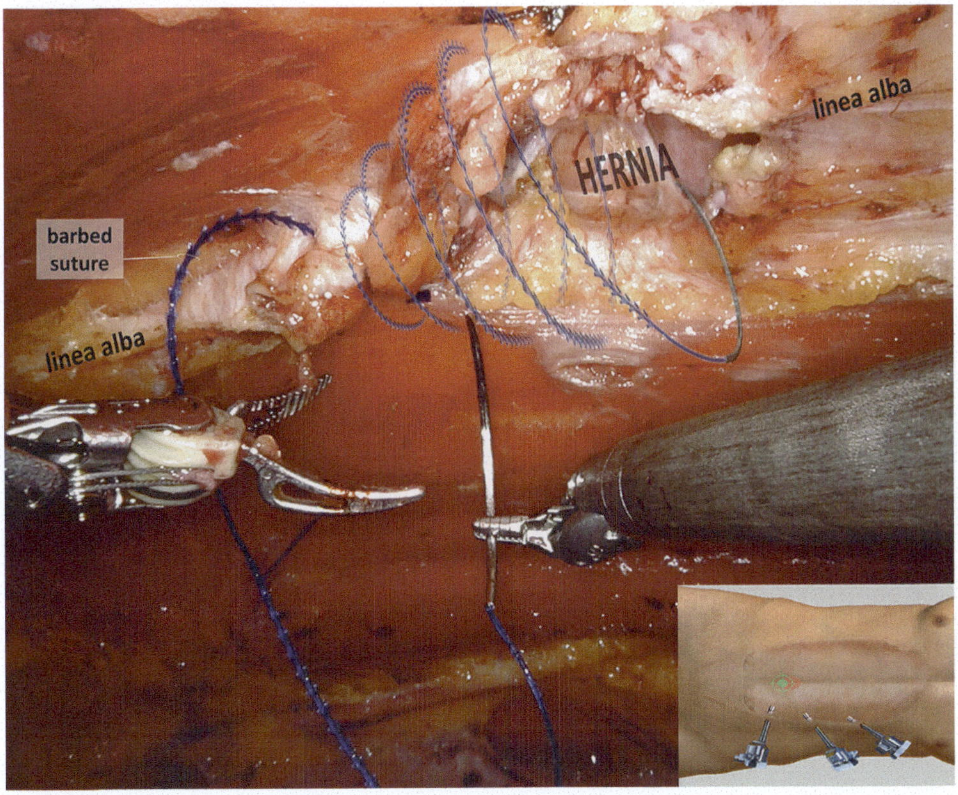


Fig. 3.31 Once retromuscular dissection is completed, the next step is to close the hernia defect. The authors prefer a small-bite suture technique in running fashion, using a long-lasting absorbable barbed suture (Stratafix™ 0 on CT-1 needle, Ethicon, Somerville, NJ, USA). Reducing $CO_2$ pressure may facilitate this step. In the case of diastasis recti, linea alba reconstruction is performed

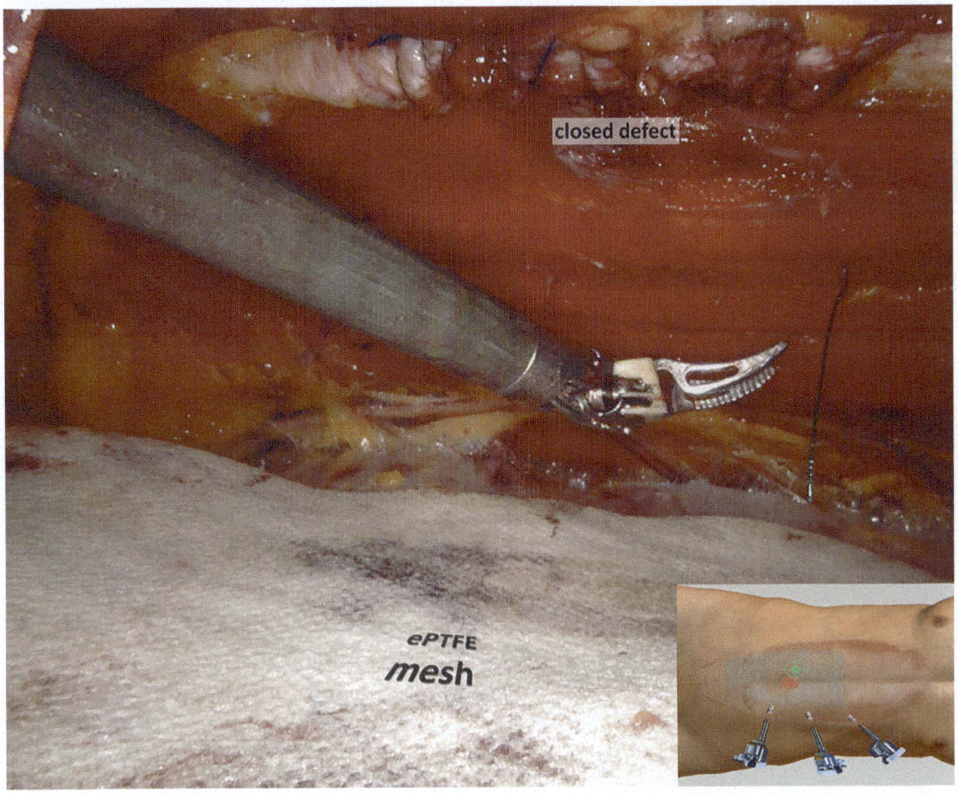


Fig. 3.32 After closing the defect, the mesh is deployed in the retrorectus space. Mesh fixation is not required generally. ePTFE expanded polytetrafluoroethylene

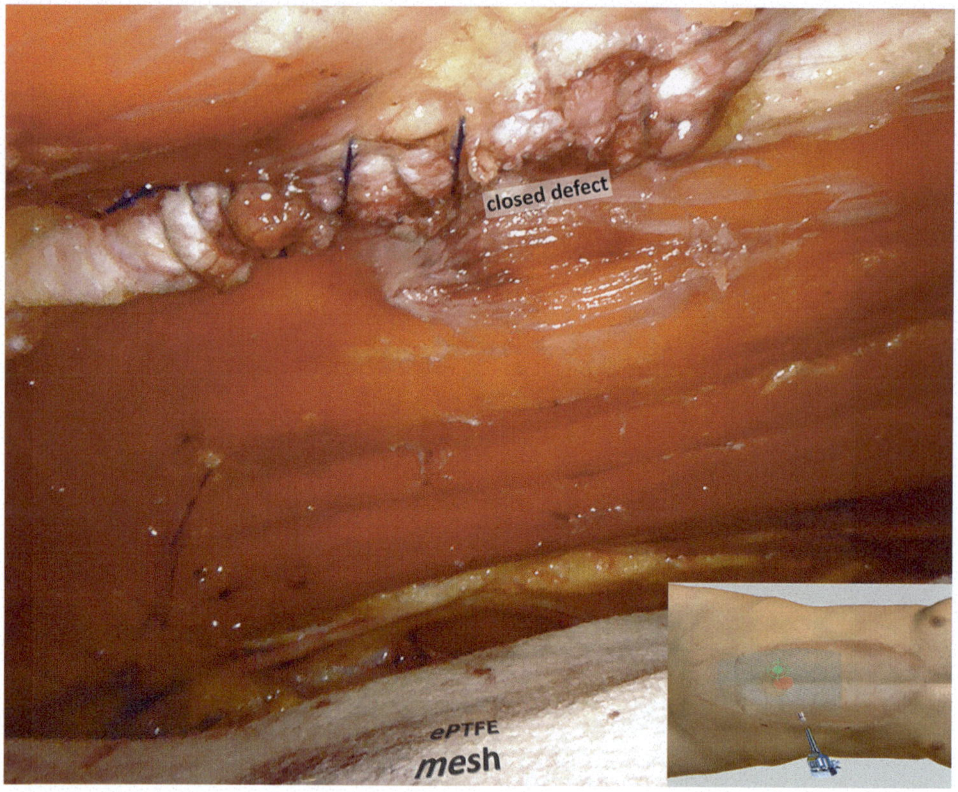


Fig. 3.33 $CO_2$ is evacuated under direct vision

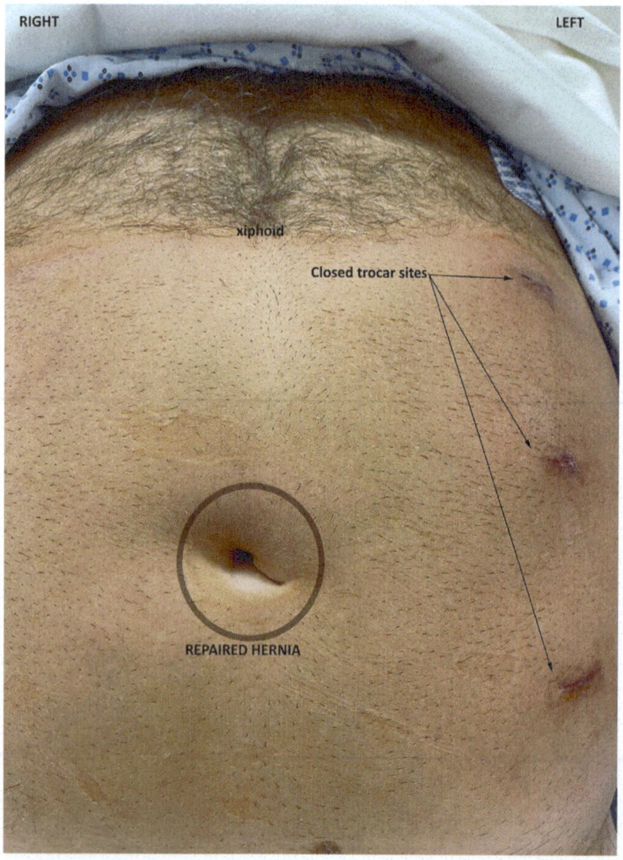


Fig. 3.34 The skin incisions are closed using an absorbable suture

## References

1. Carbonell AM. Rives-Stoppa retromuscular repair. In: Novitsky YW, editor. Hernia surgery: current principles. Cham: Springer; 2016. p. 107–15.
2. Belyansky I, Reza Zahiri H, Sanford Z, Weltz AS, Park A. Early operative outcomes of endoscopic (eTEP access) robotic-assisted retromuscular abdominal wall hernia repair. Hernia. 2018;22:837–47. https://doi.org/10.1007/s10029-018-1795-z.

# 4 Robotic Hybrid Ventral Hernia Repair: Totally Extraperitoneal (TEP)

Naseem Bou-Ayash, Fahri Gokcal, and Omar Yusef Kudsi

## Introduction

Hybrid robotic ventral hernia repair (hrVHR) has been used in minimally invasive surgery (MIS) to combine advantages of both the robotic and open approaches. In general, hrVHR is adopted for large incisional ventral hernias, which present particular difficulty in terms of dissection of attenuated anatomical layers and approximation of the fascia prior to mesh deployment. By doing so, surgeons reap the benefits of the robotic platform by obtaining precise dissection. After creating the necessary retromuscular space robotically, surgeons often struggle to manipulate the fascial edges during defect closure, risking high tension and disruption of the fascia. This is where the open approach can be implemented to help deploy a wide mesh and to facilitate defect closure. When compared with open repair, hrVHR has been shown to achieve shorter length of hospital stay (LOS) with similar rates of complication and wound morbidity [1, 2].

## Procedure: Illustrated Steps

Figures 4.1, 4.2, 4.3, 4.4, 4.5, 4.6, 4.7, 4.8, 4.9, 4.10, 4.11, 4.12, 4.13, 4.14, 4.15, 4.16, 4.17, 4.18, 4.19, 4.20, 4.21, 4.22, 4.23, 4.24, 4.25, 4.26, 4.27, 4.28, 4.29, 4.30, 4.31, 4.32, and 4.33 illustrate the technical aspects of hybrid robotic totally extraperitoneal retromuscular repair with transversus abdominis release of a large incisional hernia.

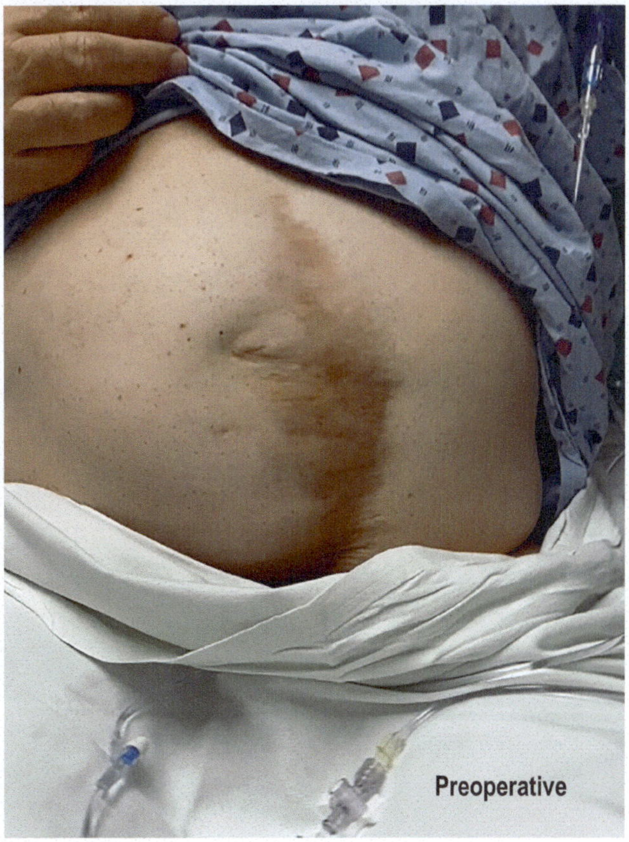


**Fig. 4.1** Preoperative incisional hernia

N. Bou-Ayash · F. Gokcal
Department of Surgery, Good Samaritan Medical Center, Brockton, MA, USA

O. Y. Kudsi (✉)
Department of Surgery, Good Samaritan Medical Center, Tufts University School of Medicine, Boston, MA, USA


O. Y. Kudsi (ed.), *Robotic Hernia Surgery*, https://doi.org/10.1007/978-3-030-46667-1_4

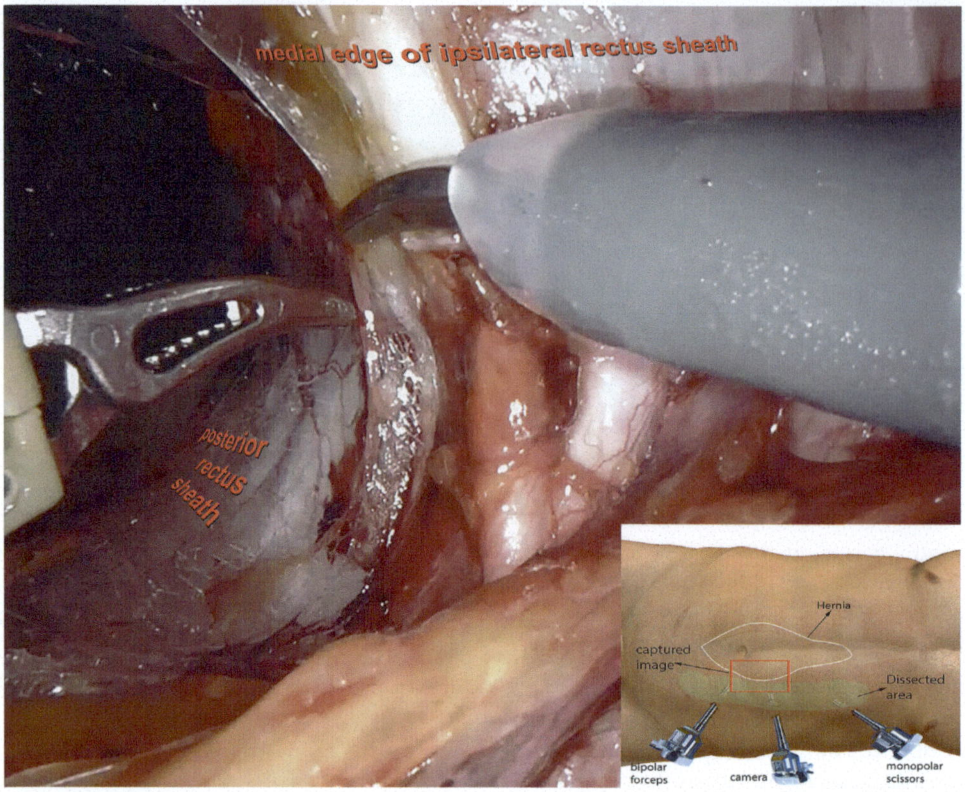


**Fig. 4.2** After TEP access (described in Chap. 3), the patient-side cart of the robot is docked and ipsilateral retrorectus dissection is performed. The sub-figure shows trocar positions, captured image, and hernia location

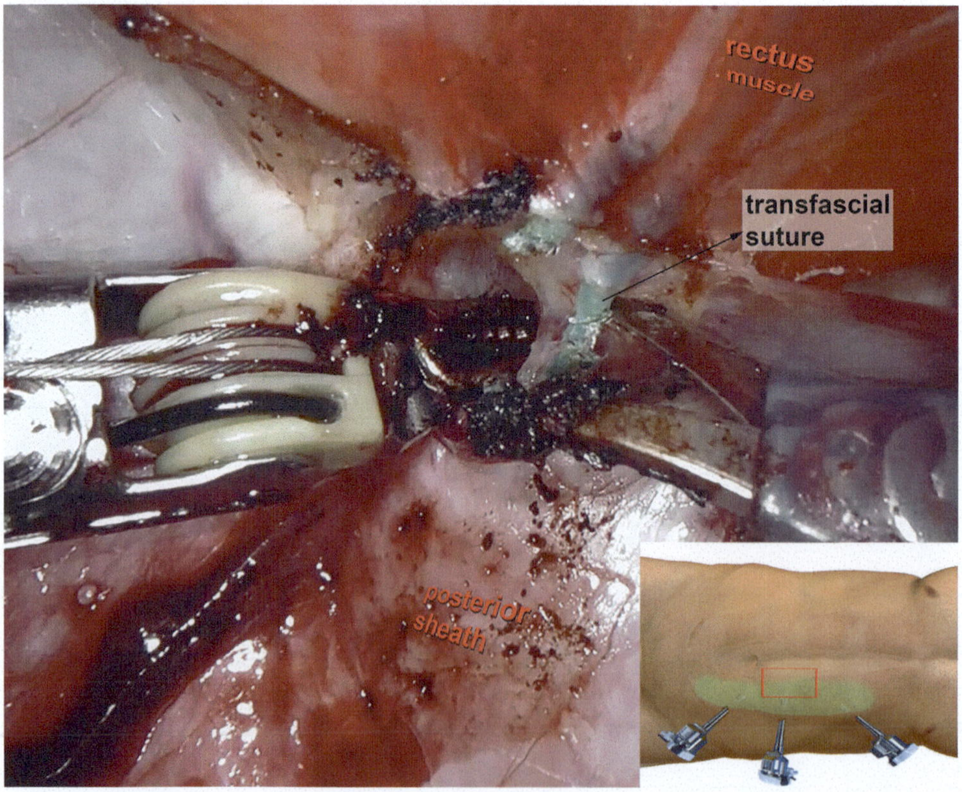


**Fig. 4.3** Once the retrorectus space is entered, ipsilateral retrorectus dissection is performed. Throughout dissection, previously placed transfascial sutures are cut as encountered

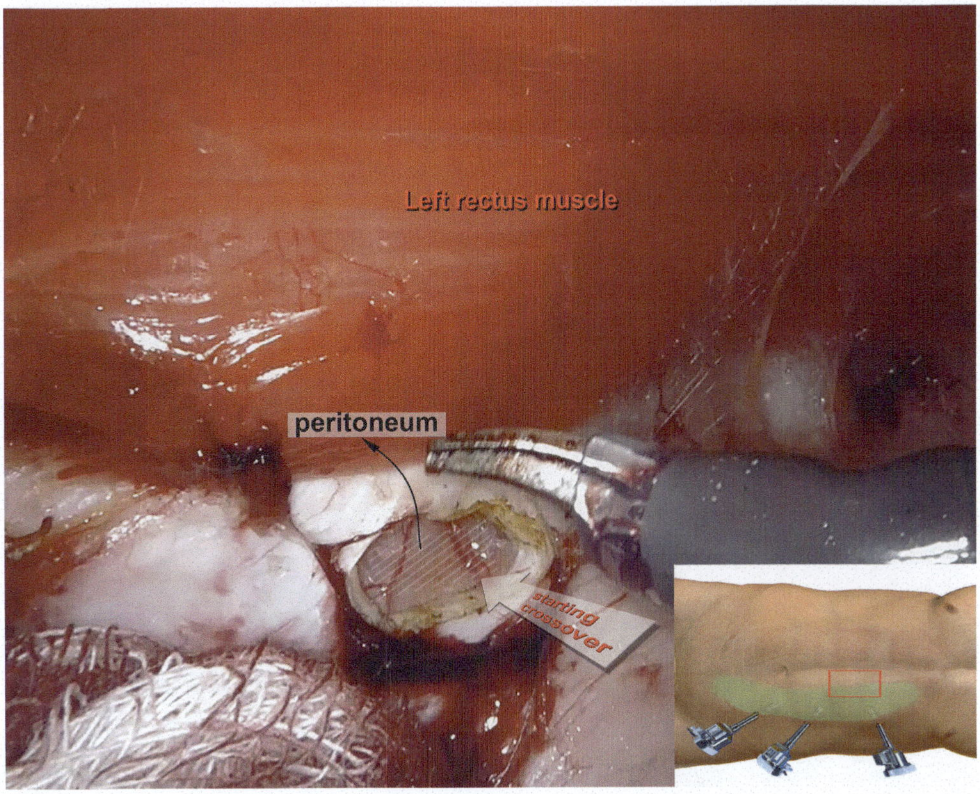


Fig. 4.4 Once ipsilateral retrorectus dissection is completed, crossover into the contralateral retrorectus space is started by incising the medial aspect of the posterior rectus sheath

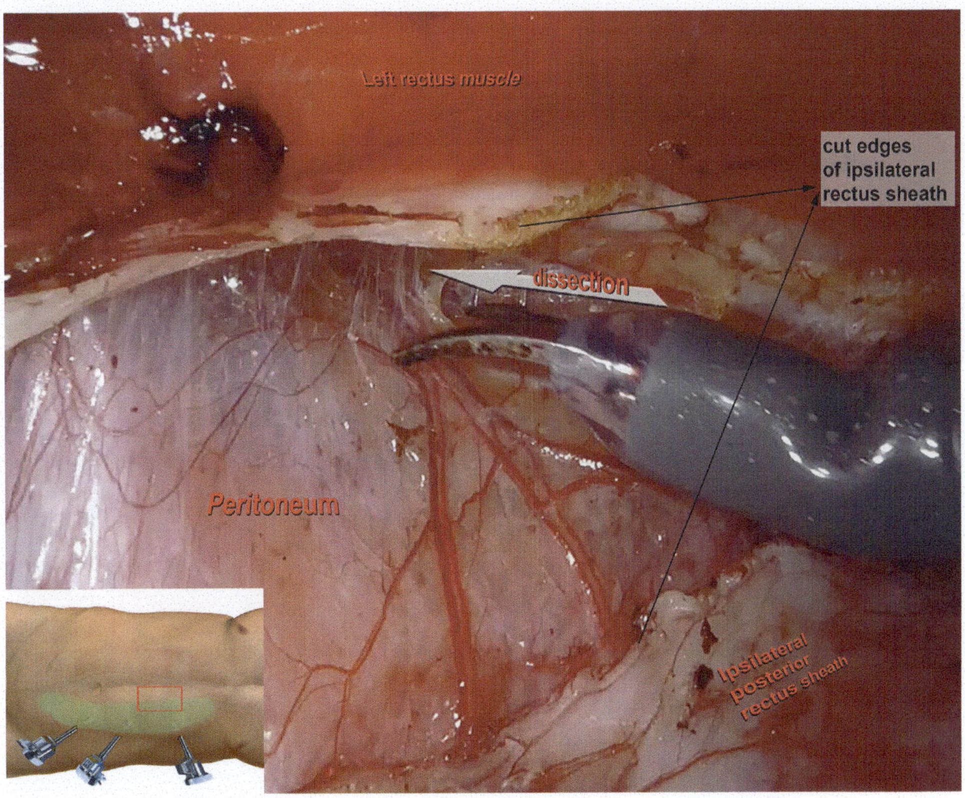


Fig. 4.5 The medial aspect of the posterior rectus sheath is divided, and preperitoneal dissection is performed inferior to the linea alba

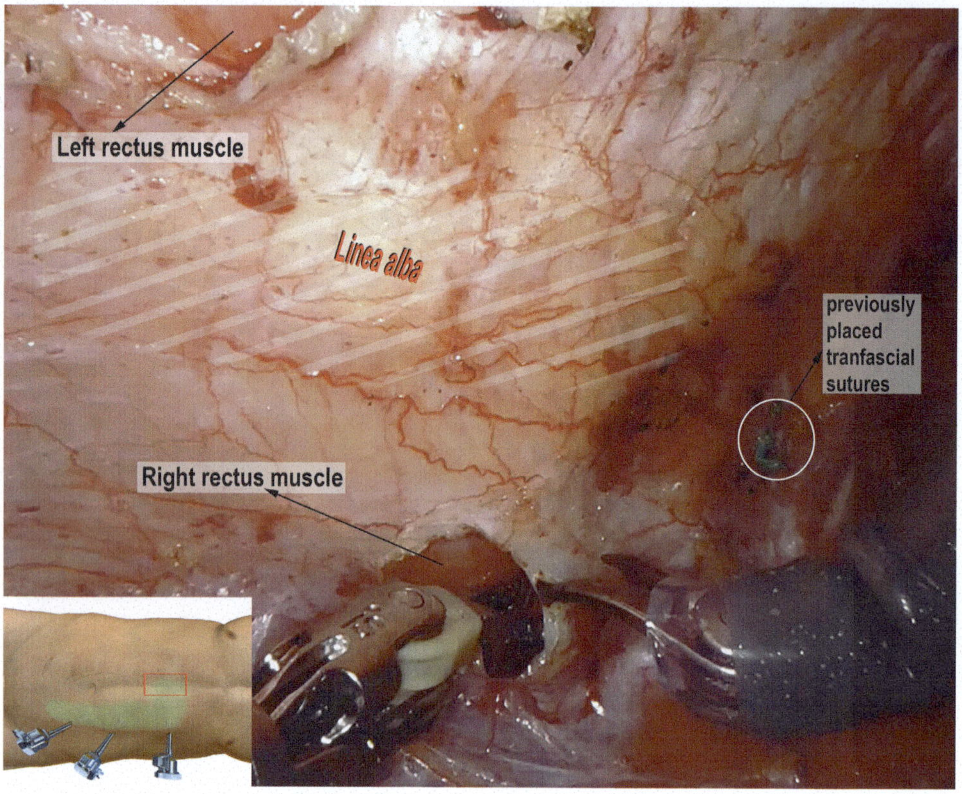


Fig. 4.6 After preperitoneal dissection, the contralateral rectus sheath is incised and entered

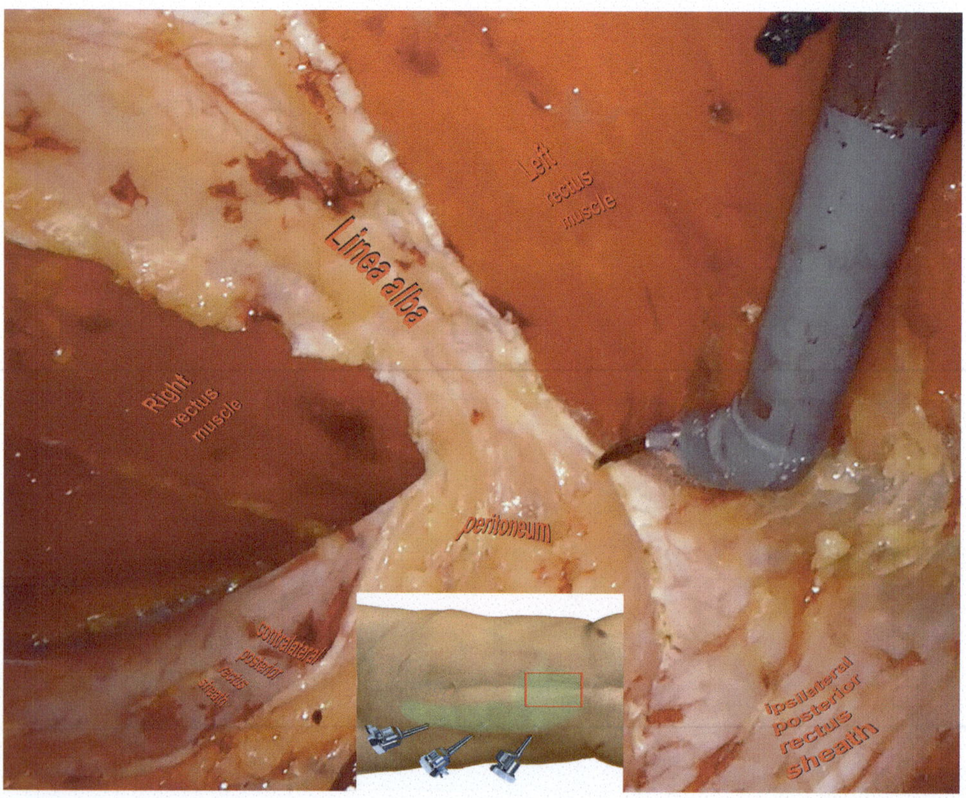


Fig. 4.7 Crossover is achieved, and both retrorectus spaces are merged into one space. The dissection is carried out towards the sub-xyphoid area

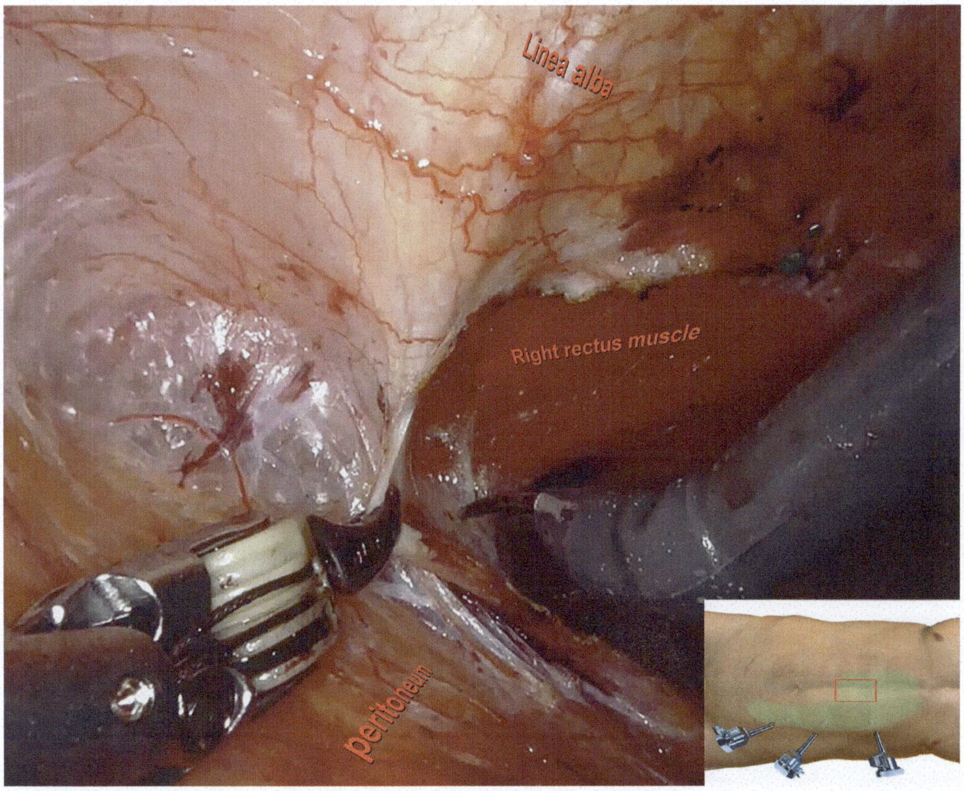


**Fig. 4.8** Initiation of crossover takes place in virgin tissue planes, followed by craniocaudal dissection towards the incisional hernia site

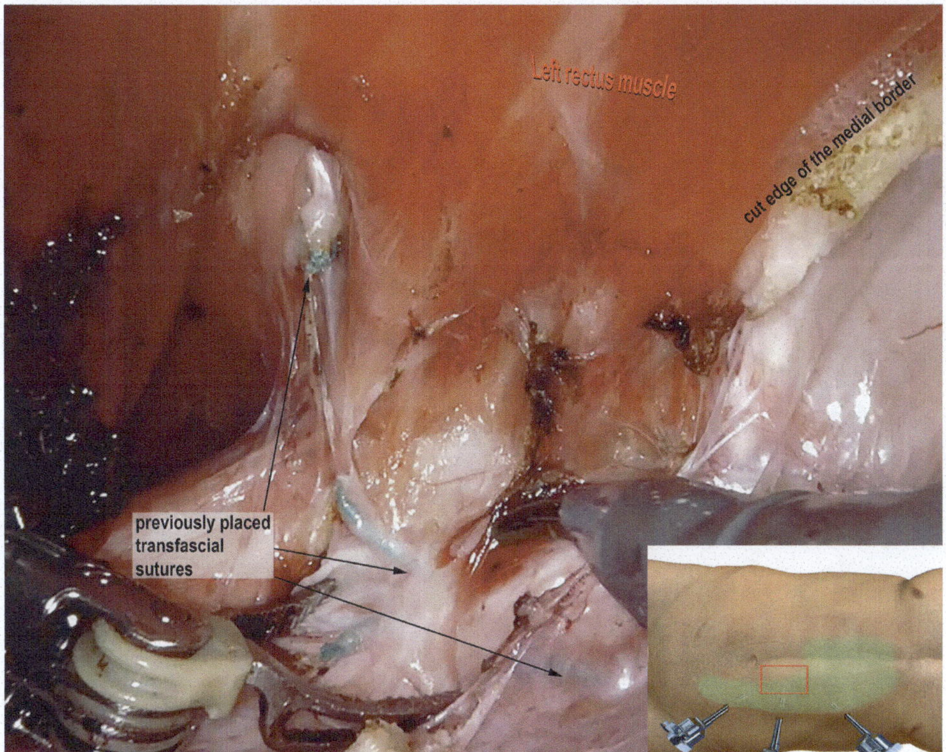


**Fig. 4.9** Upon reaching the hernia site, circumferential dissection should be performed to facilitate hernia sac reduction. A medial view of the hernia sac is shown

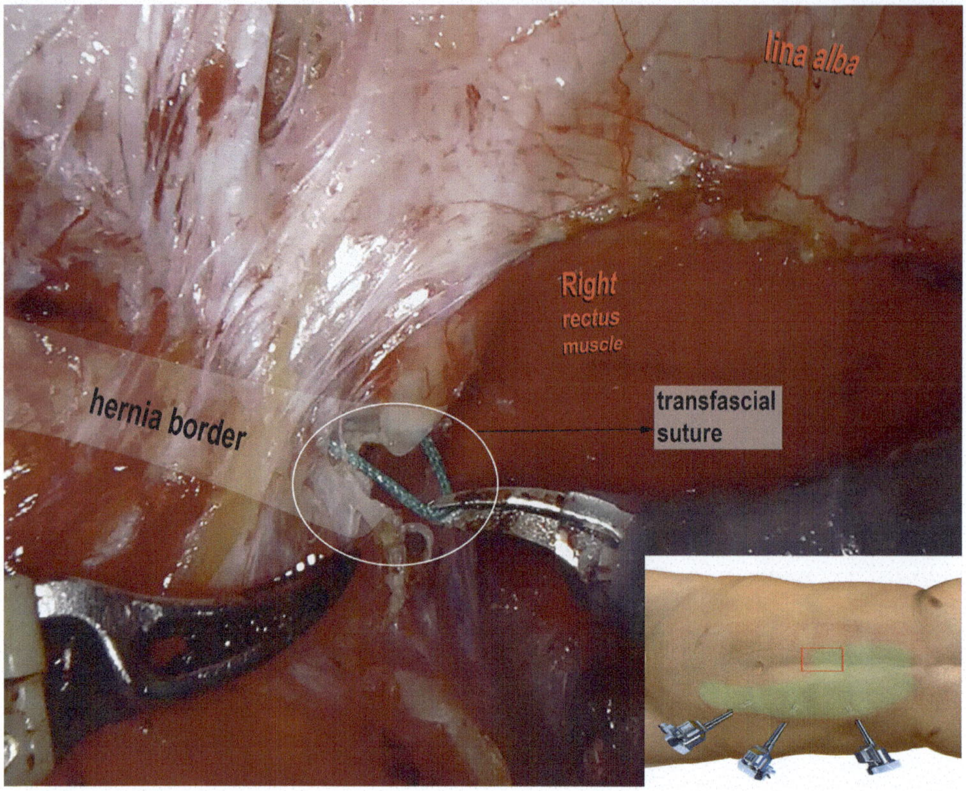


**Fig. 4.10** Circumferential dissection is continued around the superior border of the hernia sac

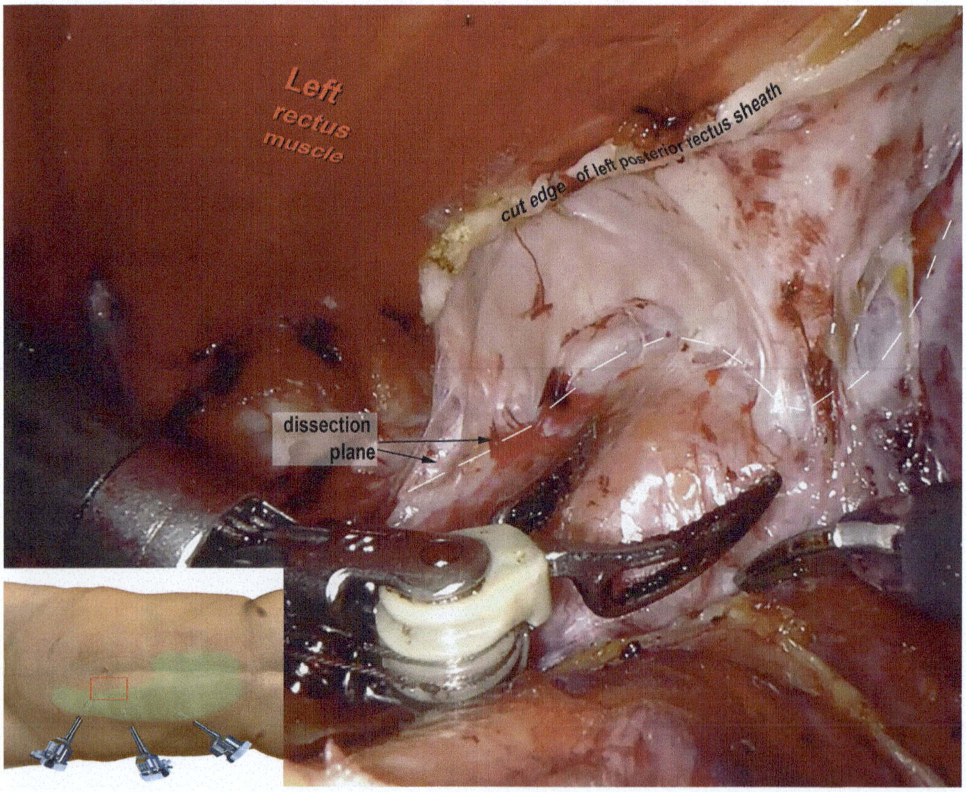


**Fig. 4.11** Soft pressure against the hernia sac reveals the dissection plane

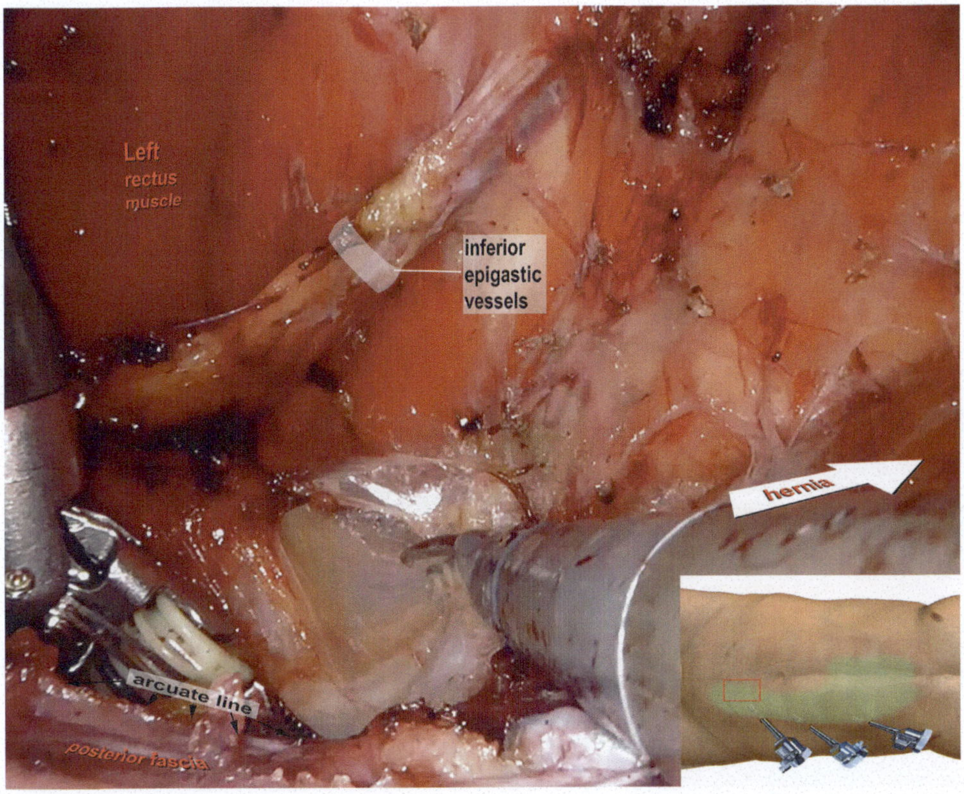


**Fig. 4.12** The medial posterior rectus sheath in the infra-umbilical region is dissected. The inferior epigastric vessels, which perforate the rectus abdominis near the arcuate line, are identified

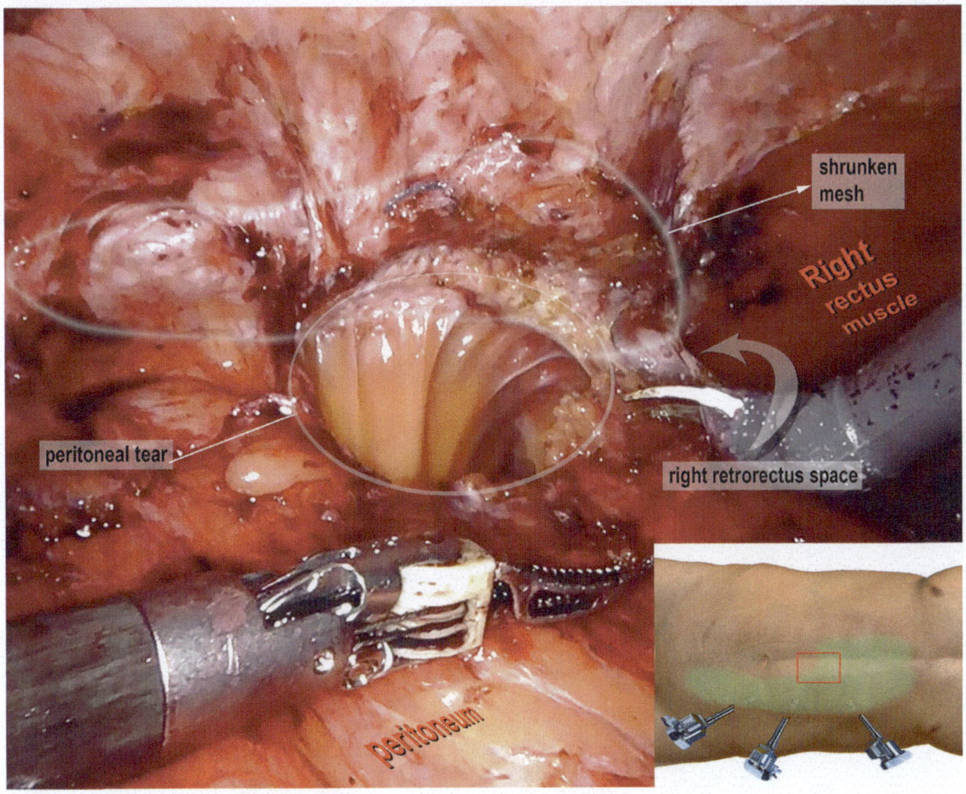


**Fig. 4.13** Delineated area showing the previously placed shrunken mesh over a peritoneal tear, which will be sutured later

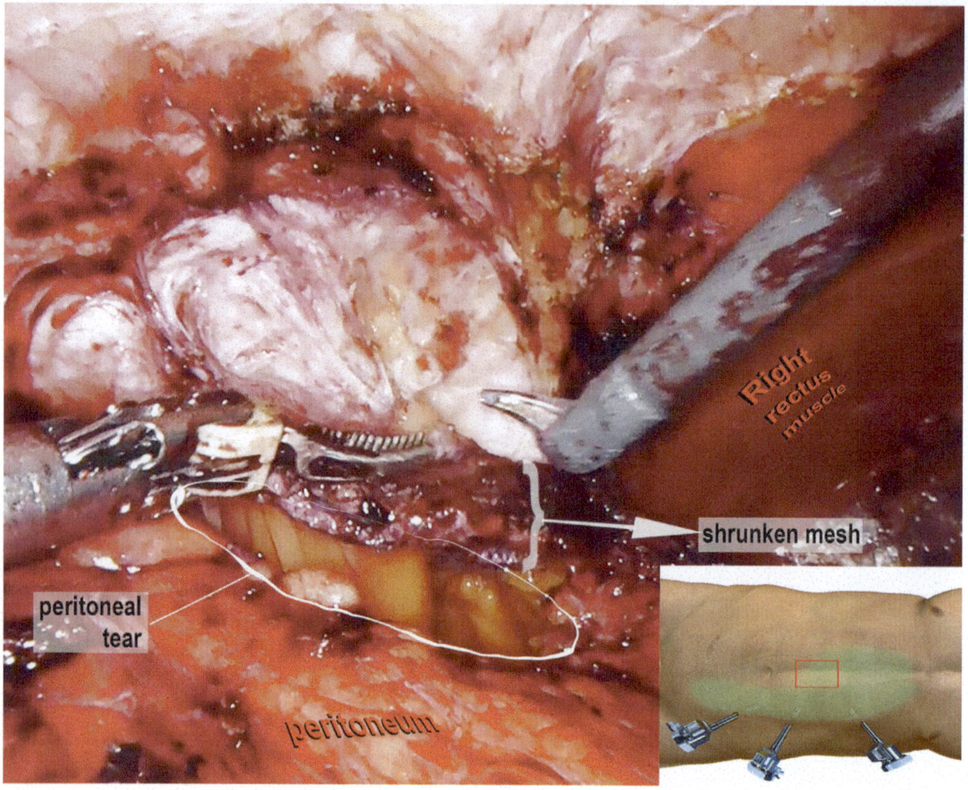


Fig. 4.14 Dissection is carried out superior to the shrunken mesh, which is left in place as part of the posterior layer

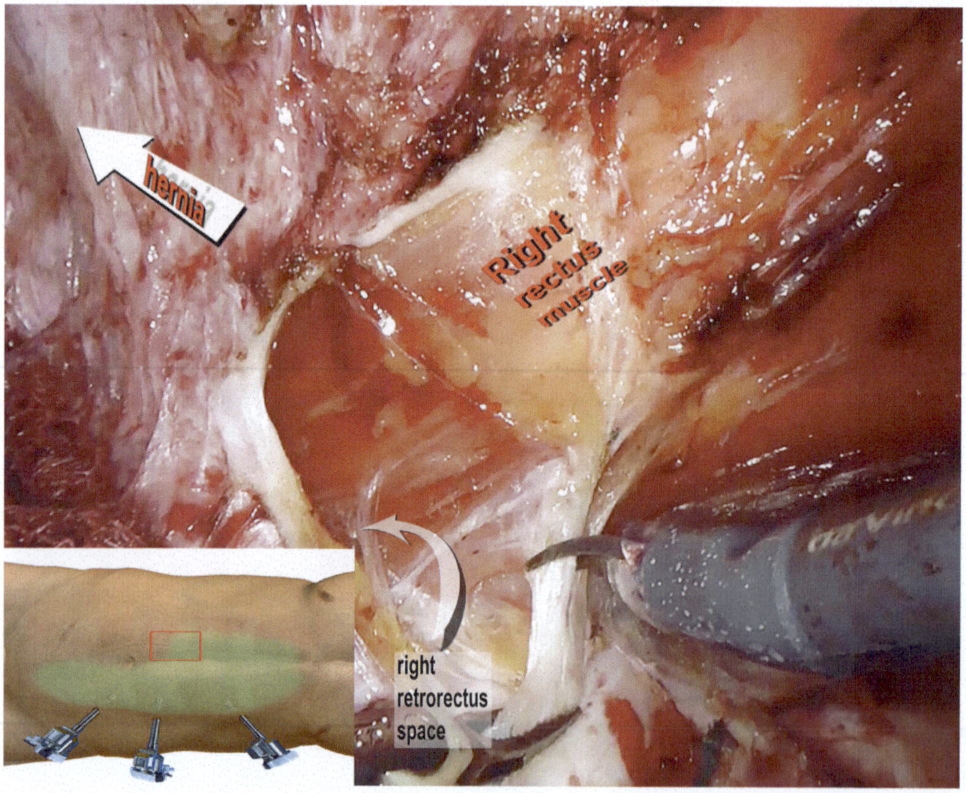


Fig. 4.15 The medial side of the contralateral rectus sheath is dissected circumferentially

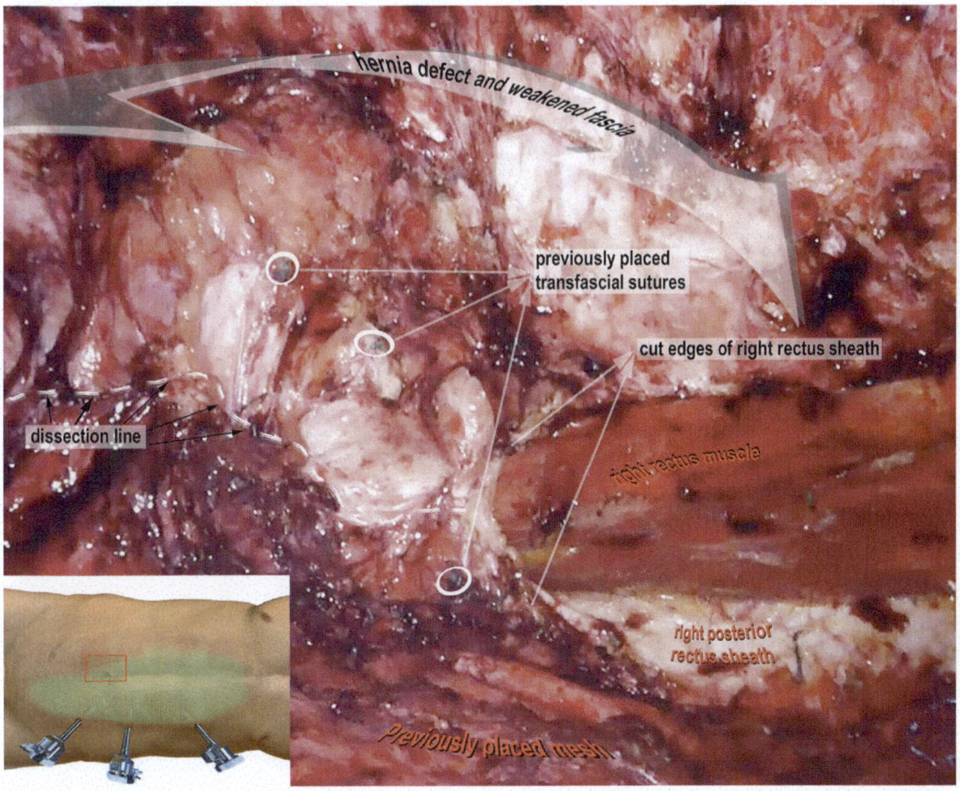


**Fig. 4.16** The previous mesh is separated from the hernia defect and weakened fascia. The dissection plane is delineated at the medial border of the right posterior rectus sheath

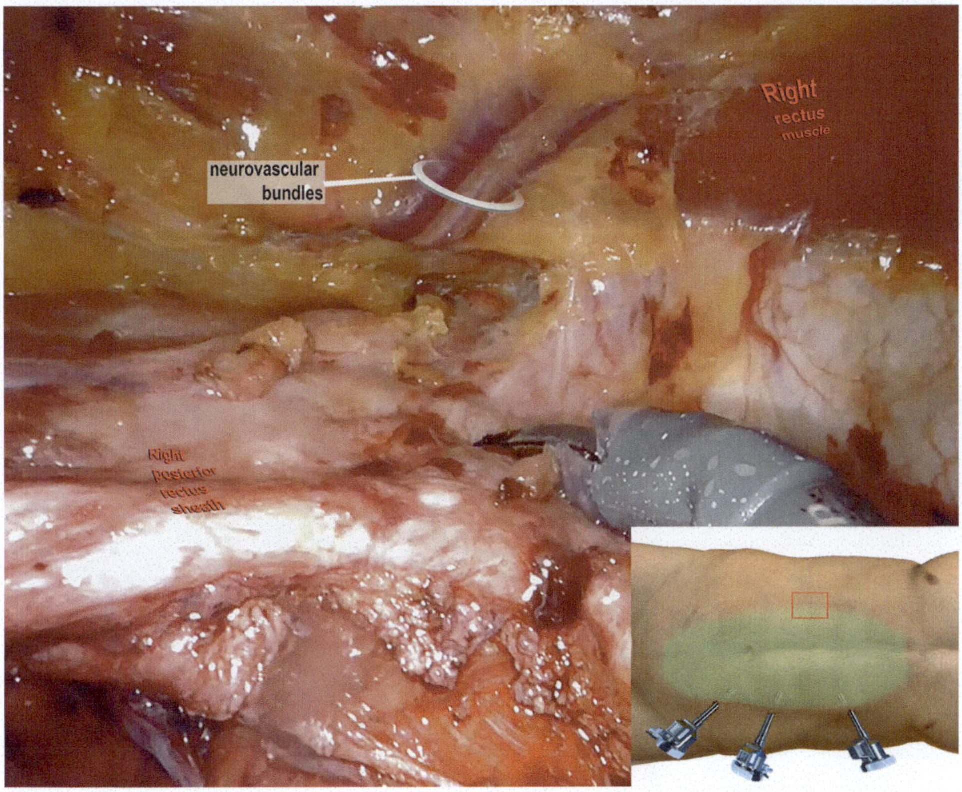


**Fig. 4.17** Identifying and preserving neurovascular bundles in the right retrorectus space

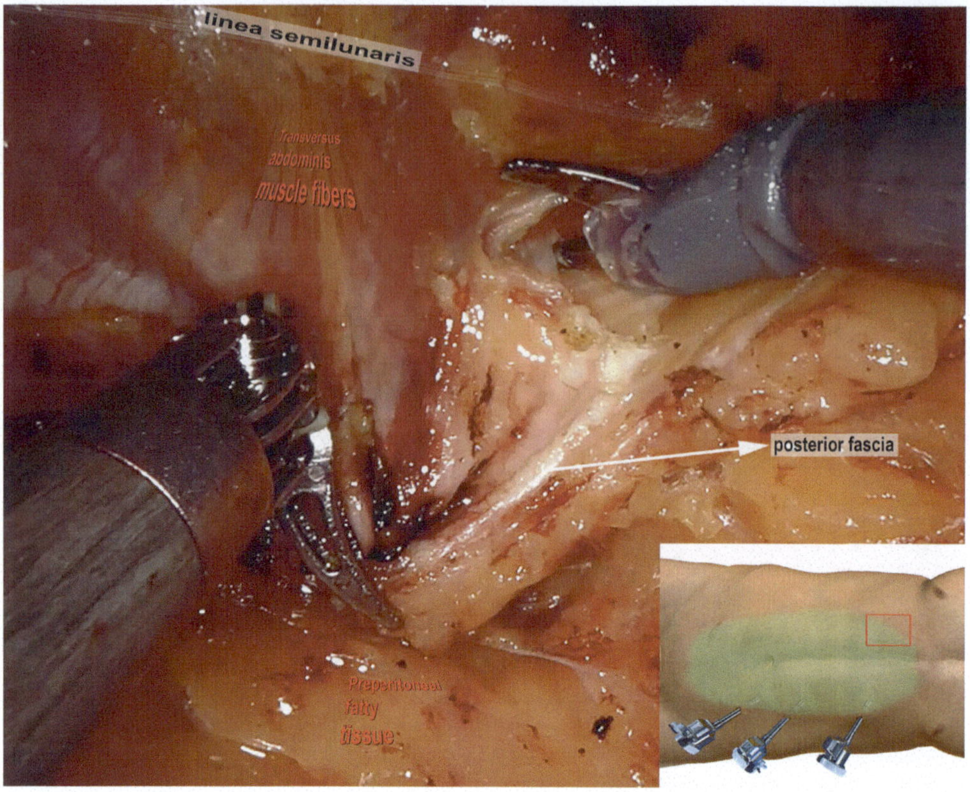


**Fig. 4.18** Once transversus abdominis fibers are visualized, dissection is initiated along the contralateral rectus sheath, parallel to the linea semilunaris

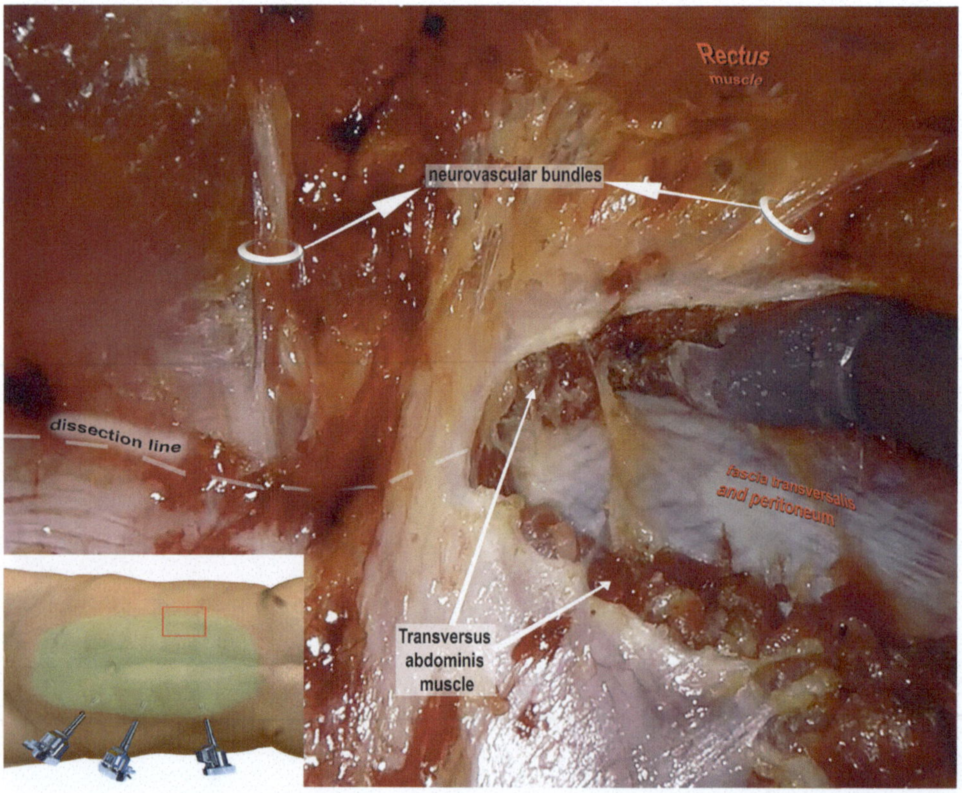


**Fig. 4.19** Transversus abdominis release (TAR) is continued while preserving neurovascular bundles

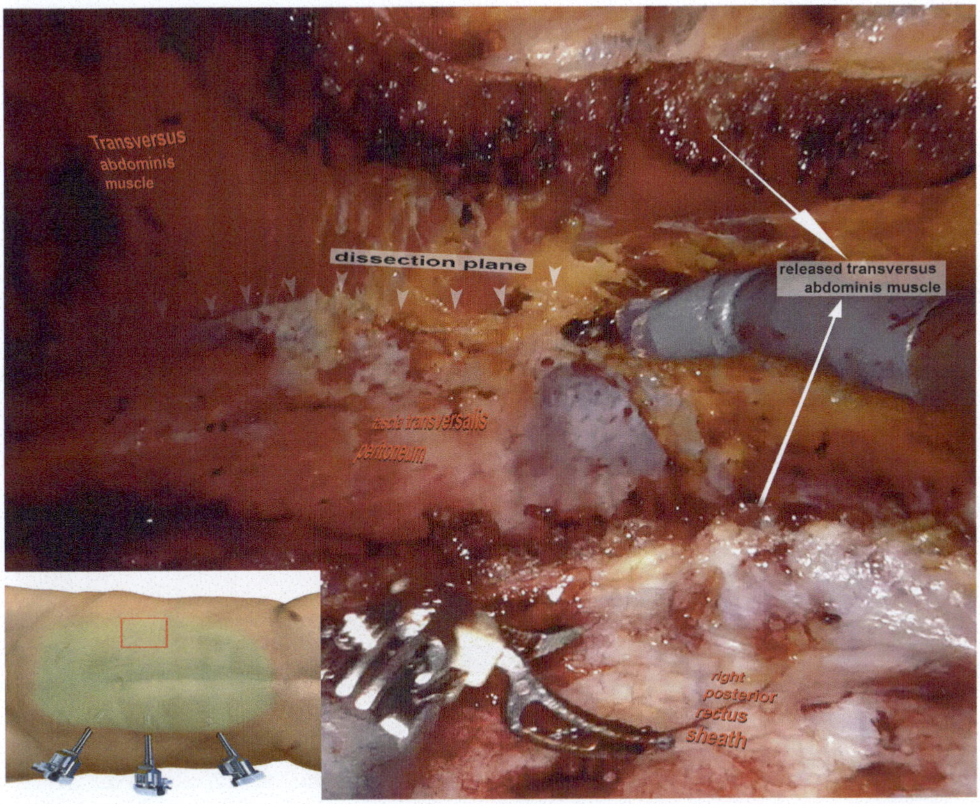


**Fig. 4.20** Once TAR has been performed, separation of the transversus abdominis muscle from the fascia transversalis is carried out along the mid-axillary line

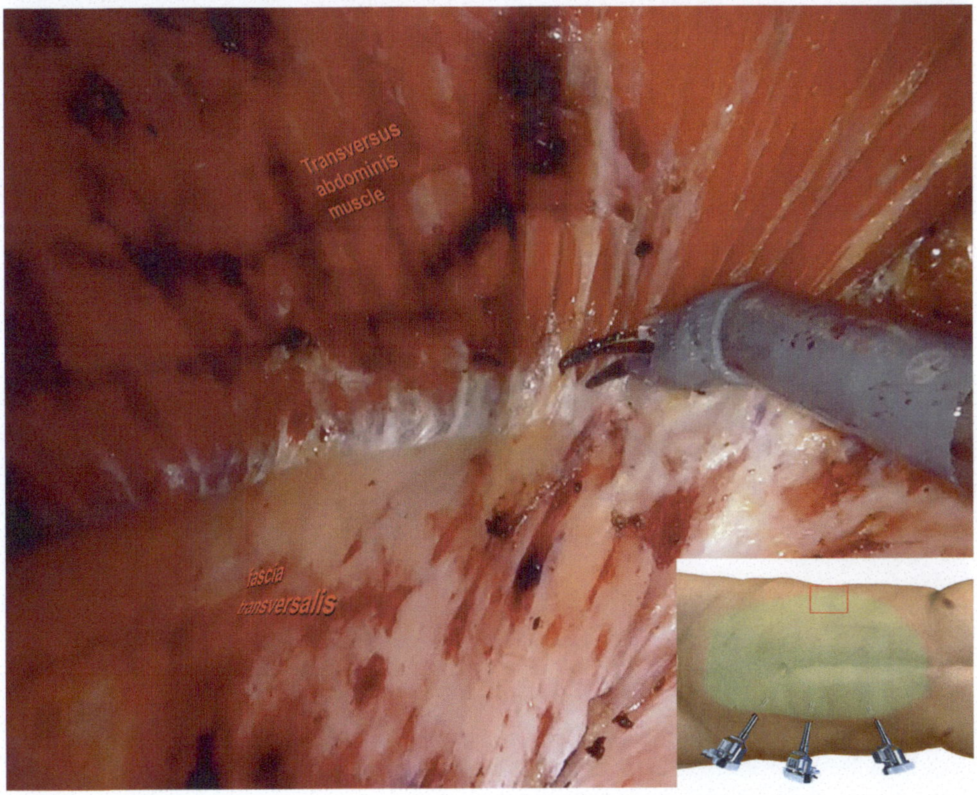


**Fig. 4.21** Gentle pressure along fascia transversalis and limited use of monopolar scissors may facilitate separation of the transversus abdominis and fascia transversalis

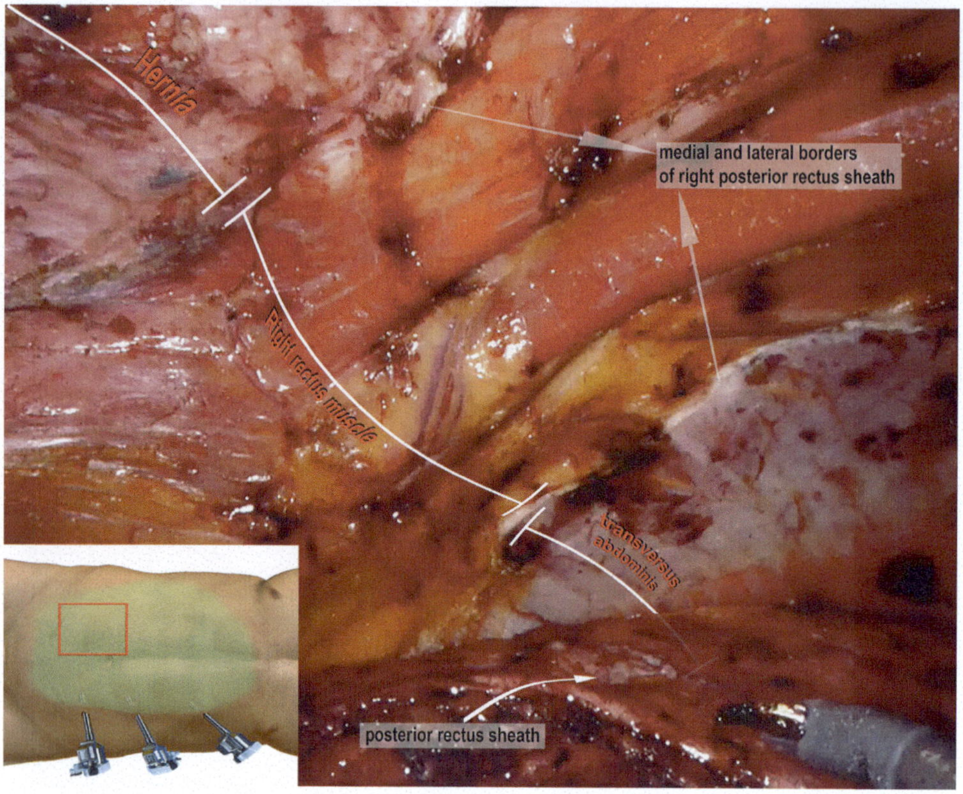


**Fig. 4.22** Right inferior view of the dissection

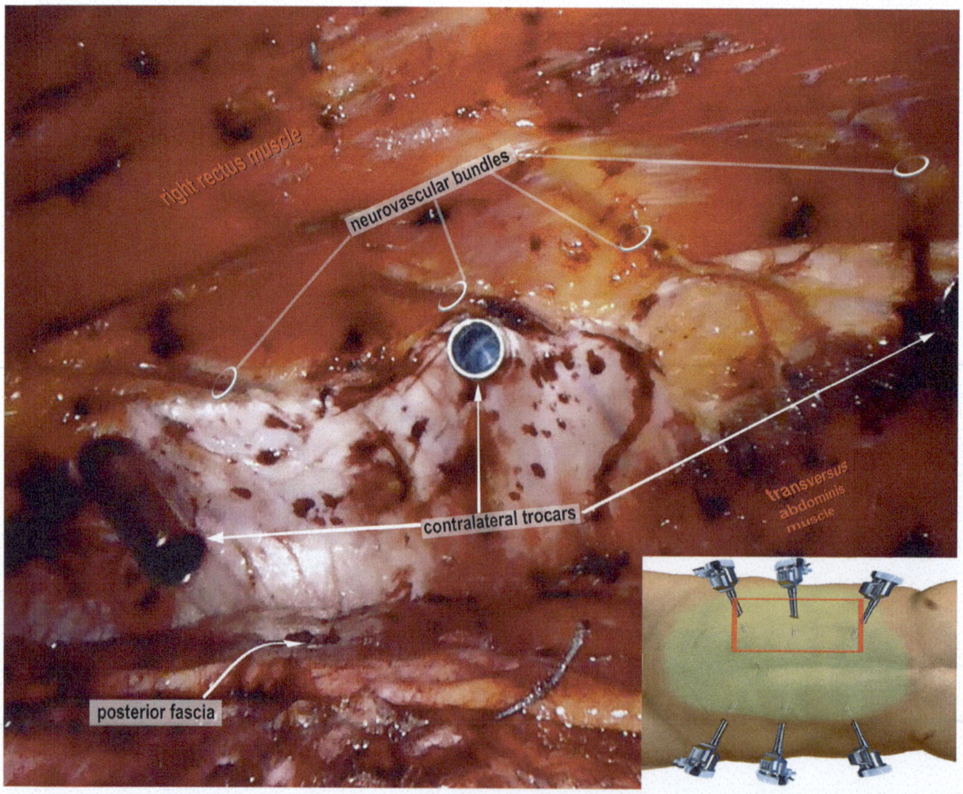


**Fig. 4.23** Contralateral trocars are inserted into the right retrorectus space under direct vision

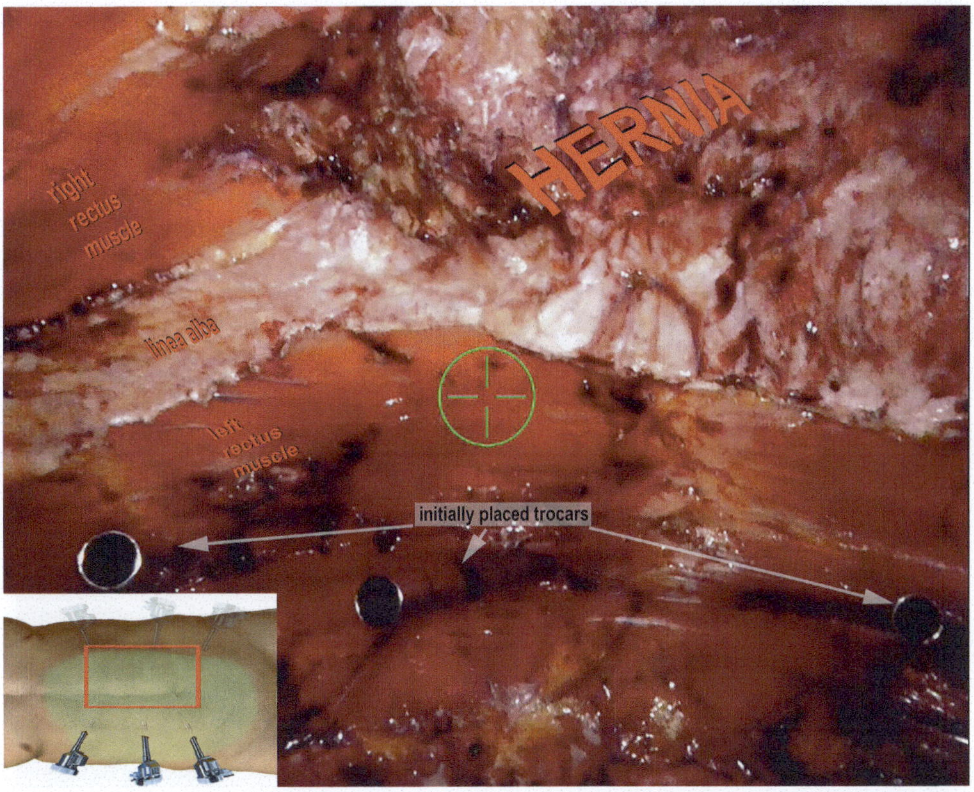


**Fig. 4.24** View of initial trocars and hernia after the patient-side cart of the robot is re-docked

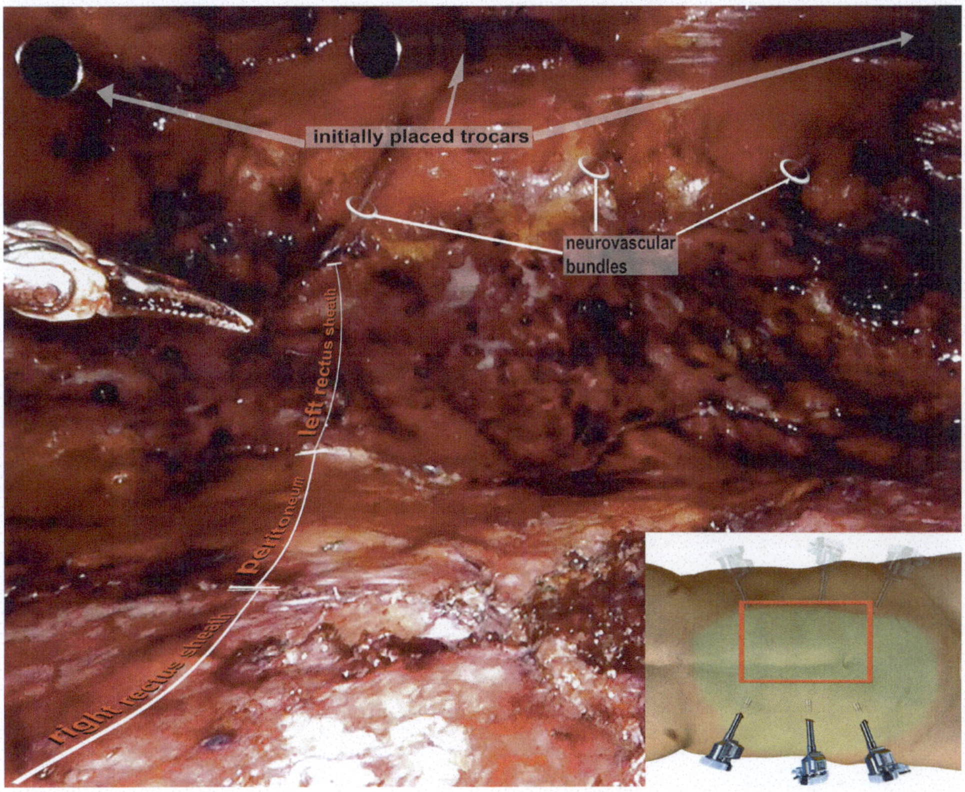


**Fig. 4.25** View of the posterior layer: right rectus sheath, peritoneum, and left rectus sheath

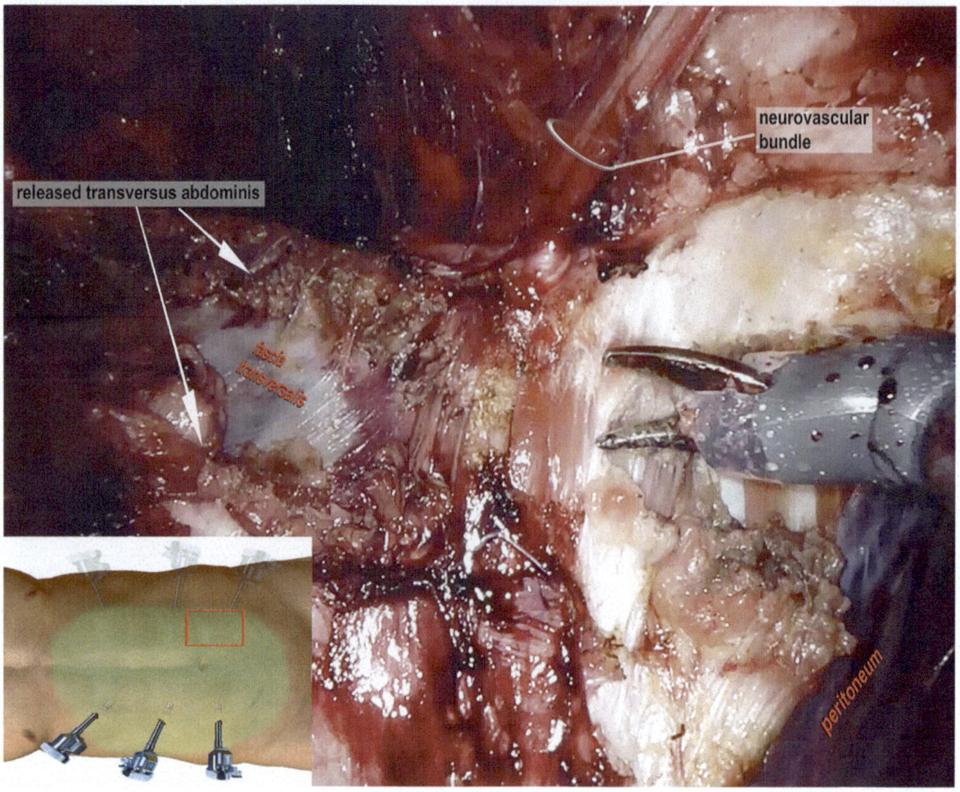


Fig. 4.26 Contralateral TAR while preserving neurovascular bundles

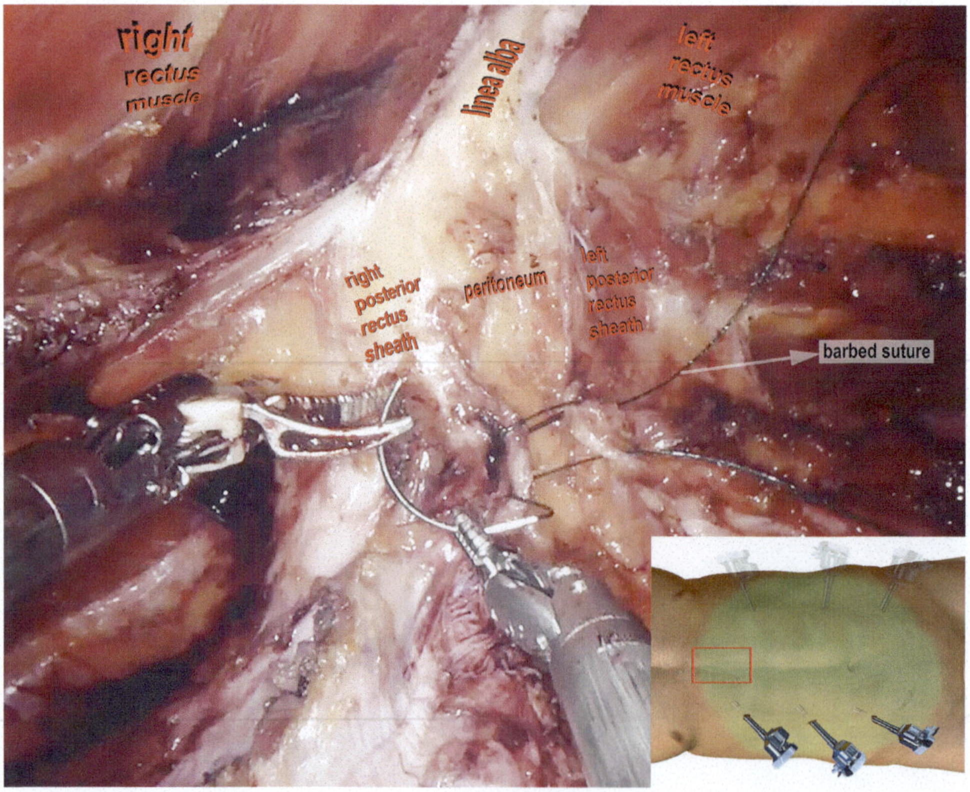


Fig. 4.27 Approximation of both sides of the posterior rectus sheath using a barbed suture

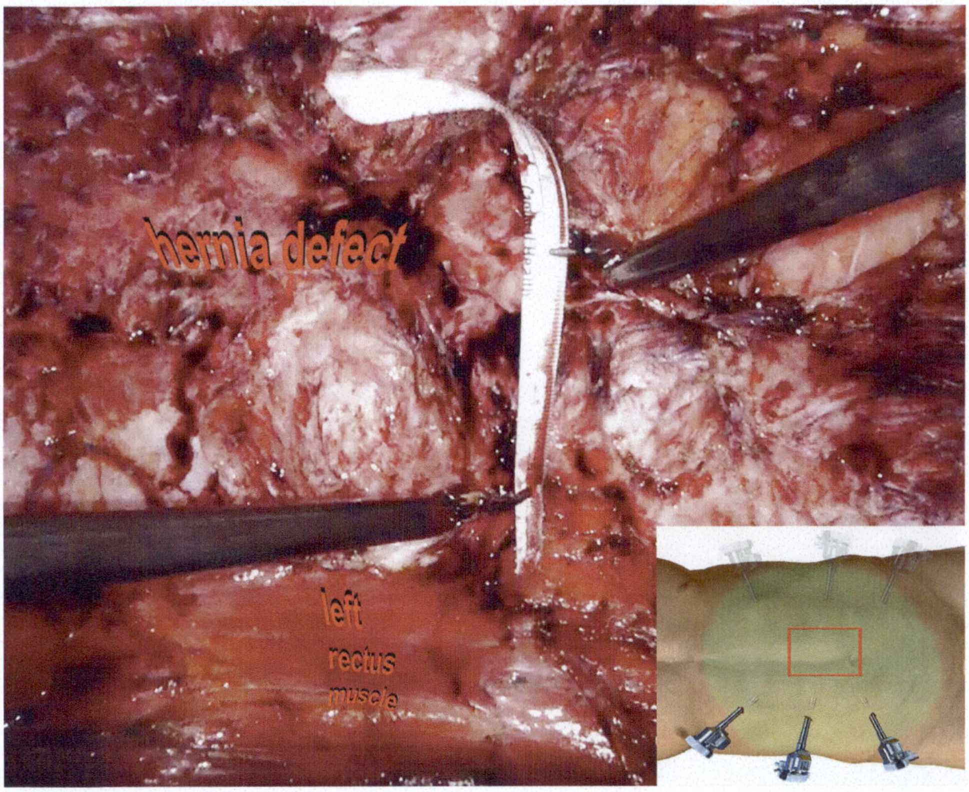


Fig. 4.28 Measurement of the hernia defect

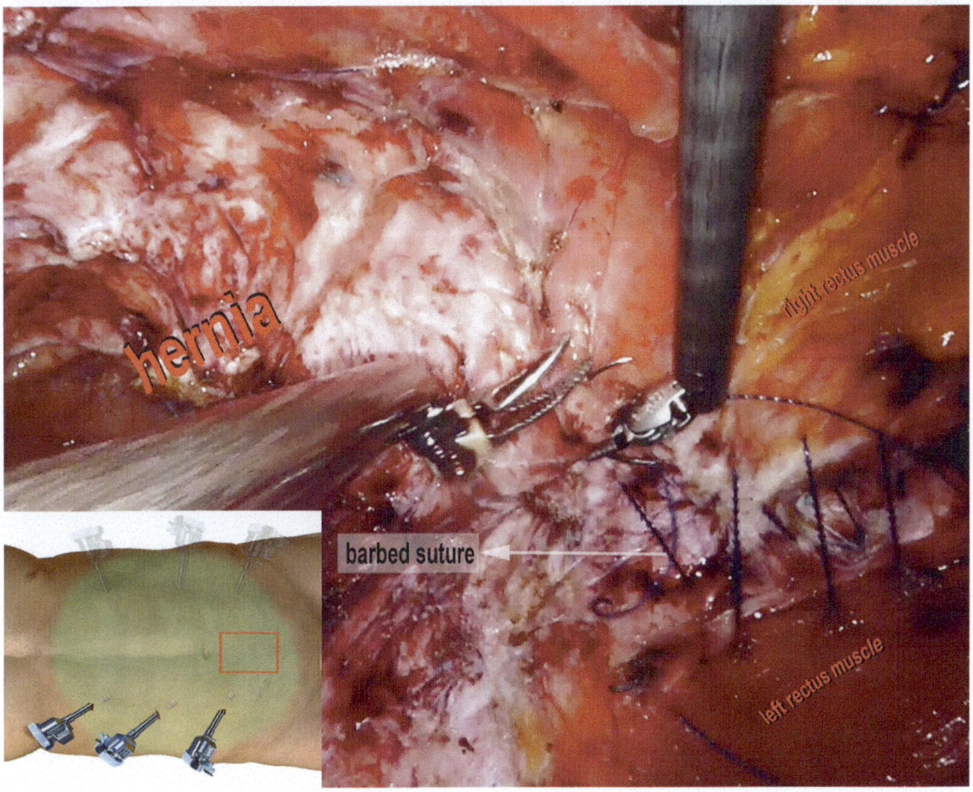


Fig. 4.29 Initiation of defect closure in the caudal-to-cranial direction, using barbed suture in a small-bite fashion

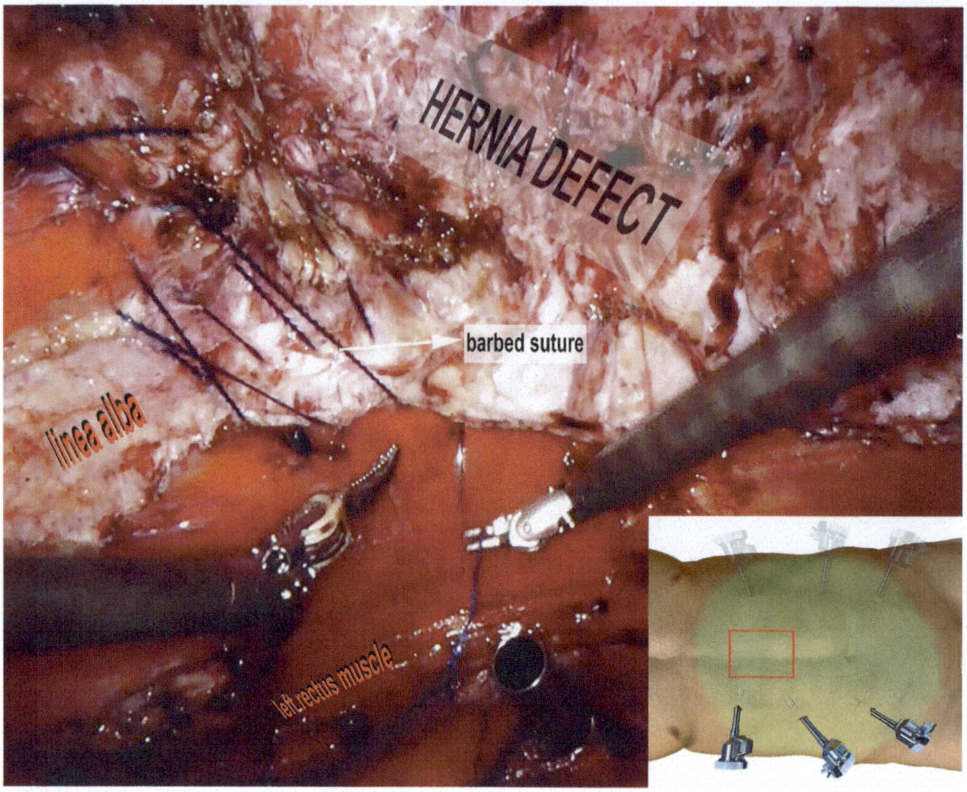


Fig. 4.30 Similarly, closure is performed in the cranial-to-caudal direction. Approximately 8 cm of the defect is left unclosed, to allow for mesh deployment via an open skin incision as part of the hybrid technique

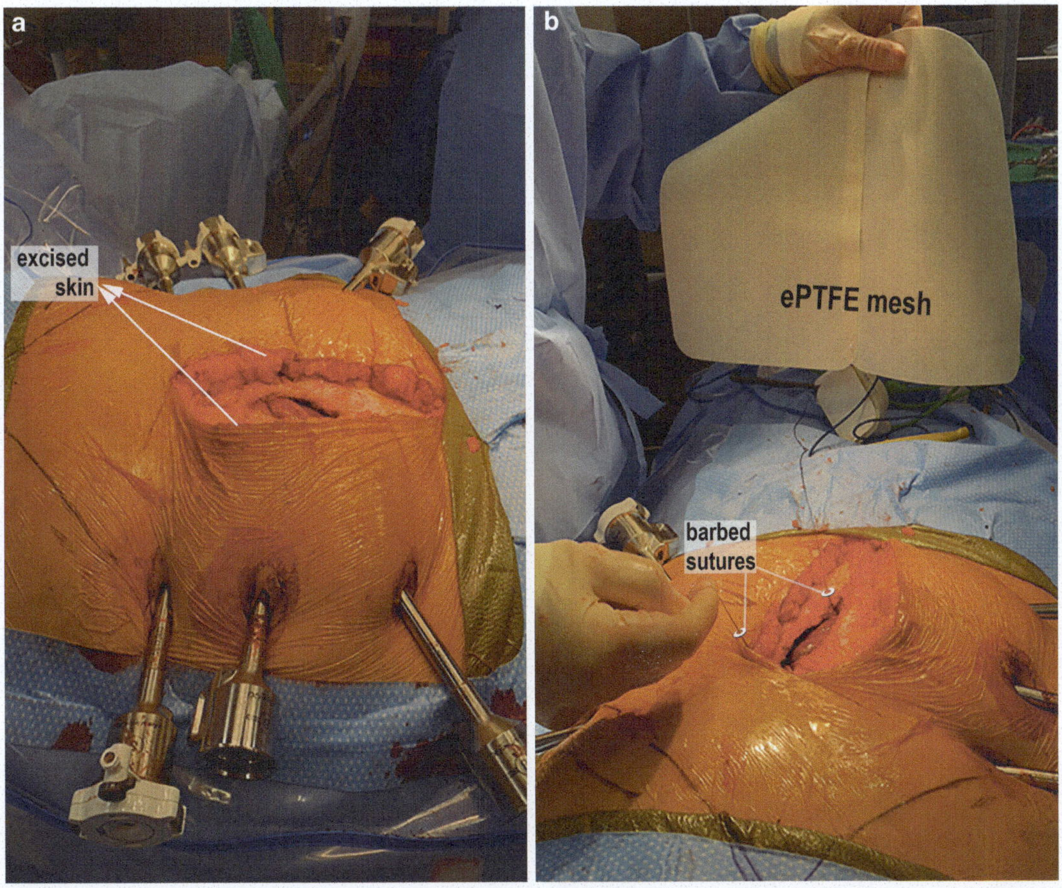


**Fig. 4.31** (**a**) A skin incision is made and is aligned over the fascial defect left behind. (**b**) Two pieces of expanded polytetrafluoroethylene (ePTFE) mesh are sewn together in order to fully occupy the dissected area

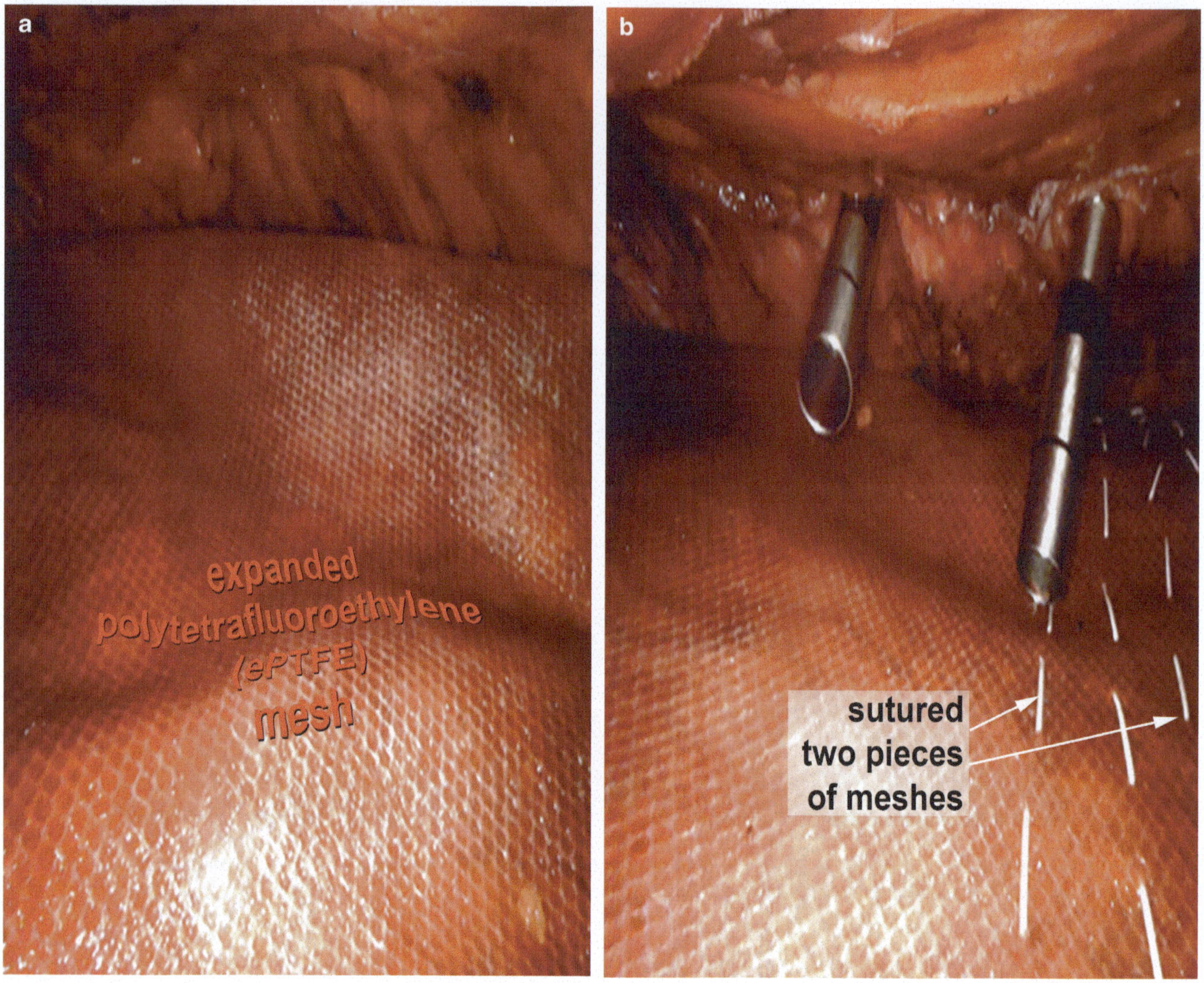


**Fig. 4.32** After manual deployment, the remaining fascial defect is closed. Shown are inferior (**a**) and lateral (**b**) laparoscopic views

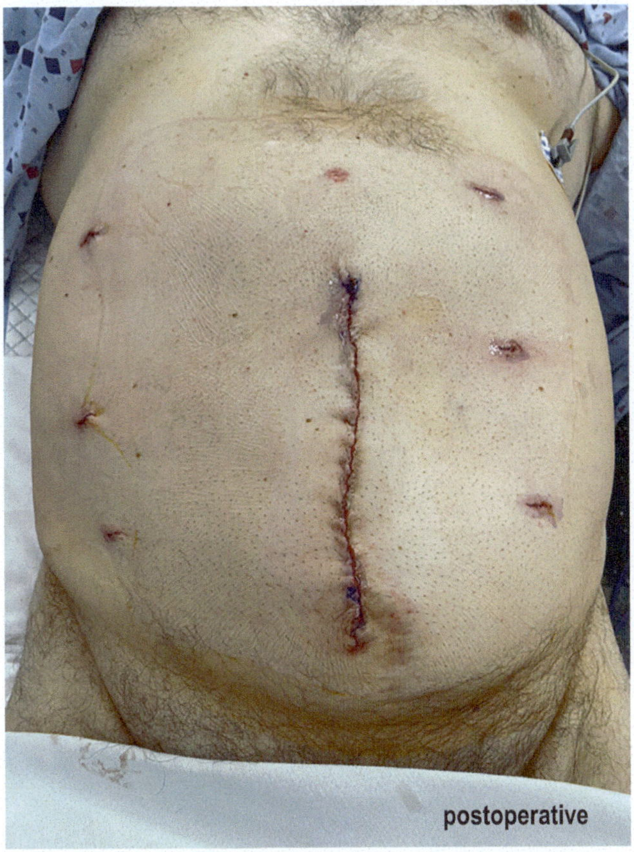


**Fig. 4.33** Removal of the trocars and closure of all skin incisions

## References

1. Halka JT, Vasyluk A, Demare A, Iacco A, Janczyk R. Hybrid robotic-assisted transversus abdominis release versus open transversus abdominis release: a comparison of short-term outcomes. Hernia. 2019;23:37–42. https://doi.org/10.1007/s10029-018-1858-1.
2. Halka JT, Vasyluk A, DeMare AM, Janczyk RJ, Iacco AA. Robotic and hybrid robotic transversus abdominis release may be performed with low length of stay and wound morbidity. Am J Surg. 2018;215:462–5. https://doi.org/10.1016/j.amjsurg.2017.10.053.

# Robotic Supra-pubic Hernia Repair: Transabdominal Preperitoneal (TAPP)

5

Flavio Malcher, Eduardo Parra-Davila, and Leandro Totti Cavazzola

The majority of supra-pubic hernias are incisional in their nature [1]. Data show that the Rives-Stoppa repair of ventral hernias is the standard of care by which open hernia repairs should be judged [2]. However, laparoscopic ventral hernia repair has been found to result in negligible wound complications and low recurrence rates [3], and it has been associated with faster recovery, fewer complications, and a lower recurrence rate than the open technique, but there continues to be a significant incidence of postoperative pain associated with the transabdominal wall sutures and tackers fixation [4–7].

Robotic ventral hernia repair (RVHR), on the other hand, offers traditional open repair techniques through minimal-access incisions by upscaling the surgeon's skills [8]. Previous reports have demonstrated the ease of intracorporeal suturing of the mesh to the abdominal wall [7, 8].

## Specific Features of the Supra-pubic Hernia

By definition, fascial defects that are located within 5 cm of the symphysis pubis are considered supra-pubic [9]. They are more common in females, often as a result of gynecologic procedures via a lower midline or Pfannenstiel approach. This corresponds to 15% of ventral hernia cases in large series [10].

F. Malcher (✉)
Montefiore Medical Center, Albert Einstein College of Medicine, Bronx, NY, USA

E. Parra-Davila
Good Samaritan Medical Center, West Palm Beach, FL, USA

L. T. Cavazzola
Department of Surgery, Universidade Federal do Rio Grande do Sul, Porto Alegre, Rio Grande do Sul, Brazil

General Surgery Section – Hospital de Clínicas de Porto Alegre, Porto Alegre, Rio Grande do Sul, Brazil

## Technique

Hernia repair techniques amenable to the robotic approach include the intra-peritoneal onlay mesh (IPOM) bridge (which is being abandoned owing to the final bridge repair), IPOM after primary closure of the defect (the so-called IPOM Plus), preperitoneal placement of mesh (transabdominal preperitoneal [TAPP] repair, as in inguinal hernia repair), or placement of retrorectus mesh with or without separation of posterior components. The retrorectus position can be achieved by a transabdominal approach (as in TAPP) or by the extended totally extraperitoneal approach (eTEP) [11]. These individual techniques are chosen based on the location of the hernia defect, the size of the defect, and perhaps most importantly, surgeon experience.

This chapter provides a full description of the TAPP technique. Robotic preperitoneal repair facilitates bladder mobilization, visualization of the pelvic rim, and creation of a large space to accommodate overlapping mesh, which is more often required for recurrent hernias or in patients with previous open prostatectomy [7, 12].

## Patient Positioning, Trocar Placement and Docking

The patient is placed in a supine modified lithotomy position. A three-way Foley catheter is inserted to allow filling of the bladder intraoperatively for identification of its borders during dissection. The patient is placed in a slight Trendelenburg position.

The camera trocar (8 mm in DaVinci [dV] Xi or 12 mm in dV Si) is placed into the camera port, which must be at least 15–20 cm from the superior aspect of the hernia defect at midline. Two or three dV 8-mm trocars are placed in line with the camera trocar at the upper abdomen and the robot is docked in between the legs. Alternatively (especially for small hernias), the patient can be positioned in supine posi-


O. Y. Kudsi (ed.), *Robotic Hernia Surgery*, https://doi.org/10.1007/978-3-030-46667-1_5

tion and the robot can be "side docked" (in Si). This can be achieved without any problem with the Xi, which allows side docking by just moving the boom accordingly.

## Adhesiolysis

Adhesiolysis of the abdominal wall to isolate the hernia defect must be performed meticulously. The dV platform facilitates adhesiolysis through its 3-D visualization, tremorless precision, and superior ergonomics [8]. For direct bowel handling, the dV fenestrated bipolar grasper results in less trauma to serosal tissue. It is important to emphasize the loss of haptic feedback when performing robotic surgery, but this shortcoming is overcome by the improved ability to see individual stretch fibers. Special attention is therefore required to prevent inadvertent bowel injury and excessive bleeding by way of atraumatic handling and judicious use of cautery. Clearing the entire abdominal wall of adhesions is mandatory to ensure complete evaluation. If adhesions are dense, the robotic harmonic scalpel may facilitate hemostasis.

After safe entrance into the abdominal cavity, trocar positioning, and docking of the robot as described above, adhesiolysis is undertaken with caution, trying not to damage the parietal peritoneum, in order to avoid contact of the mesh with the abdominal cavity. Figure 5.1 illustrates what should be the final aspect of the dissection prior to incising the peritoneum.

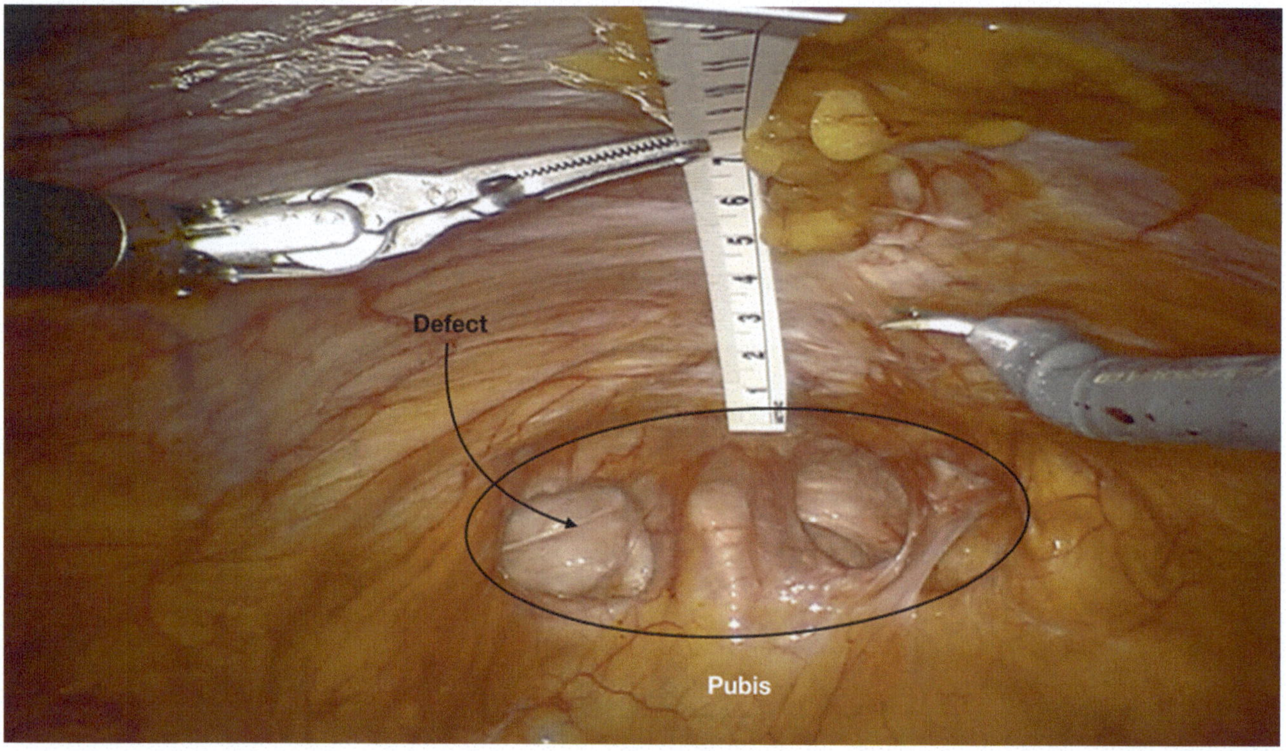


**Fig. 5.1** Initial intraperitoneal view. Suprapubic defect (*black oval*) is visualized

## Abdominal Wall Planes Dissection

Exploiting the layers of the abdominal wall is made possible by the precision afforded by the dV robot. With conventional laparoscopy, it is possible to work high on the anterior abdominal wall, but it remains technically demanding and ergonomically challenging. Placing mesh in the preperitoneal space obviates the need for a more costly tissue-separating mesh and allows the mesh to incorporate directly on the fascia, thereby decreasing the need for sutures or tack fixation, which causes postoperative pain. It also avoids complications (such as bowel erosion or fistula) that are inherent when mesh is left in the intraperitoneal position.

The robotic TAPP ventral hernia repair (VHR) was developed based on the TAPP inguinal hernia repair and involves dissection of the preperitoneal plane, reduction of the hernia sac, primary closure of the defect, placement of mesh with minimal fixation, and reperitonealization of the mesh [7].

The peritoneal incision is started. As shown in Fig. 5.2, it is very important at this time to mark the correct site of the incision by measuring in different parts of the wall, being away from the regular robotic view (which is closer to the target organ). Because with the robot we work closer to the surgical field it is common to get disoriented and turn the peritoneal incision toward the defect or even the bone structures.

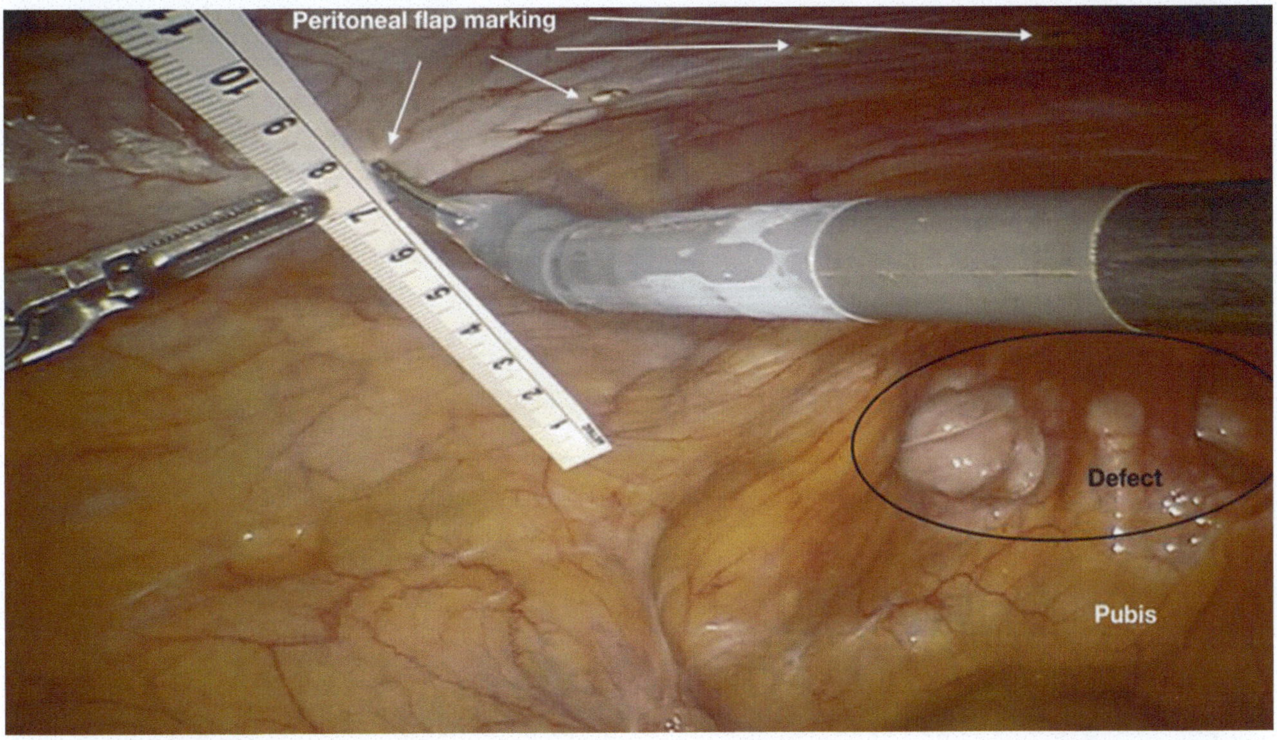


Fig. 5.2 Cautery marking of the peritoneal incision, 8 cm cranial to the superior edge of the defect

A preperitoneal plane is incised a minimum of 5 cm cephalad to the superior aspect of the hernia defect. Figure 5.3 shows the beginning of the peritoneal incision after all the markup of the desired peritoneal flap. Using a combination of sharp and blunt dissection, the retromuscular space is accessed. If this is above the linea arcuata, the posterior rectus sheath is more dense, as shown in Fig. 5.4. In lower incisions, only peritoneum and transversalis fascia will be part of this layer, and extra caution should be used to avoid tears in the posterior sheath. Because this is an avascular plane, blunt dissection can be used safely, with wider movements.

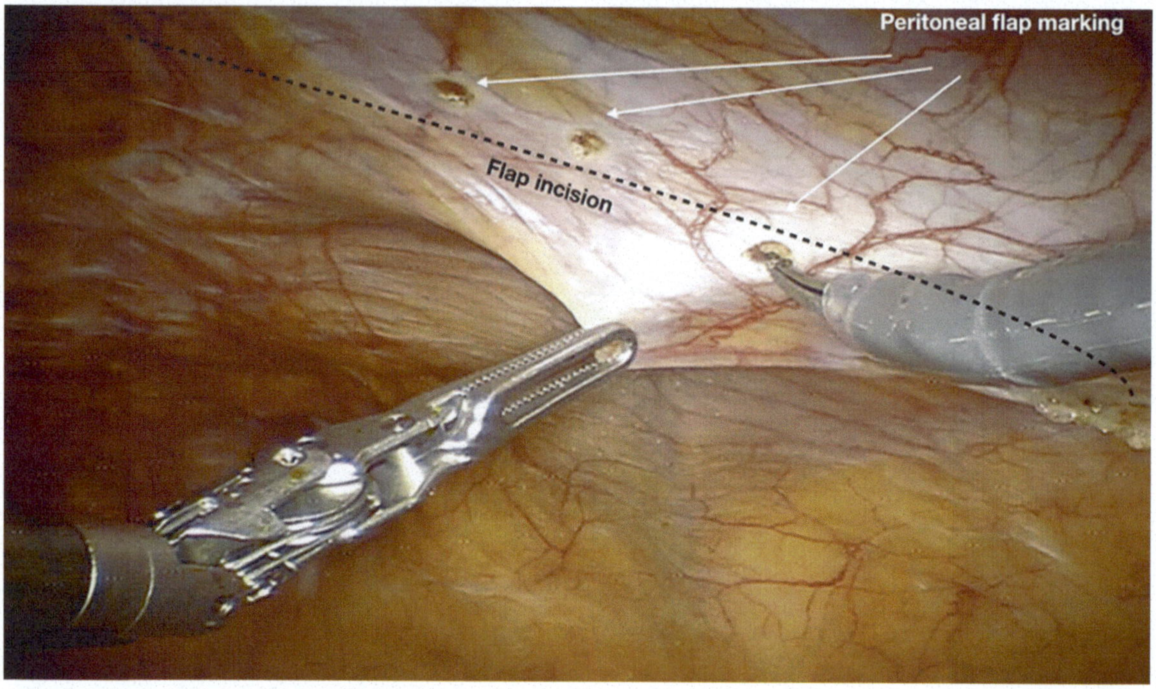


Fig. 5.3 Completed marking of the proposed peritoneal flap incision, in a closer view than Fig. 5.2

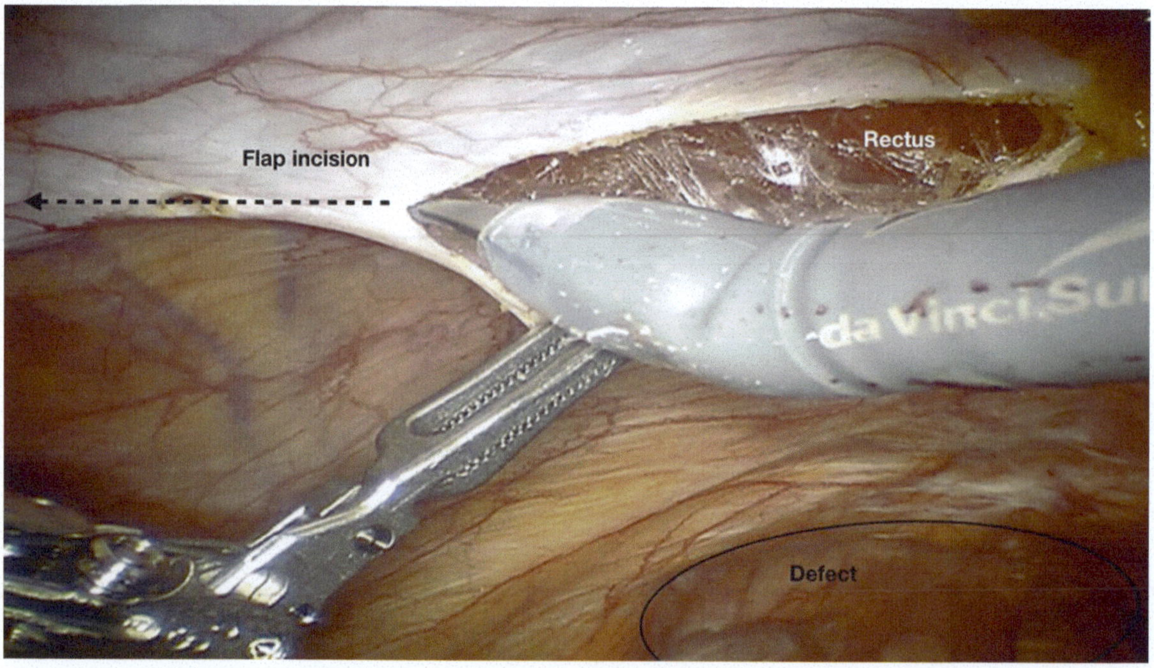


Fig. 5.4 Peritoneal incision with exposure of the rectus muscle

Figure 5.5 shows the creation of the left preperitoneal space, with identification of the important anatomic structures. Note that the only vascular structures identified here are the epigastric vessels, which should be kept on the muscle to avoid injury. Also note that traction is exerted on the posterior wall, which allows dissection with the scissors in the avascular plane behind the rectus muscle.

Both sides are dissected and the linea alba is reached, with identification of the superior aspect of the defect (Fig. 5.6). Again it is possible to see the left hand exerting traction on the posterior sheath to allow dissection with the right hand and creation of a wide space.

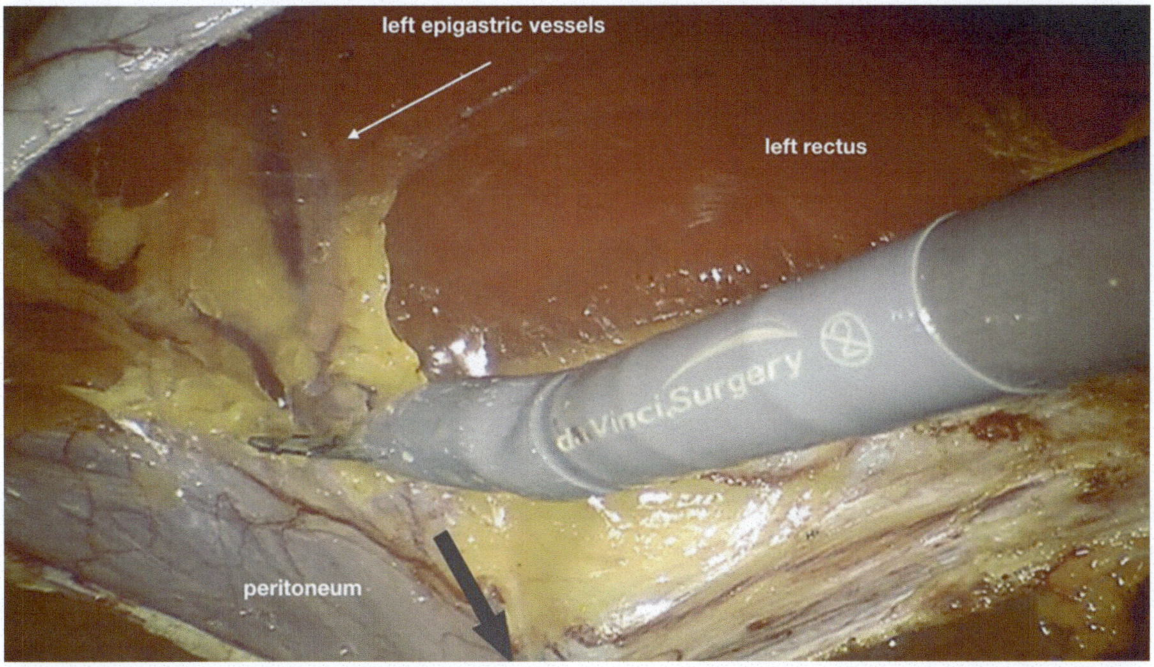


**Fig. 5.5** Preperitoneal space dissection with identification of left epigastric vessels (*white arrow*), with posterior traction of the peritoneum (*black arrow*). It is important to keep the epigastric vessels on the muscle

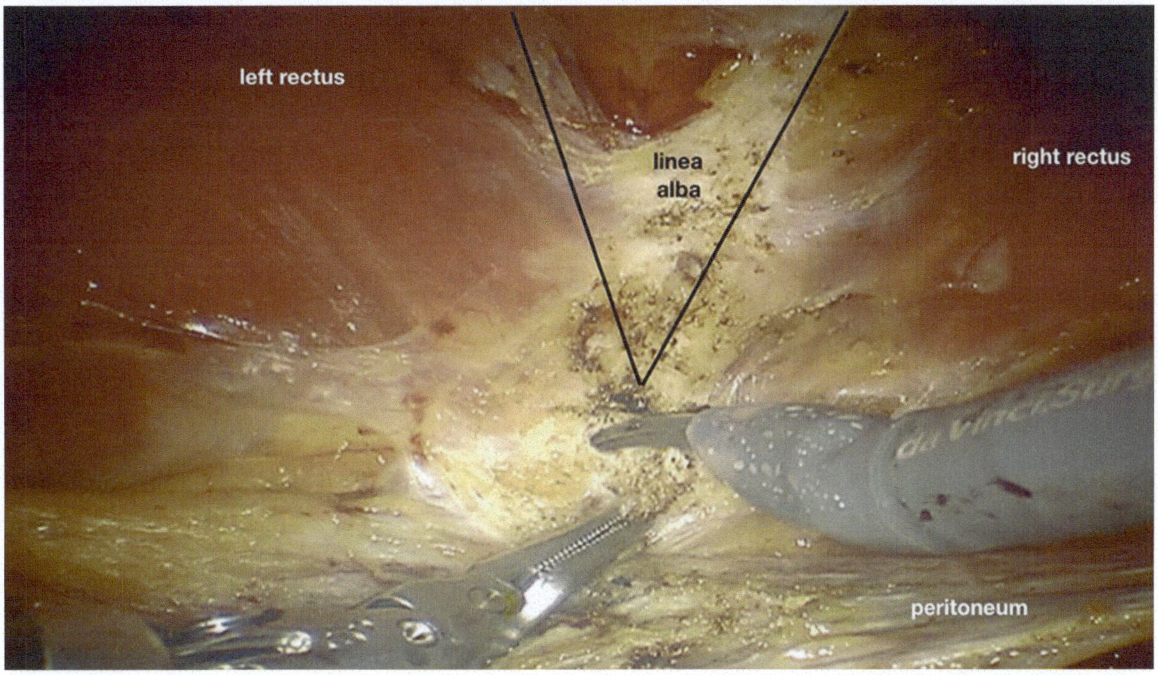


**Fig. 5.6** Preperitoneal space creation progression, reaching the superior edge of the defect and identifying the linea alba

After wide dissection of the preperitoneal space, attention is now directed to the hernia sac (Fig. 5.7). The scissors are positioned on the limit of the defect, with the left hand keeping firm traction on the hernia sac. The dissection progresses caudally. Both sides of the preperitoneal space will be enlarged until a huge pocket is developed. It is crucial to identify the anatomical structures that will guide the full space creation (the epigastric vessels in Fig. 5.8).

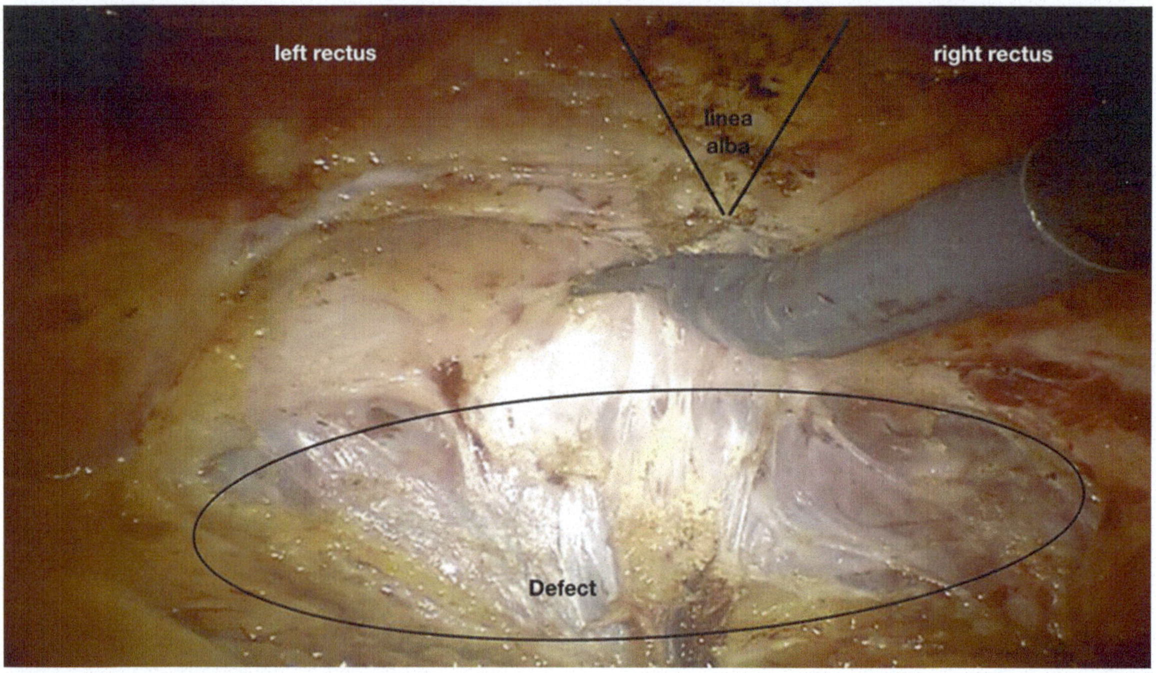


Fig. 5.7 Initial dissection of the hernia sac

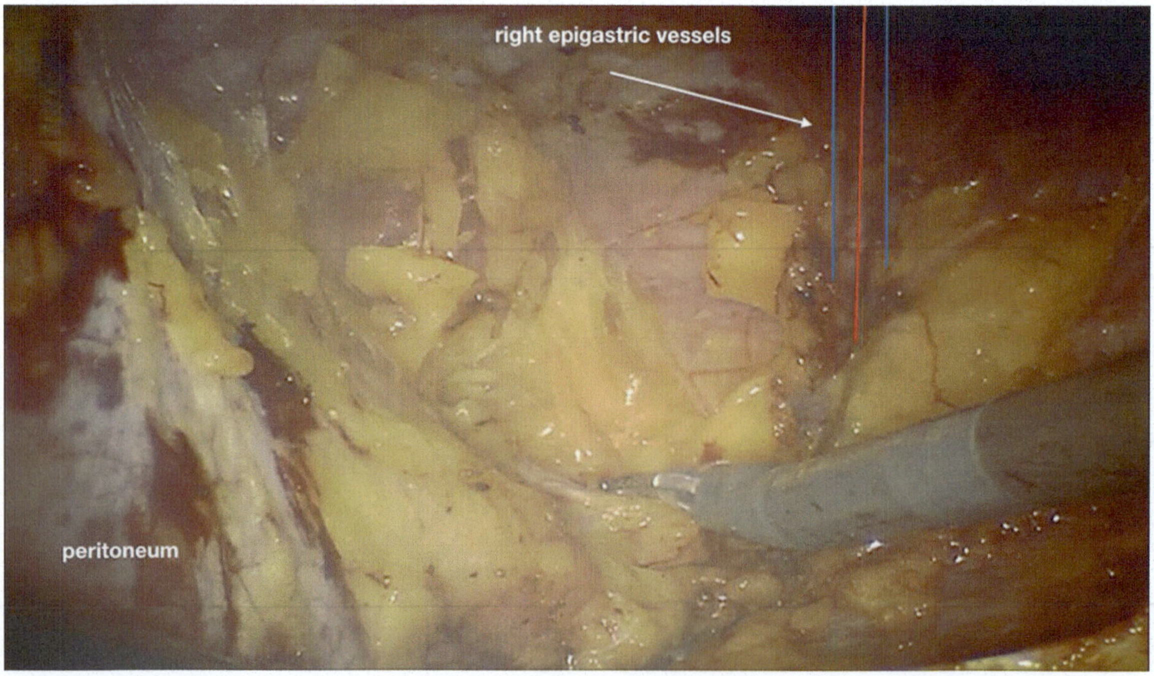


Fig. 5.8 Lateral progression of the dissection on the right, with proper identification of the right epigastric vessels

The hernia sac is reduced as much as possible to provide mesh coverage (Fig. 5.9). It is important to identify the edges of the defect, to define how much overlap will be necessary in each direction for adequate mesh size and position.

Eventually it is necessary to transect the hernia sac, to continue with the dissection toward the edge of the defect (Fig. 5.10). It is important that the holes created are closed at the end of the procedure, to avoid mesh contact with the abdominal cavity.

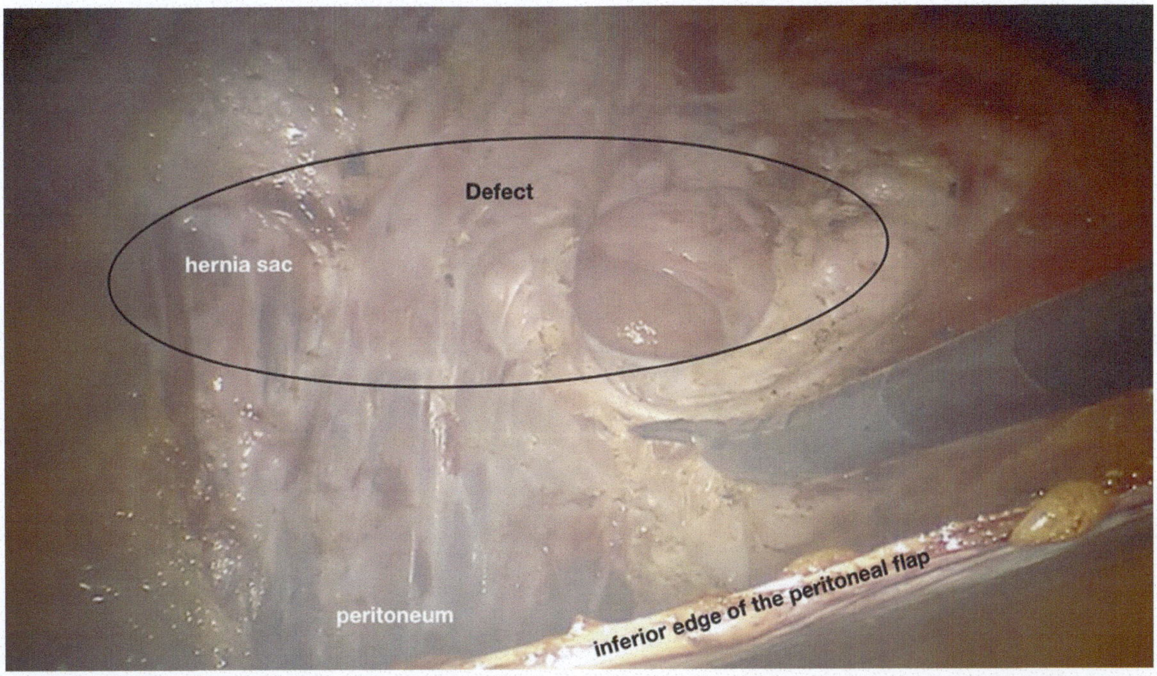


**Fig. 5.9** Reduction of the hernia sac as much as possible, with identification of the edges of the defect

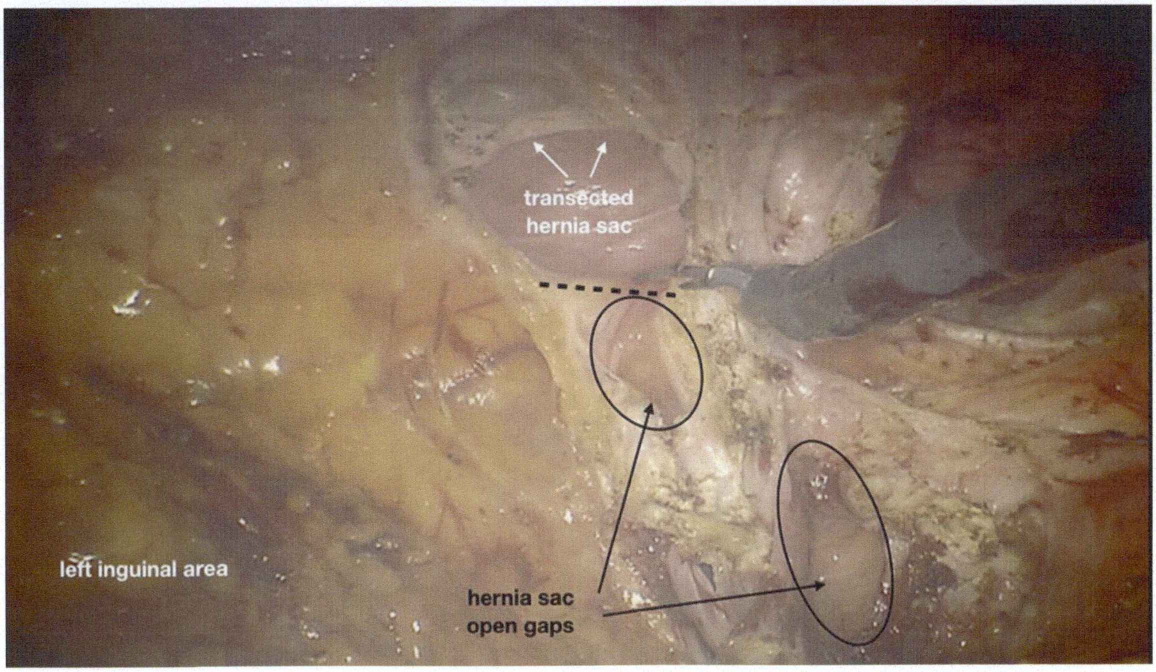


**Fig. 5.10** Transection of the hernia sac (superior edge at *white arrow*; posterior edge at *dotted black line*) to properly identify hernia defect edges

A wide plane of dissection is necessary to accommodate a large sheet of overlapping mesh. The superior dome of the bladder may occupy the hernia sac, so great care and meticulous dissection is performed to safely mobilize the bladder. This procedure is facilitated by instilling 300 cc of sterile saline into the bladder for easy identification. The retroinguinal space (space of Bogros) is developed bilaterally to expose Cooper's ligament. Caudal mobilization of the bladder reveals the space of Retzius. This space can be dissected inferiorly to ensure adequate overlap of mesh inferior to the caudal aspect of the hernia defect. Figure 5.11 shows all the important anatomic landmarks. Note the small openings in the hernia sac, which should be closed after completion of the repair.

To achieve adequate overlap on the sides of the defect, attention is directed to the inguinal region (Fig. 5.12, showing the right side). In this step of the procedure, it is important to be familiar with laparoscopic inguinal anatomy in order to avoid damaging cord structures (in men) or the round ligament.

Complete right inguinal dissection with identification of all the anatomical landmarks of the region (Fig. 5.13). The same procedure is performed on the contralateral side.

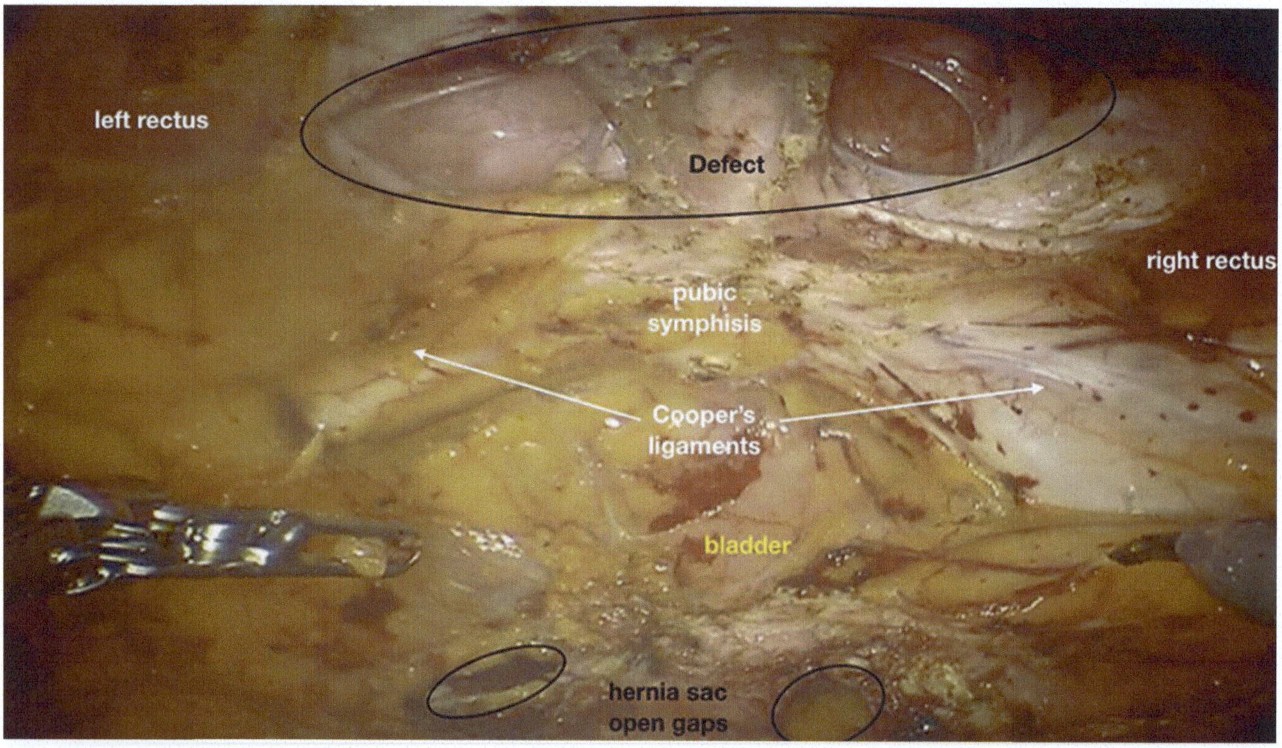


**Fig. 5.11** Full medial dissection with identification of the pubic symphysis, bilateral Cooper's ligaments, and Retzius space, with at least 2–3 cm dissection anterior to the bladder

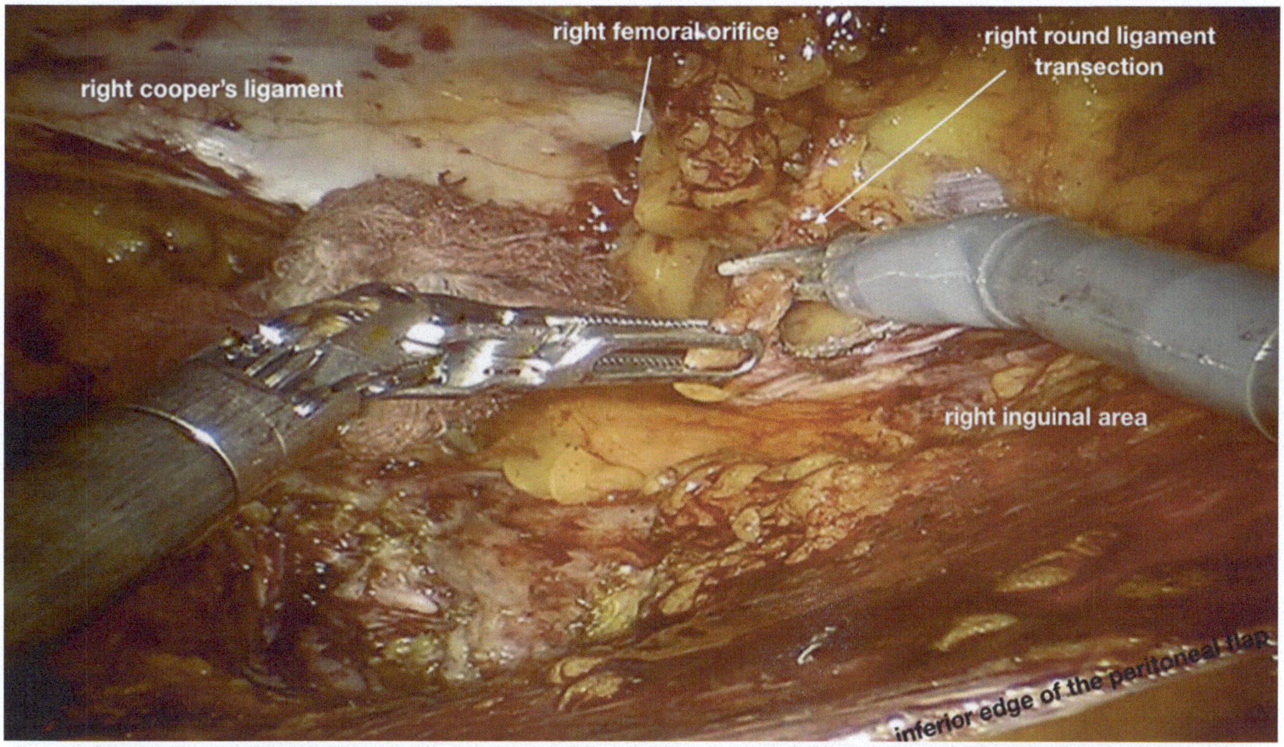


**Fig. 5.12** Right lateral dissection with transection of the right round ligament (*white arrow*). In men, the vas deferens and spermatic vessels should be identified and parietalized, as done in inguinal hernia repairs

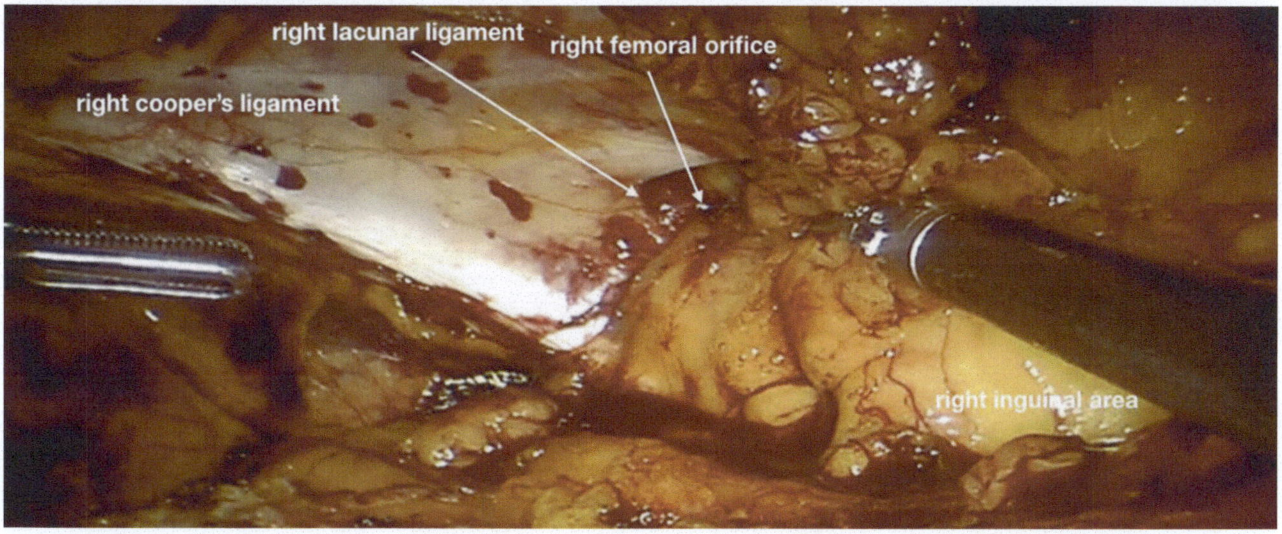


**Fig. 5.13** Full right lateral dissection with identification of the femoral orifice

## Defect Closure

Attention now is directed to defect closure, which is greatly facilitated by the use of the robot and #0 or #1 slowly absorbable or non-absorbable barbed sutures, as shown in Fig. 5.14.

The closure initially is undertaken with a loose suture, which will be tightened after four or five lines with decreased pressure (Fig. 5.15). This allows a functional closure of the defect, much more consistent than transfascial sutures could achieve. The dome of the defect also may be incorporated into the closure in order to obliterate the dead space and avoid seroma formation.

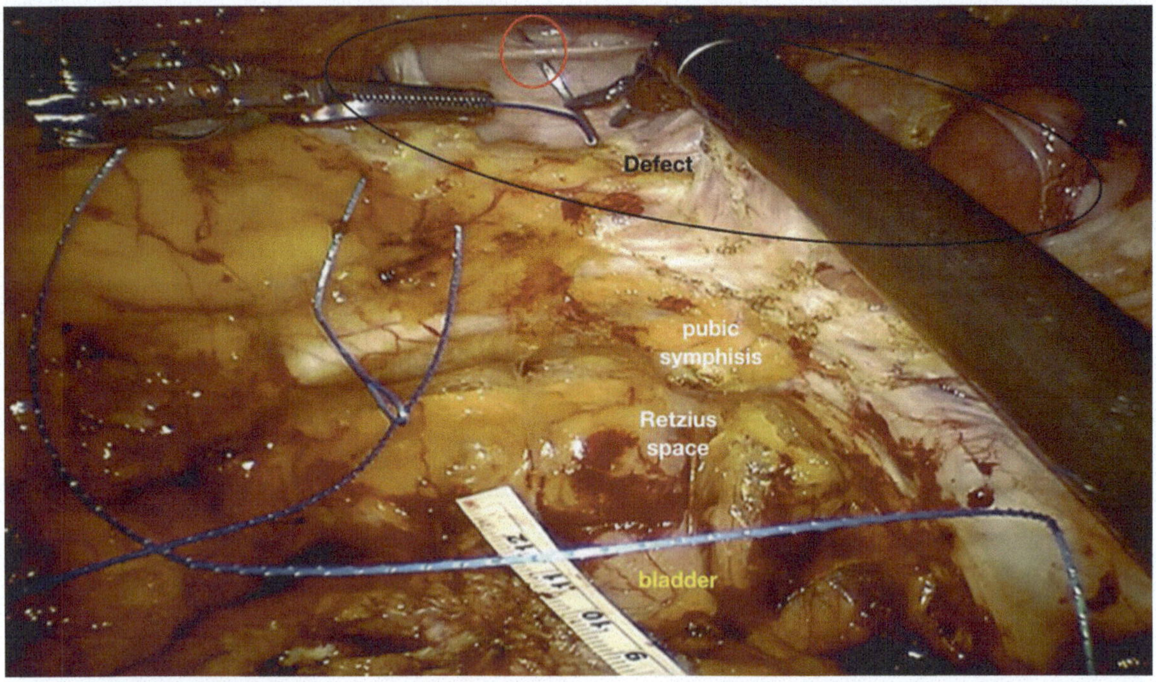


**Fig. 5.14** Defect closure with non-absorbable 0 V-Loc™ running suture (Medtronic). The *small red circle* at the top shows the bite of the hernia sac to reduce postoperative seroma formation

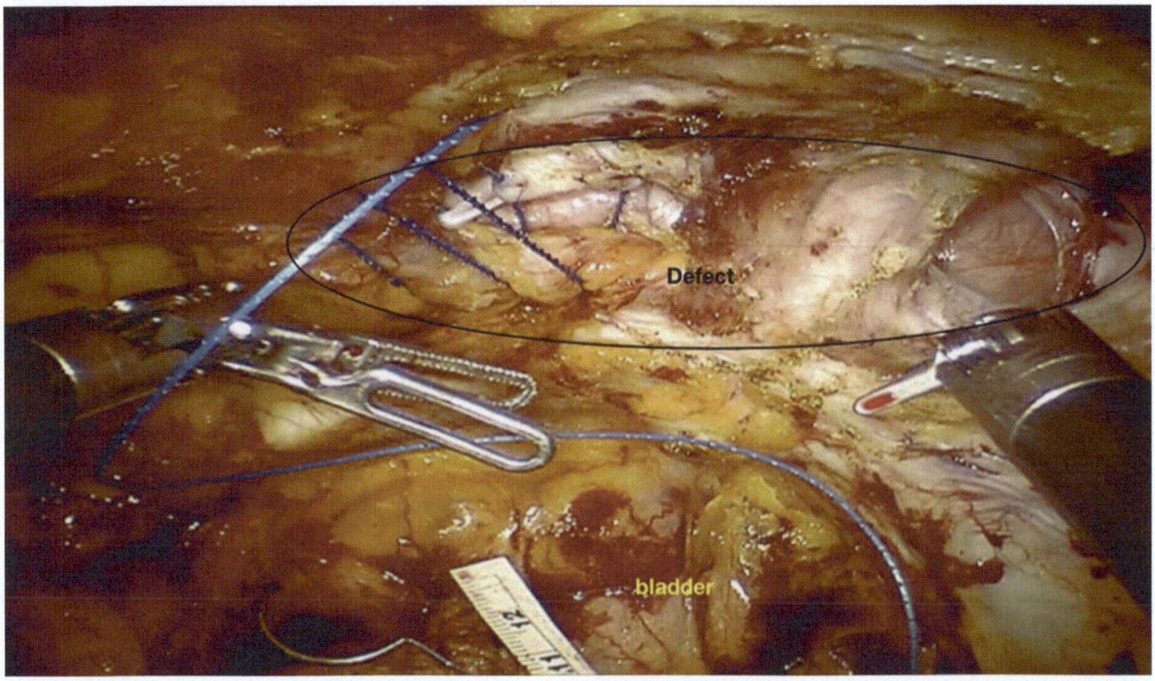


**Fig. 5.15** Progression of closure with loose suture to avoid excessive tension during the closure

Partial disinflation of the abdominal cavity may be required to adequately approximate the defect. The suture is tightened after decreasing the abdominal pressure, and always running the stitch towards the suture line (in Fig. 5.16 from lateral to medial). In this situation, it is important to avoid traction in the cranial or caudal direction, which can lead to tears in the abdominal wall.

A barbed suture allows good traction, allowing adequate defect closure (Fig. 5.17). Figure 5.18 shows the complete closure of the defect. With the use of barbed suture, it is not necessary to tie the suture, but it is important to run back two stitches so the suture can be securely locked in place to keep the defect closed safely (Fig. 5.19).

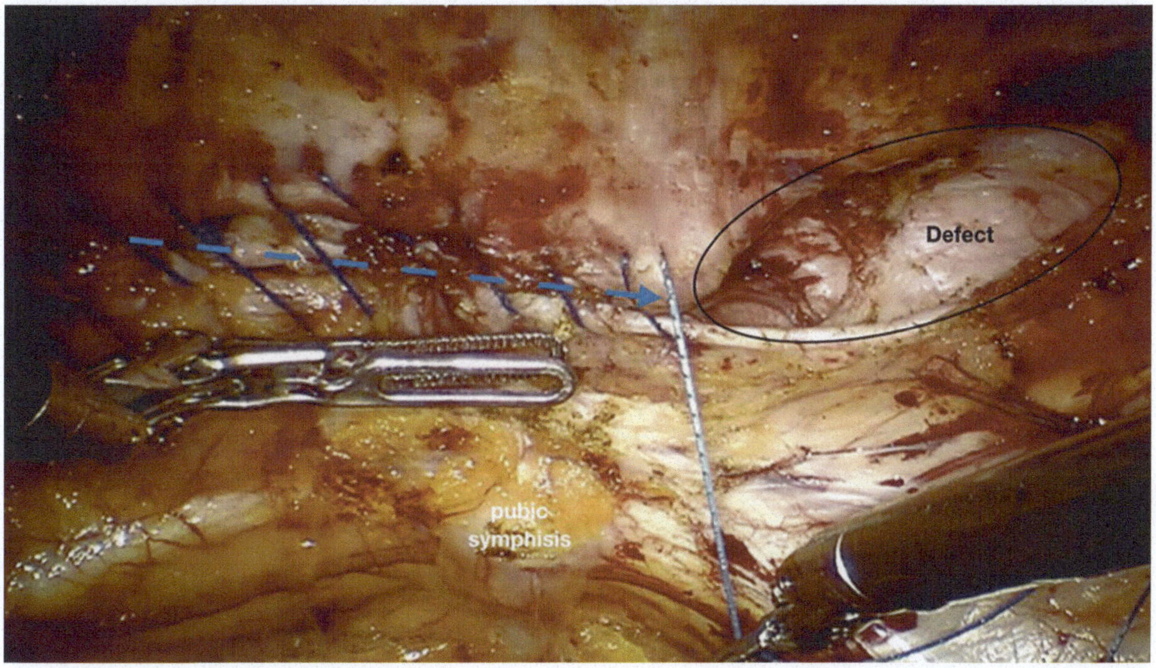


**Fig. 5.16** Progressive tightening of the suture from the corner to the medial aspect (*blue dotted arrow*)

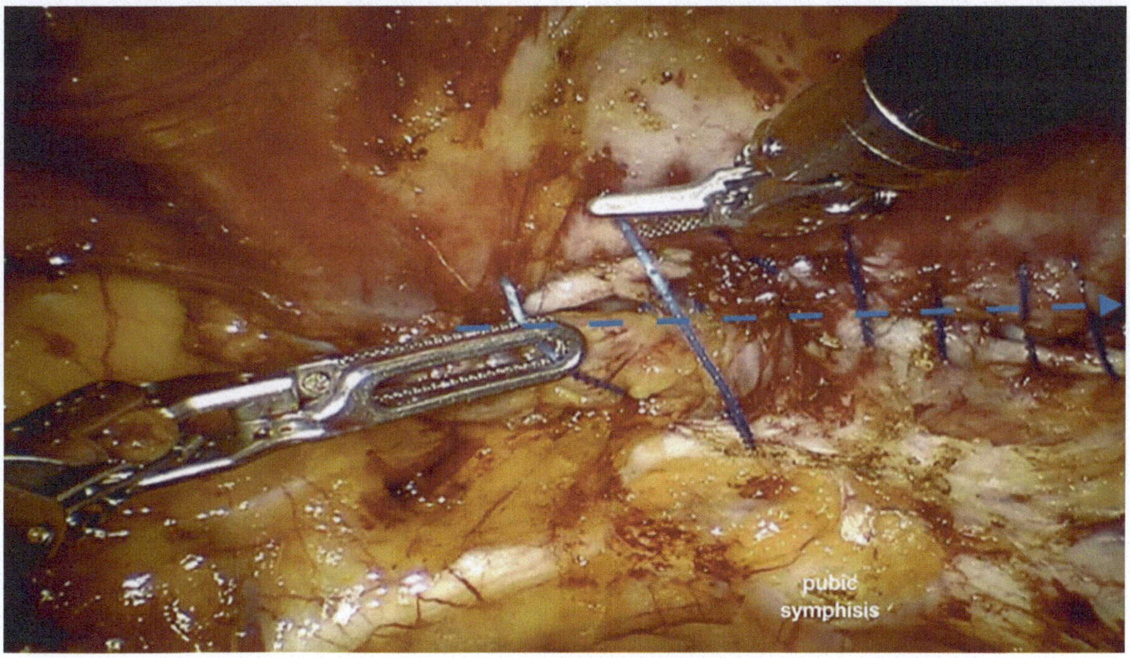


**Fig. 5.17** Progressive tightening of the suture from the corner (*blue dotted arrow*)

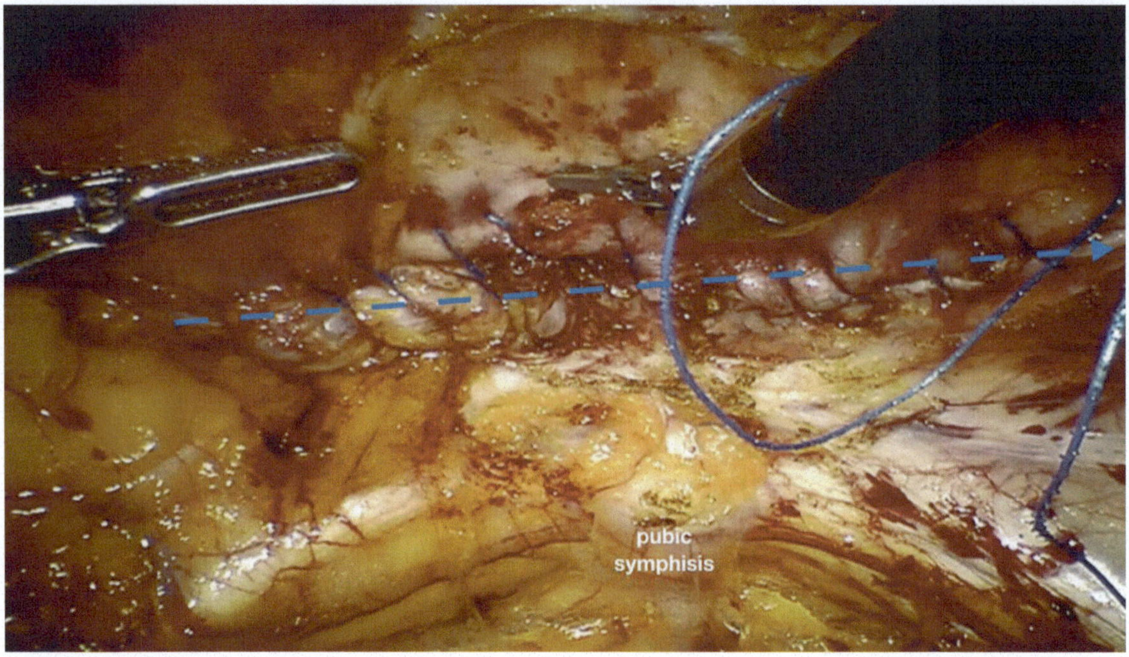


**Fig. 5.18** Final tightening of the suture after complete closure of the defect (*blue dotted arrow*)

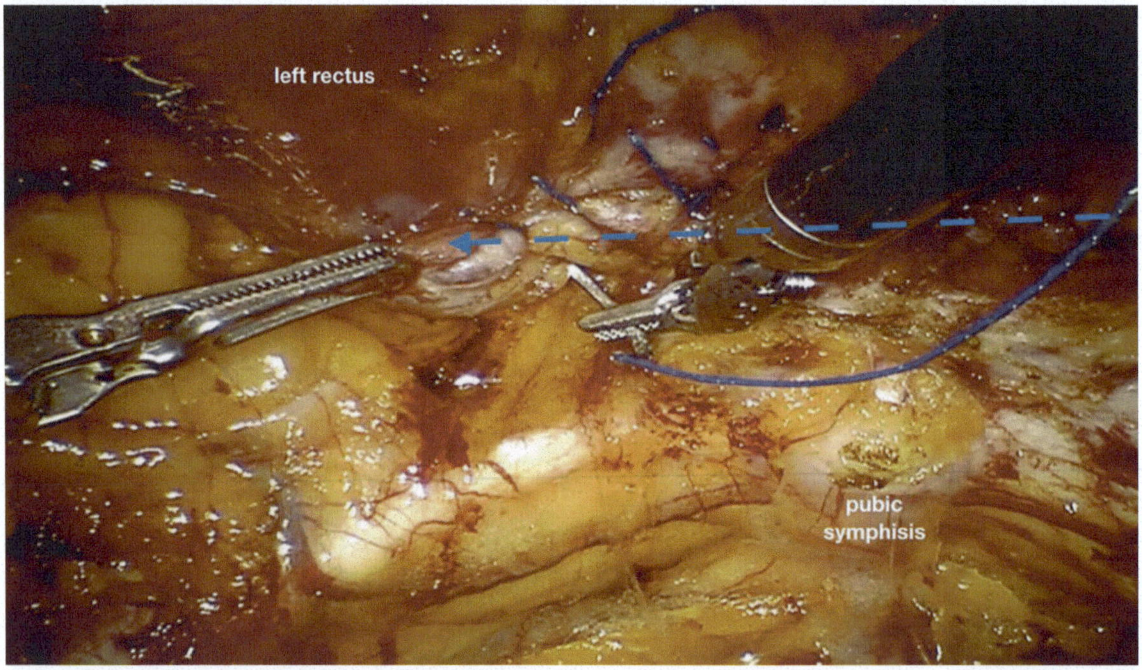


**Fig. 5.19** Back suturing with the V-Loc™ to ensure locking of the suture

## Mesh Implantation

After completion of the defect closure, a ruler is used to measure the size of the preperitoneal pocket created and the size of the mesh that will be used (Fig. 5.20). Figure 5.21 shows the latero-lateral measurement and all the important anatomic landmarks that should always be identified in order to achieve an adequate repair.

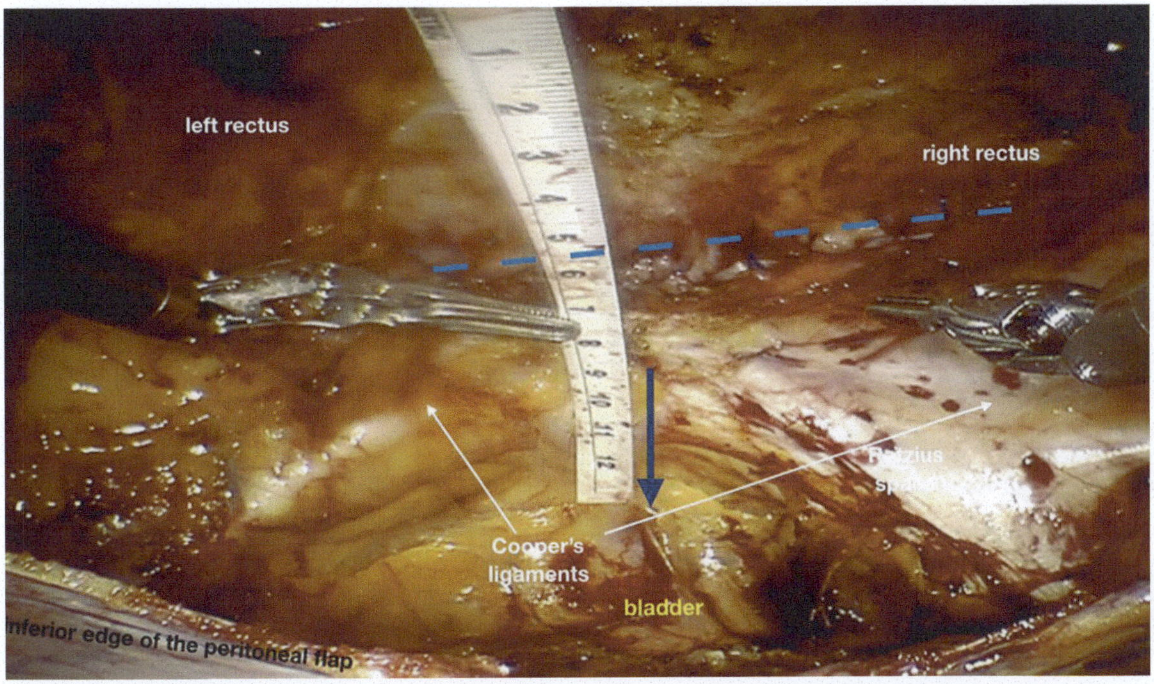


**Fig. 5.20** Cranio-caudal measurement of the space after complete defect closure (*dotted blue line*). Meshes at least 15–20 cm long are used. The caudal overlap of 2–3 cm into the Retzius space is shown (*blue arrow*)

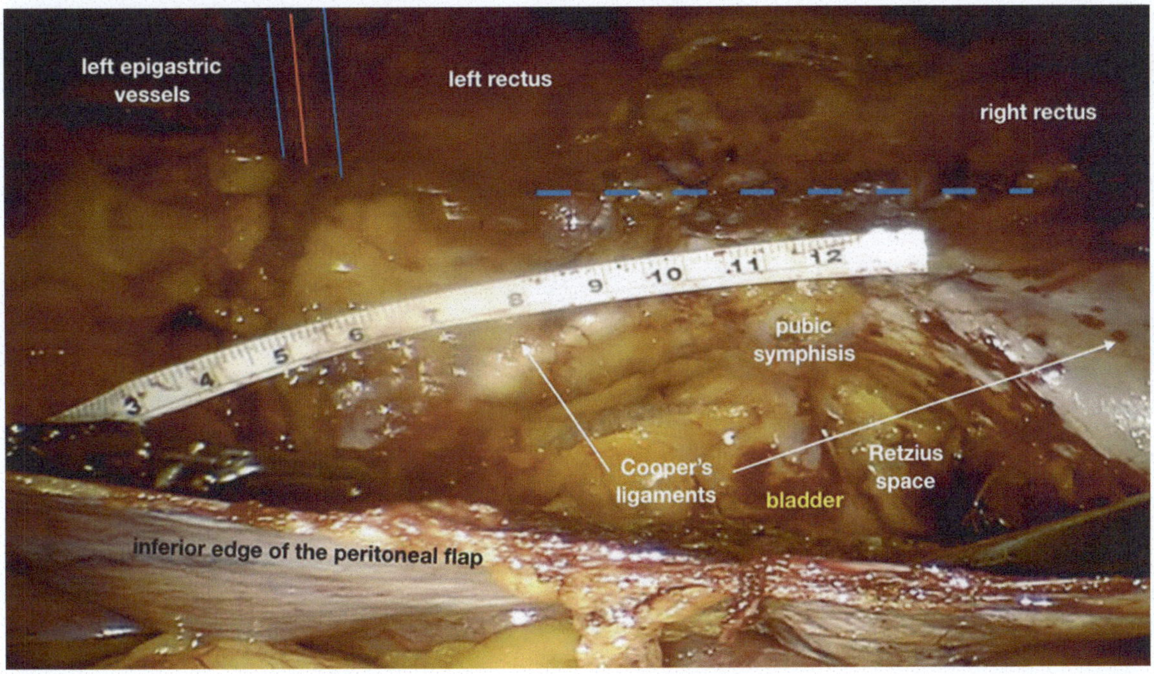


**Fig. 5.21** Latero-lateral measurement of the space; meshes at least 25–30 cm wide are used

A regular midweight polypropylene mesh is used, tailored according to the measurements previously described (Fig. 5.22). In this situation, one of the arms is undocked and the mesh is inserted in the abdominal cavity and inside the pocket created. Figure 5.23 shows complete mesh opening inside the pocket previously developed. Note that there is a huge overlap below the pubic bone. This shows the importance of the bladder dissection and the creation of a large retropubic and inguinal spaces adequate to promote mesh overlap and positioning and avoid recurrences.

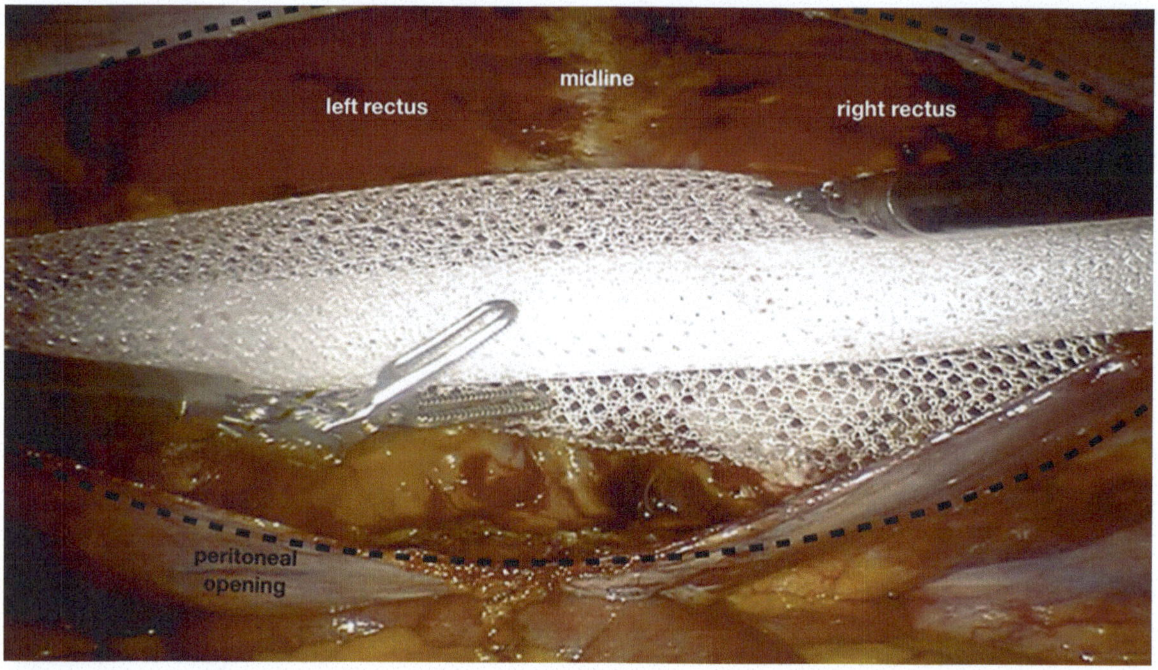


**Fig. 5.22** Initial mesh positioning inside the preperitoneal pocket. The mesh is kept rolled to facilitate orientation and positioning. The midline portion of the mesh may be marked to help

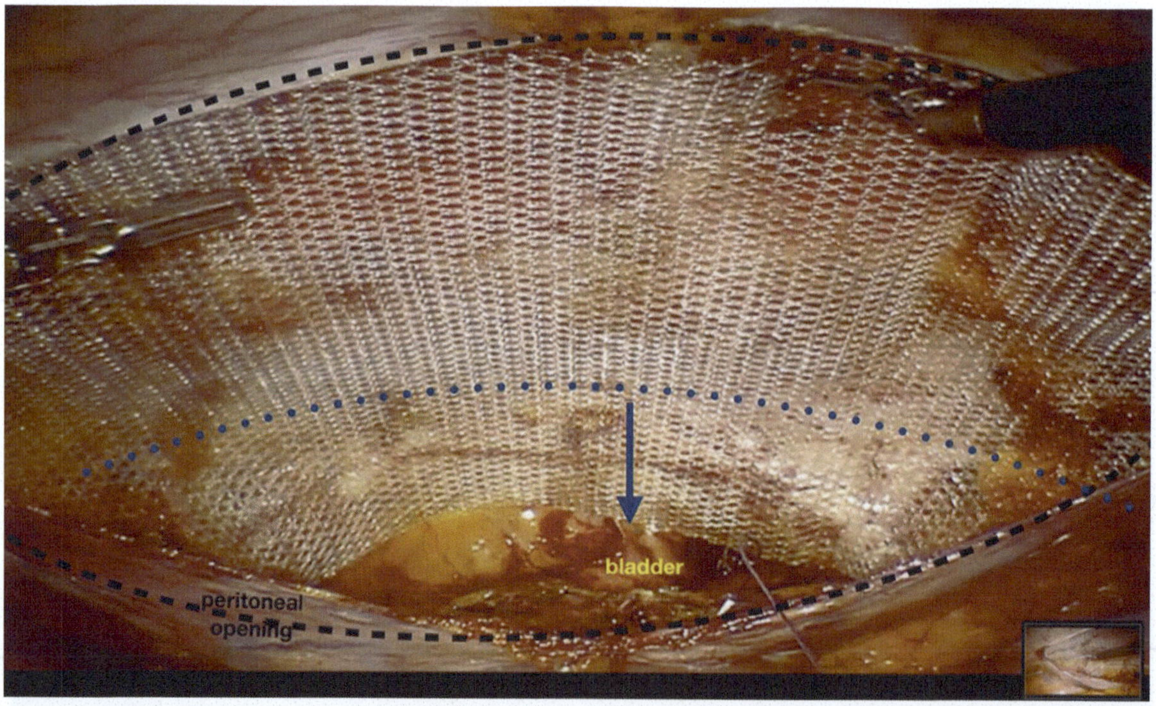


**Fig. 5.23** Full opening of the mesh with no wrinkles or folds. It is important to create a big enough preperitoneal pocket to accommodate the mesh. Note the caudal overlap into the Retzius space (*blue arrow*), below both Cooper's ligaments and the pubis. (The *dotted line* demonstrates the projection of those structures)

Mesh fixation is accomplished with interrupted sutures positioned in the cardinal points of the mesh, just to keep the mesh in position during the first days of integration (Figs. 5.24 and 5.25). The anatomical principles are respected, avoiding sutures below the iliopubic tract in the lateral aspect of the dissection.

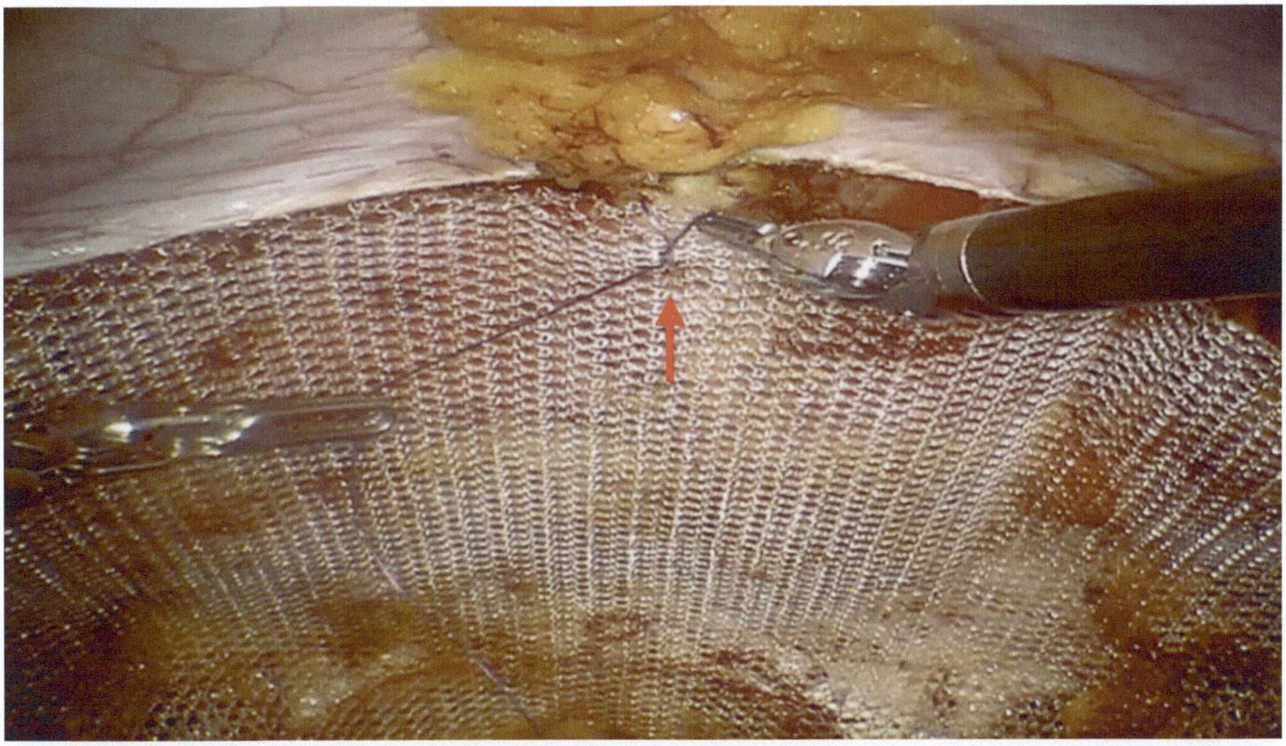

Fig. 5.24 Initial mesh fixation with midline interrupted 3–0 Vicryl suture (*red arrow*)

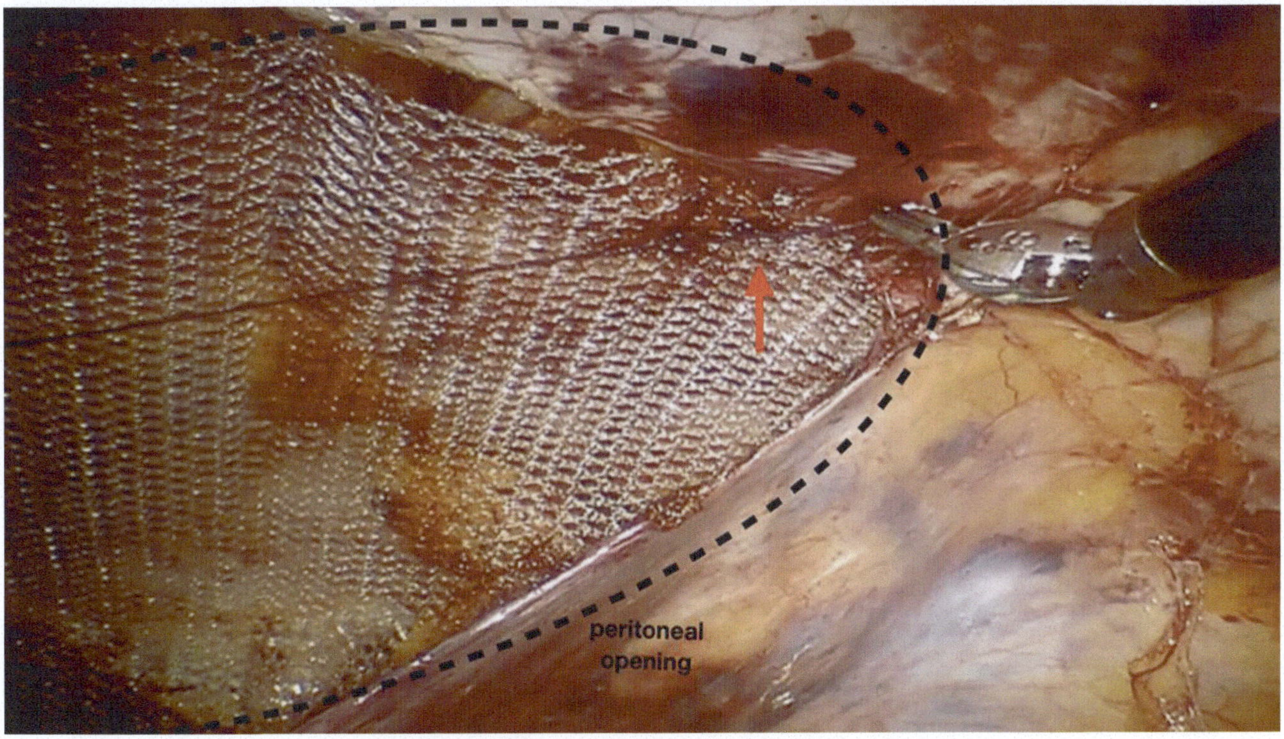


Fig. 5.25 Superior-lateral (right side) mesh fixation with midline interrupted 3–0 Vicryl suture (*red arrow*). As at an inguinal repair, the inferior lateral mesh edge is not fixated, just wide positioned into the space to avoid any nerve injury

Figure 5.26 stresses the importance of bladder mobilization to achieve adequate retropubic and infrapubic overlap to avoid recurrence. Additional sutures are placed to maintain adequate mesh positioning (Fig. 5.27). This is facilitated by the use of the robotic platform.

Cooper's ligament is used to add additional sutures in both sides of the inguinal regions (Fig. 5.28).

## Peritoneal Closure

Peritoneal flap closure is started from lateral to medial using a running suture with a barbed 3-0 absorbable V-Loc™ (Fig. 5.29). When the initial suture reaches midline, the right side of the posterior rectus sheath is completely isolated from the abdominal cavity (Fig. 5.30).

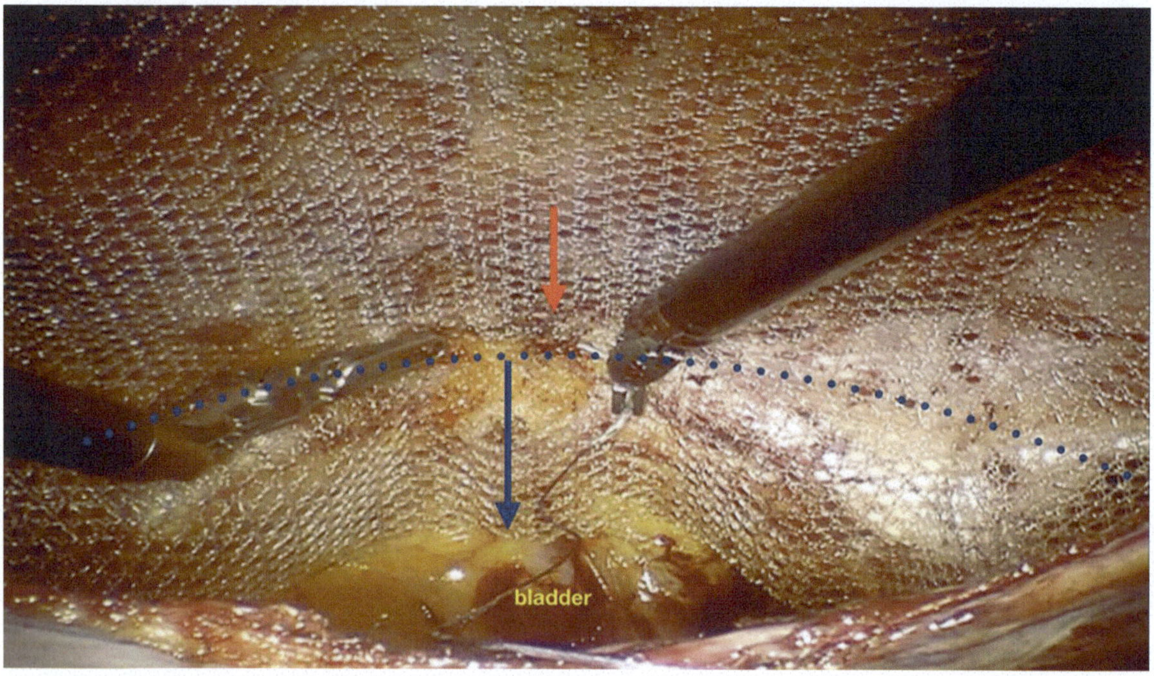


**Fig. 5.26** Mesh fixation with suprapubic interrupted 3–0 Vicryl suture (*red arrow*). Note the adequate 3 cm caudal overlap into the Retzius space (*blue arrow*)

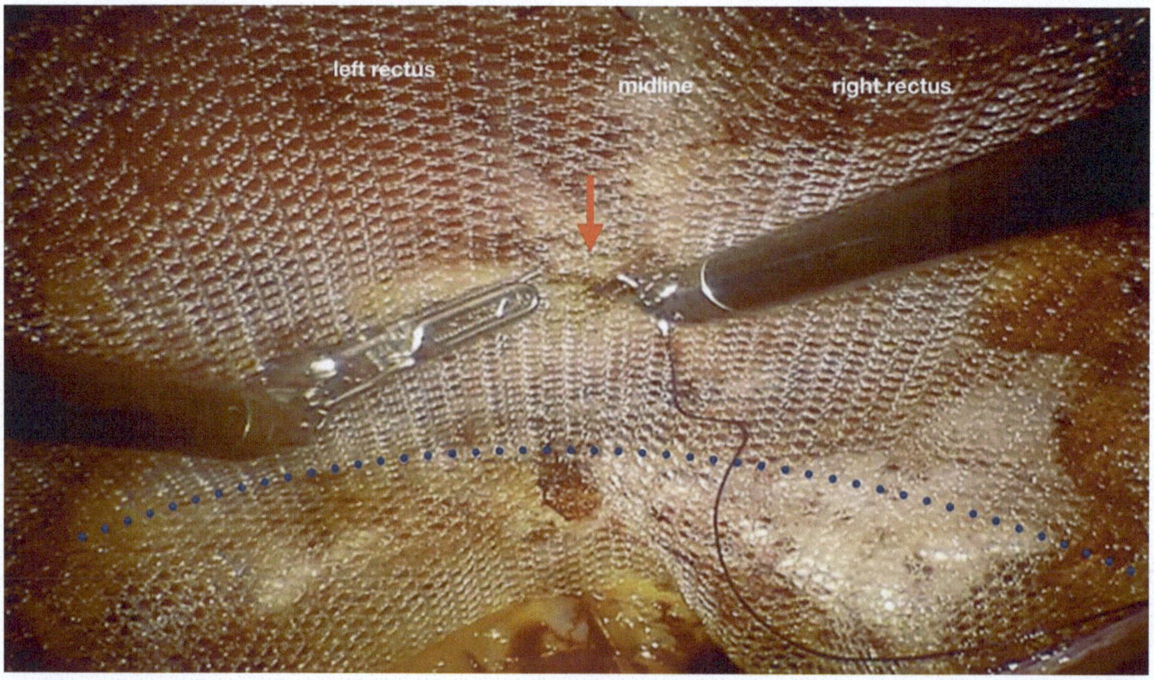


**Fig. 5.27** Additional medial mesh fixation is performed with interrupted 3-0 Vicryl suture (*red arrow*). Note the projection of the pubis and Cooper's ligaments (*dotted blue line*)

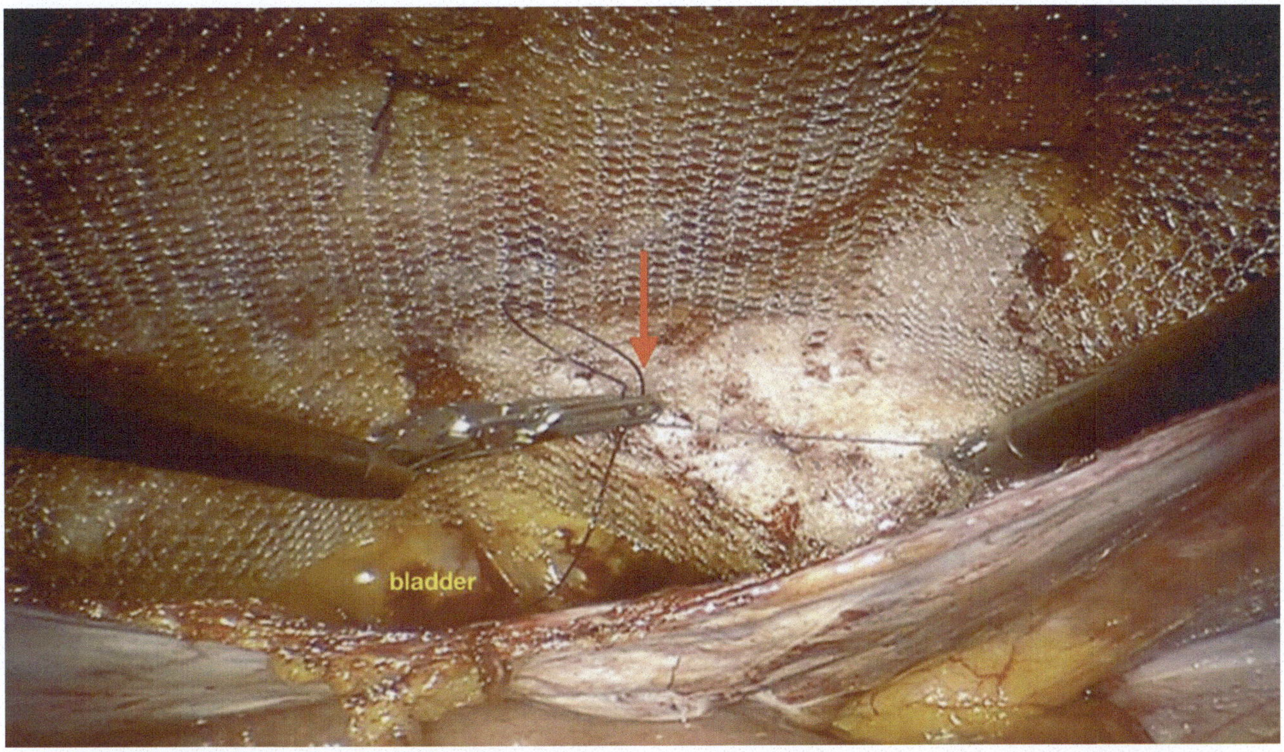


**Fig. 5.28** Mesh fixation with interrupted 3-0 Vicryl suture into both Cooper's ligaments (*red arrow*)

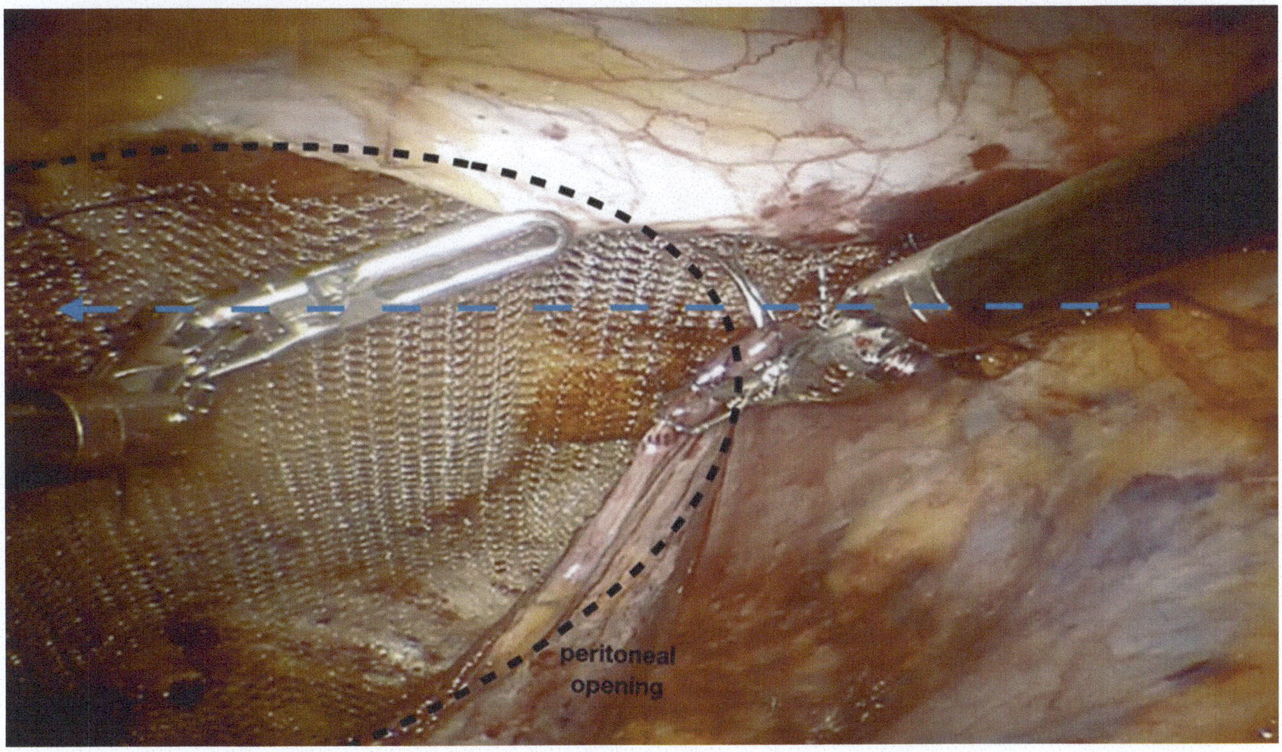


**Fig. 5.29** Initial peritoneal flap closure with 3-0 V-Loc™ from lateral to medial (*dotted blue arrow*)

Another suture is performed in the same way at the left side, closing the defect and avoiding contact between the mesh and abdominal contents (Fig. 5.31). Note the mattress suture that is performed to close the peritoneum. This is important to avoid exposing the abdominal contents to the barbs of the sutures.

The peritoneal holes are closed with interrupted absorbable sutures to avoid contact of the mesh with the viscera (Fig. 5.32).

Ports are removed under direct vision to ensure hemostasis, 12 mm ports are closed with 0 Vicryl and skin is closed properly.

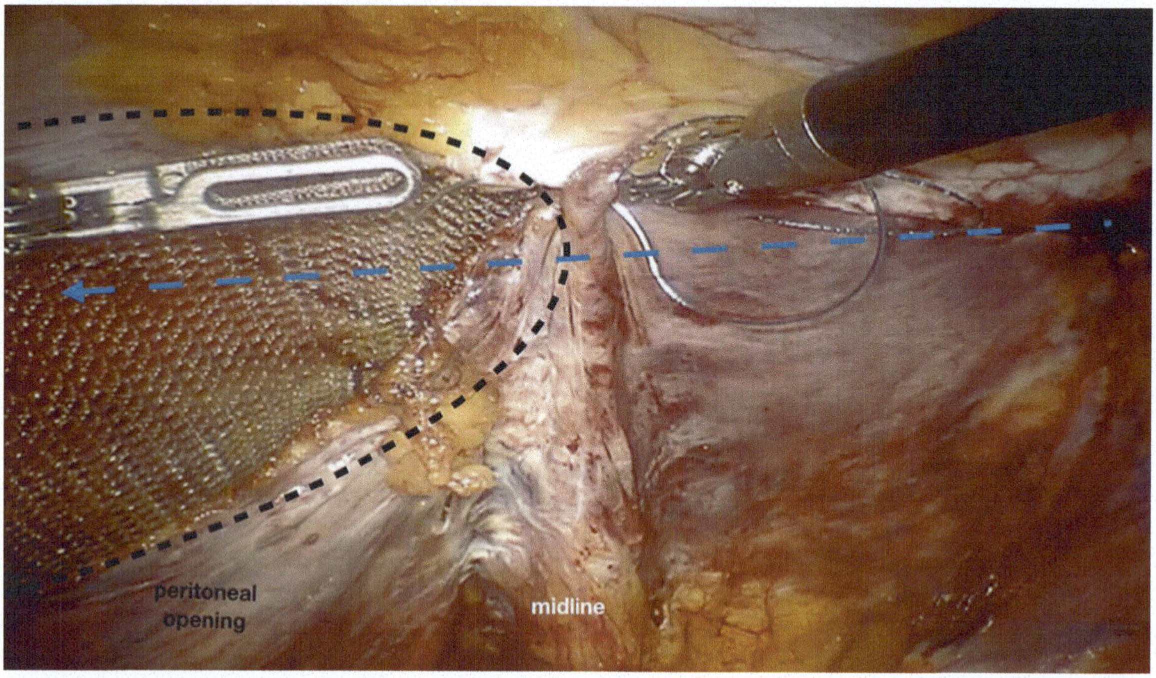


**Fig. 5.30** Peritoneal flap closure with 3-0 V-Loc™ reaches midline (*dotted blue arrow*)

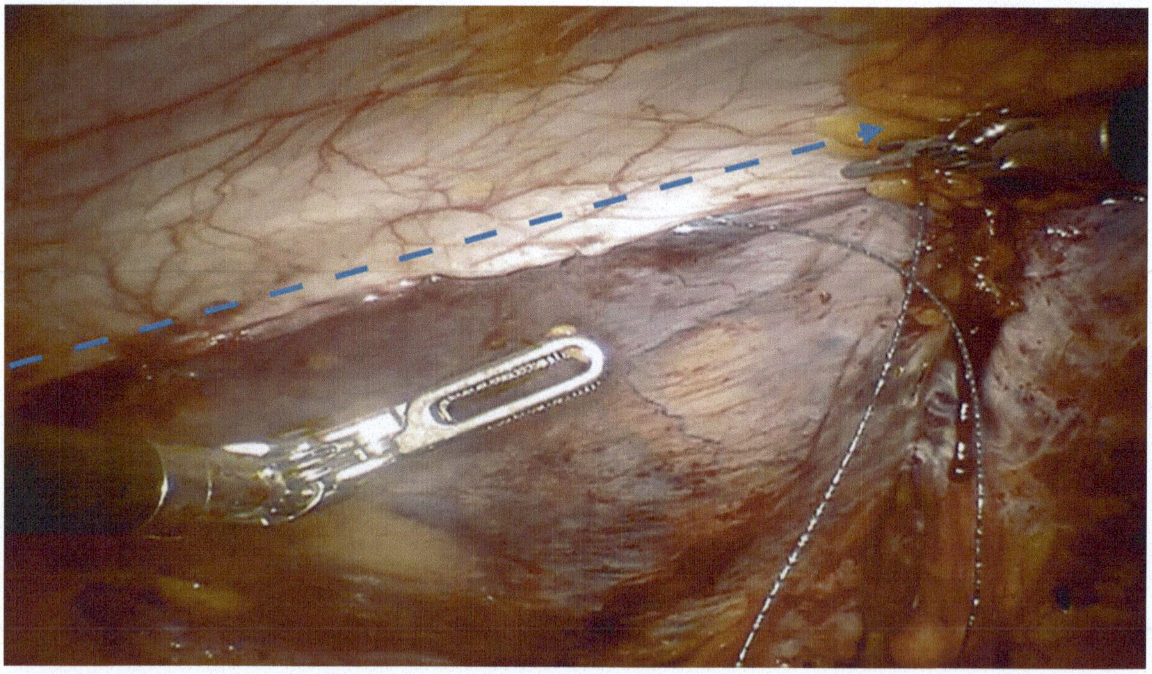

**Fig. 5.31** Final aspect of peritoneal flap closure with 3-0 V-Loc™ (*dotted blue arrow*) with horizontal mattress suture, which hides the barbed suture from the viscera

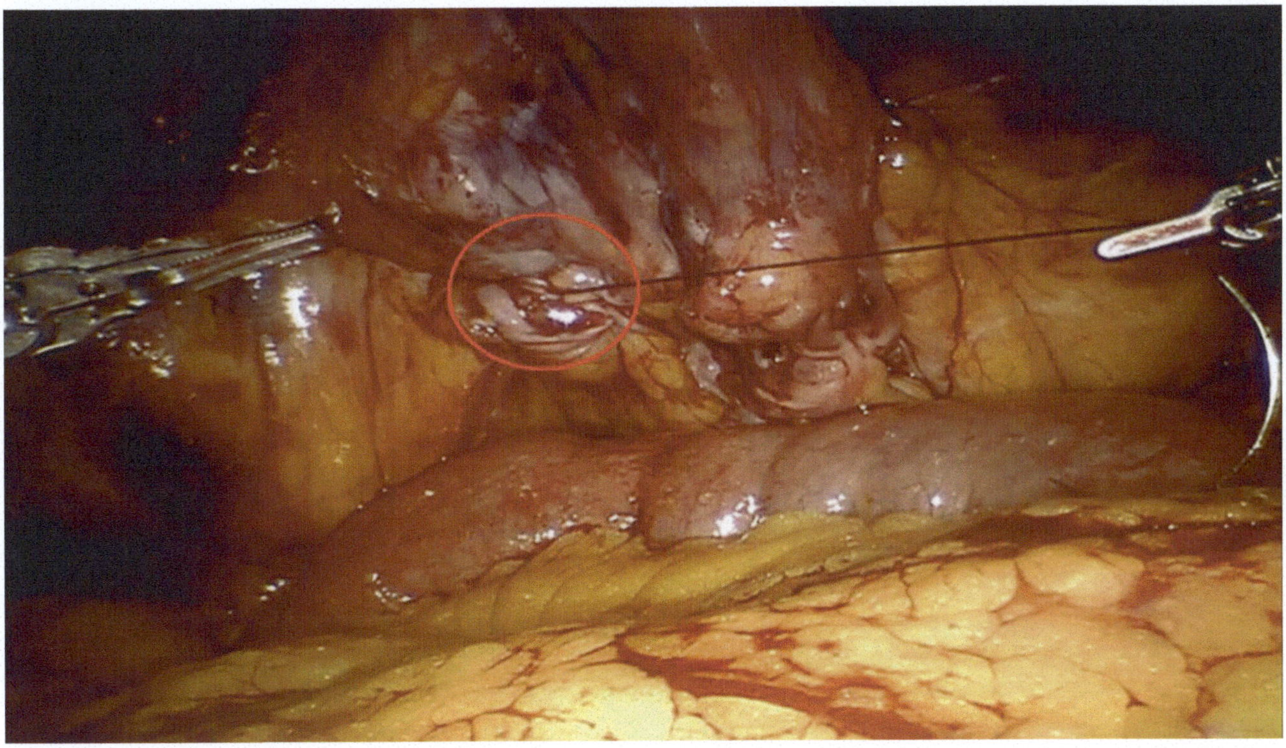

**Fig. 5.32** All hernia sac openings are closed with interrupted 3-0 Vicryl sutures (*red circle*)

## Summary

The technique of robotic ventral TAPP incisional hernia repair in the supra-pubic area with intracorporeal closure of the fascial defect and mesh fixation is feasible, can reduce wound morbidity, allows good mesh overlap and fixation in the retropubic space, and may reduce postoperative pain by eliminating transfascial suture. Further evaluation is needed, and long-term data are lacking to assess the benefit to the patient.

## References

1. Cobb WS. Laparoscopic subxiphoid and suprapubic hernia repair. In: Novitsky YW, editor. Hernia surgery. Cham: Springer International Publishing; 2016. p. 253–60. https://doi.org/10.1007/978-3-319-27470-6_24.
2. Malcher F, Cavazzola LT, Kingsnorth A. Open repair. In: KA LB, Kingsnorth A, Sanders DL, editors. Management of abdominal hernias. Cham: Springer; 2018. p. 365–79. https://doi.org/10.1007/978-3-319-63251-3_25.
3. Heniford BT, Park A, Ramshaw BJ, Voeller G. Laparoscopic repair of ventral hernias: nine years' experience with 850 consecutive hernias. Ann Surg. 2003;238:391–400.
4. Earle D, Seymour N, Fellinger E, Perez A. Laparoscopic versus open incisional hernia repair: a single-institution analysis of hospital resource utilization for 884 consecutive cases. Surg Endosc. 2006;20:71–5.
5. McKinlay RD, Park A. Laparoscopic ventral incisional hernia repair: a more effective alternative to conventional repair of recurrent incisional hernia. J Gastrointest Surg. 2004;8:670–4.
6. Jin J, Rosen MJ. Laparoscopic versus open ventral hernia repair. Surg Clin North Am. 2008;88:1083–100, viii. https://doi.org/10.1016/j.suc.2008.05.015.
7. Parra-Davila E, Malcher F, Hartmann C. Robotic repair of lower abdomen defects. In: Abdalla RZ, Costa TN, editors. Robotic surgery for abdominal wall hernia repair. Cham: Springer International Publishing; 2018. p. 35–47. https://doi.org/10.1007/978-3-319-55527-0.
8. Ballecer C, Jarvis Walters J, Prebil BE. Masters program hernia pathway: Robotic ventral hernia repair. In: Patel AD, Oleynikov D, editors. The SAGES manual of robotic surgery. The SAGES University Masters Program Series. Cham: Springer International Publishing; 2018. p. 67–84. https://doi.org/10.1007/978-3-319-51362-1.
9. Muysoms FE, Miserez M, Berrevoet F, Campanelli G, Champault GG, Chelala E, et al. Classification of primary and incisional abdominal wall hernias. Hernia. 2009;13:407–14. https://doi.org/10.1007/s10029-009-0518-x.
10. Carbonell AM, Kercher KW, Matthews BD, Sing RF, Cobb WS, Heniford BT. The laparoscopic repair of suprapubic ventral hernias. Surg Endosc. 2005;19:174–7.
11. Malcher F, Cavazzola LT, Belyansky I. Robotic retro-rectus repairs. In: LeBlanc K, editor. Robotic assisted hernia repair. Cham: Springer; 2019. p. 331–49. https://doi.org/10.1007/978-3-030-23025-8.
12. Dolan P, Dakin G. Challenging hernias: spigelian, flank hernias, suprapubic, and subxiphoid. In: Davis Jr S, Dakin G, Bates A, editors. The SAGES manual of hernia surgery. Cham: Springer; 2019. p. 343–58. https://doi.org/10.1007/978-3-319-78411-3.

# 6 Robotic Posterior Component Separation

Ibnalwalid Saad and Alfredo M. Carbonell

## Introduction

The open transversus abdominis release (TAR) has been described as a lateral extension of the Rives-Stoppa retromuscular repair to provide a tension-free closure of the hernia defect, place the mesh in the retrorectus space, and avoid the creation of large subcutaneous flaps needed for performing anterior component separation. Our robotic approach is essentially a replica of the open technique with the added advantage of shorter hospital stay and lower wound morbidity when compared with the open approach.

## Selection Criteria

This minimally invasive technique is particularly useful for patients with increased risk for wound complications such as diabetics, smokers, and morbidly obese patients. Preoperative assessment with imaging and a physical examination to assess the defect size and the compliance of the abdominal wall are essential to predict the ability to close the defect robotically and appropriately select candidates for this technique.

## Operative Technique

Figures 6.1, 6.2, 6.3, 6.4, 6.5, 6.6, 6.7, 6.8, 6.9, 6.10, 6.11, 6.12, 6.13, and 6.14 illustrate the technique we use for robotic transversus abdominis release (TAR).

I. Saad · A. M. Carbonell (✉)
Department of Surgery, Prisma Health-Upstate, University of South Carolina School of Medicine, Greenville, Greenville, SC, USA
e-mail: Alfredo.carbonell@prismahealth.org


O. Y. Kudsi (ed.), *Robotic Hernia Surgery*, https://doi.org/10.1007/978-3-030-46667-1_6

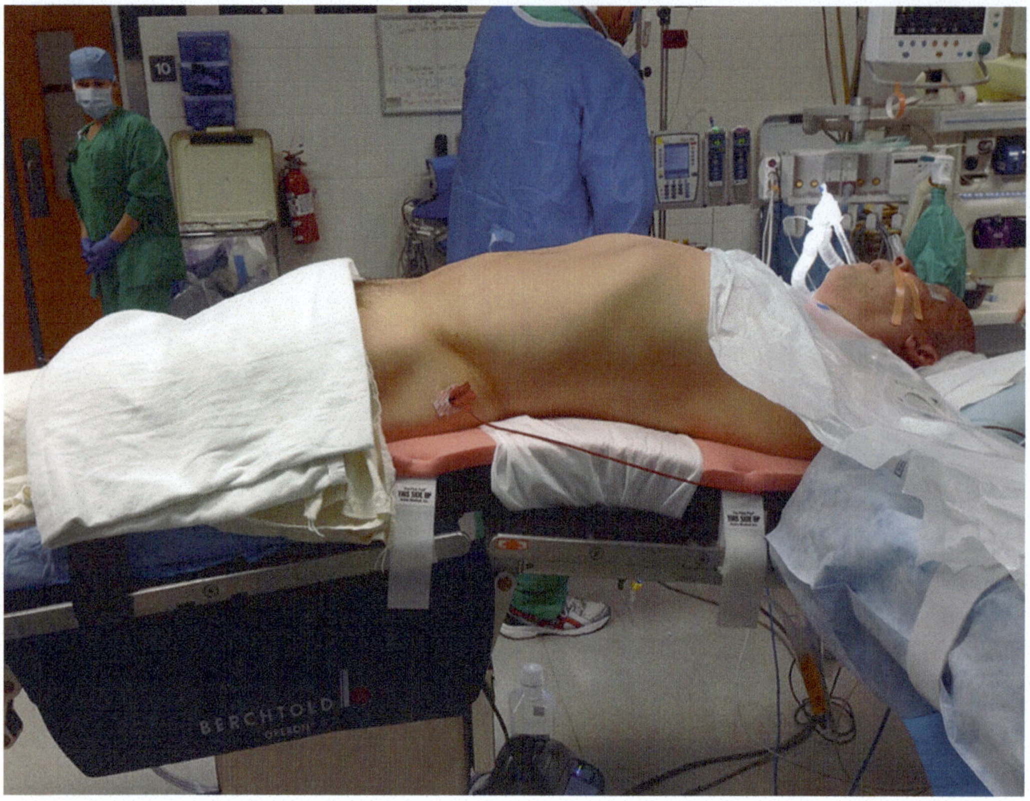


**Fig. 6.1** Patient positioning. The patient is placed in a supine position with the table flexed at the level of the umbilicus to increase the distance between the costal margin and the iliac crest, allowing for widely spaced trocars and avoiding robotic arm collision. The patient's arms are not tucked, to give more range of motion for the robotic arms

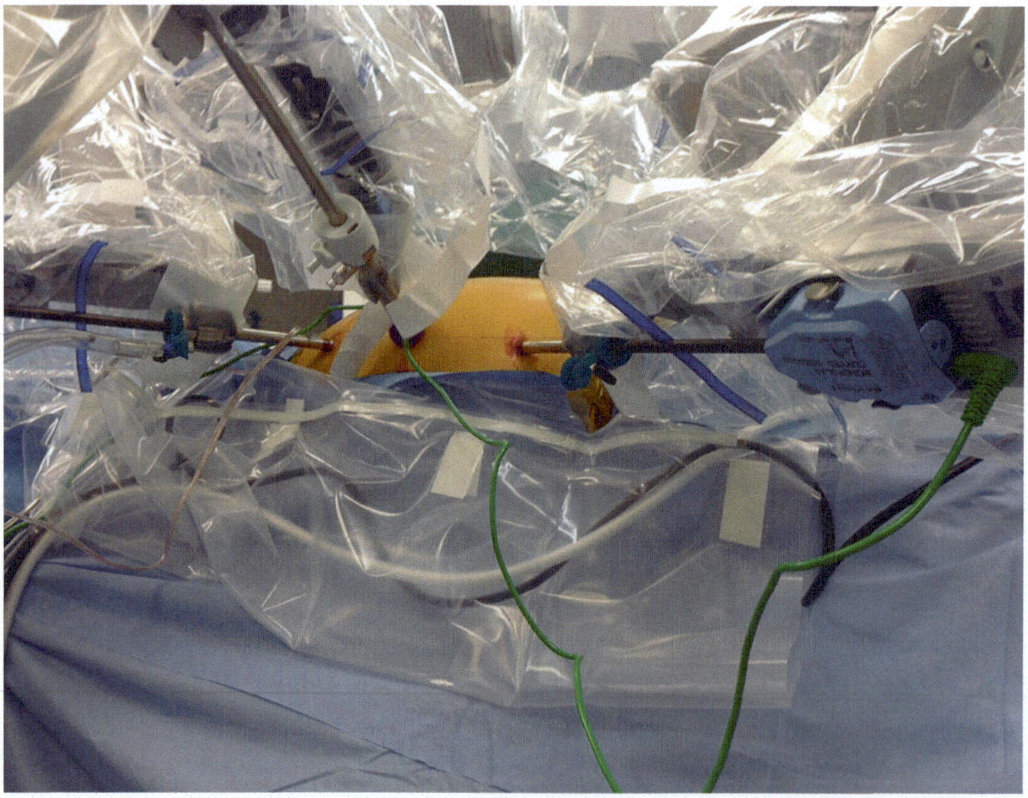

**Fig. 6.2** Trocar placement. The peritoneal cavity is accessed in the right upper quadrant using a 5-mm optical trocar followed by two more lateral ports. The 5-mm port is switched to a robotic trocar under laparoscopic vision

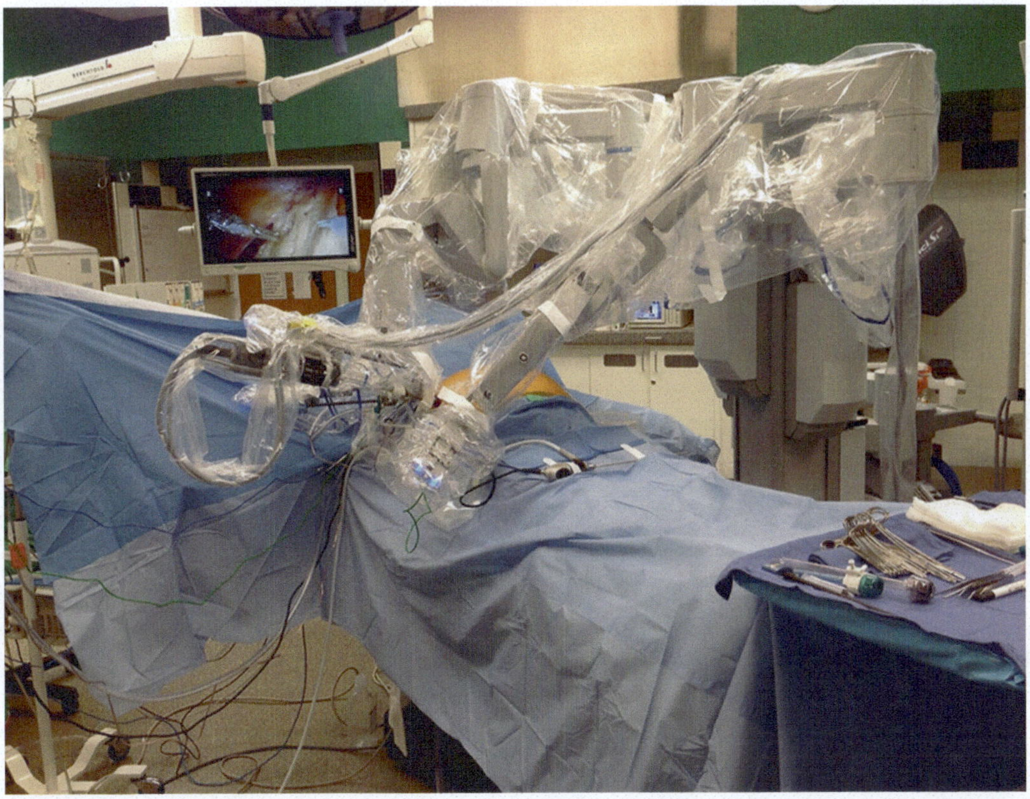

**Fig. 6.3** The robot is docked from the right side, with the side cart perpendicular to the patient bed. The center column is aligned with the anterior superior iliac spine; this position gives room for the assistant to stand between the cart and the right arm. For dissection, we use HotShears™ curved scissors in the right arm and ProGrasp™ forceps in the left arm (Intuitive Surgical; Sunnyvale, CA, USA); for suturing, we use a large needle driver

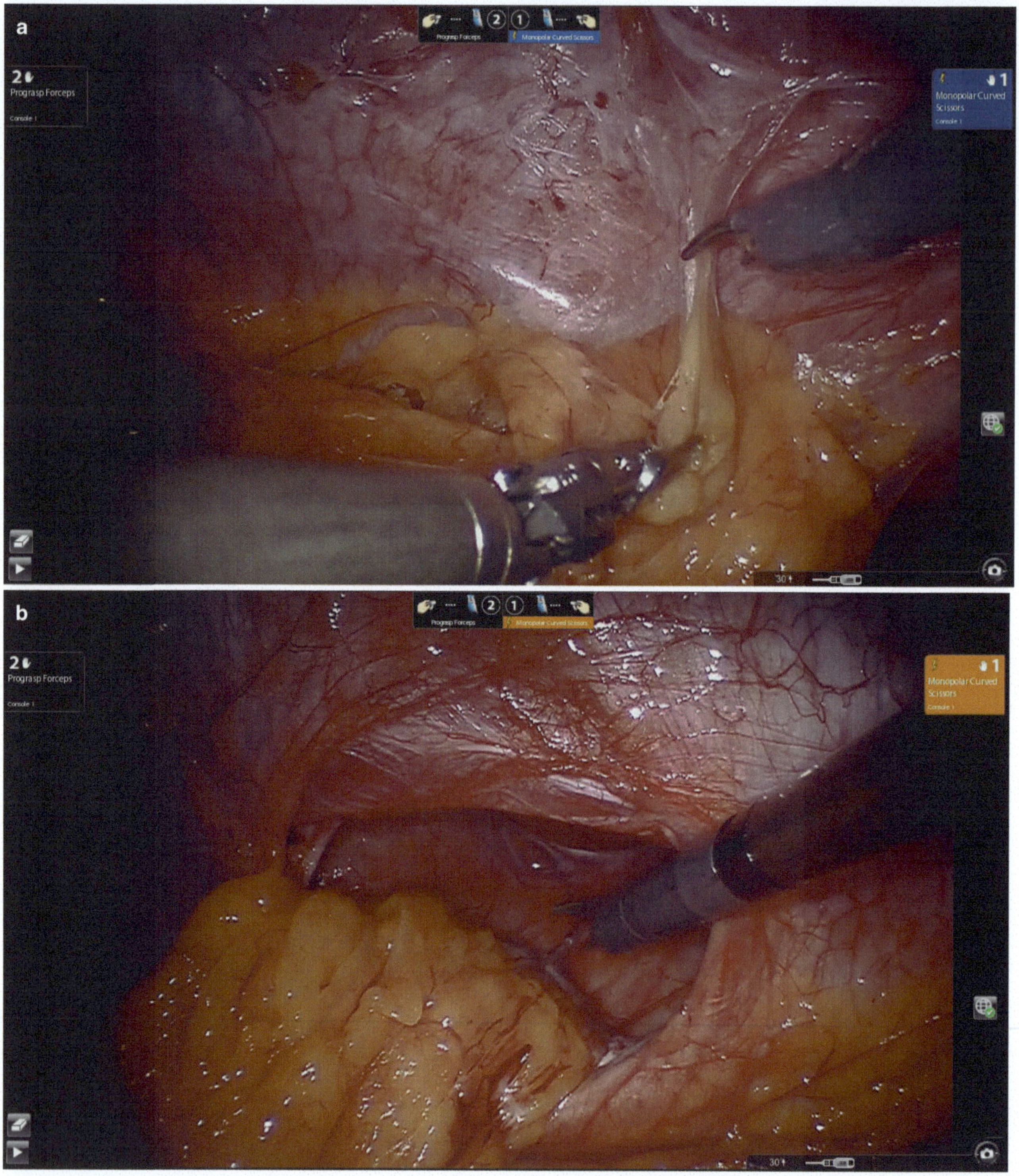


**Fig. 6.4** (**a**) Lysis of adhesions is performed (laparoscopically, if needed) until there is 2–3 cm of a clear zone in front of the robotic instruments; then the rest can be completed robotically. Care should be taken to avoid injury to the peritoneum to maintain a barrier between the future mesh and the viscera and also to prevent the development of an interparietal hernia. (**b**) The hernia sac contents are reduced. External pressure on the hernia by a bedside assistant can improve visualization when taking down the attachments between the hernia sac and its contents

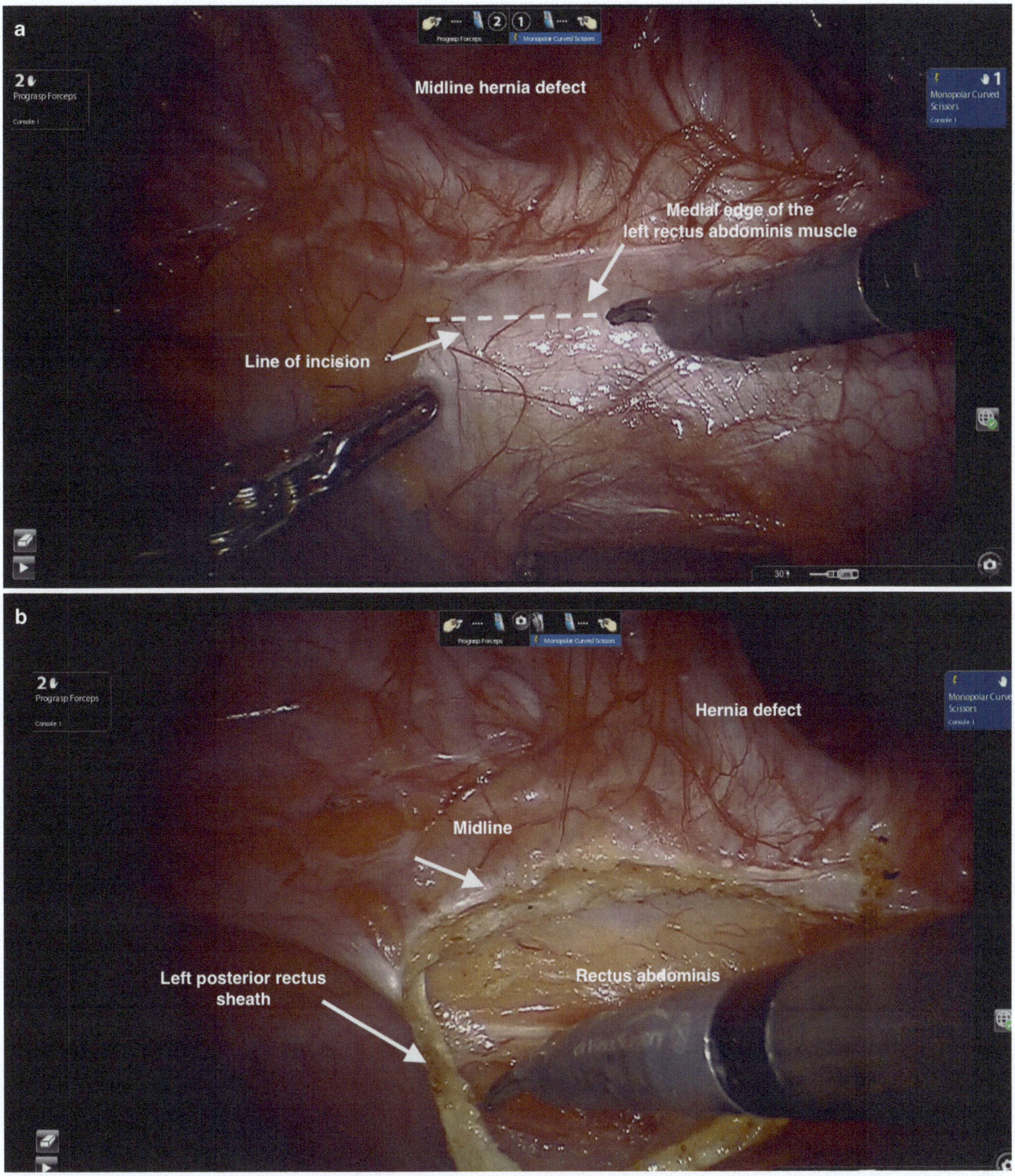


**Fig. 6.5** (**a**) and (**b**) The hernia defect is identified and measured; then the Rives-Stoppa dissection is started by incising the left posterior rectus sheath close to the hernia defect (using cut mode). The dissection is continued 5–7 cm above and below the defect to get enough overlap. The posterior rectus sheath is dissected from the rectus muscle up to the semilunar line and the segmental innervation to the rectus muscle. (**c**) Care should be taken to preserve the segmental innervation to the rectus muscle

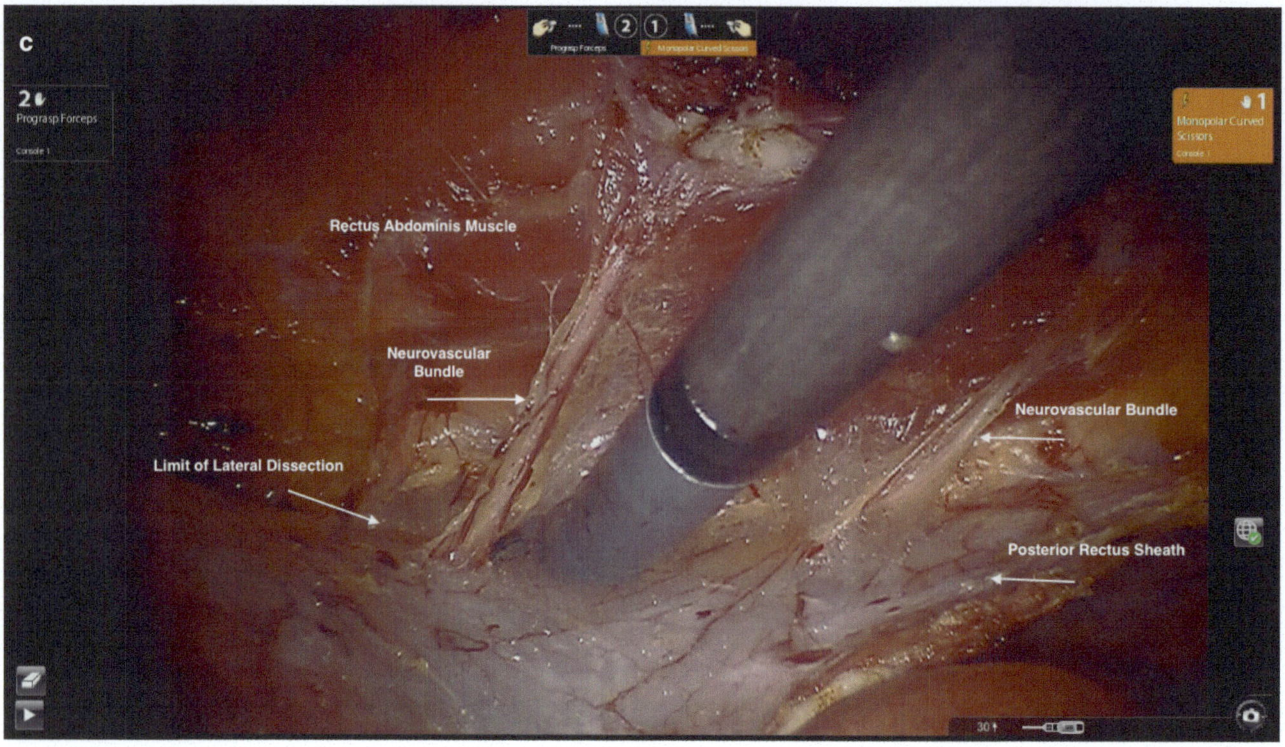


Fig. 6.5 (continued)

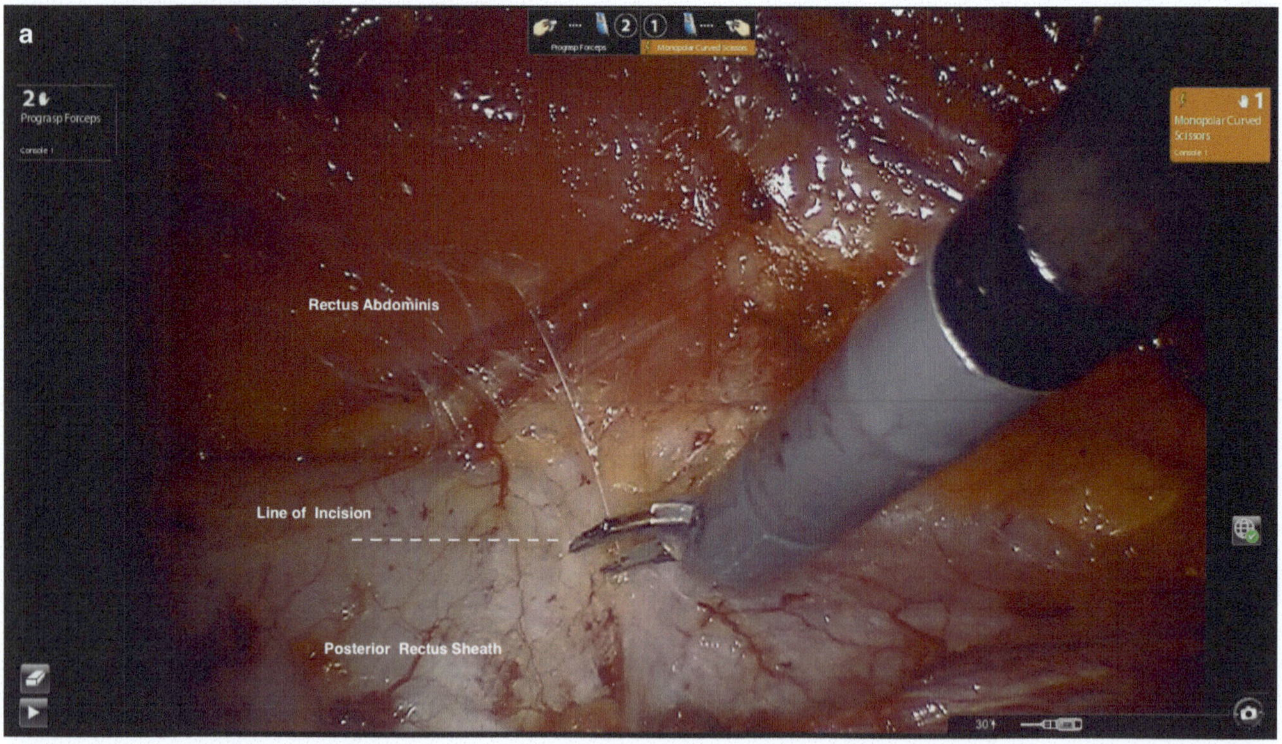


Fig. 6.6 Starting the transversus abdominis release (TAR). (**a**) The left TAR is started by dividing the transversus abdominis muscle (TAM). This can be started superiorly or inferiorly, but it is easier to perform in the upper abdomen, as the TAM is more robust closer to the costal margin and more aponeurotic in the lower abdomen. (**b**) Once the muscle is divided, the peritoneum and transversalis fascia can be identified. (**c**) Further dissection can be carried out in the preperitoneal plane or between the transversalis fascia and TAM

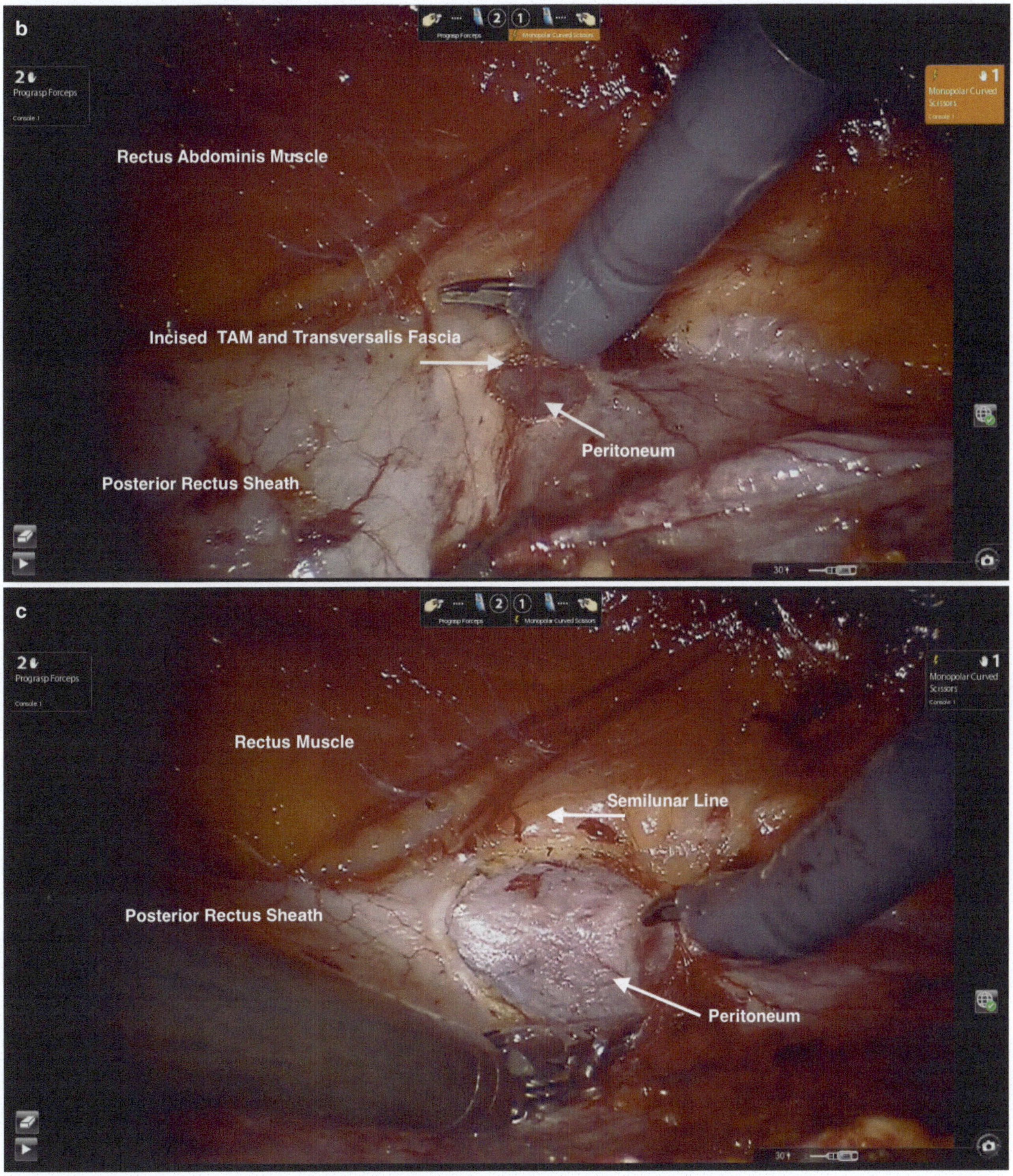


**Fig. 6.6** (continued)

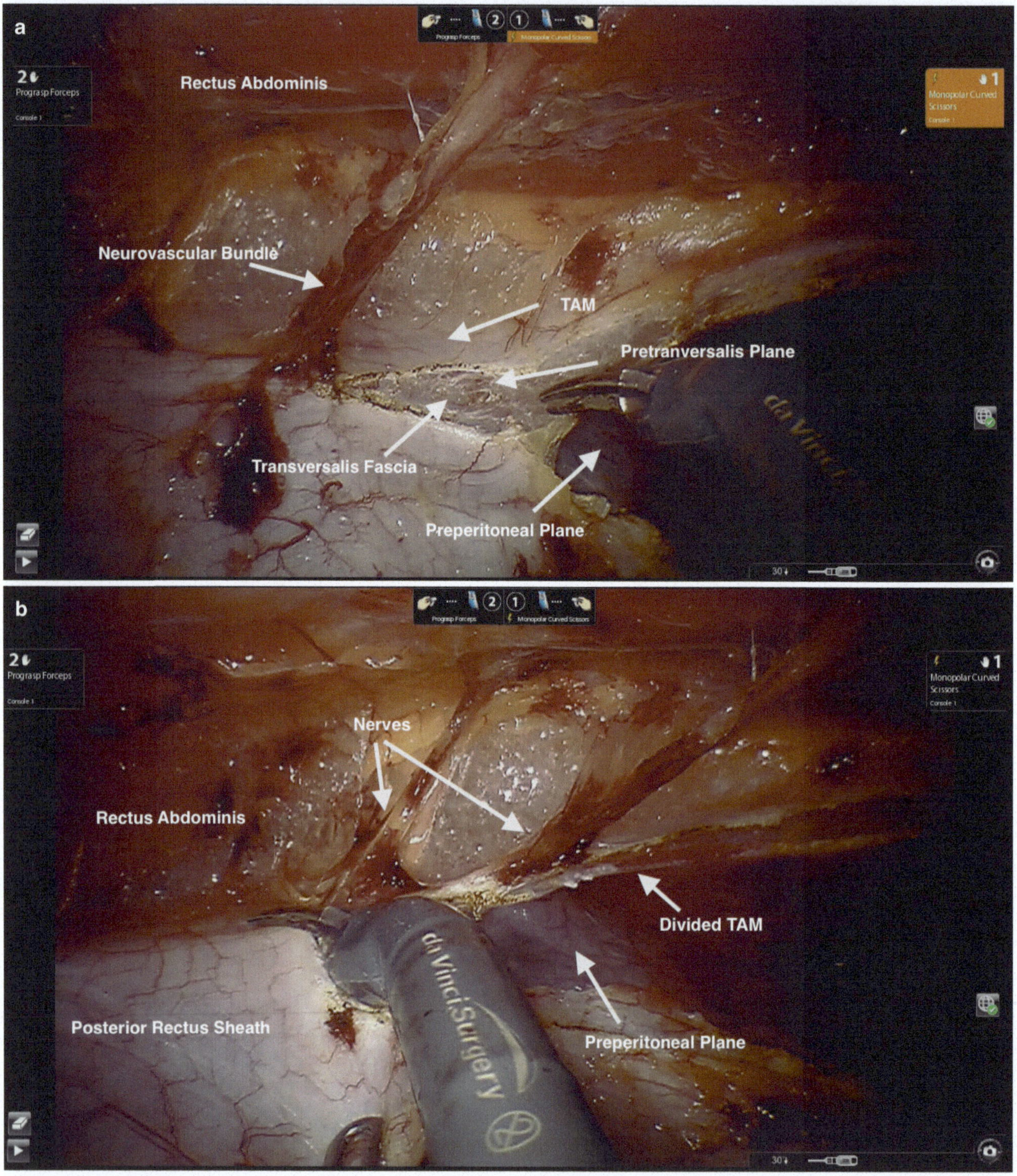


**Fig. 6.7** (**a**) The line of division must remain medial to the neurovascular bundle. It is easier to develop the preperitoneal plane, but sometimes the peritoneum is very thin and can tear easily. In that case, the pretransversalis plane is preferred, though it is a bit more of an adherent plane which can be harder to develop. (**b**) and (**c**) The preperitoneal space is dissected bluntly and sharply from medial to lateral until the peritoneum and posterior rectus sheath rest on the viscera with no tension

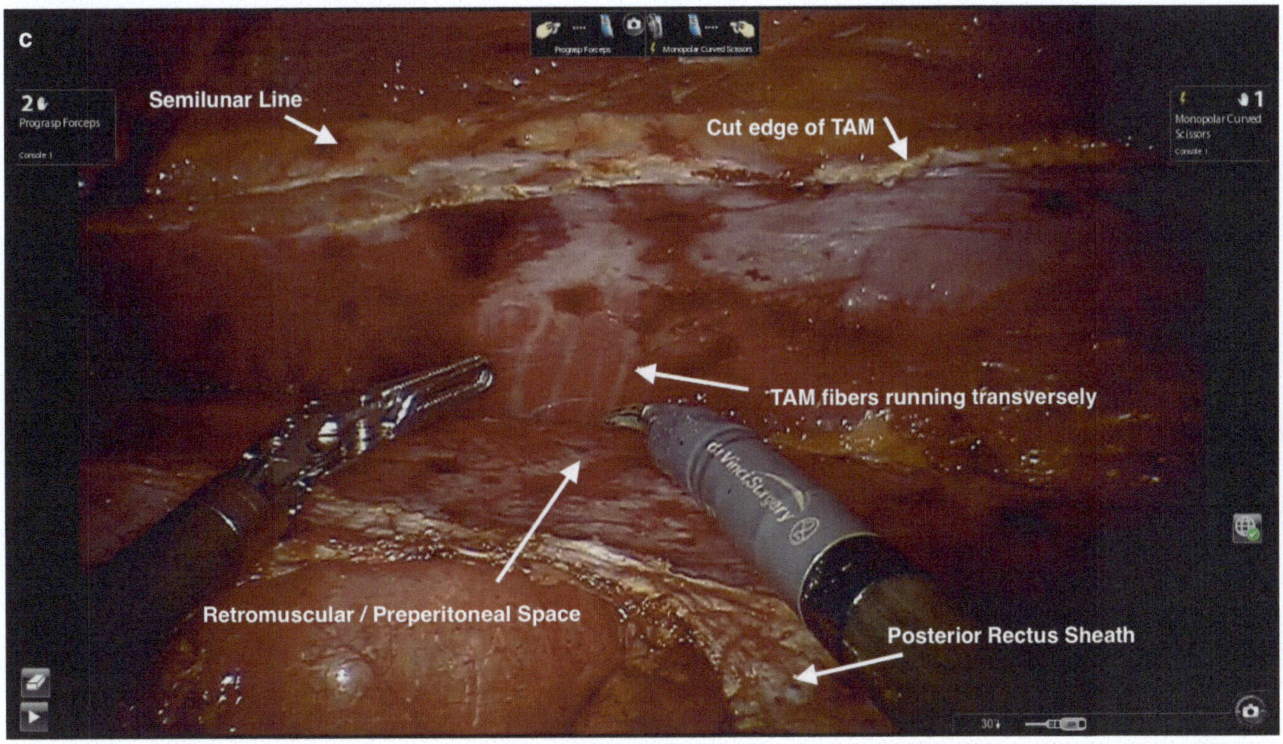


**Fig. 6.7** (continued)

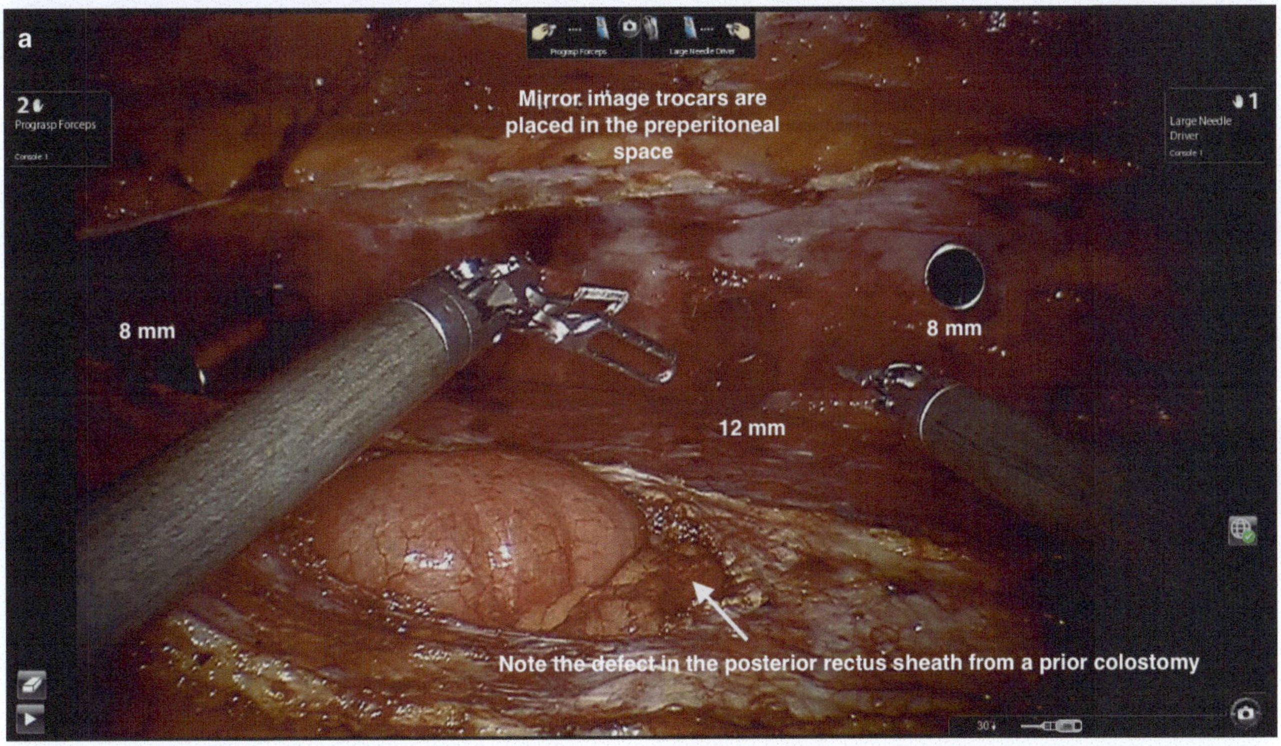


**Fig. 6.8** (**a**) Mirror image trocars are placed on the contralateral side. They are not placed intraperitoneally, but rather into the retromuscular or preperitoneal space, depending on the plane of dissection. (**b**) The length of the dissected space is measured by placing a ruler on the anterior abdominal wall; this is going to be the length of the mesh. About 5–7 cm of dissection is needed above and below the defect to provide a good overlap. (**c**) Since half of the width of the dissection is done at this point, the width of the dissected peritoneal flap will be measured as half of the width of the mesh

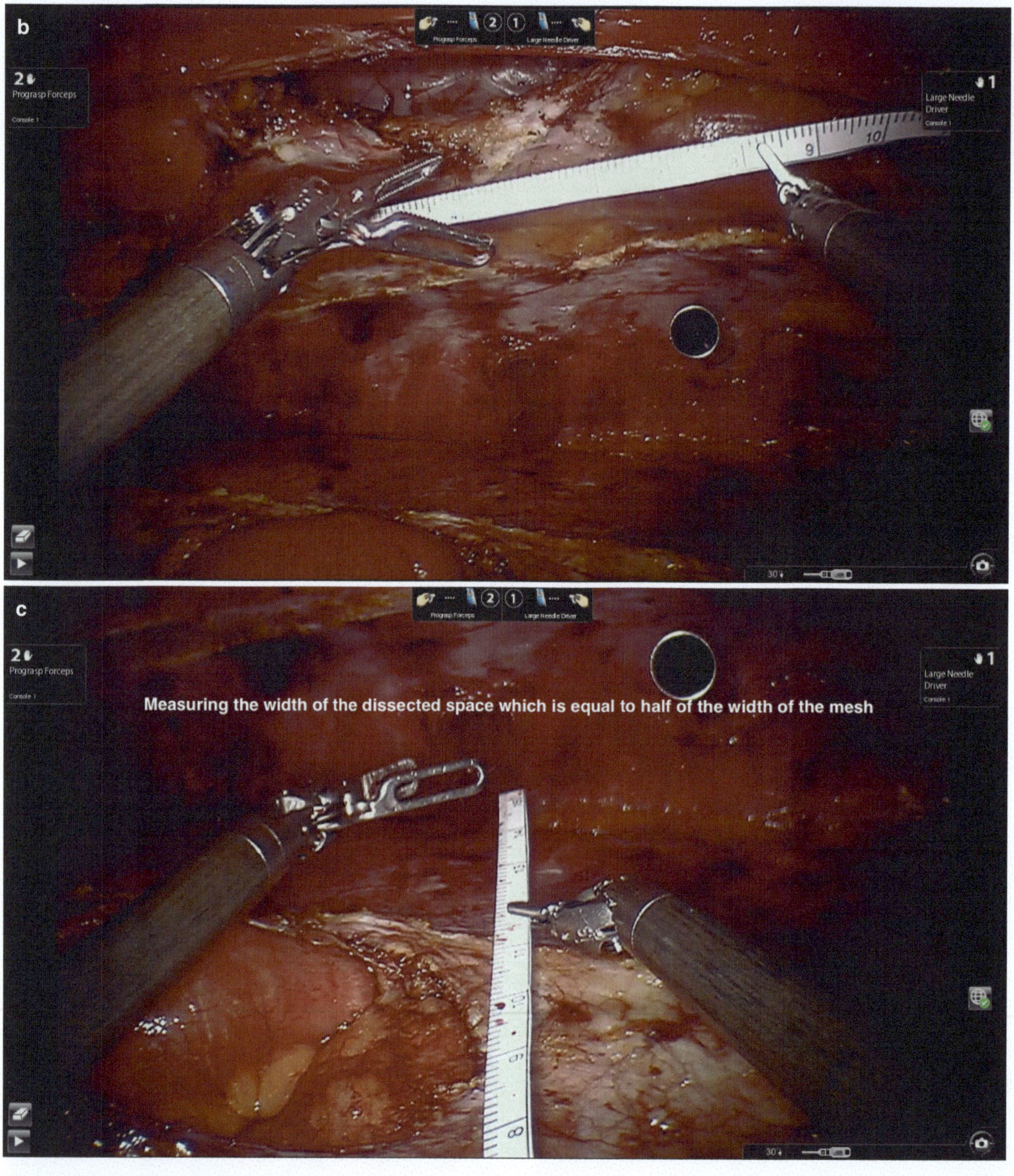


**Fig. 6.8** (continued)

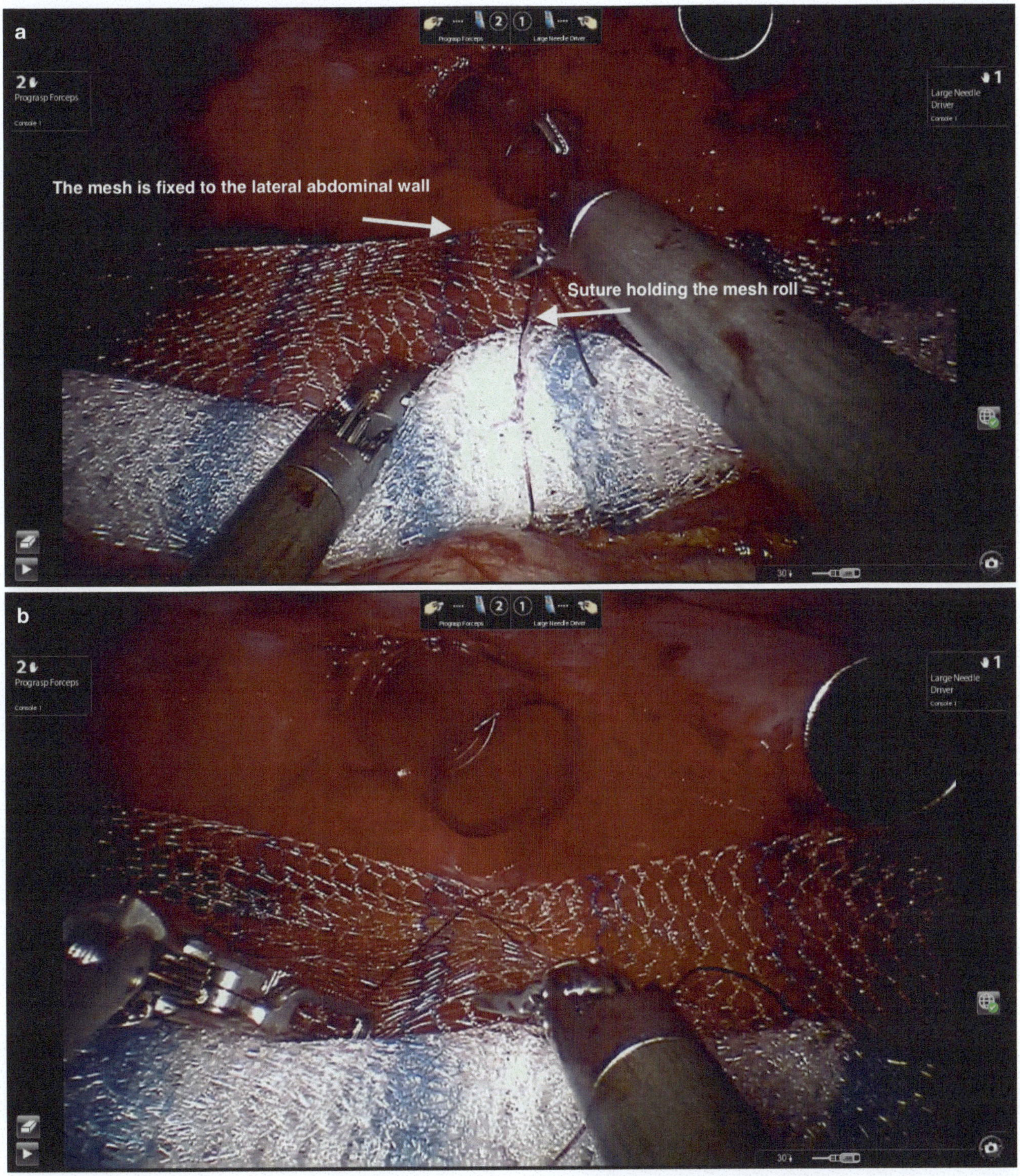


Fig. 6.9 (**a**) The mesh is introduced into the space though the contralateral 12-mm trocar. The mesh is rolled along its long axis, leaving a 2-cm portion of the mesh unrolled; the roll is maintained by placing a loose temporary stitch. (**b**) The free edge is fixed laterally with a single absorbable suture. (**c**) The mesh is tucked under the contralateral trocars with the unrolled edge toward the lateral abdominal wall

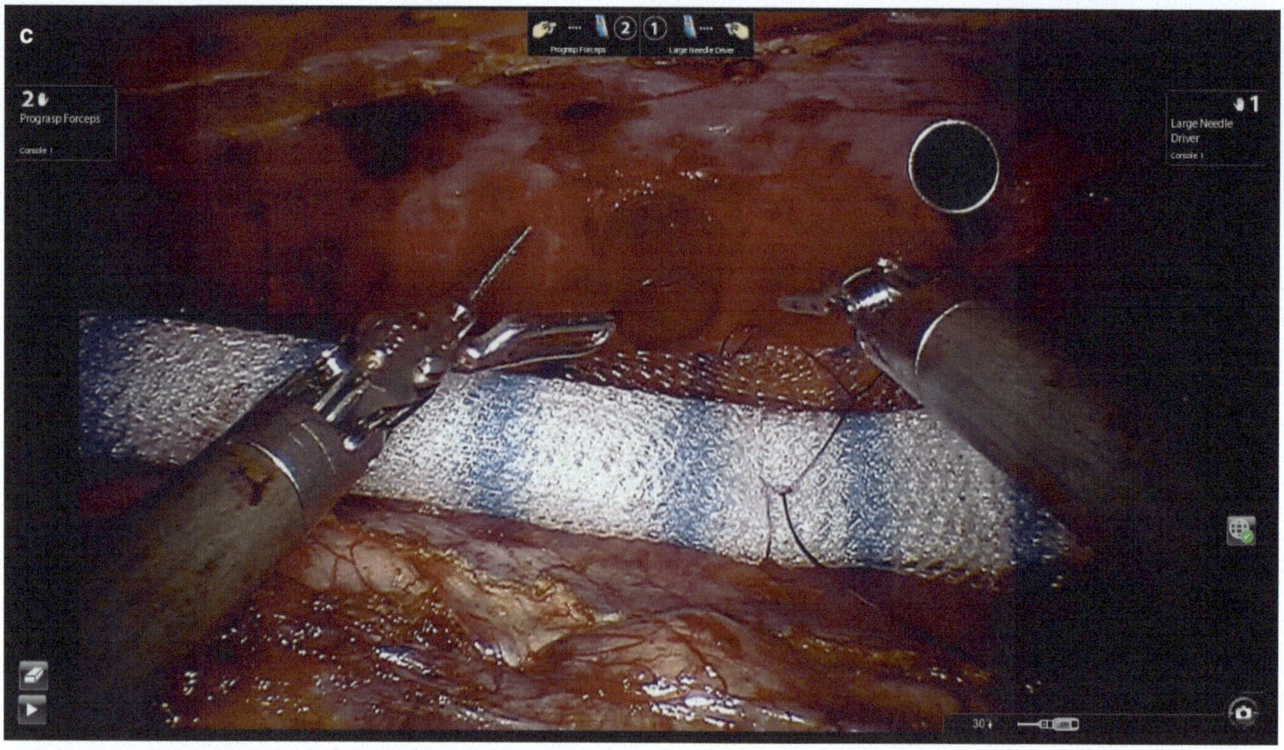


**Fig. 6.9** (continued)

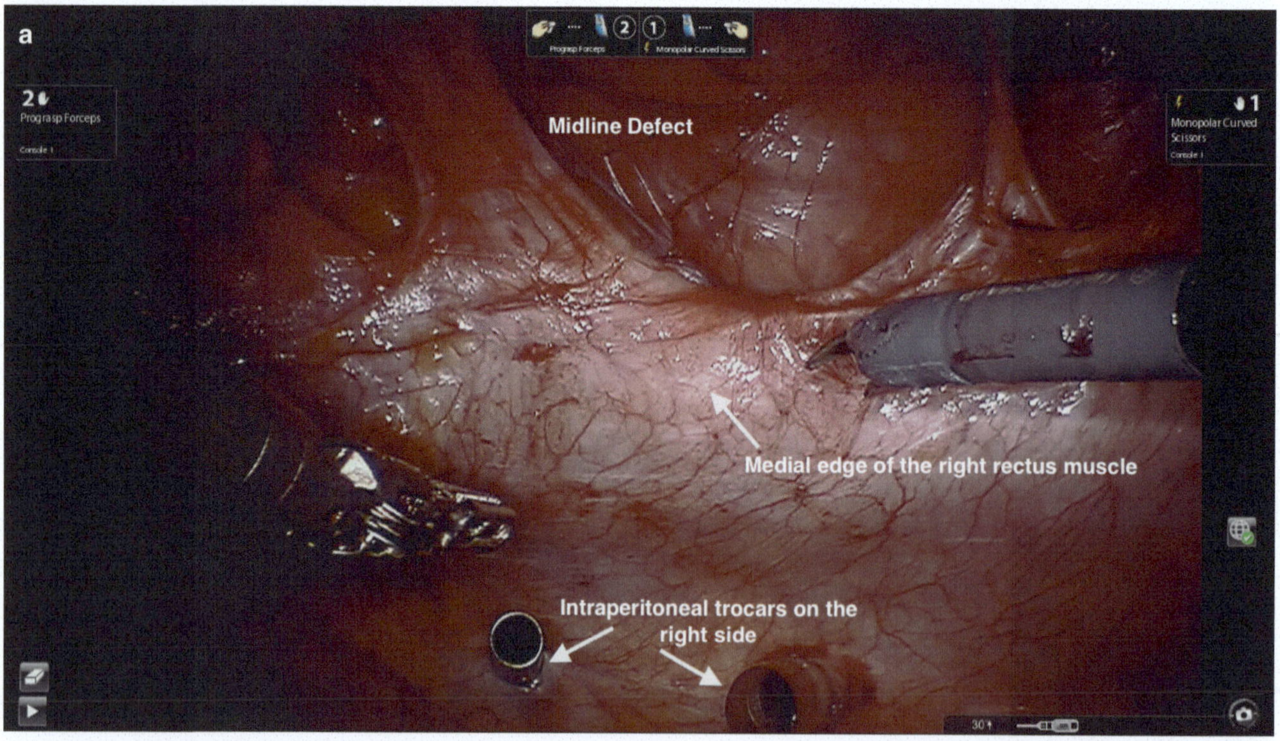


**Fig. 6.10** The robot is undocked and re-docked on the left side. The bed is moved as needed. (**a**–**c**) The retrorectus TAR dissection is repeated on the right side, starting at the right edge of the defect

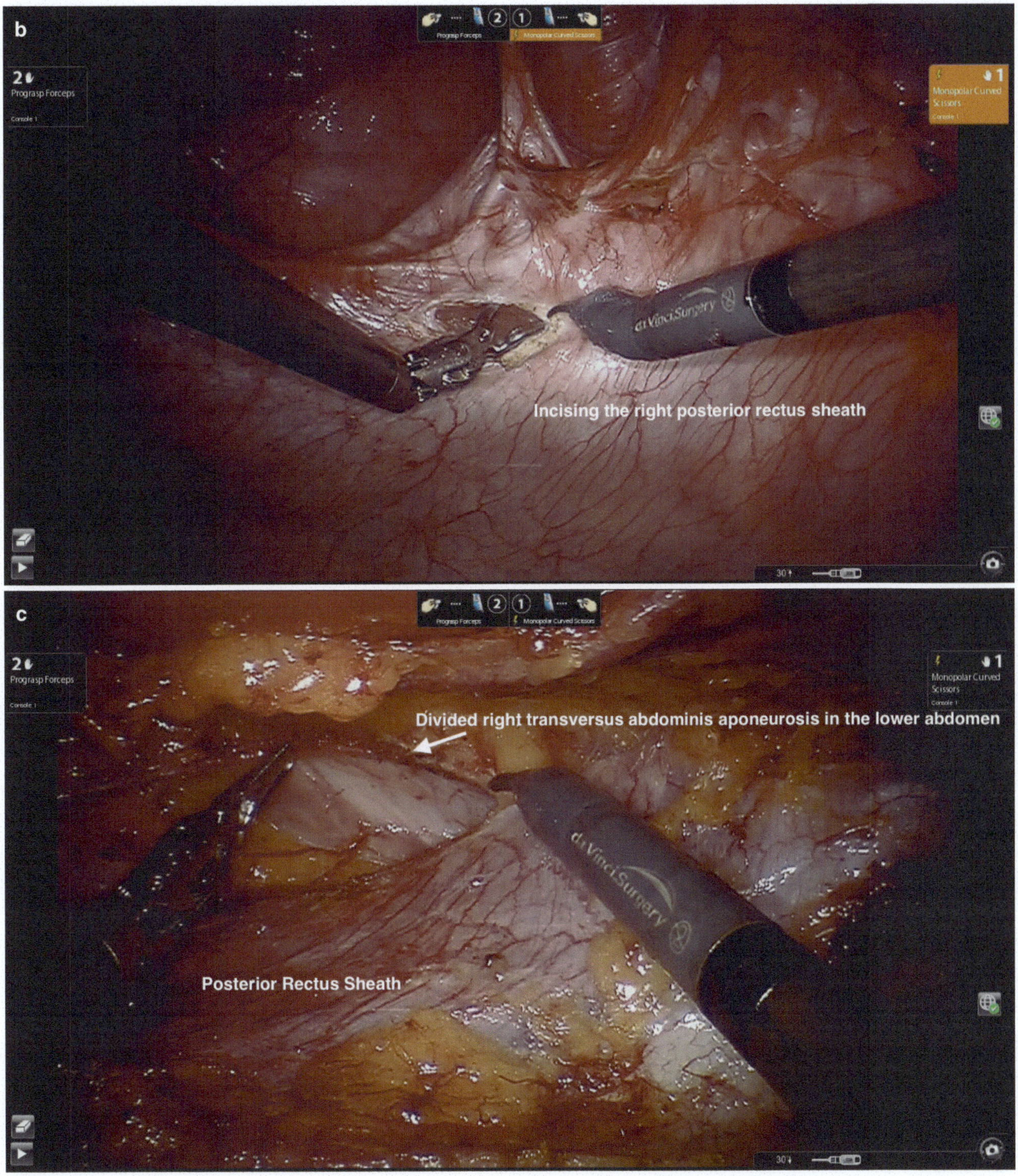


**Fig. 6.10** (continued)

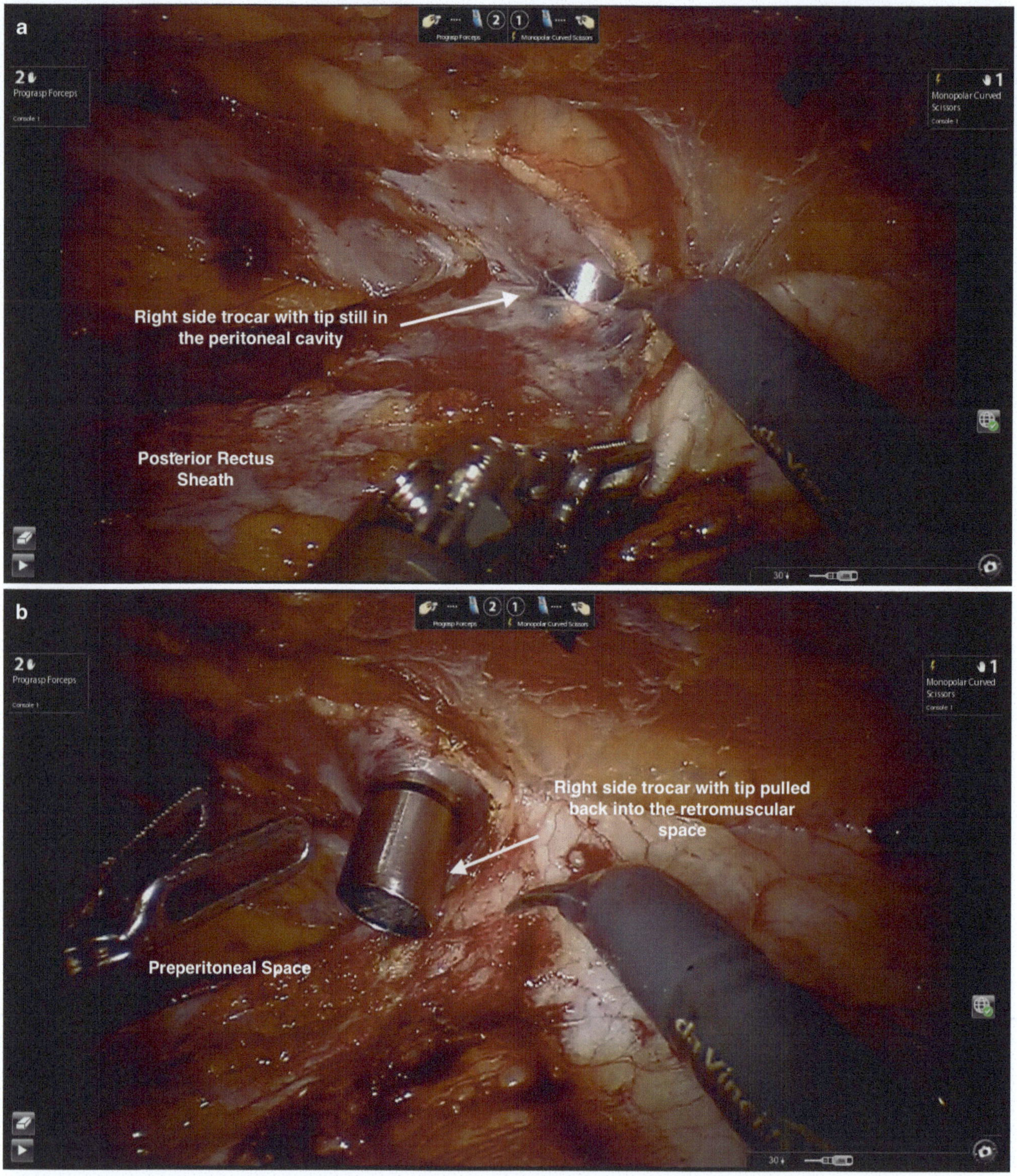


**Fig. 6.11** (**a**) and (**b**) The dissection is continued until the intraperitoneal trocars that were used in the beginning of the case are encountered and brought into the preperitoneal space. (**c**) Once the dissection is completed similar to the left side, the dissection is concluded

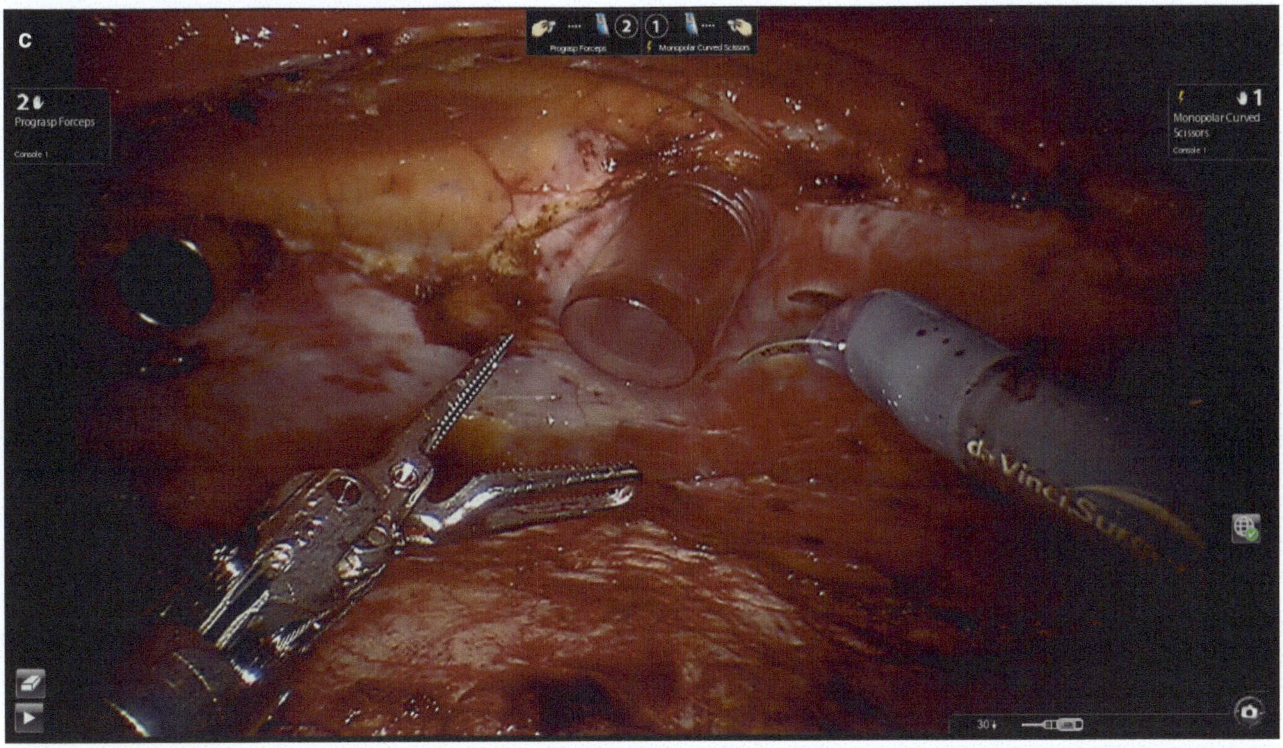


**Fig. 6.11** (continued)

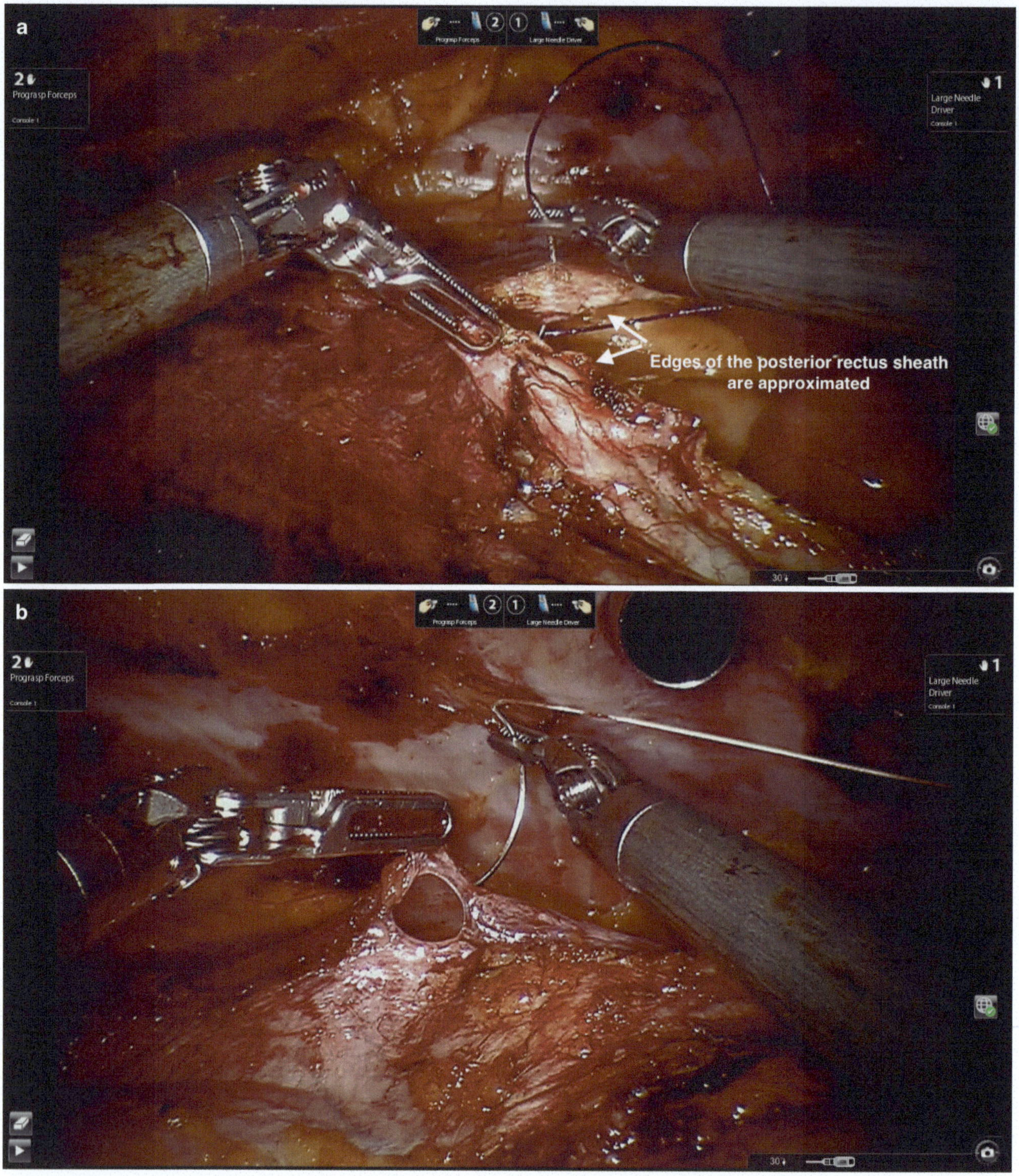


**Fig. 6.12** (**a**) The posterior rectus sheath is now closed in the midline using a 2-0, absorbable, barbed, self-fixating suture. (**b**) Any tears in the peritoneum are closed with simple 2-0 absorbable sutures

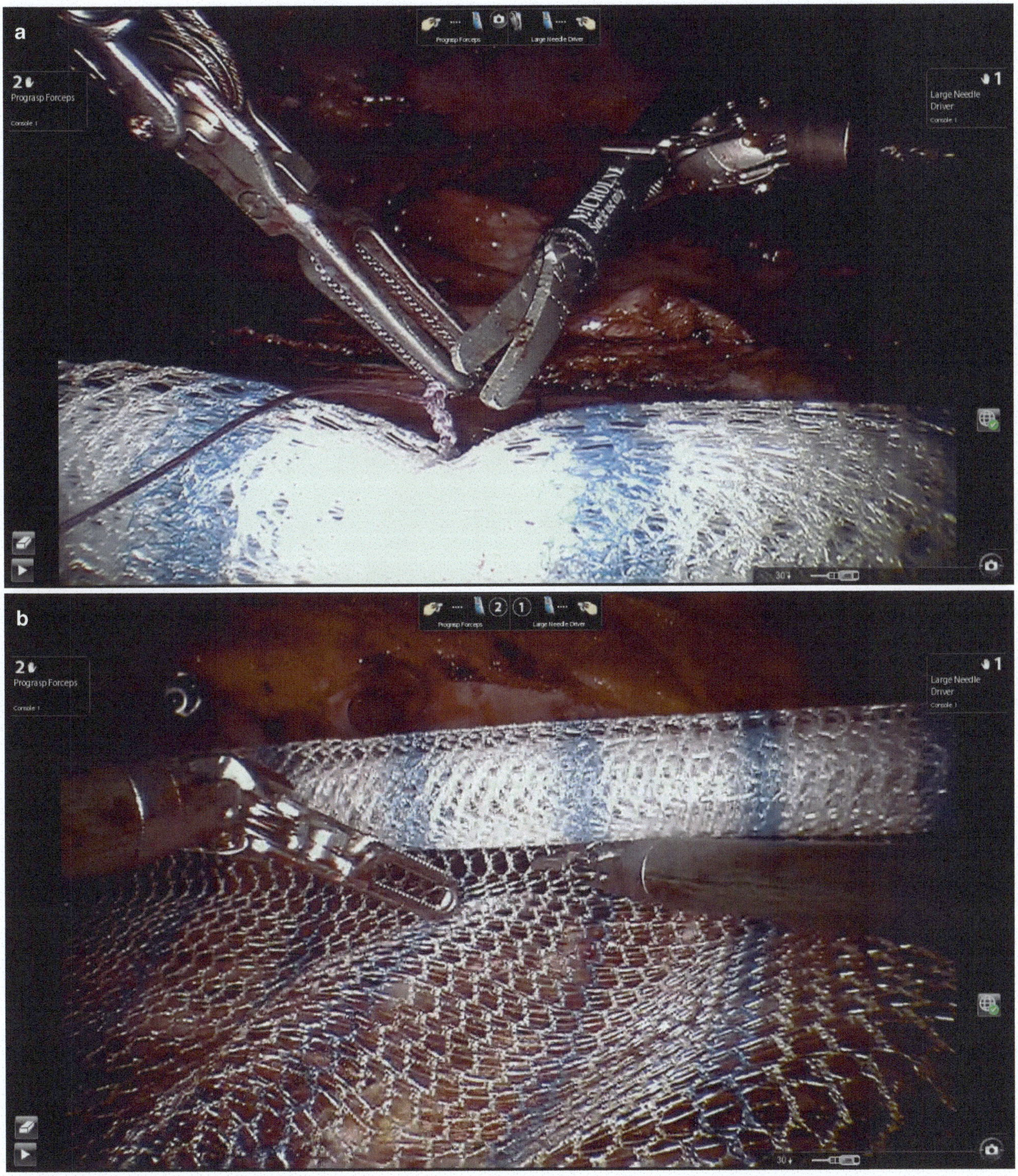


**Fig. 6.13** (**a**) and (**b**) The loose suture holding the mesh is cut and the mesh is unrolled toward the right side and laid flat over the closed posterior rectus sheath. The right edge of the mesh is fixed to the right abdominal wall similar to the left side. Superior and inferior fixation is optional

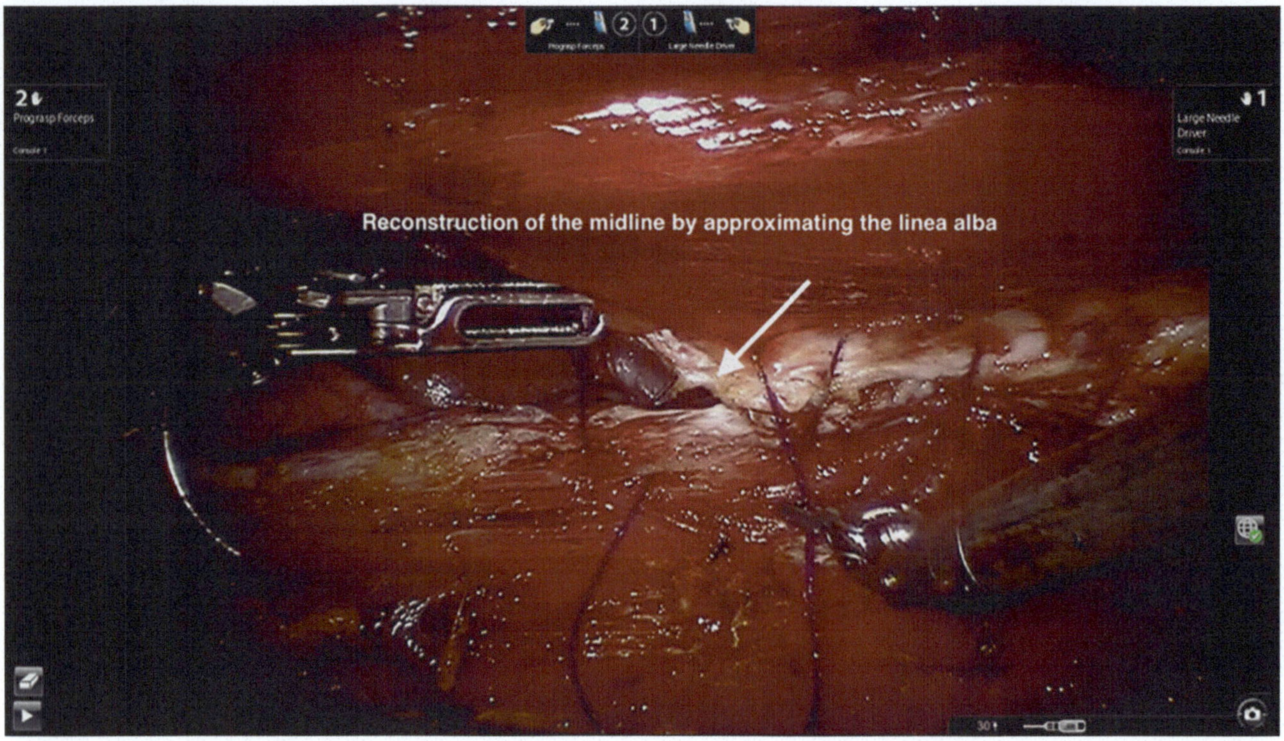


**Fig. 6.14** The linea alba is reconstructed by suturing the anterior abdominal wall in the midline using a 45-cm, #1, absorbable, barbed self-fixating suture. If there is excessive tension while suturing, the pneumoperitoneum can be reduced to 8–10 mmHg. Figure-eight sutures placed by a bedside assistant using a suture passer may also help to reduce tension and temporarily keep the edges together while suturing. The robot is undocked, and a laparoscope is used to inspect the mesh to ensure that it is lying flat. Since the mesh extends past the fascial defects, the trocar sites do not require closure

## Suggested Reading

Bittner JG, Alrefai S, Vy M, Mabe M, Del Prado PAR, Clingempeel NL. Comparative analysis of open and robotic transversus abdominis release for ventral hernia repair. Surg Endosc. 2017;16(2):179–8.

Carbonell AM, Warren JA, Prabhu AS, Ballecer CD, Janczyk RJ, Herrera J, et al. Reducing length of stay using a robotic-assisted approach for retromuscular ventral hernia repair: a comparative analysis from the Americas Hernia Society Quality Collaborative. Ann Surg. 2018;267(2):210–7.

Gokcal F, Morrison S, Kudsi OY. Robotic retromuscular ventral hernia repair and transversus abdominis release: short-term outcomes and risk factors associated with perioperative complications. Hernia. 2019;23(2):375–85.

Martin-del-Campo LA, Weltz AS, Belyansky I, Novitsky YW. Comparative analysis of perioperative outcomes of robotic versus open transversus abdominis release. Surg Endosc. 2017;204(2):709–6.

Warren JA, Cobb WS, Ewing JA, Carbonell AM. Standard laparoscopic versus robotic retromuscular ventral hernia repair. Surg Endosc. 2017;31(1):324–32.

# Robotic Midline Ventral Hernia Repair: Totally Extraperitoneal (TEP)

7

Sora Ely, Azure Adkins, and Rockson Liu

## Introduction

The overall incidence of incisional hernias is greater than 10% [1–3], and recurrence rates following repair range from 5% to 70%, depending on the technique used and the size and complexity of the hernia [4]. The use of mesh has greatly decreased recurrence rates, but its efficacy varies significantly with its anatomic placement. The retromuscular (and for ventral hernias, specifically retrorectus) mesh sublay Rives-Stoppa (RS) technique, with only minor modifications over the 50 years since it was introduced, has now become accepted as the gold standard for surgical management of large ventral hernias [4–6]. The RS ventral hernia repair (VHR) has been adapted to laparoscopy through the extended totally extraperitoneal (eTEP) approach with at least equivalent long-term outcomes, plus decreases in length of stay and wound complications. Its widespread utilization is hindered by the advanced technical skill required, however, and there is more variability—and debate—in the technical details of laparoscopic eTEP VHR.

Recently, RS repairs have been performed robotically, and the popularity of this method has risen rapidly. Although long-term outcomes are as yet unknown, robotic surgery may facilitate the adoption of minimally invasive approaches to VHR, allowing more patients to benefit from its advantages over open repair. Described techniques for robotic VHR include modifications to port placement and other aspects of the approach based on case factors, but we have found that a consistent approach facilitates learning and implementation. This chapter illustrates our standardized approach for robotic eTEP RS midline incisional hernia repair.

S. Ely
Department of General Surgery, University of California San Francisco East Bay, Highland Hospital, Oakland, CA, USA

A. Adkins · R. Liu (✉)
Alta Bates Summit Medical Center, Epic Care, Oakland, CA, USA

## Selection Criteria

In addition to the usual patient characteristics of interest during the preoperative work-up for elective hernia repair, a few additional considerations are pertinent in judging the ease and feasibility specifically of a robotic eTEP approach. Several characteristics are ideal:

- Patient slightly overweight (BMI ~30)
- Patient height > 5′8″
- Midline, periumbilical hernia location
- Hernia size 3–4+ cm
- No history of stoma
- Wide rectus muscles

Two key principles underlie these ideal selection criteria. The first is ensuring the adequacy and accessibility of the extraperitoneal space (the bilateral retrorectus spaces plus the intervening preperitoneal space underlying the linea alba), especially the left retrorectus space, which will be the first area of surgical access. The second concerns the logistical constraints of this approach with larger or more lateralized hernias, due to the proximity of the ports to the hernia defect.

## Procedure: Illustrated Steps

1. Position the patient supine with arms tucked. The bed may be slightly flexed if the patient (or their torso) is short. Slight Trendelenburg may also be helpful for hernias in the lower (inferior) midline. Re-examine the hernia under anesthesia with ultrasound and manual palpation (Fig. 7.1a–c), and mark the usual anatomical landmarks: hernia border, linea semilunaris, linea alba (including its diastatic borders), costal margin, iliac crest (Fig. 7.1d). Remember that this information will also reveal the width of the rectus muscles, i.e., the size of the potential retrorectus space in which the operation is conducted (highlighted with red shading in Fig. 7.1b).


O. Y. Kudsi (ed.), *Robotic Hernia Surgery*, https://doi.org/10.1007/978-3-030-46667-1_7

The preoperative cross-sectional imaging (Fig. 7.1e, f) may be reviewed as well, but the authors use only the measurements obtained on the day of surgery preoperatively during this step and intraoperatively in Step 11 for final decision-making.

2. Precise knowledge of these anatomical boundaries is necessary to correctly site the ports relative to these structures. Our standardized placement consists of three 8-mm ports along the patient's left side, just medial (~1 cm) to the linea semilunaris (Fig. 7.2a). We always begin with the left upper quadrant port, as the anatomy is most consistent there. This first port is placed approximately 2 cm below the costal margin, and the next two ports are placed 6 cm farther inferior along the linea semilunaris; we mark these measurements and planned port sites at the start of the case (Fig. 7.2b, with green arrowheads denoting planned port sites).

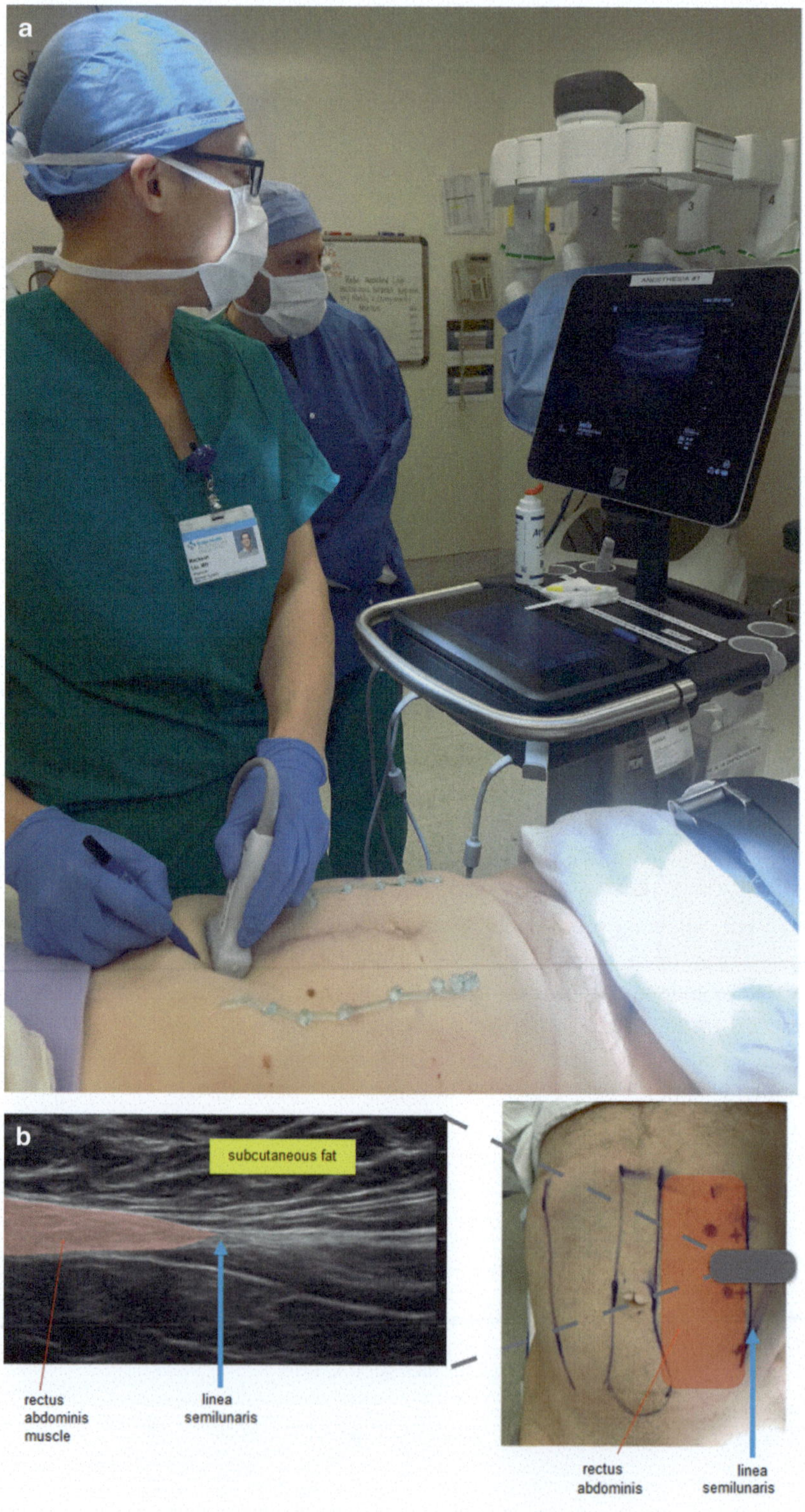


**Fig. 7.1** (**a**–**c**) Physical and ultrasound examination of the hernia, with the potential retrorectus space highlighted (*red shading*) in (**b**). (**d**) Marking of the anatomical landmarks. (**e**) and (**f**) Preoperative CT scans

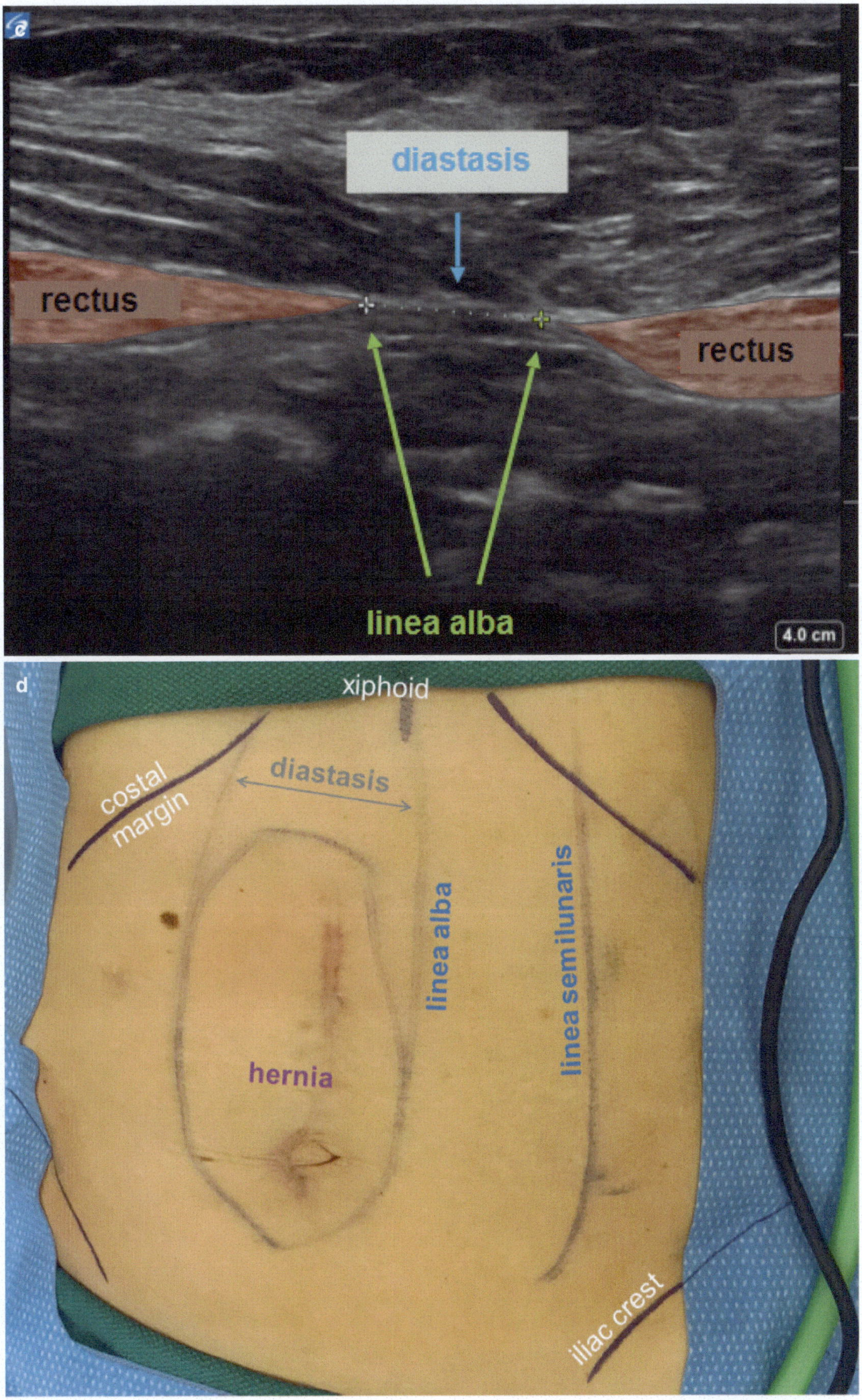


**Fig. 7.1** (continued)

**Fig. 7.1** (continued)

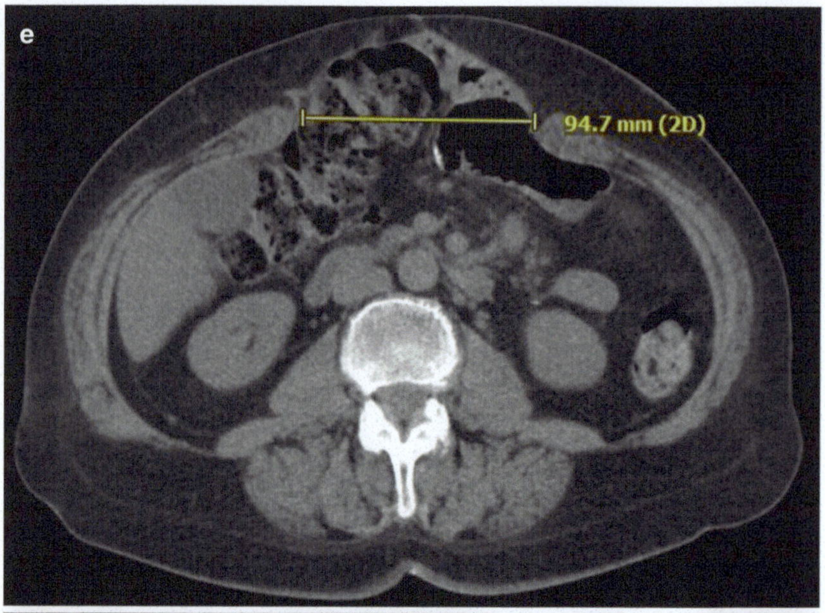


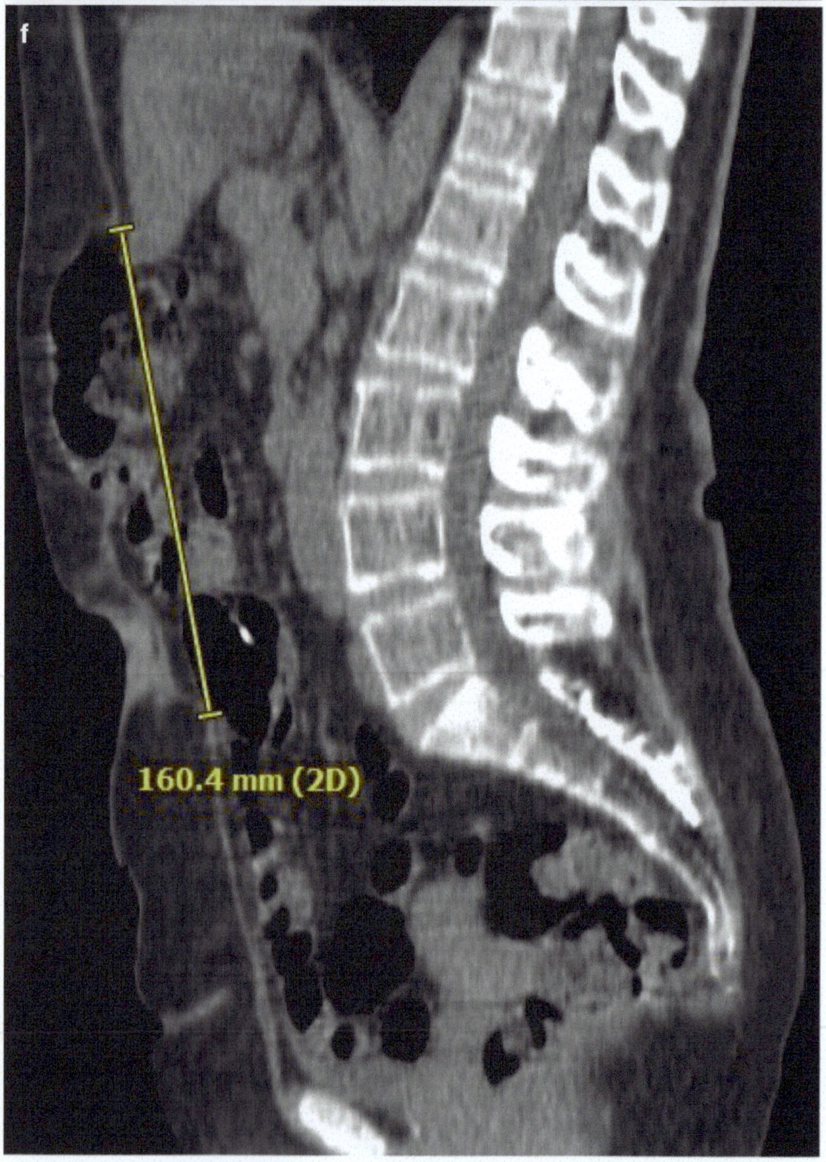

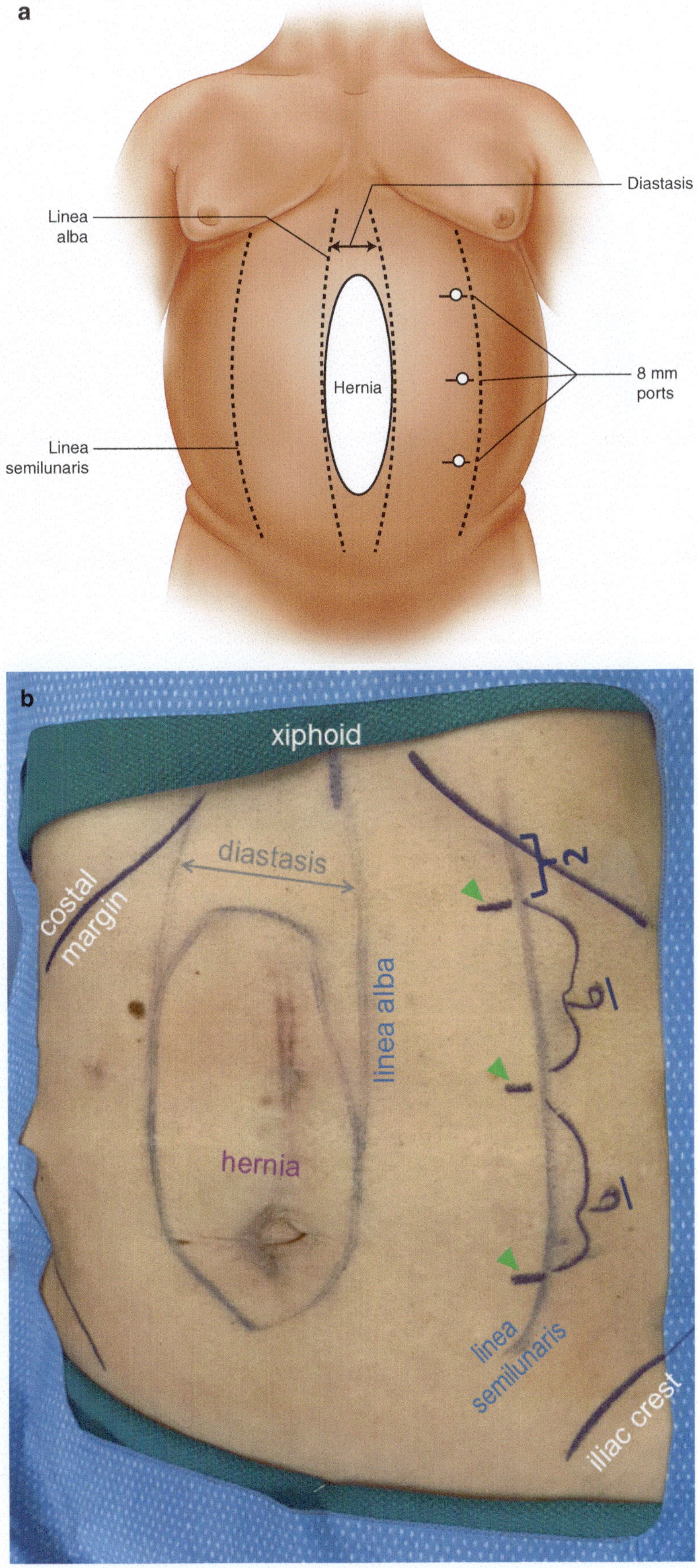


**Fig. 7.2** (**a**) and (**b**) Planned port sites (*green arrowheads*)

3. We employ an optical entry technique (with an Applied Medical Kii Fios optical trocar and 5-mm 0° laparoscope), because this allows us to utilize the gas insufflation to help with the initial dissection and opening of the potential space. We enter the soft tissues in usual fashion, and once the eyelet in the trocar tip has passed through the anterior rectus sheath and into the rectus muscle (Fig. 7.3a), we pause to insufflate to 15 mmHg. The $CO_2$ dissects into the layer of areolar fat that lies posterior to the rectus muscle (Fig. 7.3b), usually between this fatty layer and the posterior rectus sheath (Fig. 7.3c), thus opening the operative space (Fig. 7.3d).

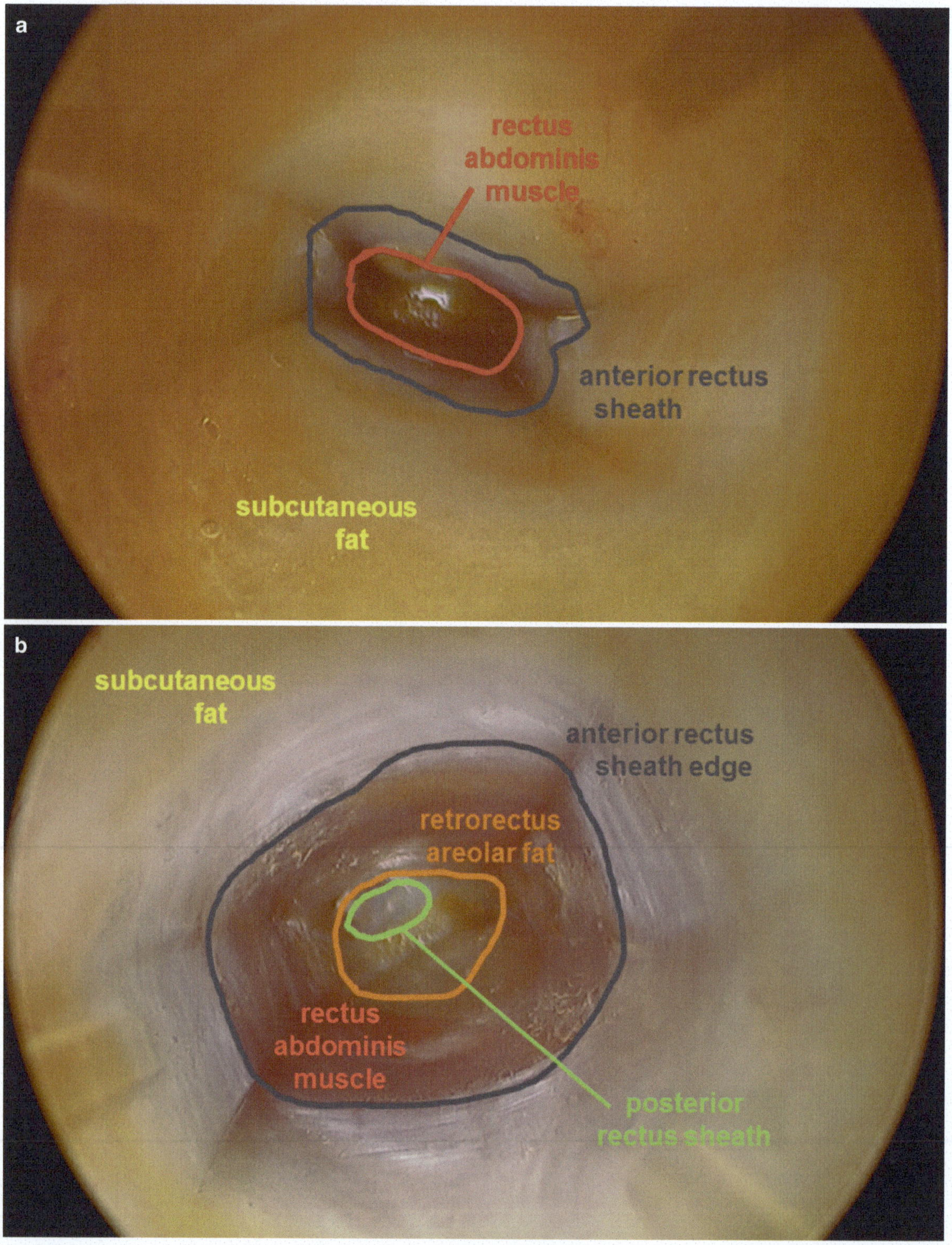


**Fig. 7.3** (**a–d**) Optical entry technique

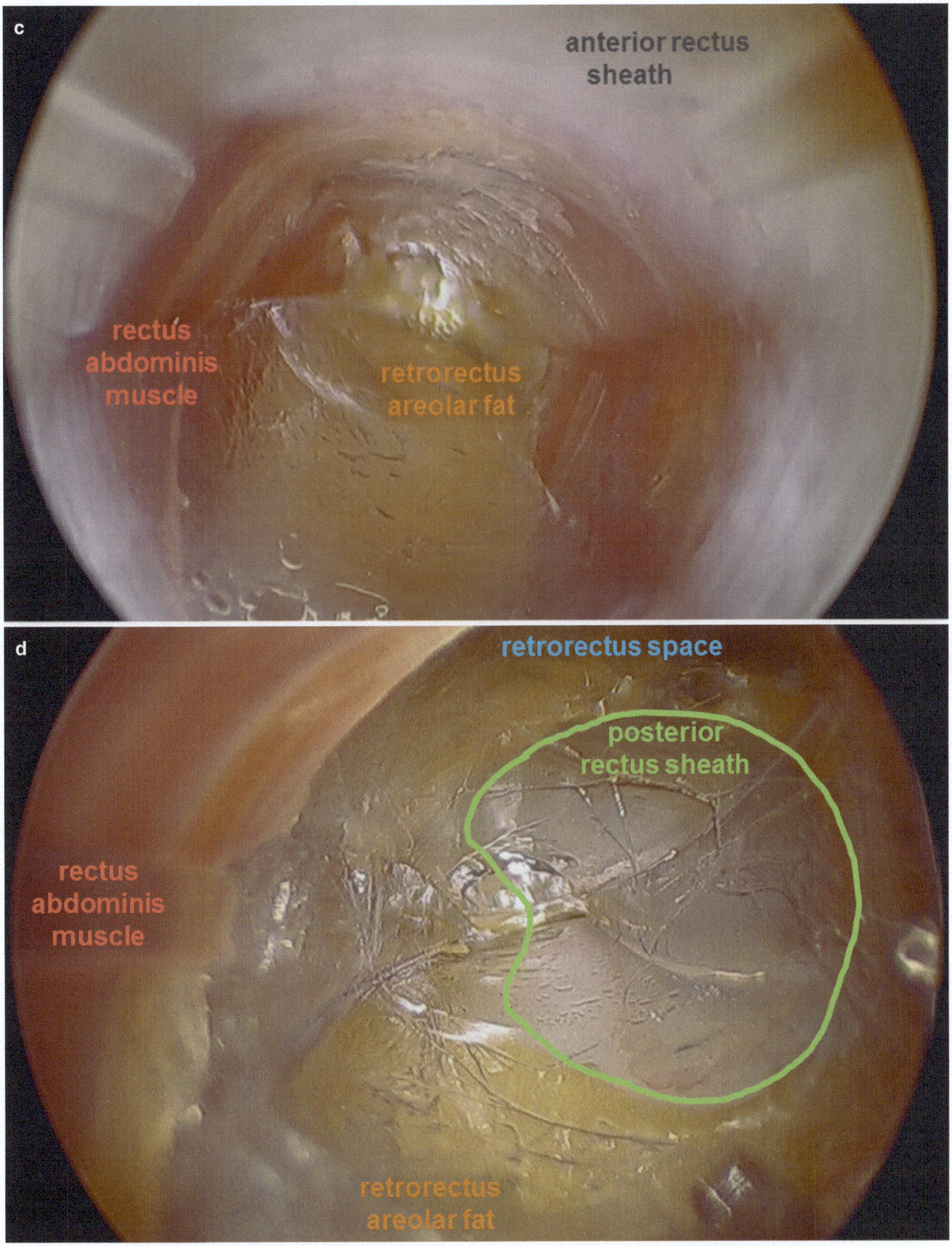


**Fig. 7.3** (continued)

4. We keep the obturator in place even after insufflating, and use it to further dissect the areolar tissue plane via side-to-side sweeping movements (Fig. 7.4a and b, with the purple arrow denoting the direction of the trocar through the tissues). This gentle, blunt dissection posterior to the retrorectus fat, just "above" the posterior rectus sheath, minimizes bleeding and nerve injury because the neurovascular bundles typically travel within the fat layer. We preserve these where possible, sweeping them "up" (anteriorly) and out of the field (Fig. 7.4c). The gas and blunt dissections are usually sufficient to develop the retrorectus potential space into a true space (as seen in Fig. 7.4d with the optical port obturator still in place, and in Fig. 7.4e through the normal laparoscopic view) that is large enough to insert the remaining two ports under visualization.

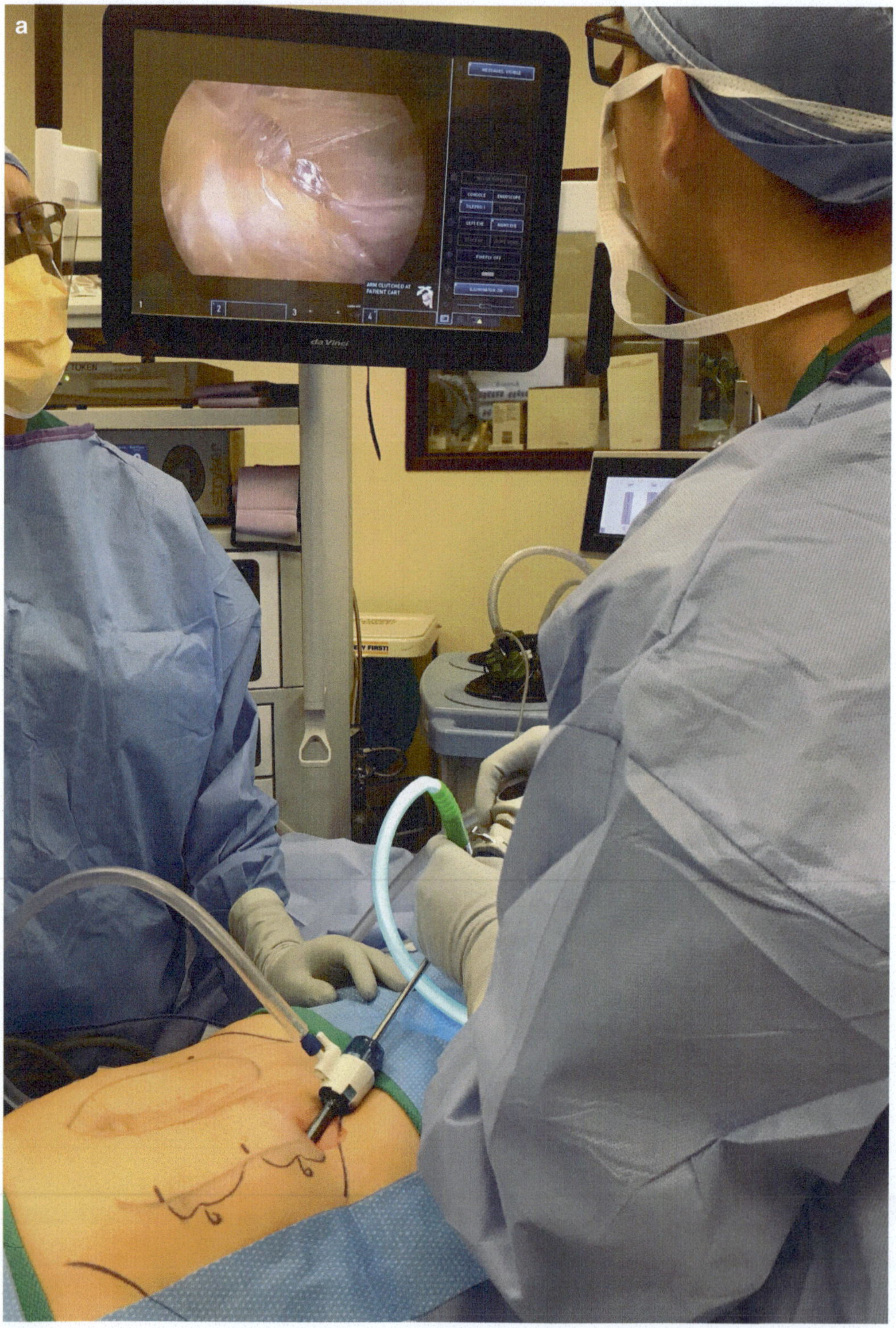


**Fig. 7.4** (**a–d**) Dissection of the retrorectus space with the obturator still in place. (**e**) Dissection of the retrorectus space after removal of the obturator

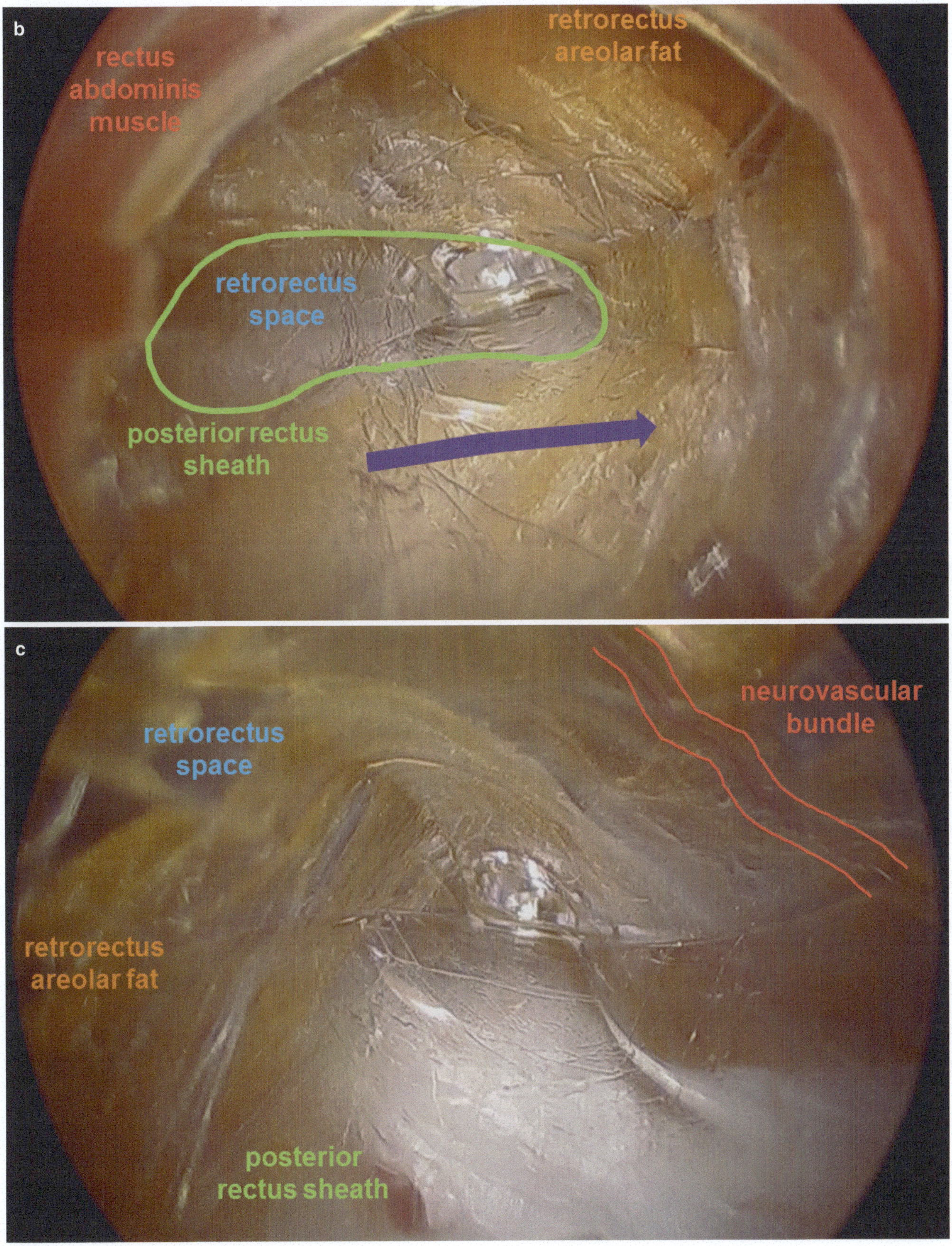


**Fig. 7.4** (continued)

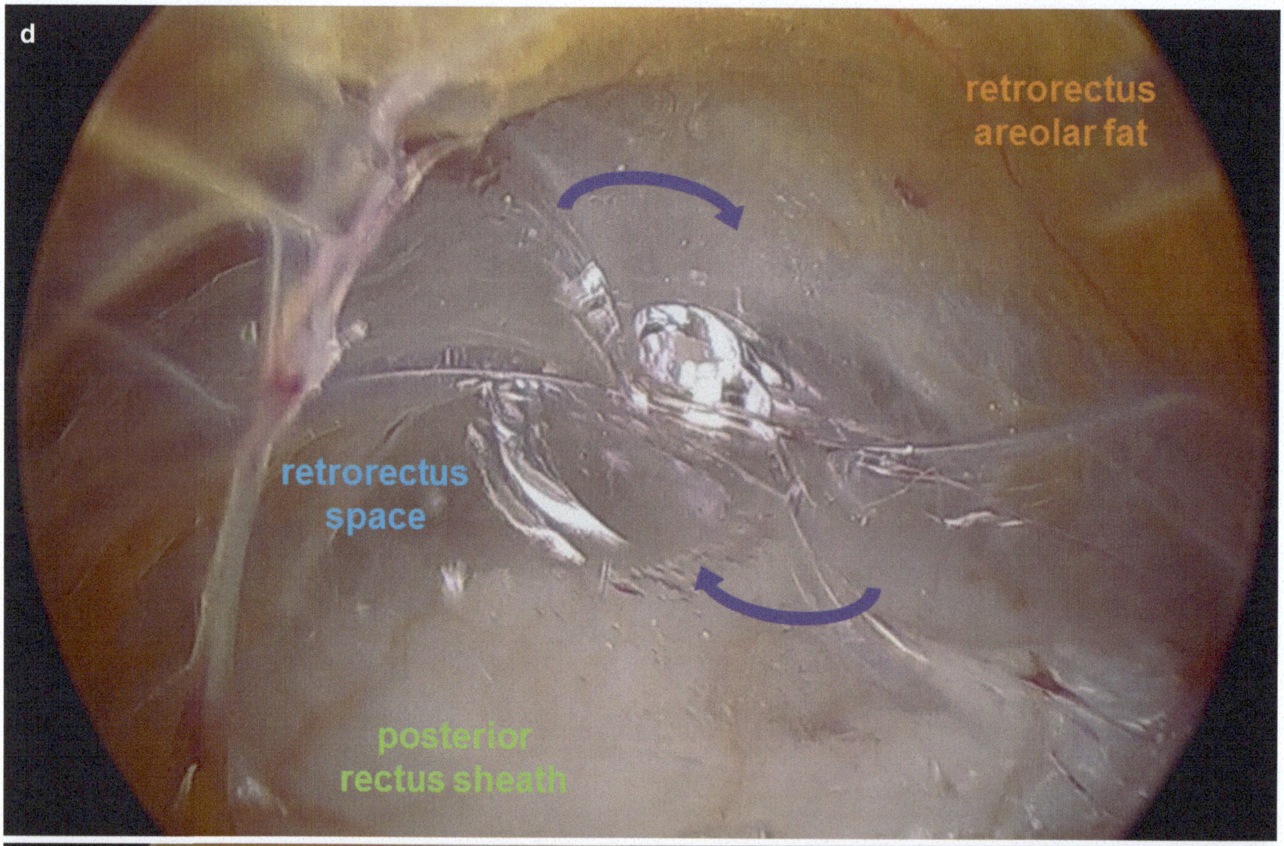


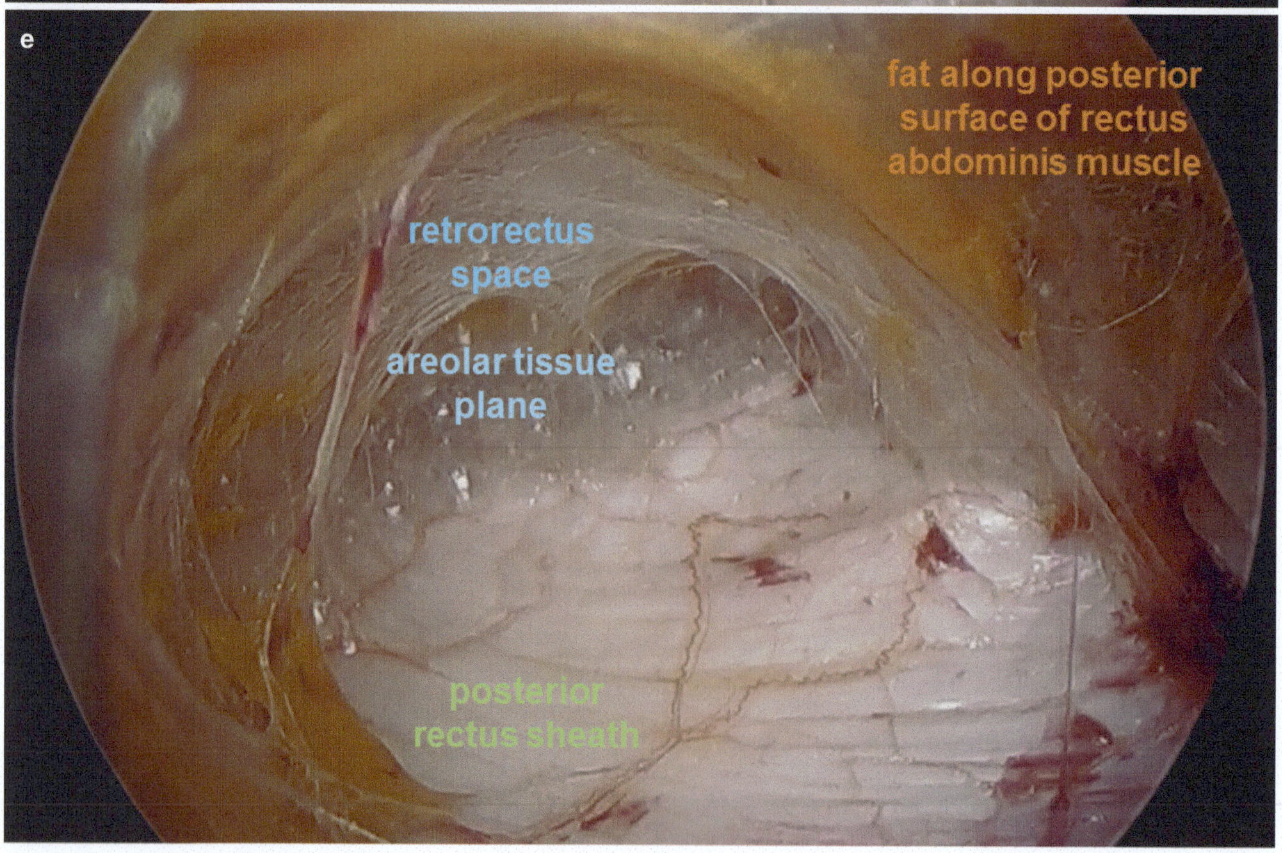


**Fig. 7.4** (continued)

5. Next we place the second port, again just medial to the linea semilunaris, 6 cm inferior to the first port and into this retrorectus space, guided by needle localization (Fig. 7.5a and b). This and any subsequent ports placed during the case should be 8-mm robotic ports. [*Note that these technical details are compatible only with the Da Vinci robot Xi model—We recommend using 8 cm spacing between the ports for the Si model.*]

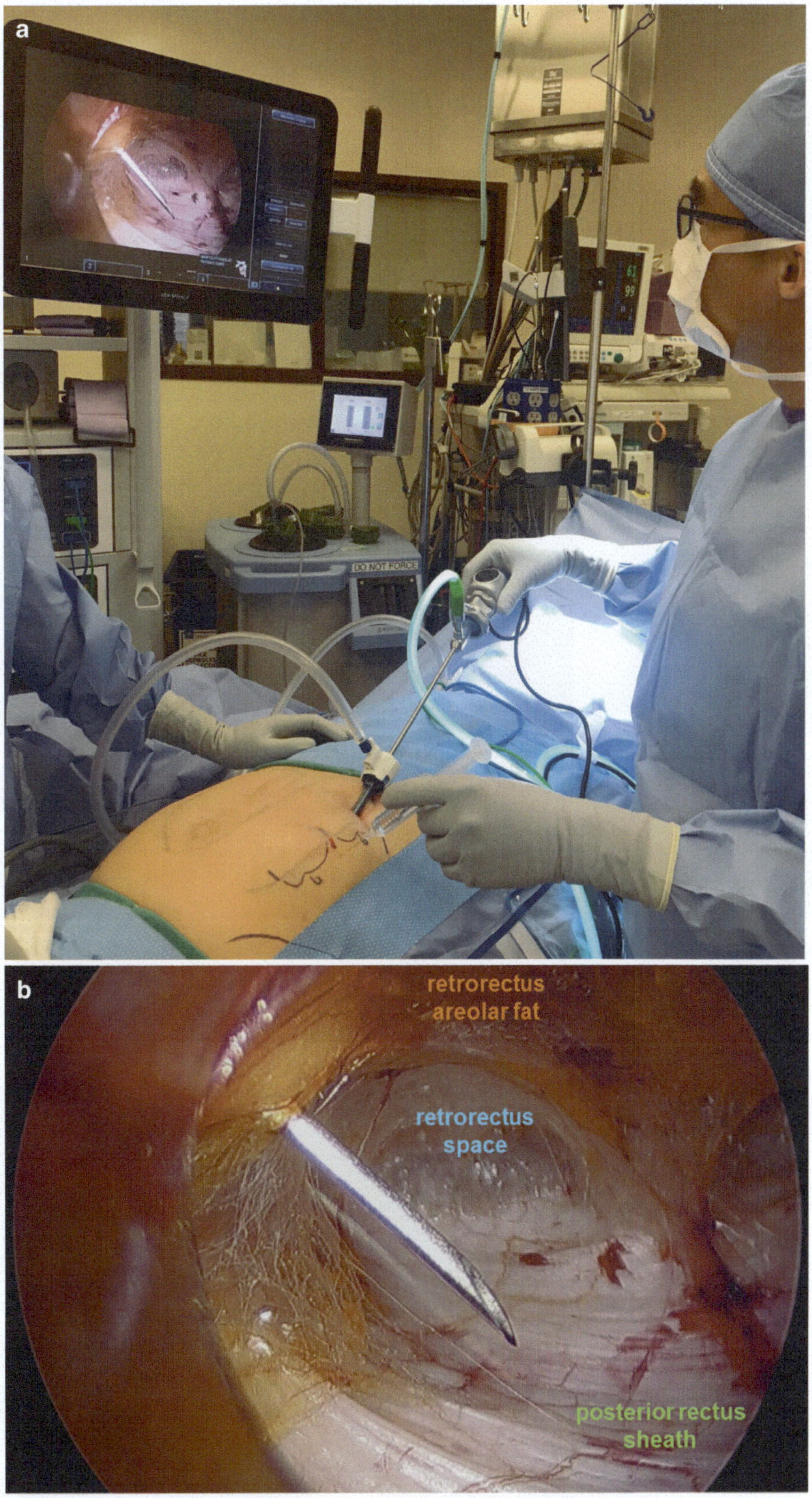


**Fig. 7.5** (**a**) and (**b**) Placement of the second port

6. If needed, dissection is continued just enough to place the third and last mandatory port, again just medial to the linea semilunaris and 6 cm inferior to the second port, with needle localization (Fig. 7.6). When placing ports in this area, be aware of the location of the inferior epigastric vessels, as well as their large branches and tributaries. In most cases, the ports will need to be inserted lateral to the inferior epigastric vessels.
7. Move the camera to the most inferior (3rd) port temporarily, to replace the laparoscopic (1st) port with a robot port (8-mm) under direct visualization. After this, the camera will be placed through the middle (2nd) port, so that working instruments are on either side of it. Figure 7.7 shows the final port configuration after the optical port has been replaced by a robotic port.
8. Dock the robot as shown in Fig. 7.8a–c. Ideally, in advance of the case, the operating room should be set up as in Fig. 7.8d to best facilitate this setup.

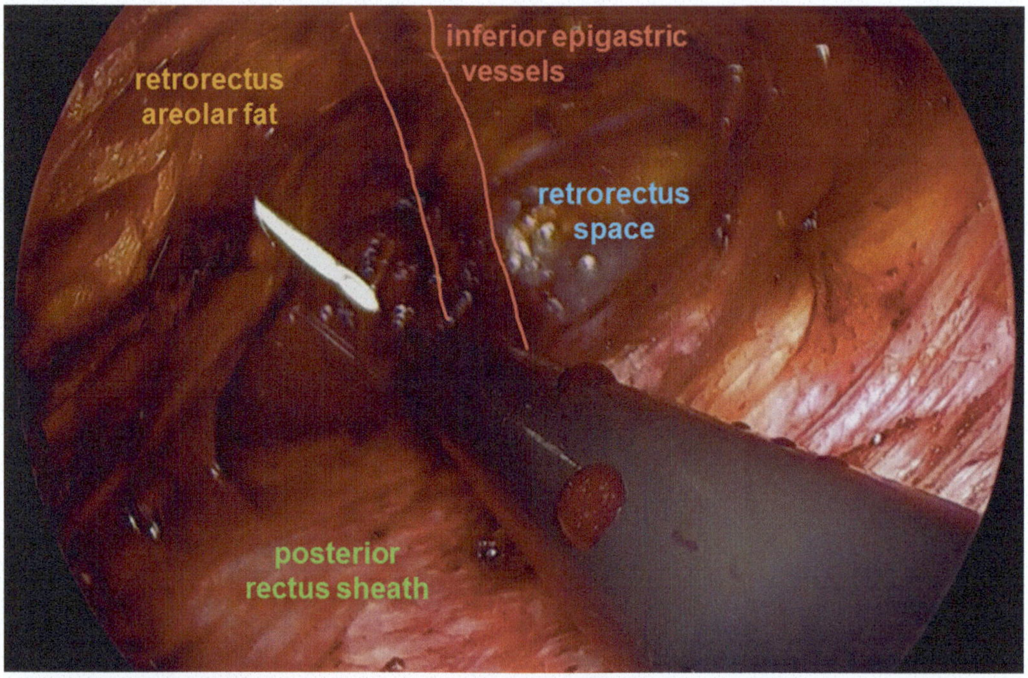


**Fig. 7.6** Placement of the third port

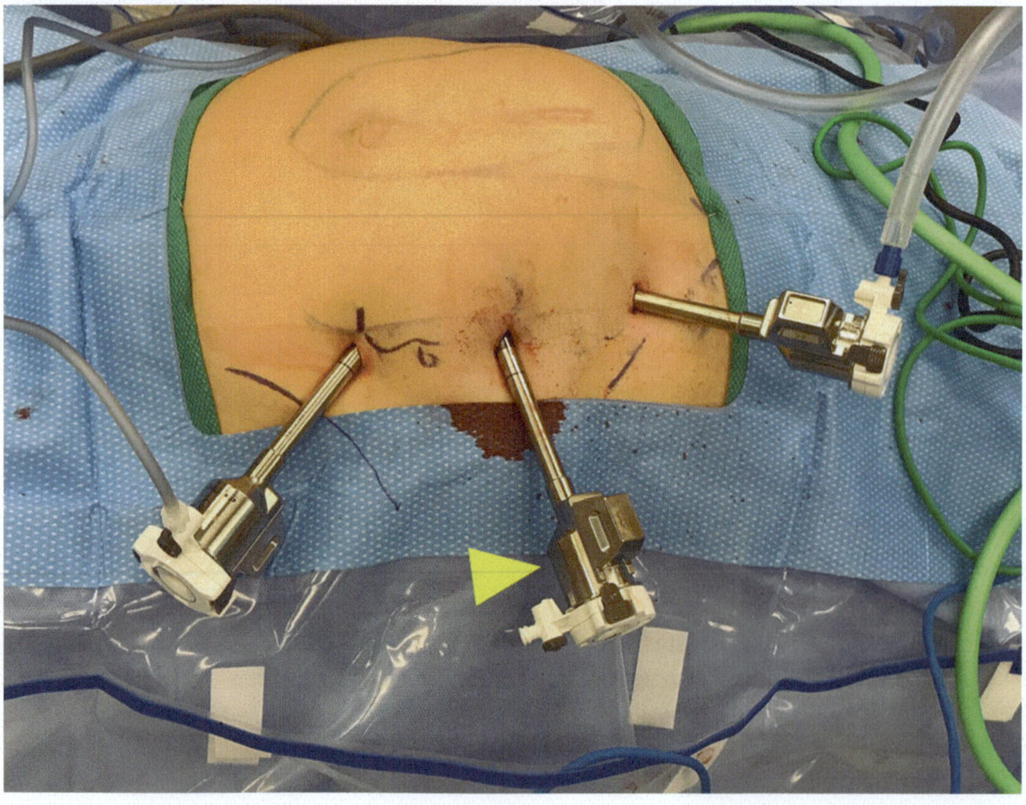

**Fig. 7.7** Final port configuration; the *yellow arrowhead* denotes the camera port

a

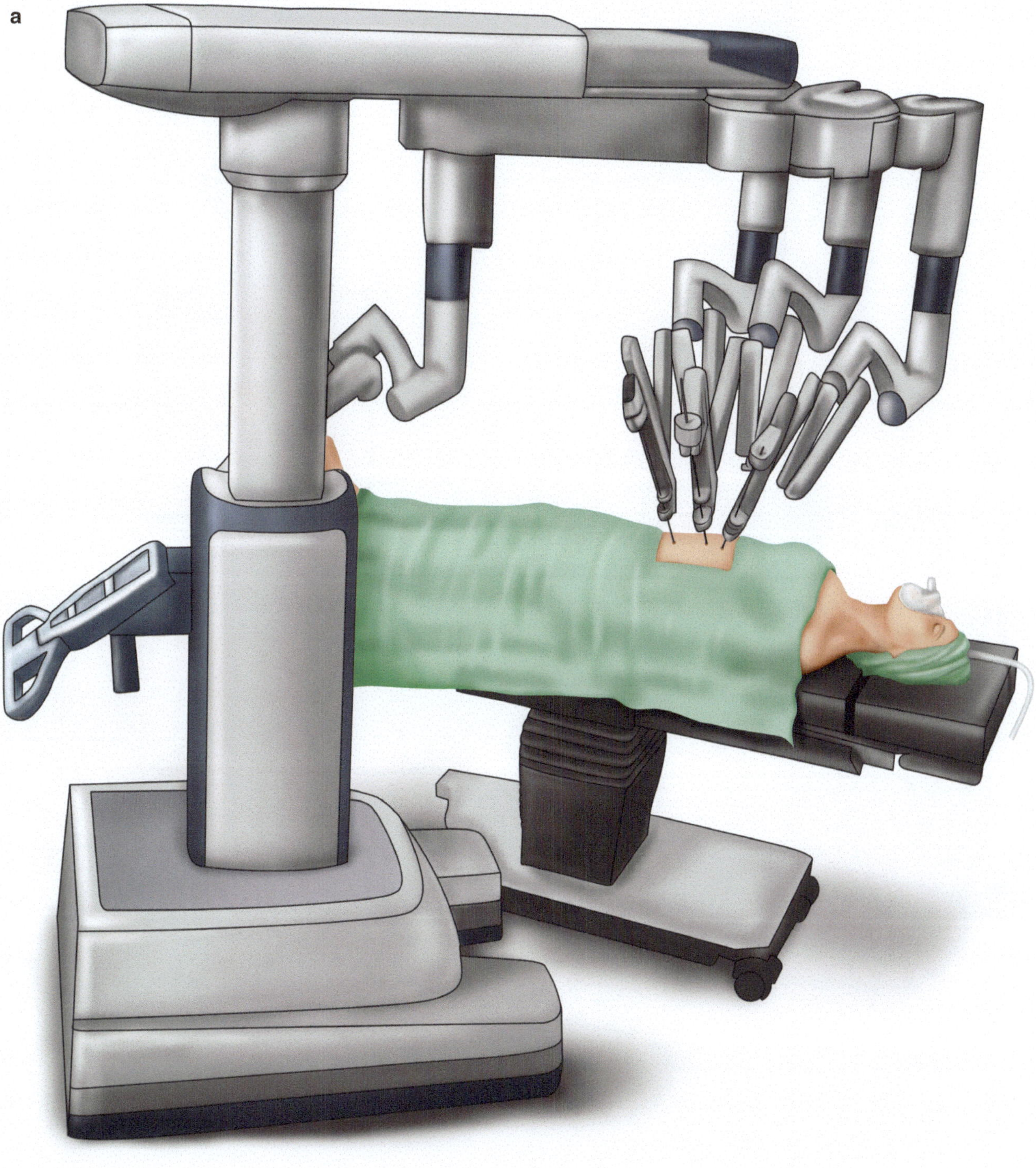

**Fig. 7.8** (**a**–**c**) Docking of the robot. (**d**) Operating room setup

b

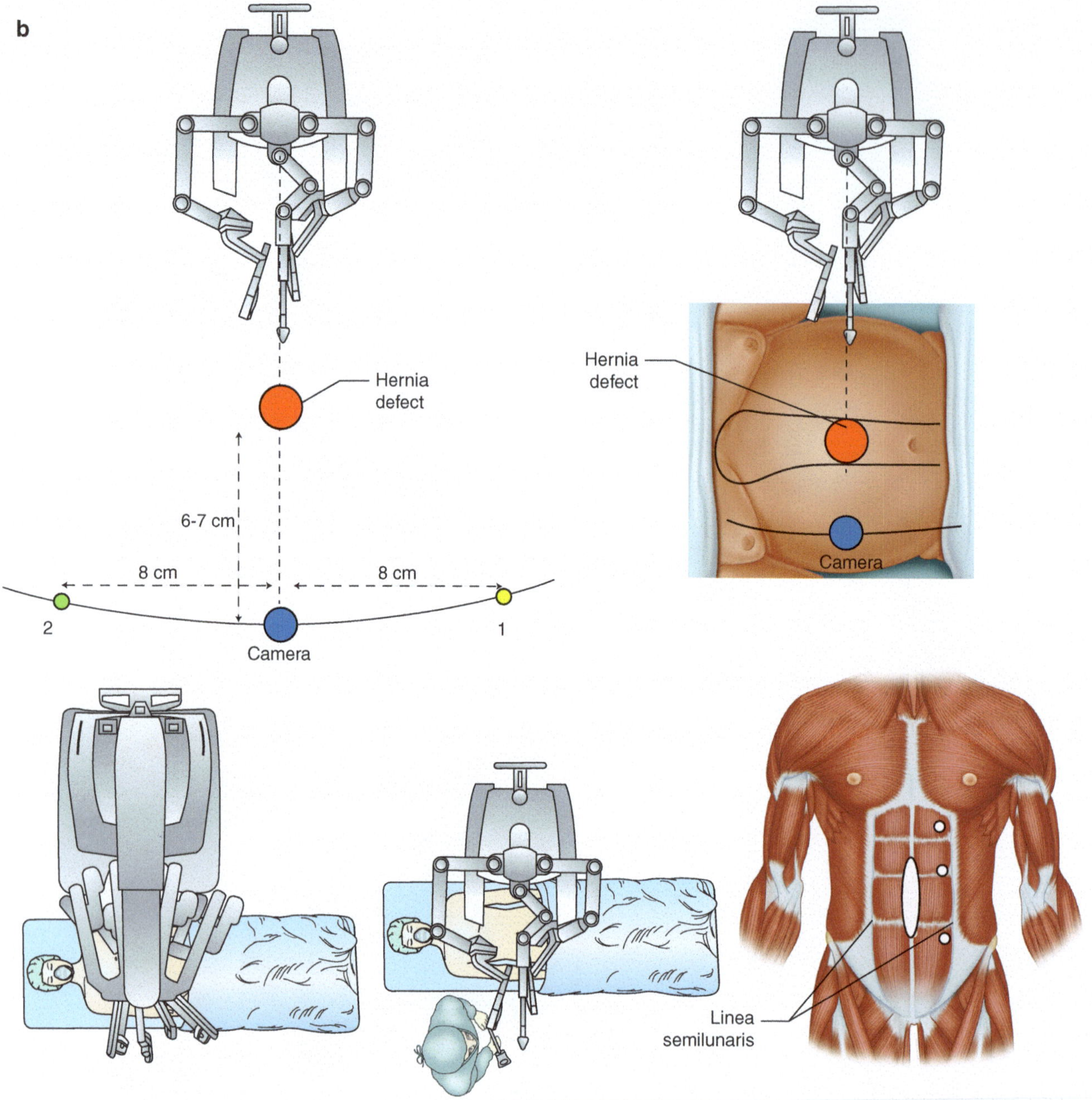


**Fig. 7.8** (continued)

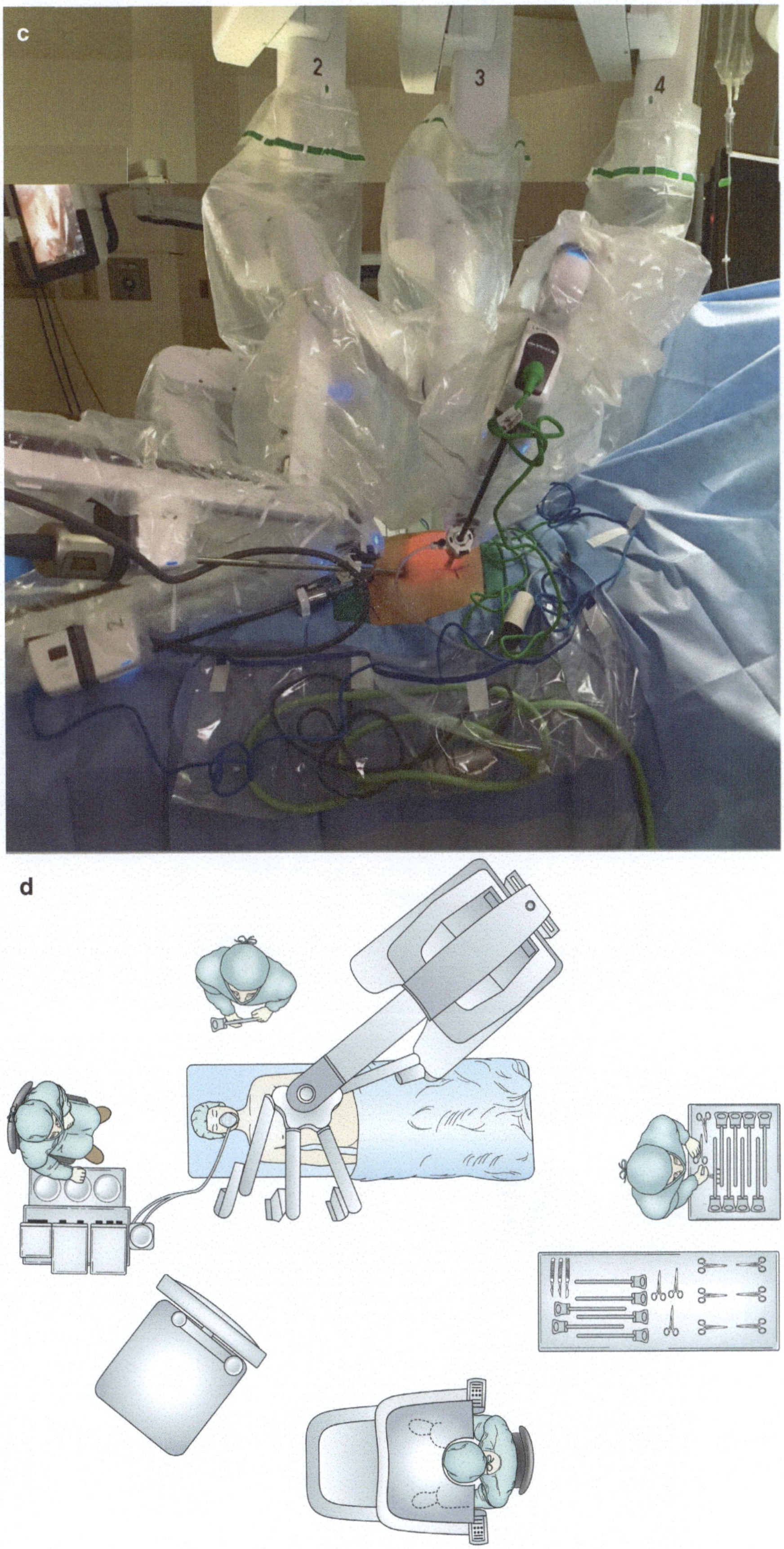


**Fig. 7.8** (continued)

9. Once the camera is in place in the middle port, introduce the instruments. We typically use the scissors, or needle-driver when called for, in the right hand and a grasper such as the bipolar in the left hand. Figure 7.9 illustrates the options we suggest.
10. Begin dissection by stages (corresponding to anatomic spaces). As Fig. 7.10a and b show, we will start in stage 1 in the left retrorectus space. Stage 2 corresponds to the preperitoneal space, which will be accessed once we are ready to incise the ipsilateral (left) posterior rectus sheath. Stage 3 corresponds to the contralateral retrorectus space, which we will enter after clearing the preperitoneal space of the hernia sac and contents by incising the contralateral posterior rectus sheath.

We recommend completing the dissection entirely at each stage before moving on to the next stage/space, in order to minimize anatomic disorientation or confusion and to ensure an optimal workspace. Moving to another stage can alter the field so that tasks in prior spaces become much more difficult.

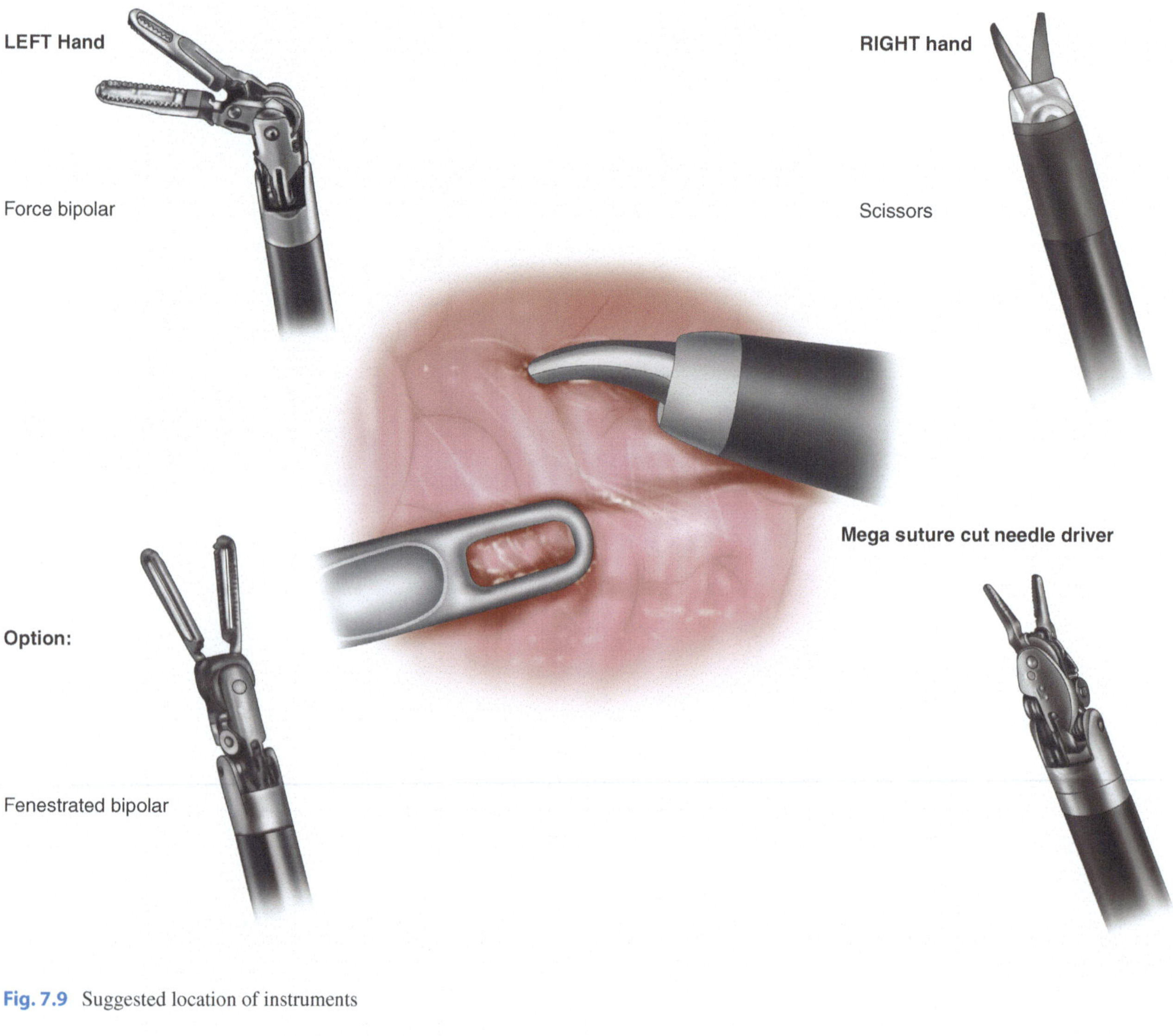


**Fig. 7.9** Suggested location of instruments

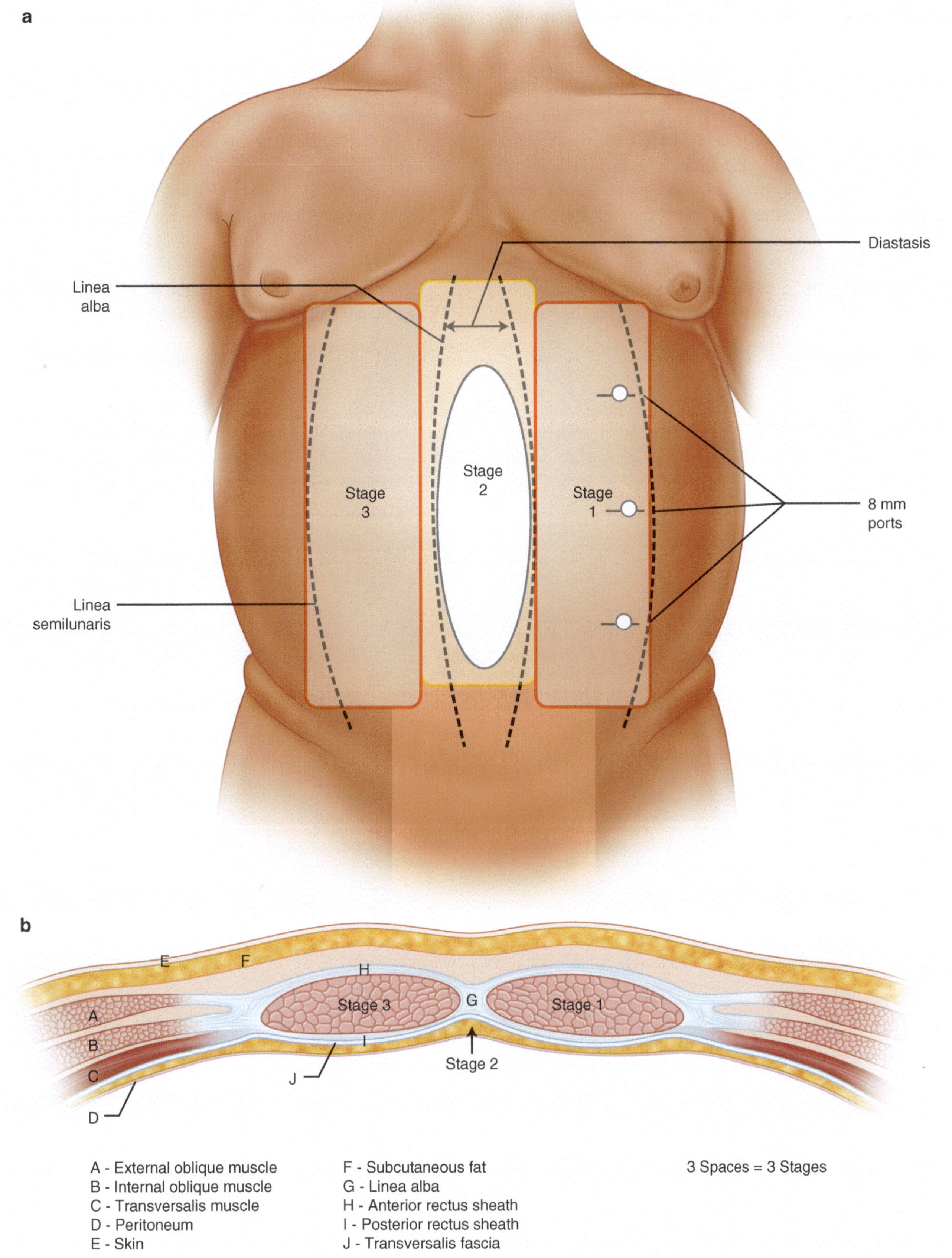


**Fig. 7.10** (**a**) and (**b**) The three stages of dissection. Stage 1: the ipsilateral retrorectus space (relative to the ports/camera). Stage 2: the preperitoneal space (and, usually, the hernia). Stage 3: the contralateral retrorectus space

**Stage 1: Ipsilateral Retrorectus Space** (Fig. 7.11)

(i). Complete the dissection of the ipsilateral (left) retrorectus space by clearing the remainder of the areolar tissue plane (Fig. 7.12a). Sweep the areolar and retrorectus fat tissues "up" (anteriorly) to expose the posterior sheath towards the linea alba (Fig. 7.12b and c). The goals in this stage are to create enough space for mesh overlap later and to identify the entire length of the linea alba before crossing over into the preperitoneal space. Remember that the retrorectus space is developed by lifting/sweeping the retrorectus fat, areolar tissue, and neurovascular bundles "up" anteriorly, off the posterior rectus sheath, as was done at the start of the case. Note that very medial neurovascular bundles are usually smaller and can be divided electrosurgically, but the larger neurovascular bundles near the linea semilunaris laterally should be preserved. (Many of the medial bundles can be preserved as well, as seen in Fig. 7.12d.) This stage should finish developing the retrorectus space but ultimately proceeds toward the linea alba.

Positively identify the linea alba to avoid inadvertently injuring it during posterior rectus sheath incision. Ideally, this is accomplished by exposing it along its entire length within the retrorectus space, but at minimum, a long portion of it should be clearly exposed before incising the posterior rectus sheath and proceeding to the next stage. Figure 7.12e shows the landmarks and planned incision within a widely-cleared field.

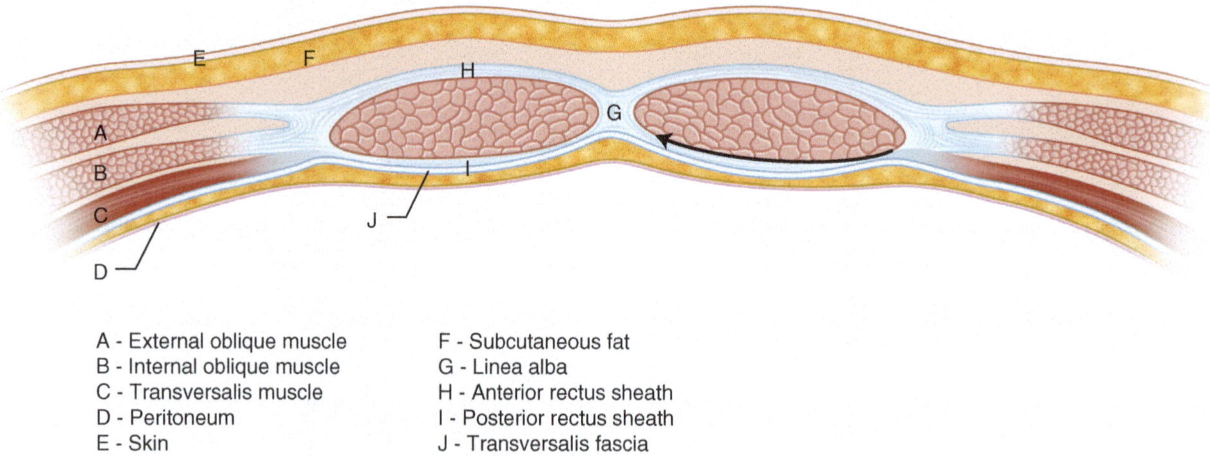


**Fig. 7.11** Ipsilateral (left) retrorectus space (Stage 1)

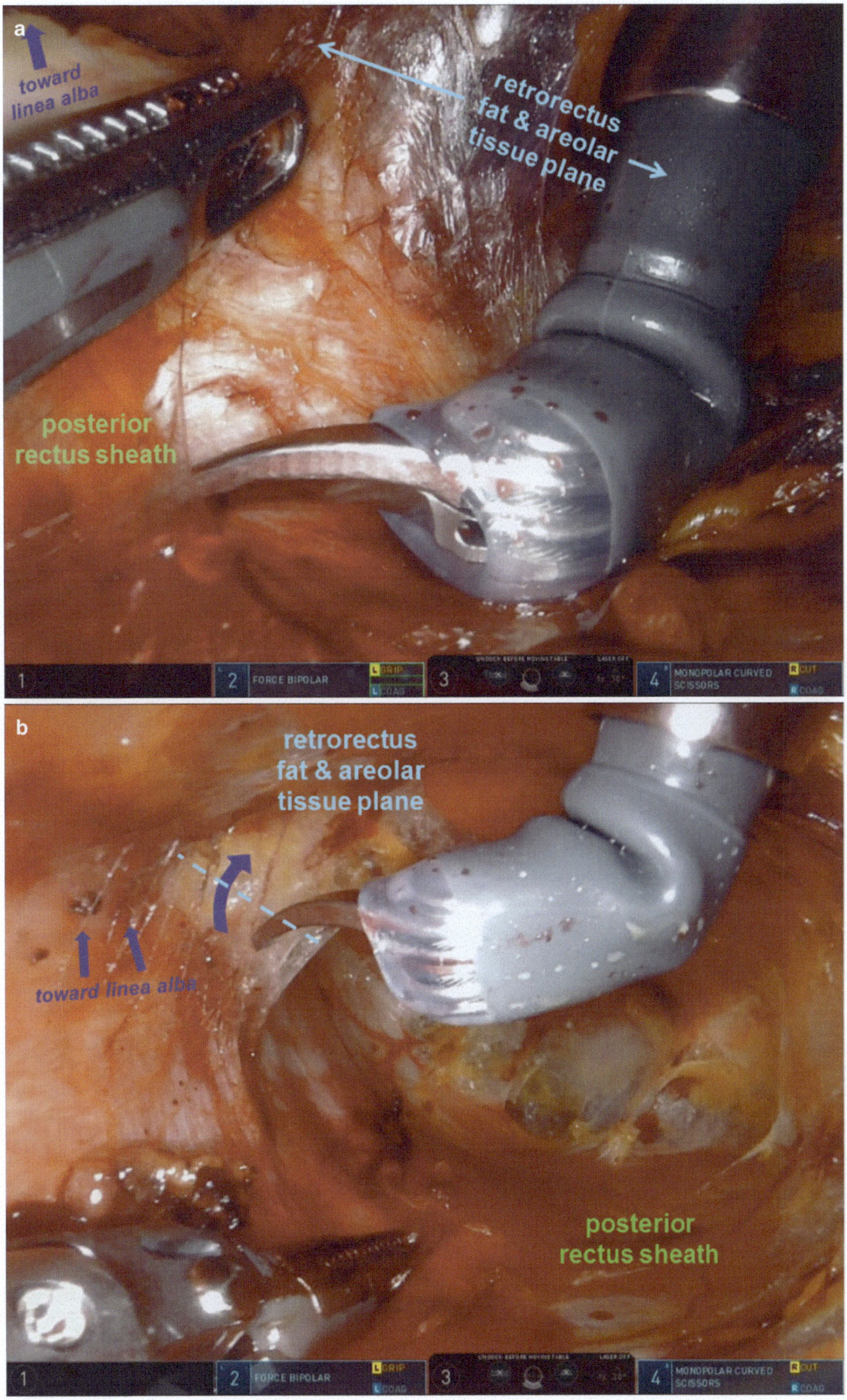


**Fig. 7.12** (**a**) Continued dissection of the retrorectus areolar tissue plane. (**b**) and (**c**) Approaching the linea alba. (**d**) Preservation of medial neurovascular bundles. (**e**) Planned linea alba incision with key landmarks

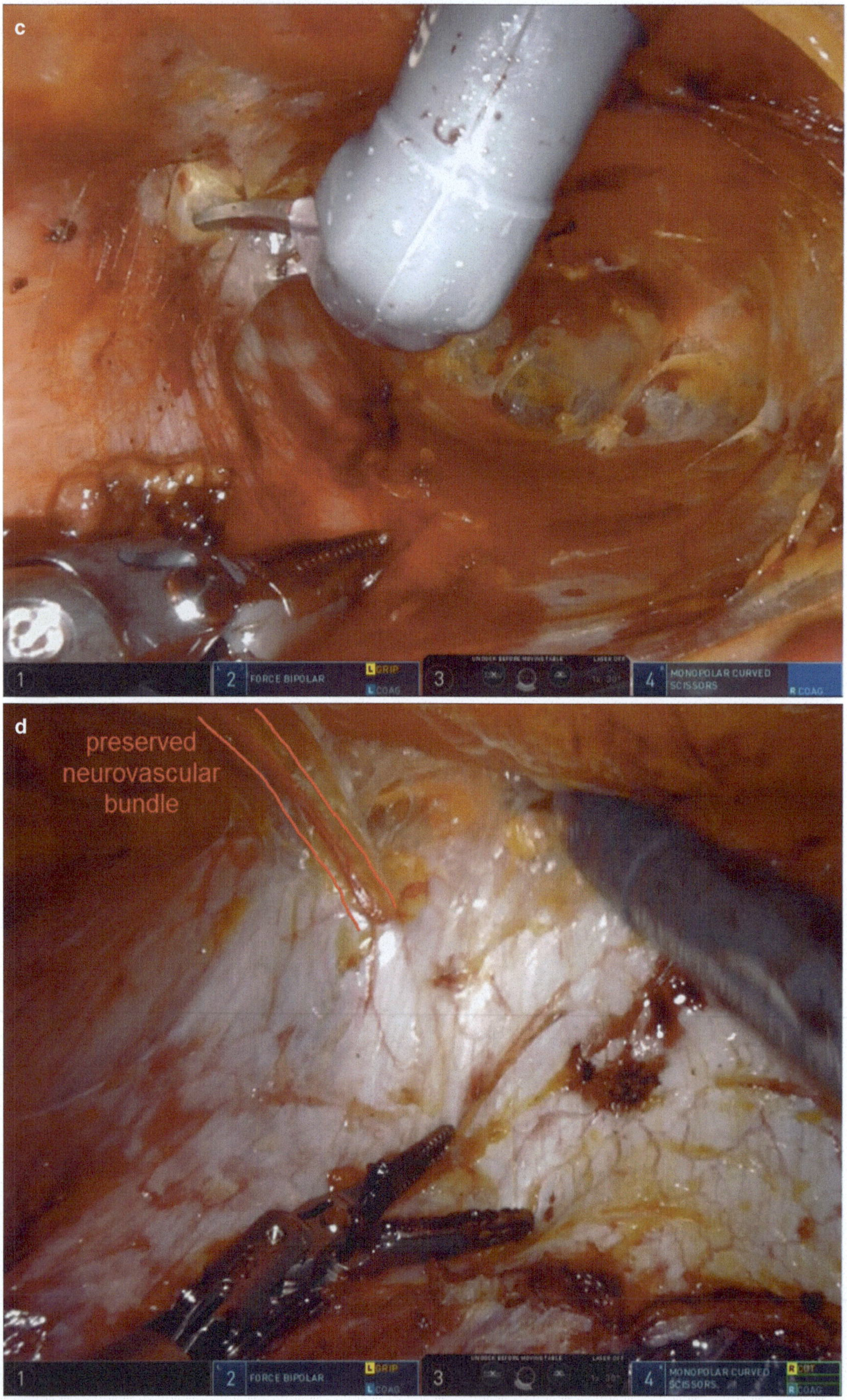


**Fig. 7.12** (continued)

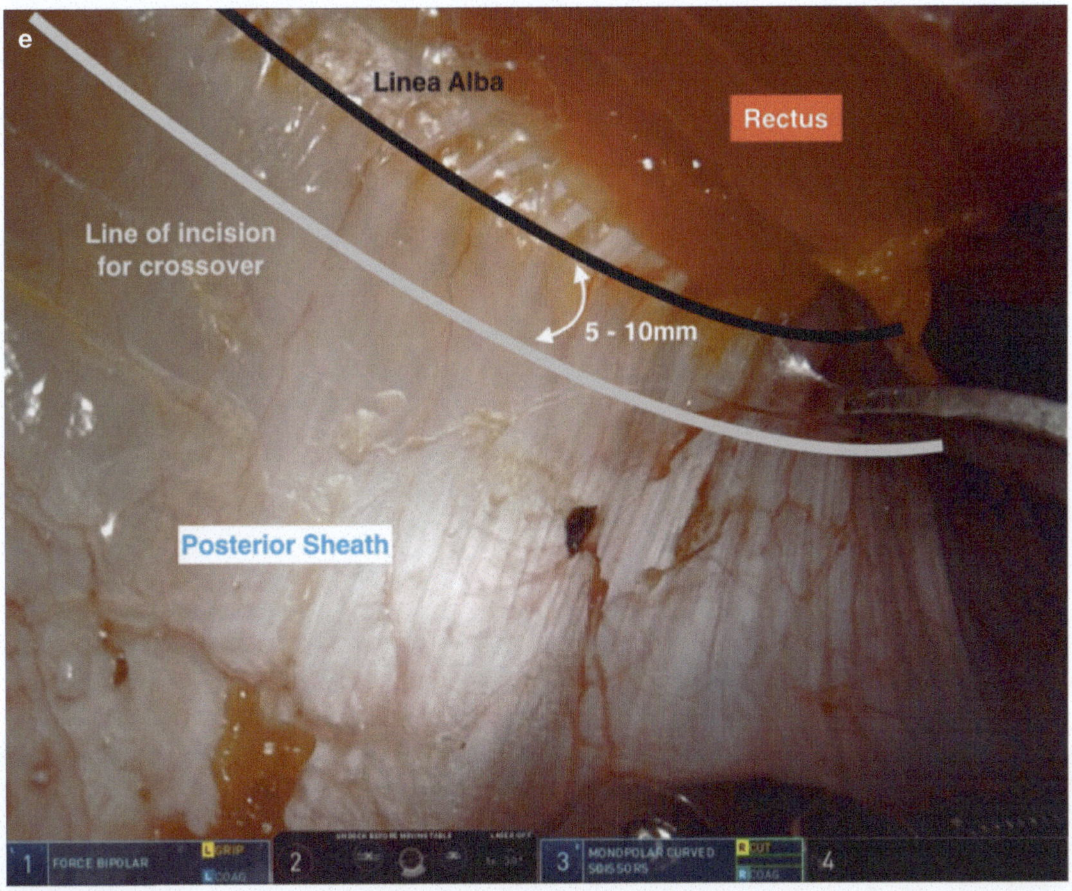


**Fig. 7.12** (continued)

(ii). Stage 1 is completed by fully opening the ipsilateral posterior rectus sheath (Fig. 7.13a), which should be incised 5–10 mm away from the linea alba. The initial incision should be made away from the hernia if possible, and without energy. Figure 7.13b–f illustrate these principles, beginning with a sharp division of the posterior rectus sheath at the appropriate distance from the linea alba and continuing with extension of the incision in both directions, taking care to ensure the fascia is clear of the hernia medially. Frequently check the location of the linea alba while incising.

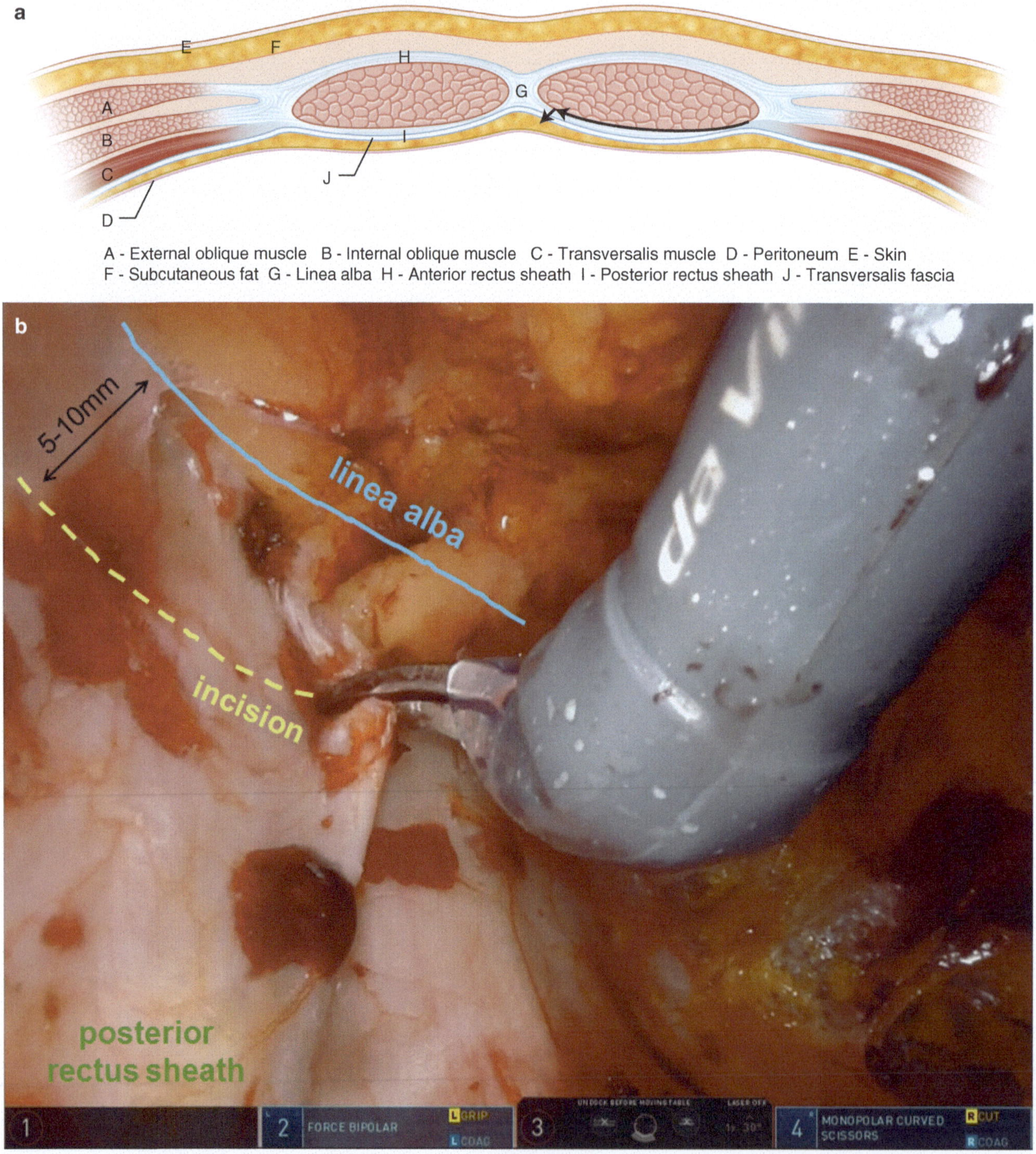


**Fig. 7.13** (a–f) Opening of the ipsilateral (patient's left) posterior rectus sheath

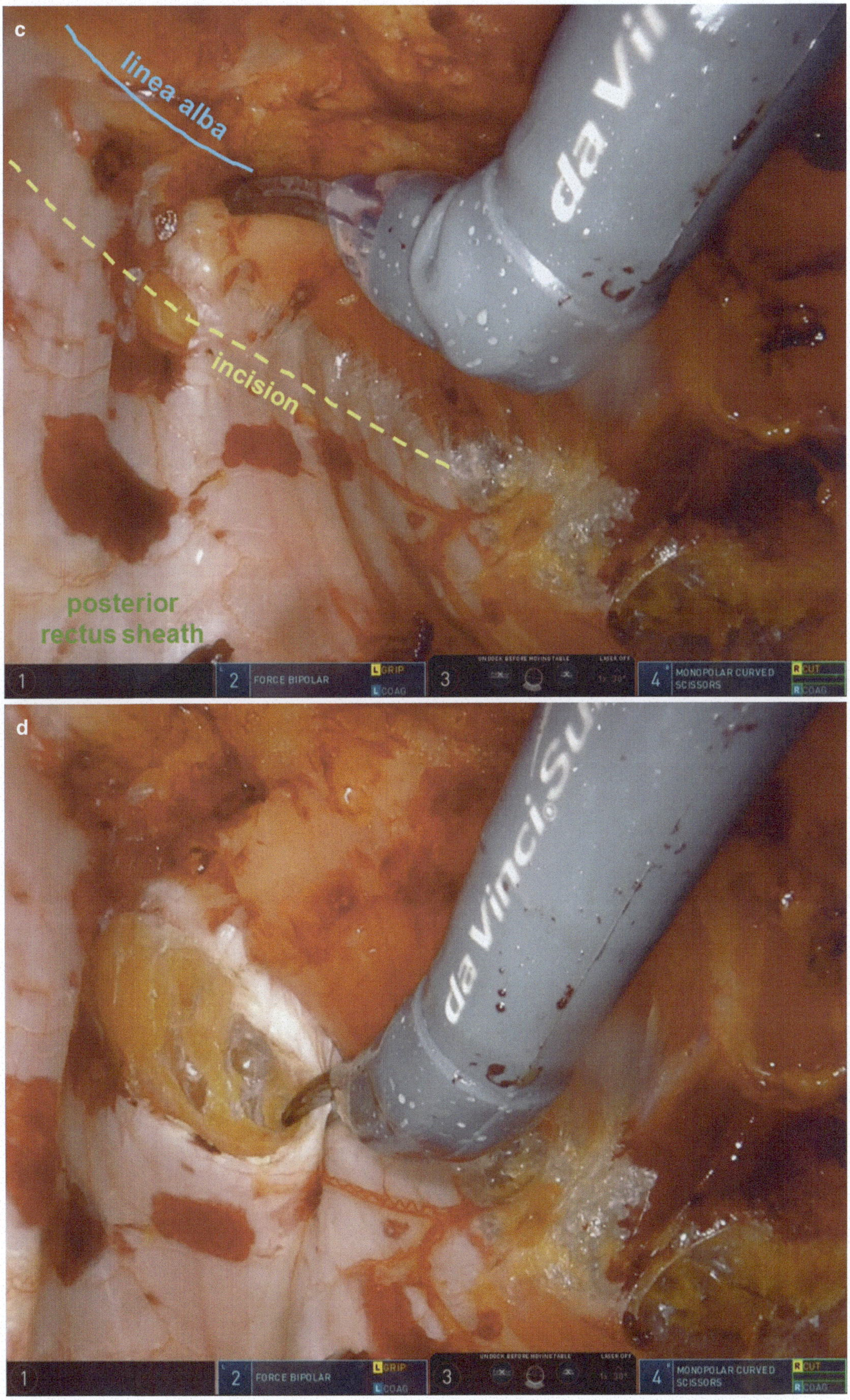


**Fig. 7.13** (continued)

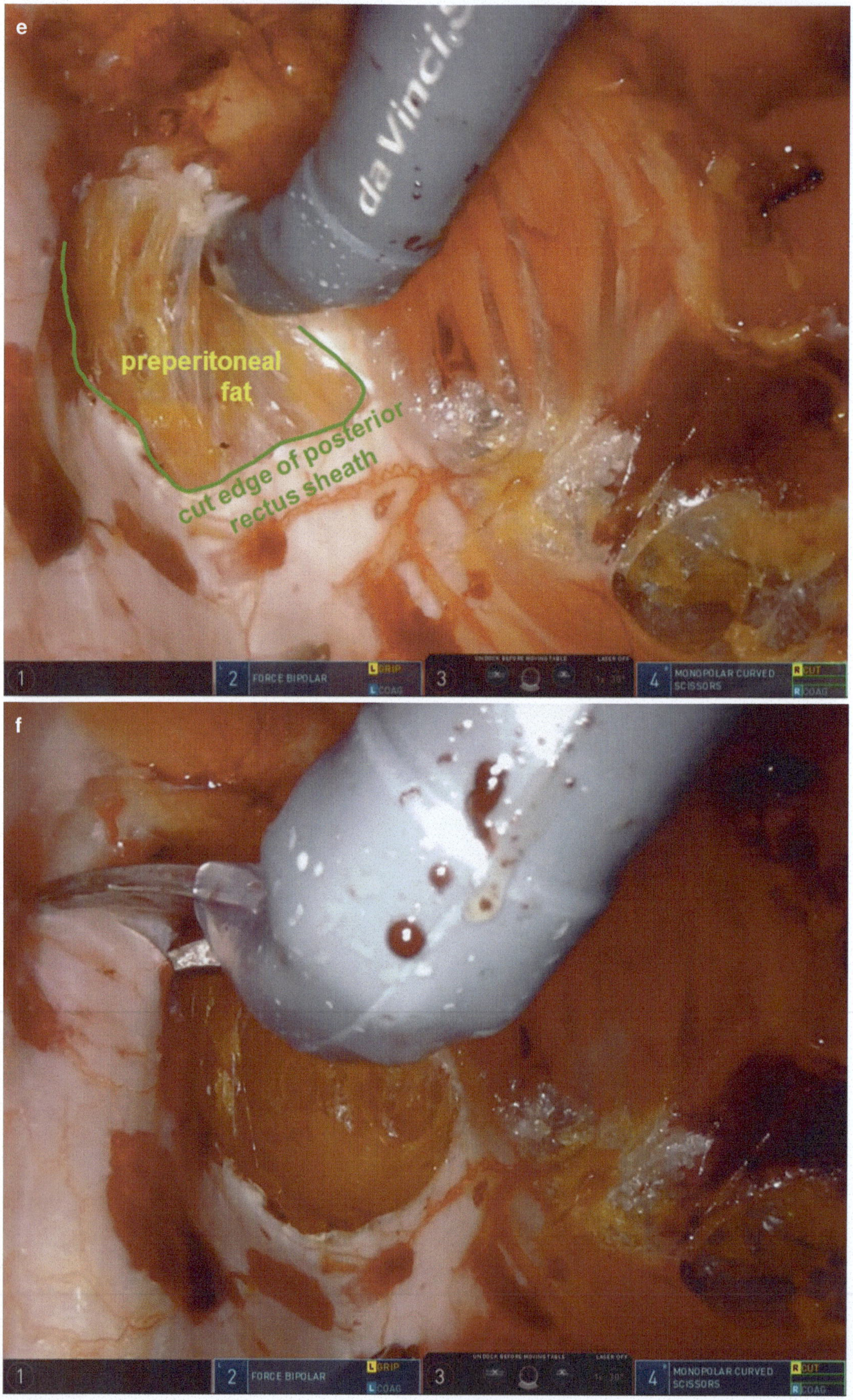


**Fig. 7.13** (continued)

(iii). When the posterior rectus sheath terminates at the arcuate line (Fig. 7.14a), the transversalis fascia must be incised instead to enter that portion of the preperitoneal space (Fig. 7.14b and c).

(iv). Once the ipsilateral posterior rectus sheath and transversalis fascia are fully opened, the ipsilateral retrorectus stage (Stage 1) is complete, and the preperitoneal space is now accessible for Stage 2. (Figure 7.15 shows what has been accomplished and the next space.)

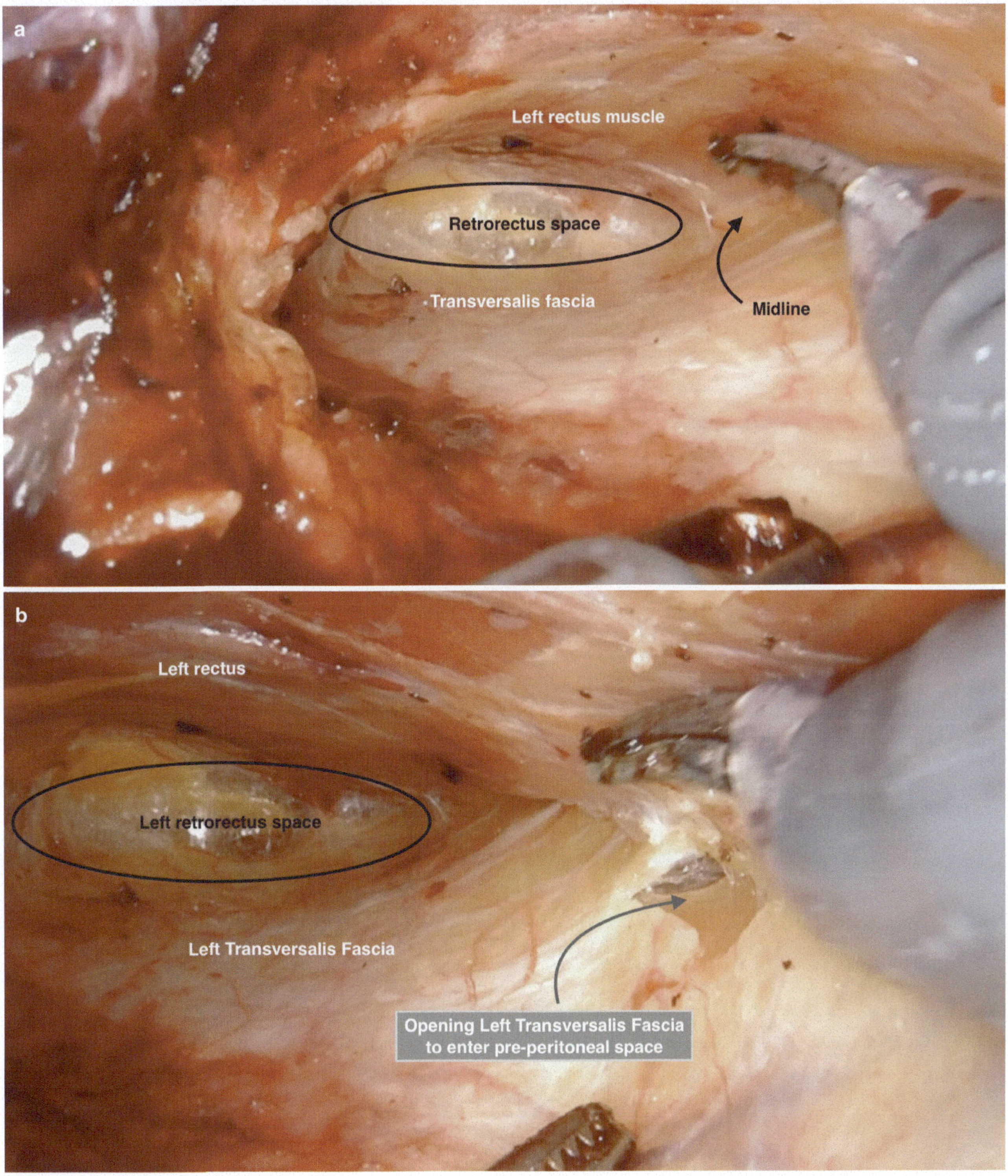


**Fig. 7.14** (**a**) Posterior rectus sheath terminating at the arcuate line. (**b**) and (**c**) Incision of the transversalis fascia to enter the preperitoneal space below the arcuate line

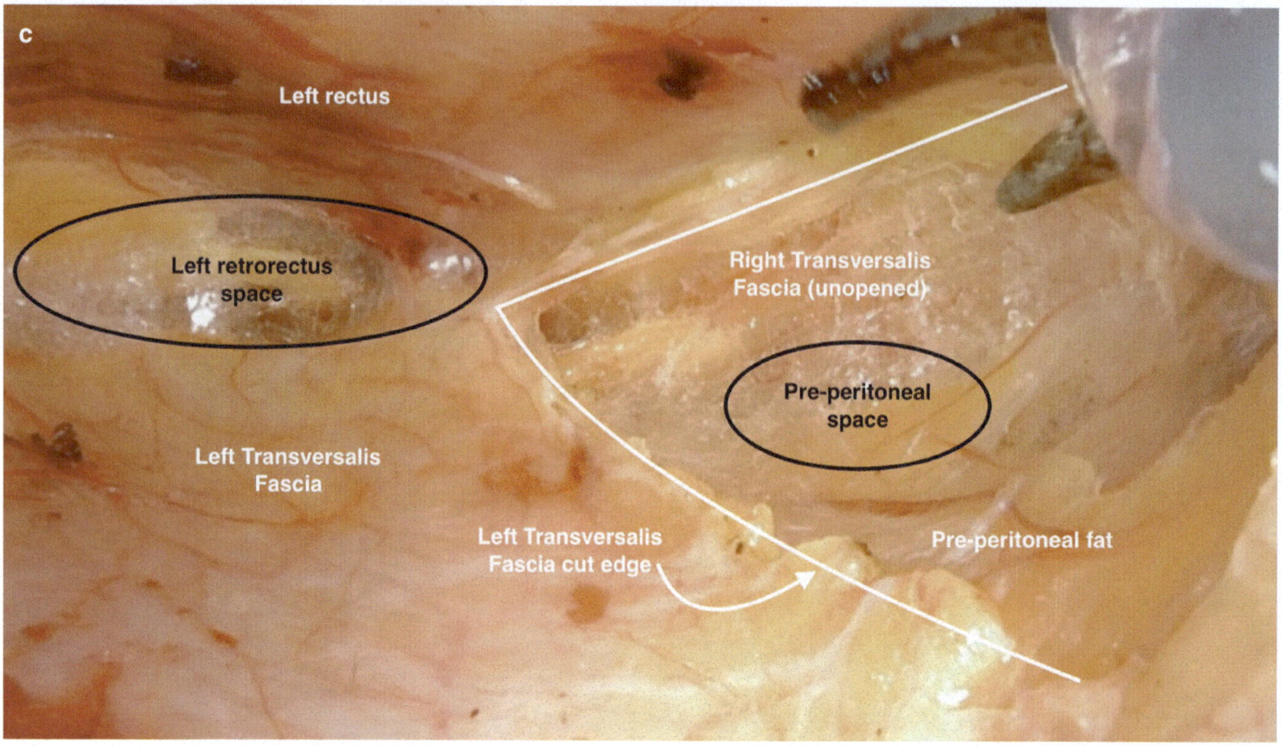


**Fig. 7.14** (continued)

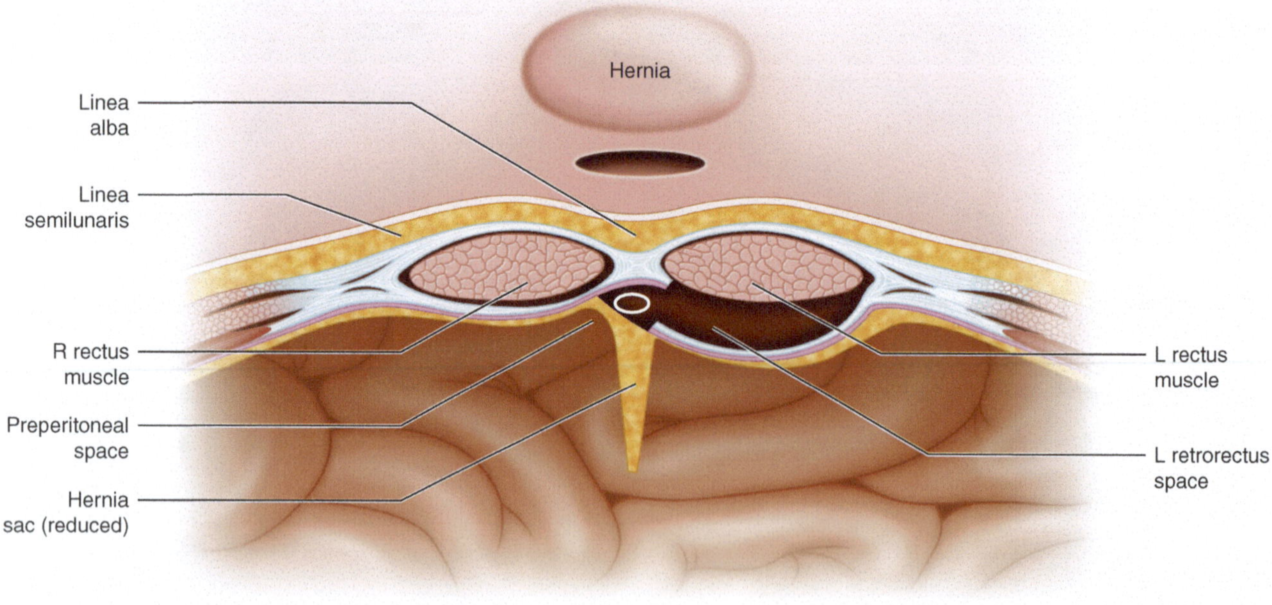


**Fig. 7.15** Completion of Stage 1 (ipsilateral rectus sheath), ready for Stage 2 (preperitoneal space)

**Stage 2: Preperitoneal Space** (Fig. 7.16)

(i). Start your dissection of the preperitoneal space away from the hernia. Instead of sweeping the fat "up" anteriorly, you will now push the fat "down" posteriorly/intra-abdominally (Fig. 7.17a and b). Try to stay between the umbilical ligaments (falciform, medial, median) and the anterior fascia (diastatic linea alba).

(ii). Then dissect free the hernia sac (Fig. 7.18a and b) and clear the fascial edges (Fig. 7.18c–e). Reduce as much hernia sac or pseudosac as possible to provide material for patching larger peritoneal defects later, if needed. If small holes are made in the peritoneum, they can be closed with 3–0 V-loc 180 (Medtronic), with or without pseudosac.

(iii). Dissect any remaining preperitoneal space, superficial to the preperitoneal fat plane. With large hernias, the dissection may be mostly completed in the course of freeing the hernia completely. Just as with Stage 1, the linea alba must be cleared (though from a medial rather than a lateral direction) to allow for safe incision of the contralateral posterior rectus sheath. Once the primary goals of this stage (completely reducing the hernia sac, clearing the diastatic linea alba, and exposing the contralateral linea alba and posterior rectus sheath) have been achieved, the contralateral posterior rectus sheath must be incised (Fig. 7.19) in a similar manner to that in Stage 1 to enter the contralateral retrorectus space.

(iv). Incise the contralateral (right) posterior rectus sheath 5–10 mm lateral to the contralateral border of the linea alba to open the contralateral retrorectus space. Figure 7.20a–e illustrate opening the contralateral posterior rectus sheath despite some distortion in the anatomy from the hernia. You can see the linea alba more clearly superiorly, where it is not so diastatic, with both rectus muscles (Fig. 7.20e). Also, the transversalis fascia will again be encountered at the inferior portion (Fig. 7.20f). Completion of the crossover is sometimes easiest at the level of the arcuate line; alternatively, a hypodermic needle can be inserted by the bedside assistant at the external linea alba marking to identify the border internally. We strongly recommend the spreading-prior-to-cutting technique shown in these figures. Figure 7.20g illustrates what has been accomplished in this stage, as well as the entry into the next space.

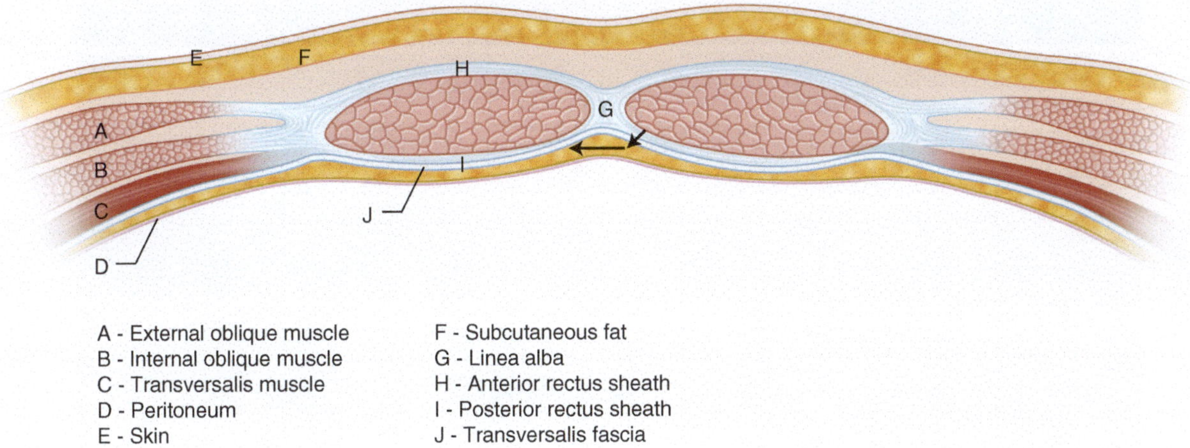


**Fig. 7.16** Preperitoneal space (Stage 2)

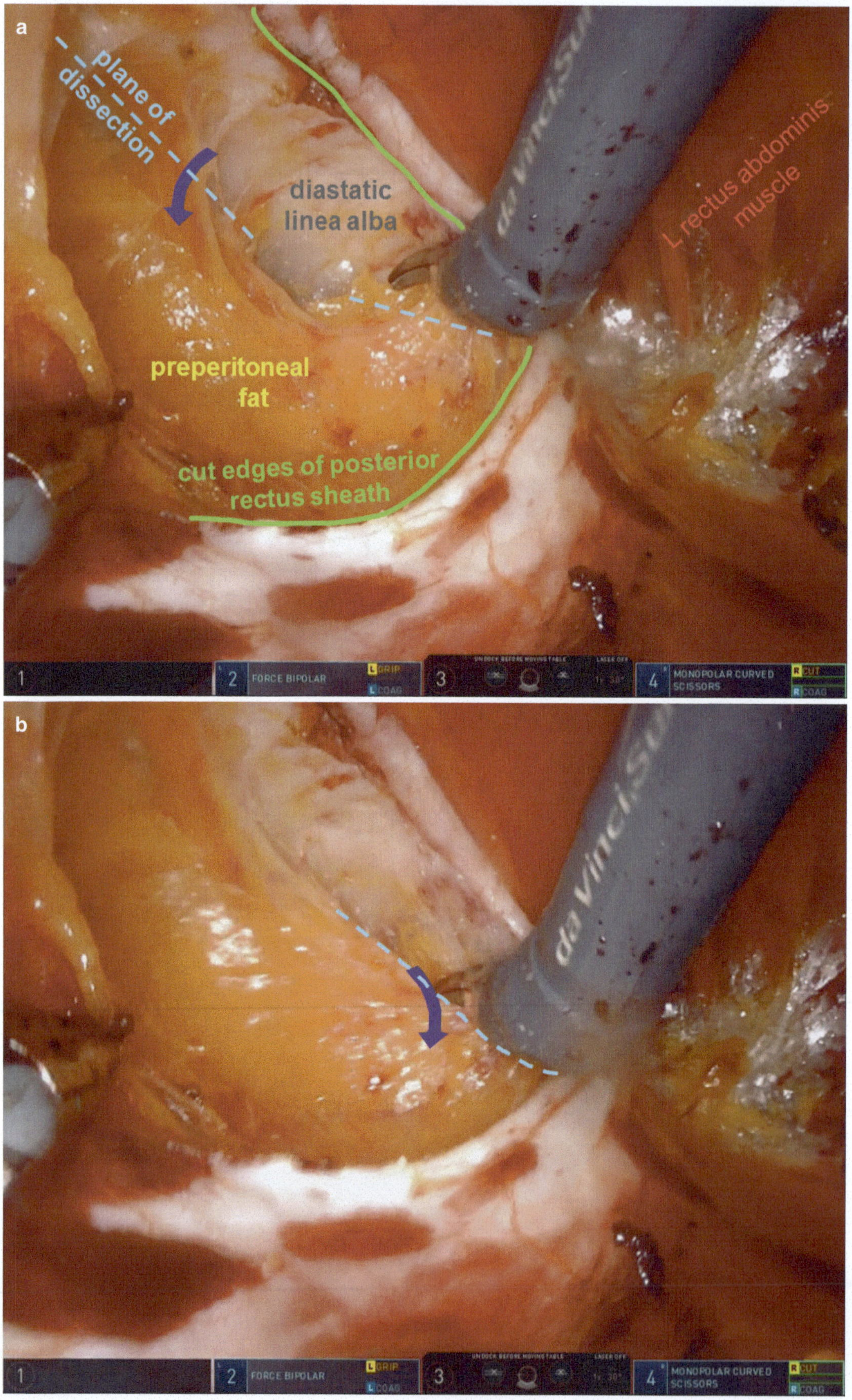


**Fig. 7.17** (**a**) and (**b**) Dissection of the preperitoneal space, pushing the fat "down" (*purple arrows*)

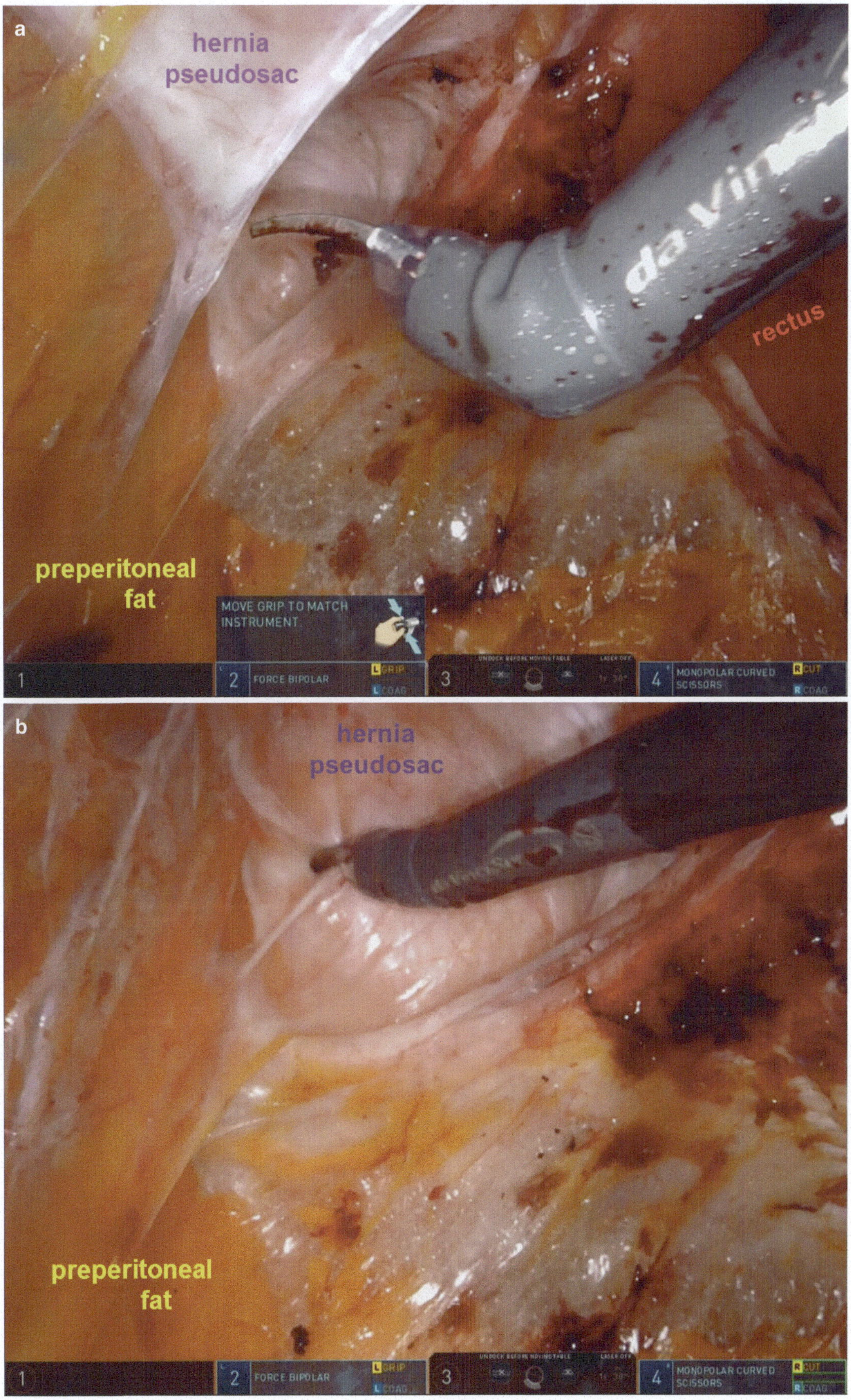


**Fig. 7.18** (**a**) and (**b**) Dissecting free the hernia sac. (**c**–**e**) Clearing the fascial edges

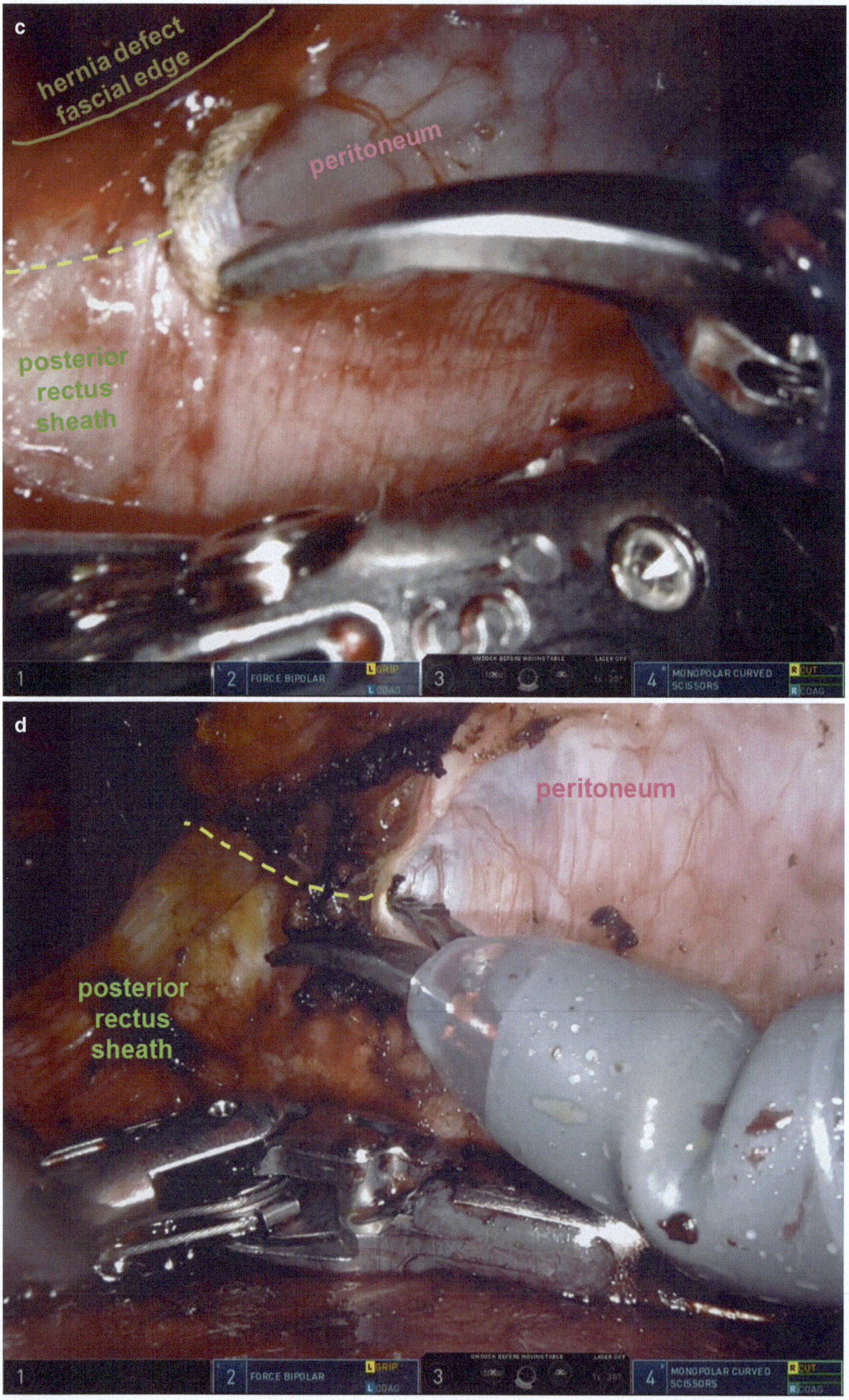


**Fig. 7.18** (continued)

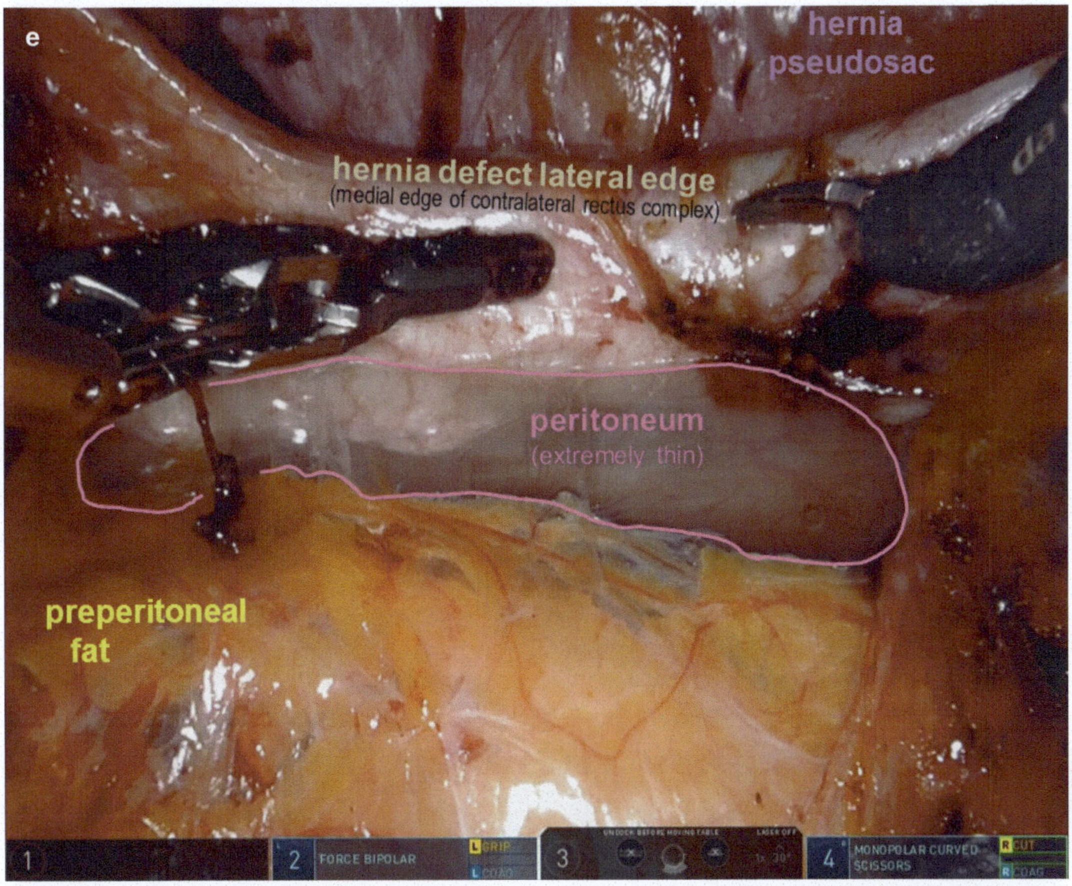


**Fig. 7.18** (continued)

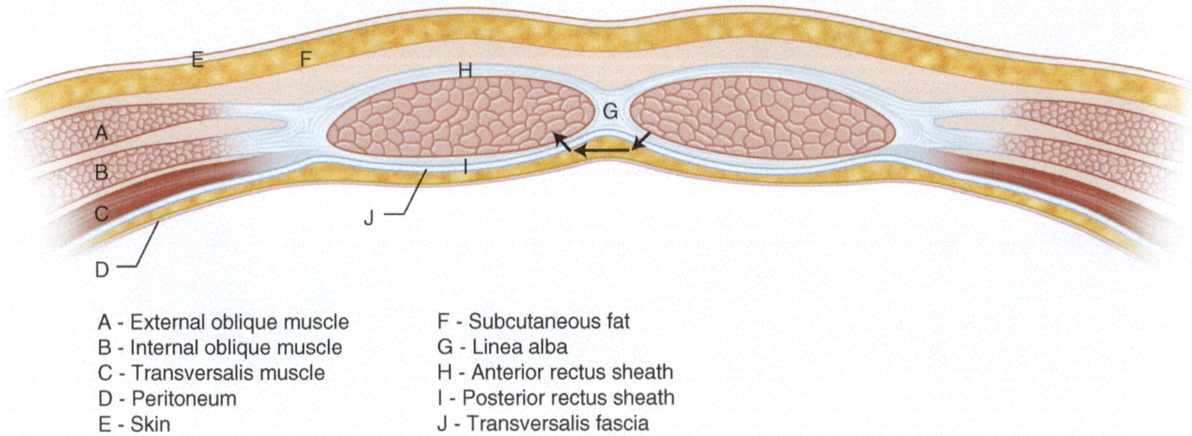


**Fig. 7.19** Incising the contralateral posterior rectus sheath

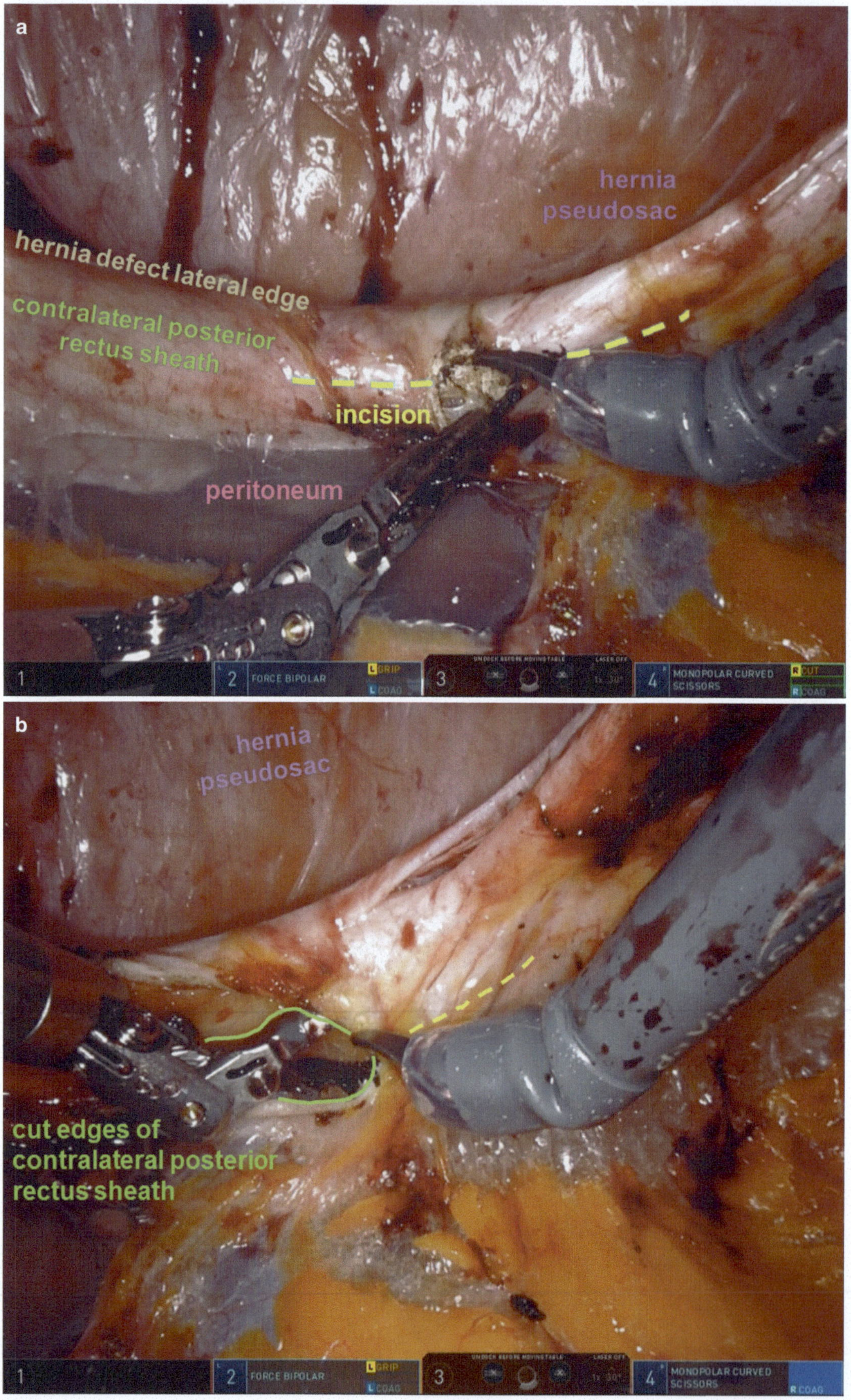


**Fig. 7.20** (**a–e**) Opening the contralateral (right) posterior rectus sheath. (**f**) The transversalis fascia is encountered at the inferior portion. (**g**) Completion of Stage 2, ready for Stage 3

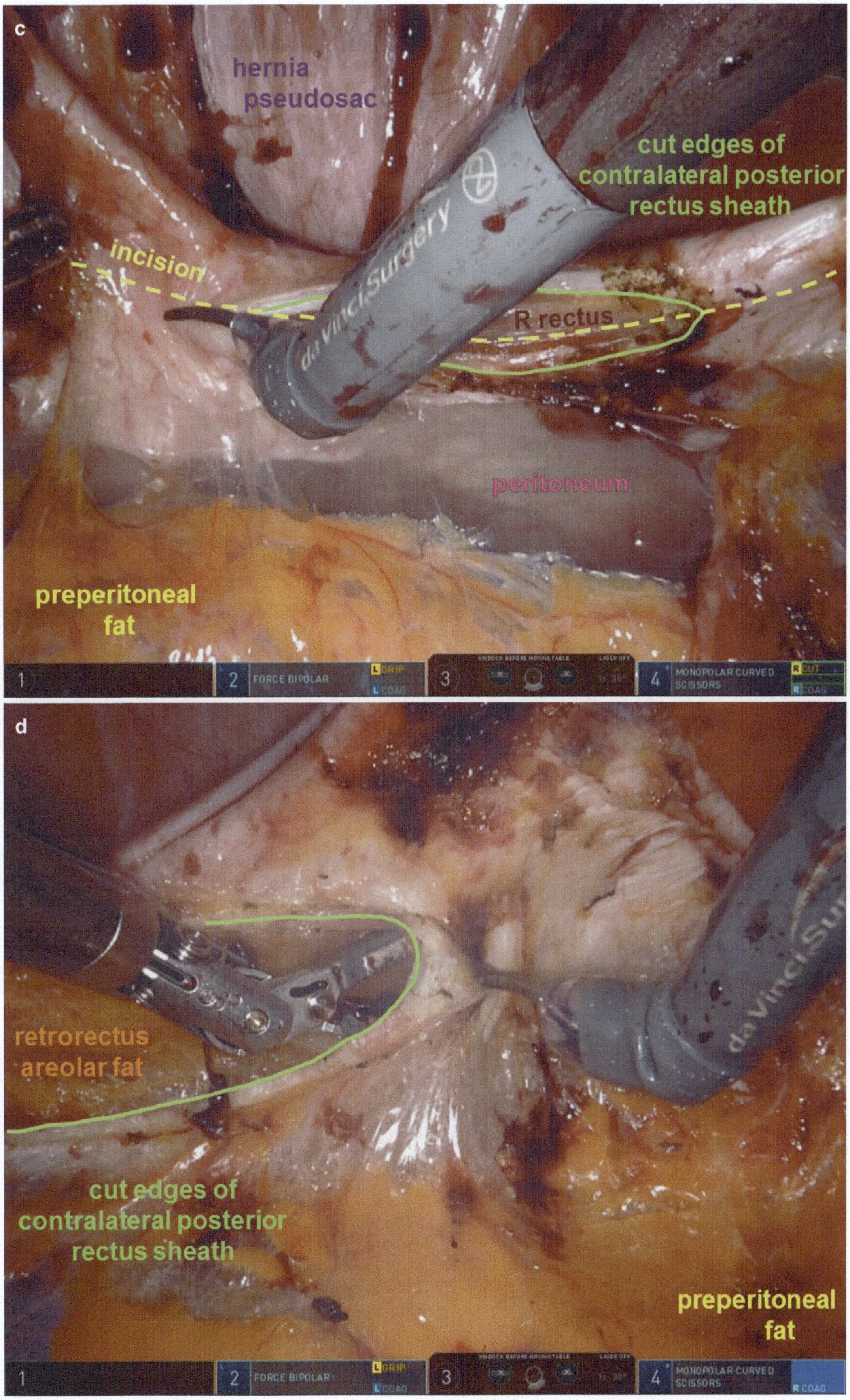


**Fig. 7.20** (continued)

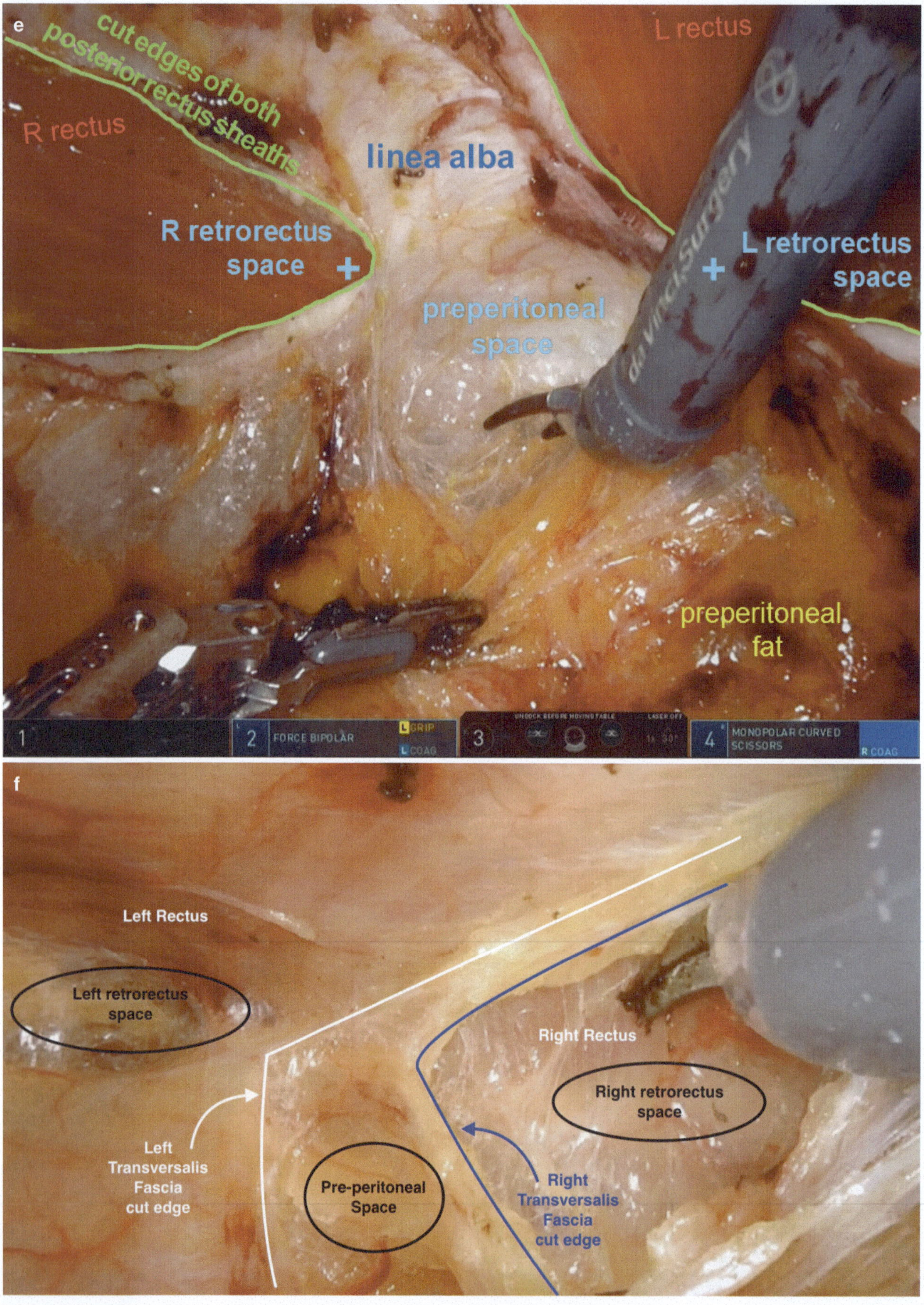


**Fig. 7.20** (continued)

g

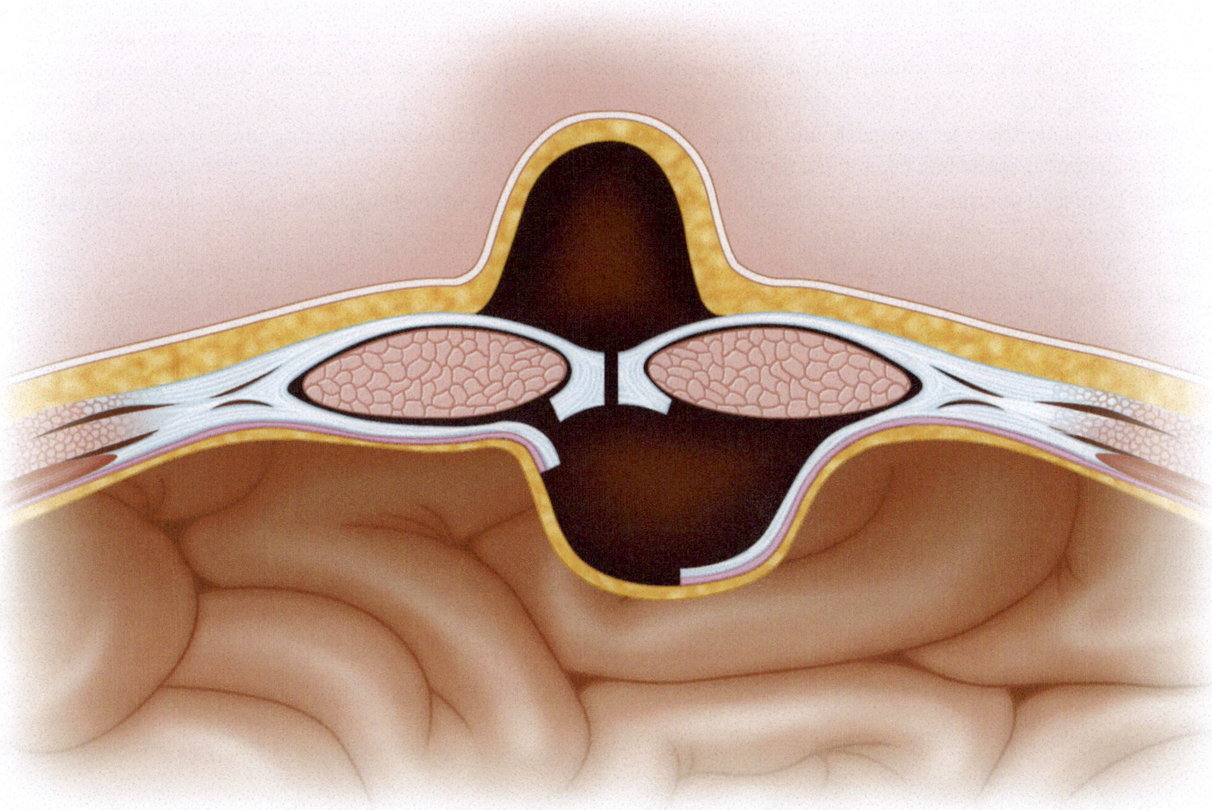

Fig. 7.20 (continued)

**Stage 3: Contralateral Retrorectus Space** (Fig. 7.21)

(i). Again, the retrorectus space is developed by lifting/sweeping the retrorectus fat, areolar tissue, and neurovascular bundles "up" anteriorly, off the posterior rectus sheath (Fig. 7.22a–c), and similarly done below the arcuate line (Fig. 7.22d). At this point, the primary goal is to create adequate space for the mesh, and a large, unified, extraperitoneal space has been created (Fig. 7.23). Ports may be placed contralaterally at this point only if a bilateral transversus abdominis release (TAR) is required. (A discussion of a robot TAR would likely warrant its own chapter.) *Note:* We do not routinely close the posterior rectus sheath, as the peritoneum serves to exclude the mesh. We strongly recommend against re-approximating the posterior rectus sheath without performing a TAR.

11. Measure the hernia defect in the superior-inferior and lateral dimensions. For very large hernias, we use the "two ruler technique" (Fig. 7.24): We place one ruler craniocaudal and leave it in place, then use a second ruler to measure the lateral width at several points along the hernia defect to get a more accurate assessment of hernia size and thus the mesh size and shape needed.
12. Close the defect/diastasis, thus re-approximating the anterior rectus sheath.
    (1) Start sewing the defect/diastasis closed from one end with 18-inch #0 V-loc 180 suture (Medtronic) on a GS21 needle. Sew "up" and toward yourself, form the contralateral edge to ipsilateral edge, as illustrated in Fig. 7.25a–d.

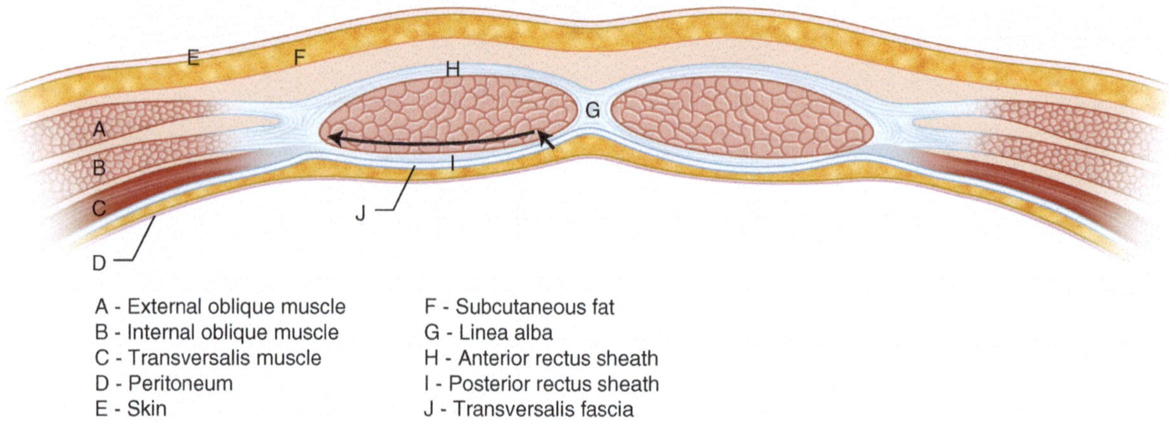


**Fig. 7.21** Contralateral retrorectus space

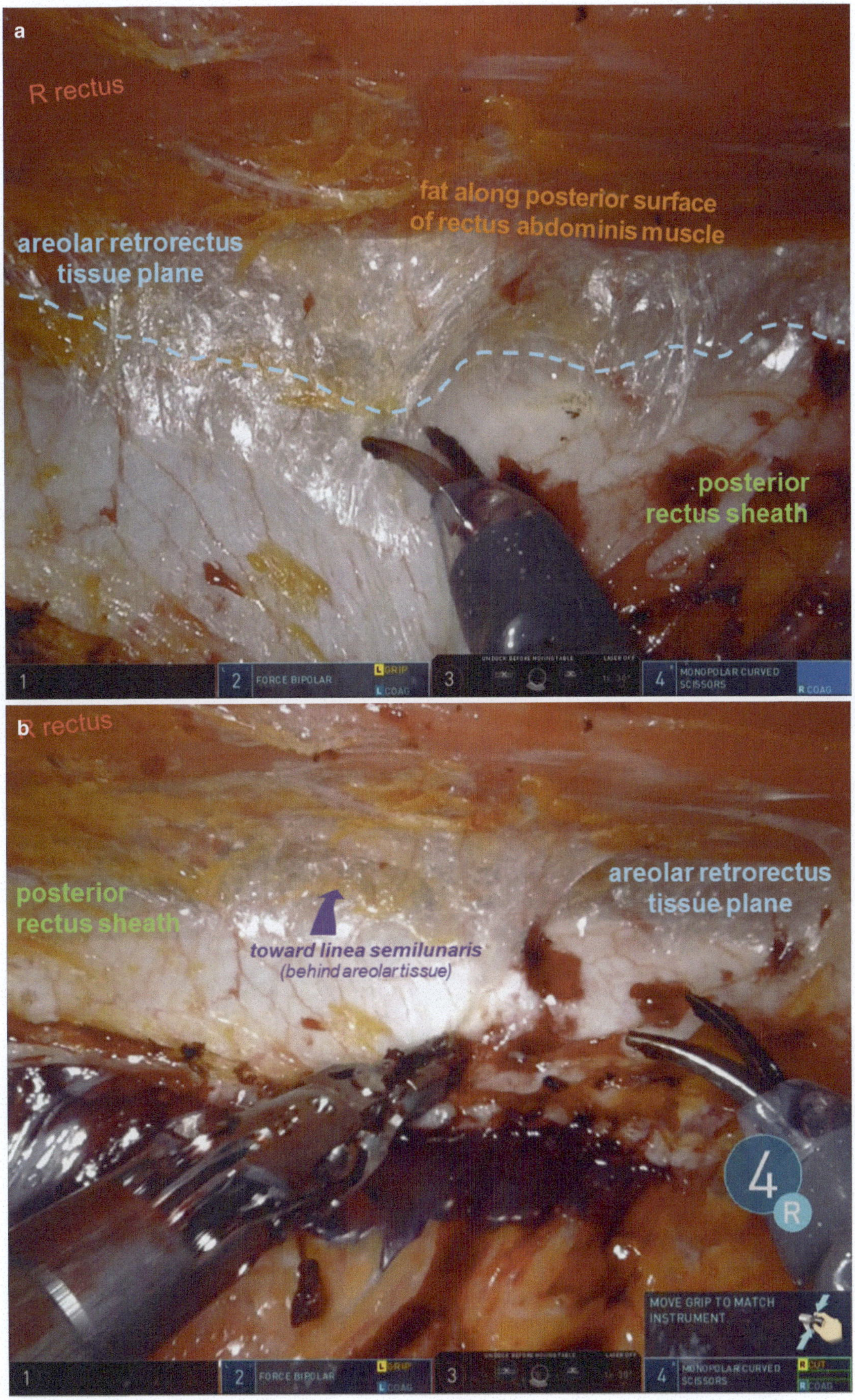


**Fig. 7.22** Developing the contralateral retrorectus space along the posterior rectus sheath above (**a–c**) and below (**d**) the arcuate line

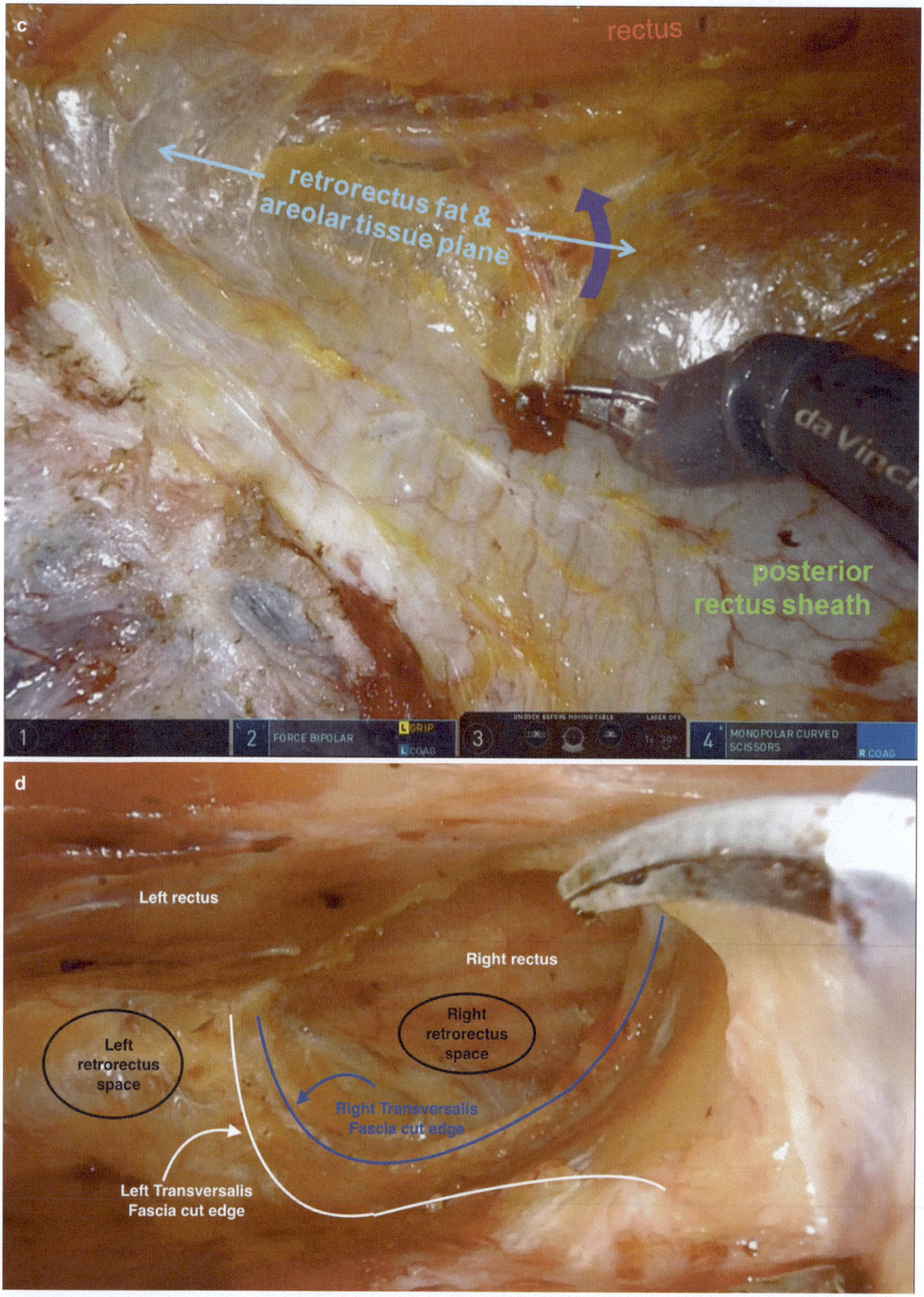


**Fig. 7.22** (continued)

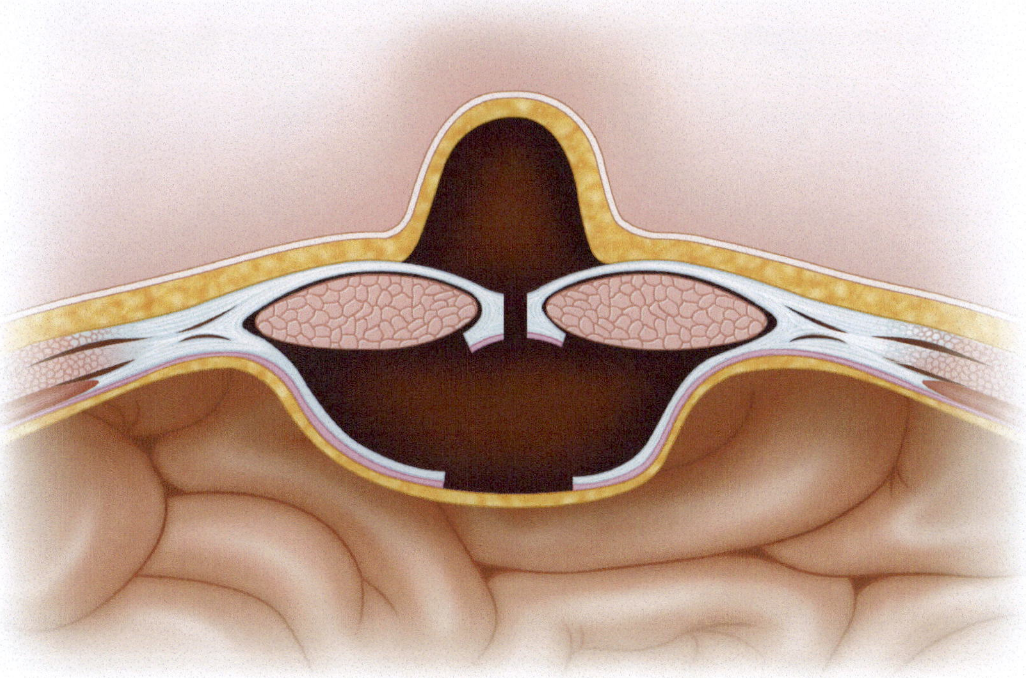

**Fig. 7.23** The large, unified, extraperitoneal space created for placement of the mesh

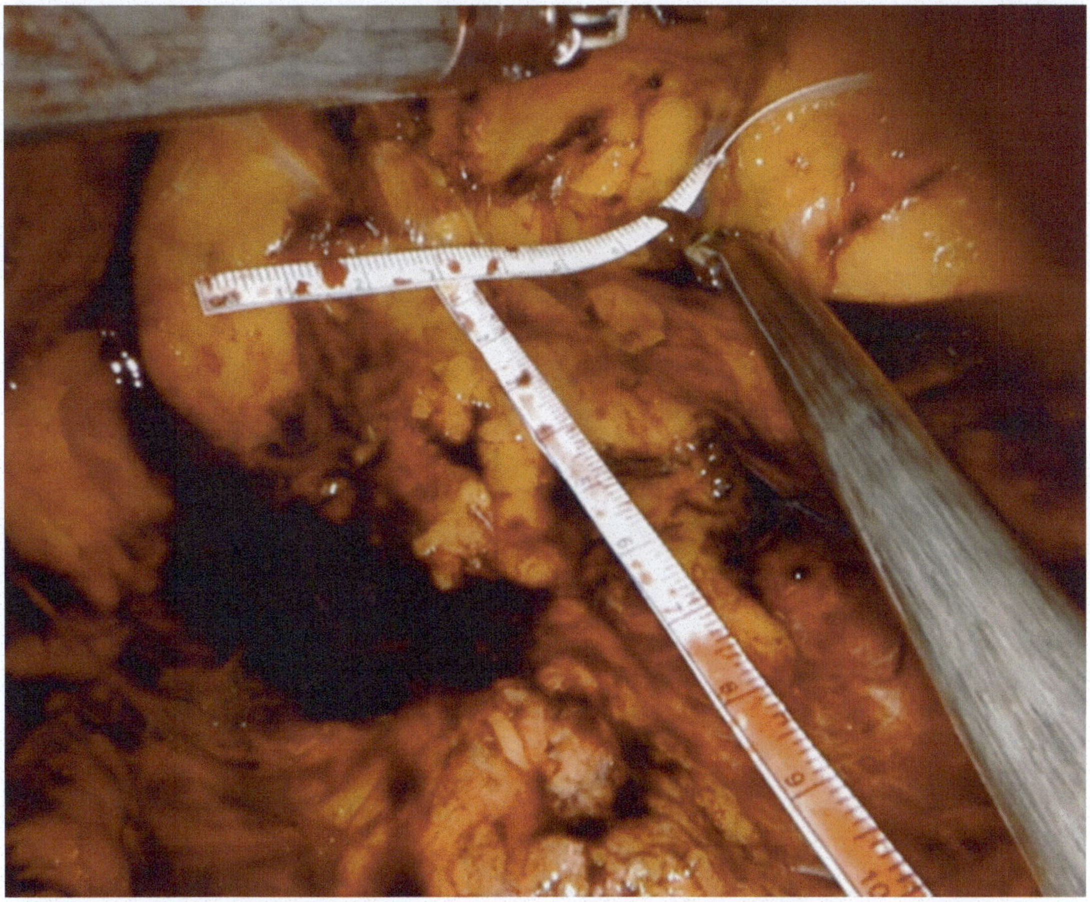

**Fig. 7.24** The "two ruler technique" for measuring large hernia defects

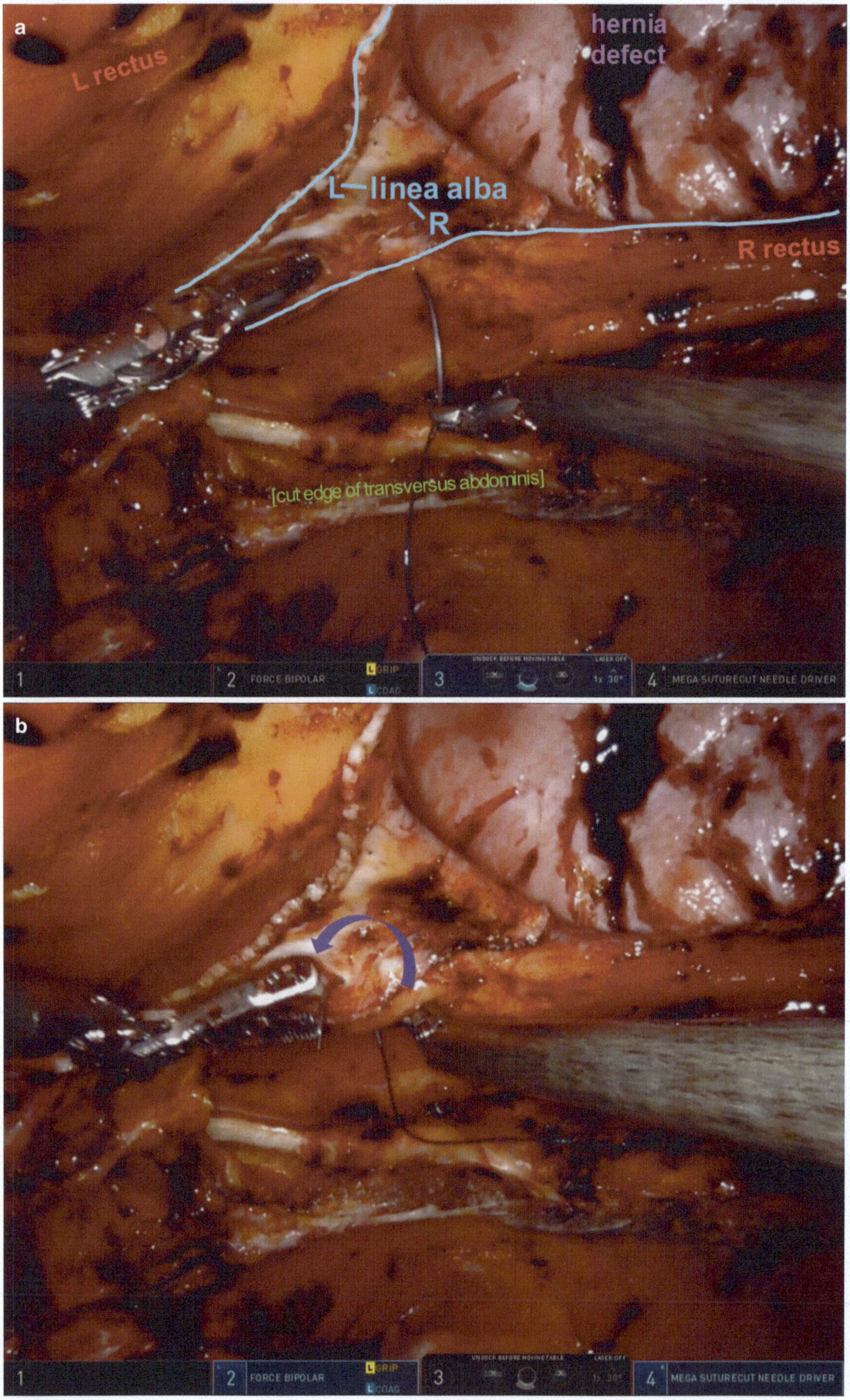


**Fig. 7.25** (**a**–**d**) Closure of the defect/diastasis, re-approximating the rectus sheath

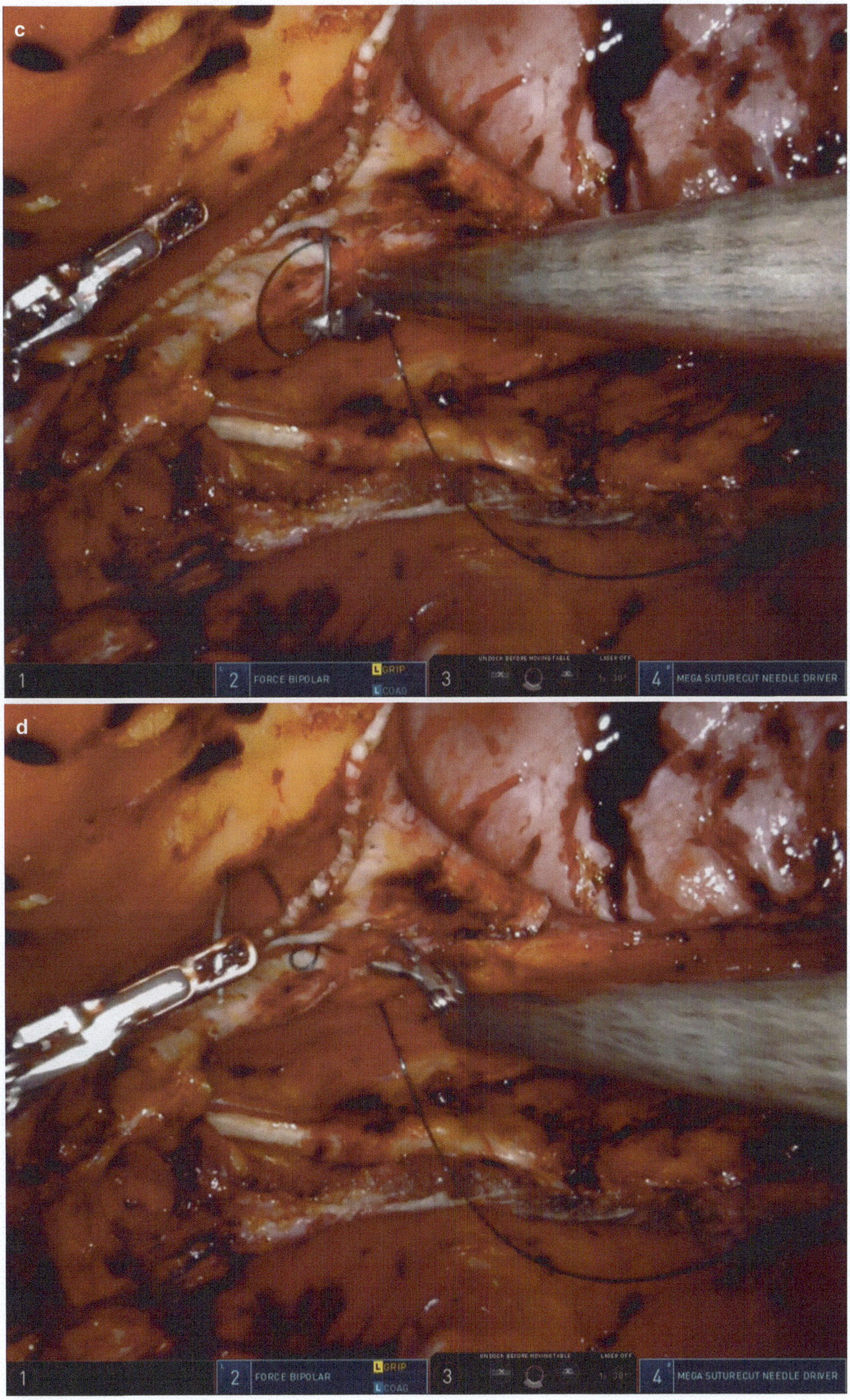


**Fig. 7.25** (continued)

(2) Place the stitches but do not tighten them at this point. When the sutures inevitably run out of length (at least a few will be required), keep track of the sharps by tucking the needle into soft tissue where the sewing was stopped (Fig. 7.26a–c). Leave a small gap between sutures, as you will be able to extend the suture into the gap once cinching begins, gradually distributed over all the sutures. Figure 7.26b and c also illustrate the incorporation of small bites of the hernia pseudosac, we prefer to do during closure of larger defects, in order to reduce the incidence of symptomatic seromas.

(3) Tighten the sutures gradually/sequentially (Fig. 7.27a), and extend suturing into the gap as more suture is freed (Fig. 7.27b and c). Burp the ports periodically to release tension and allow the abdominal wall to medialize.

(4) Now the abdominal wall integrity has been restored by the anterior rectus sheath re-approximation (Fig. 7.28a), and the extraperitoneal space is ready for the retromuscular mesh (Fig. 7.28b).

13. Introduce rolled medium-weight macroporous polypropylene mesh via the 8-mm port, cut to size per measurements from earlier in the case (Fig. 7.29a). (For larger pieces, the port seal cap must be removed.) Note that the ratio of mesh to the hernia area should be 16:1. For the mesh to pass all the way through the port, larger meshes will require pushing by the bedside assistant or technician, as well as pulling from the interior by the surgeon (Fig. 7.29b). Unfurl the mesh (Fig. 7.29c), and suture-fixate it at the edges only if necessary to properly unfurl and situate it. If sutures are required, we use two or three simple interrupted 3-0 Vicryl (Ethicon) stitches (Fig. 7.29d and e). Note that these are secured to small bites of soft tissue only; we do not use transfascial anchoring sutures. The mesh should cover the entire space's surface and sit on the "floor" posteriorly (Fig. 7.29f).

14. Placement of a drain is optional. The authors use drains only when a bilateral TAR has been performed. In those cases, we use a 19Fr Blake drain, exiting through a port site (Fig. 7.30).

15. We do not close the fascia at 8-mm port sites. Skin is closed with 4-0 Monocryl (Ethicon) subcuticular stitches plus skin glue. No dressing is placed (except for a BioPatch in cases with a drain), but the patient is given an abdominal binder (Fig. 7.31).

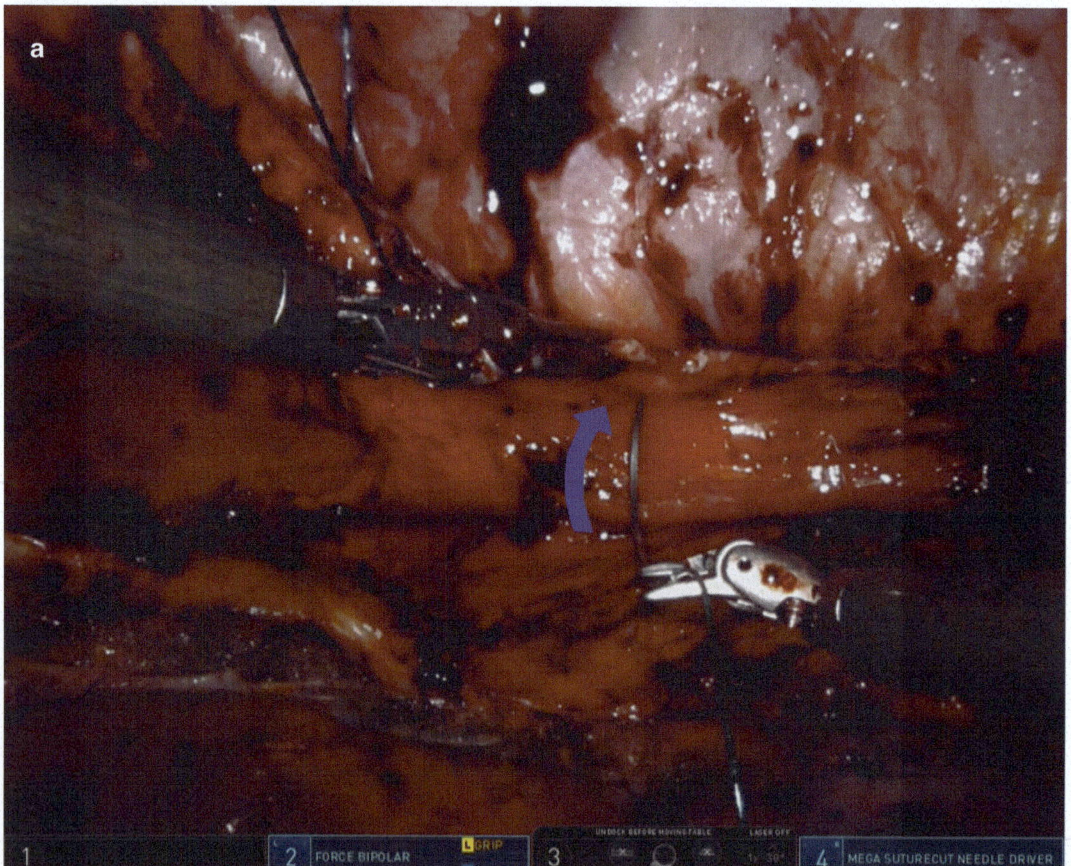


**Fig. 7.26** (**a**) Suture and needle organization by temporarily storing the needles from spent suture in the soft tissue. (**b**) and (**c**) Incorporating small bites of the hernia pseudosac to reduce the incidence of symptomatic seromas (*dotted circles*)

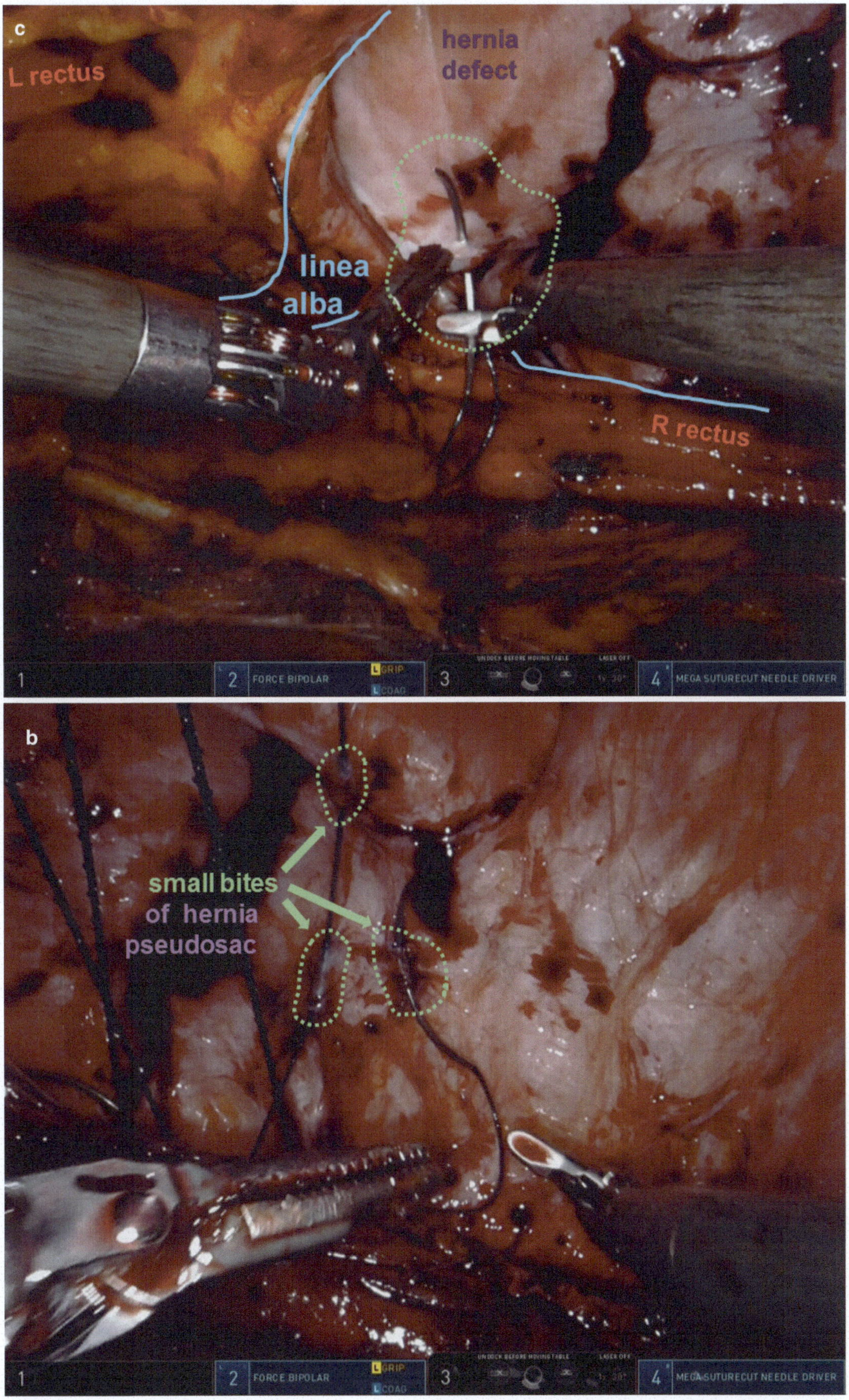


**Fig. 7.26** (continued)

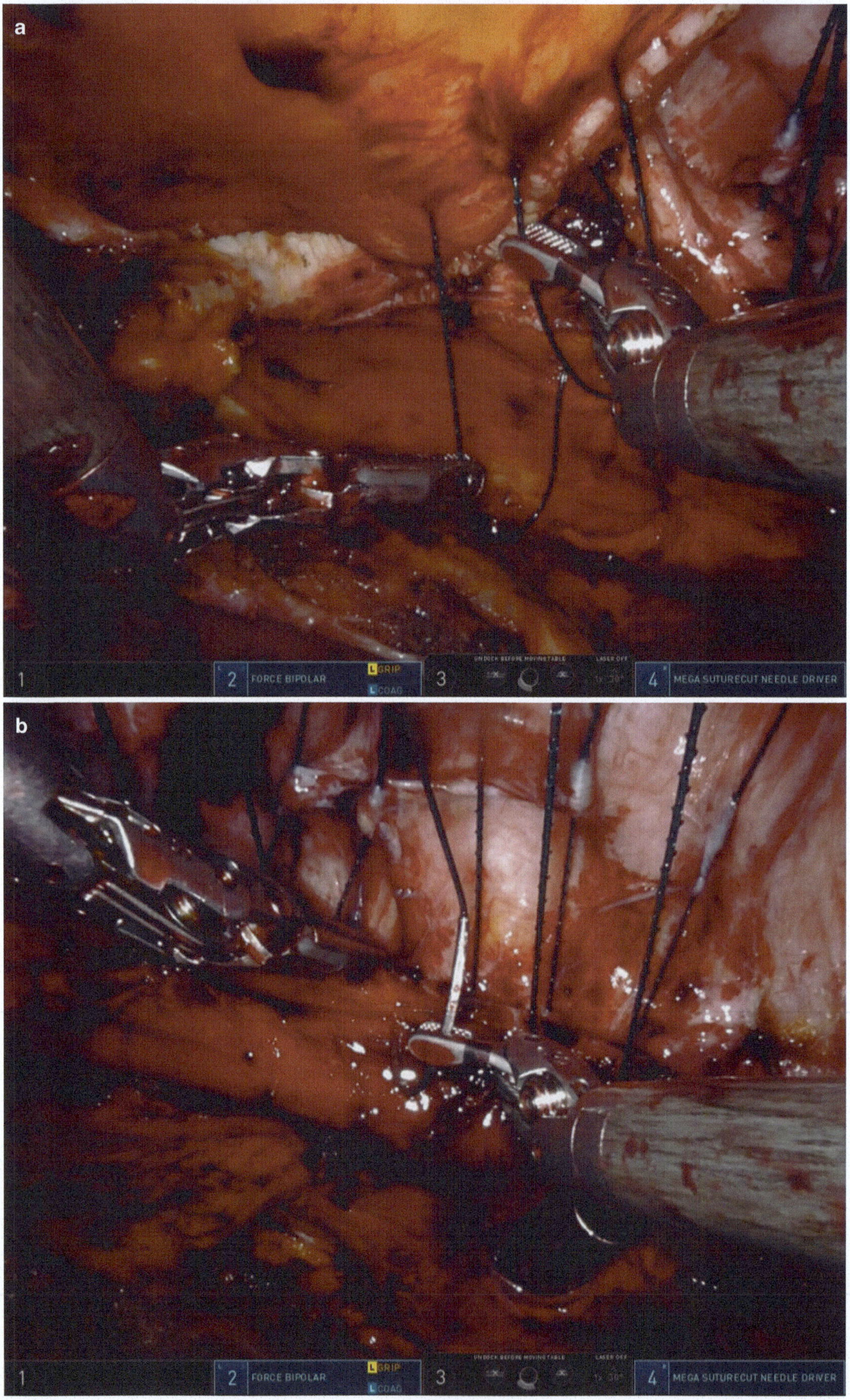


**Fig. 7.27** (**a**–**c**) Cinching of the sutures and extending suturing into the gaps

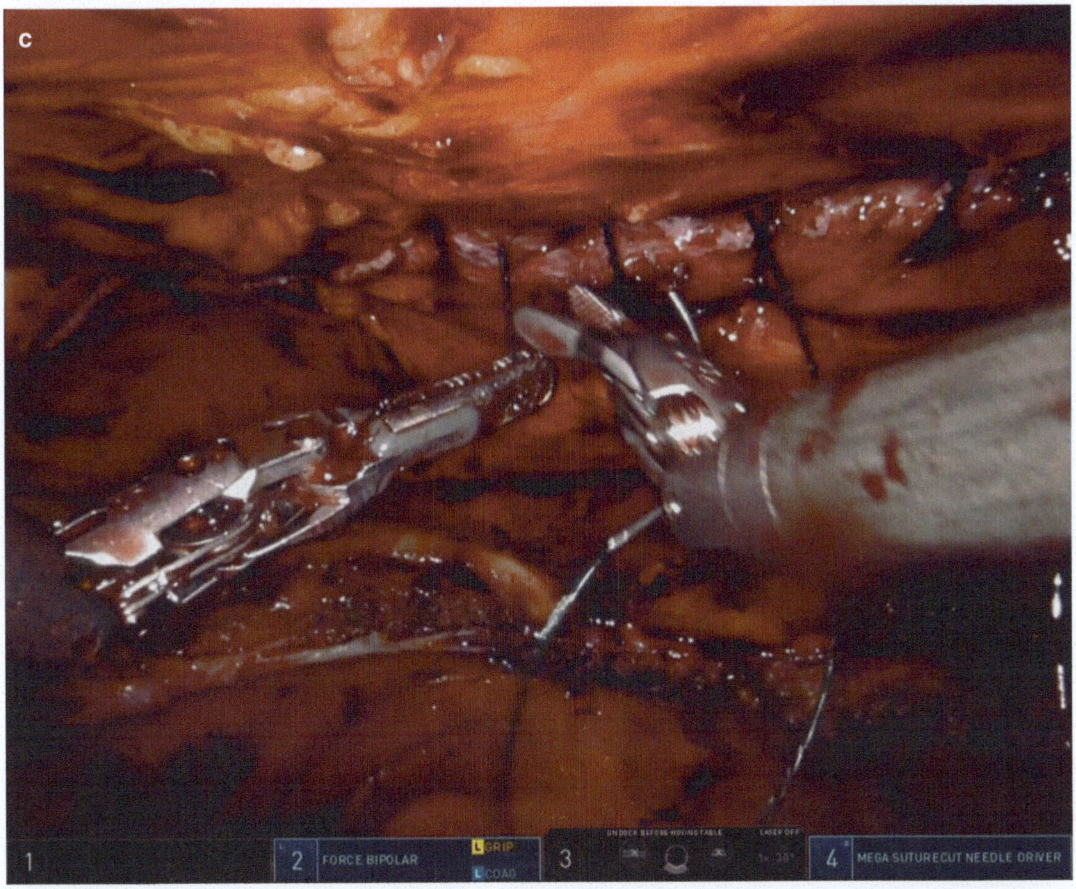


**Fig. 7.27** (continued)

a

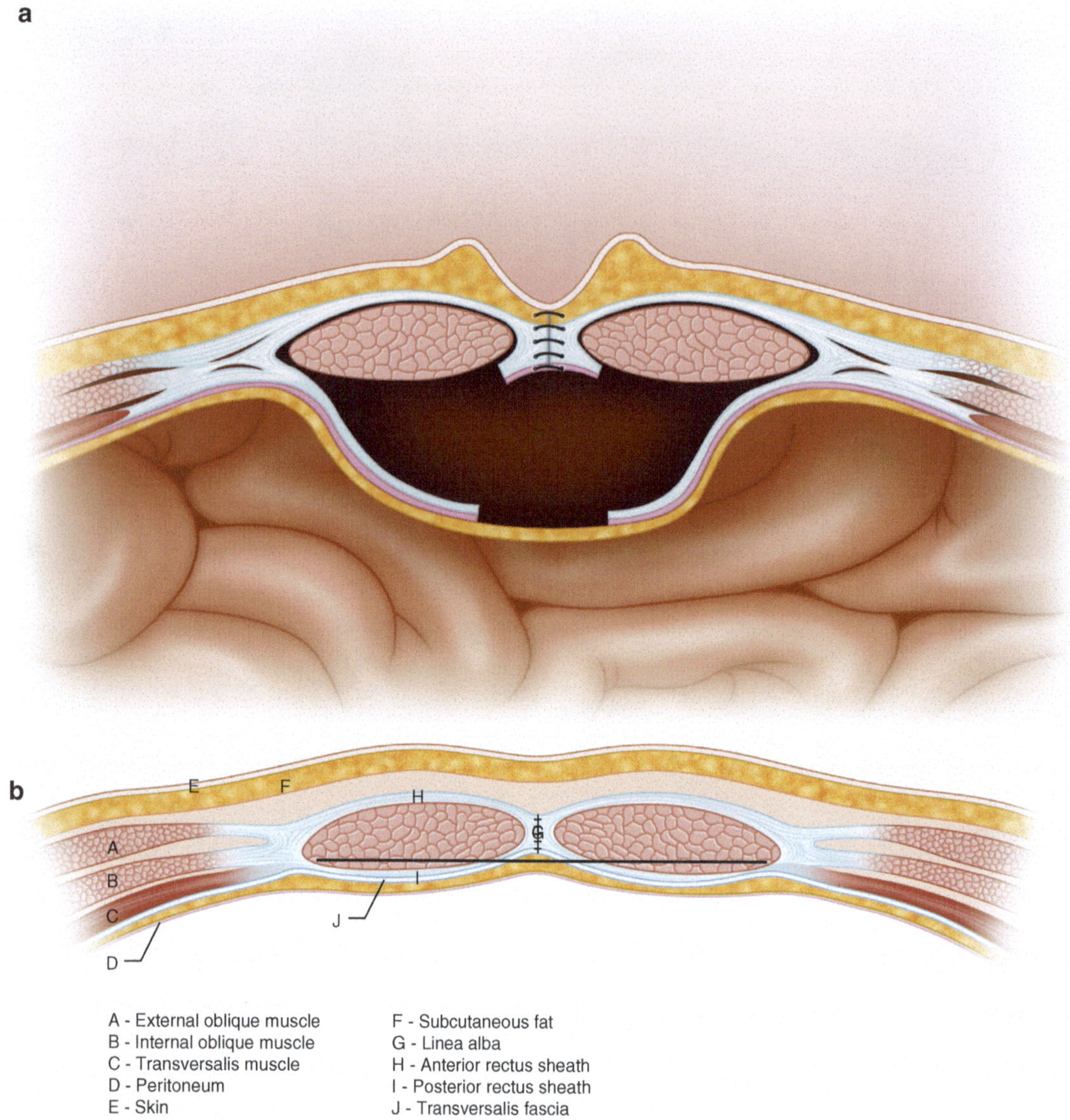


**Fig. 7.28** (**a**) Anterior rectus sheath re-approximation. (**b**) Extraperitoneal space ready for the retromuscular mesh. Note that the contralateral ports seen in some of these photos were placed in order to perform a bilateral transversus abdominis release (TAR) in this case and are otherwise unnecessary for the technique we describe

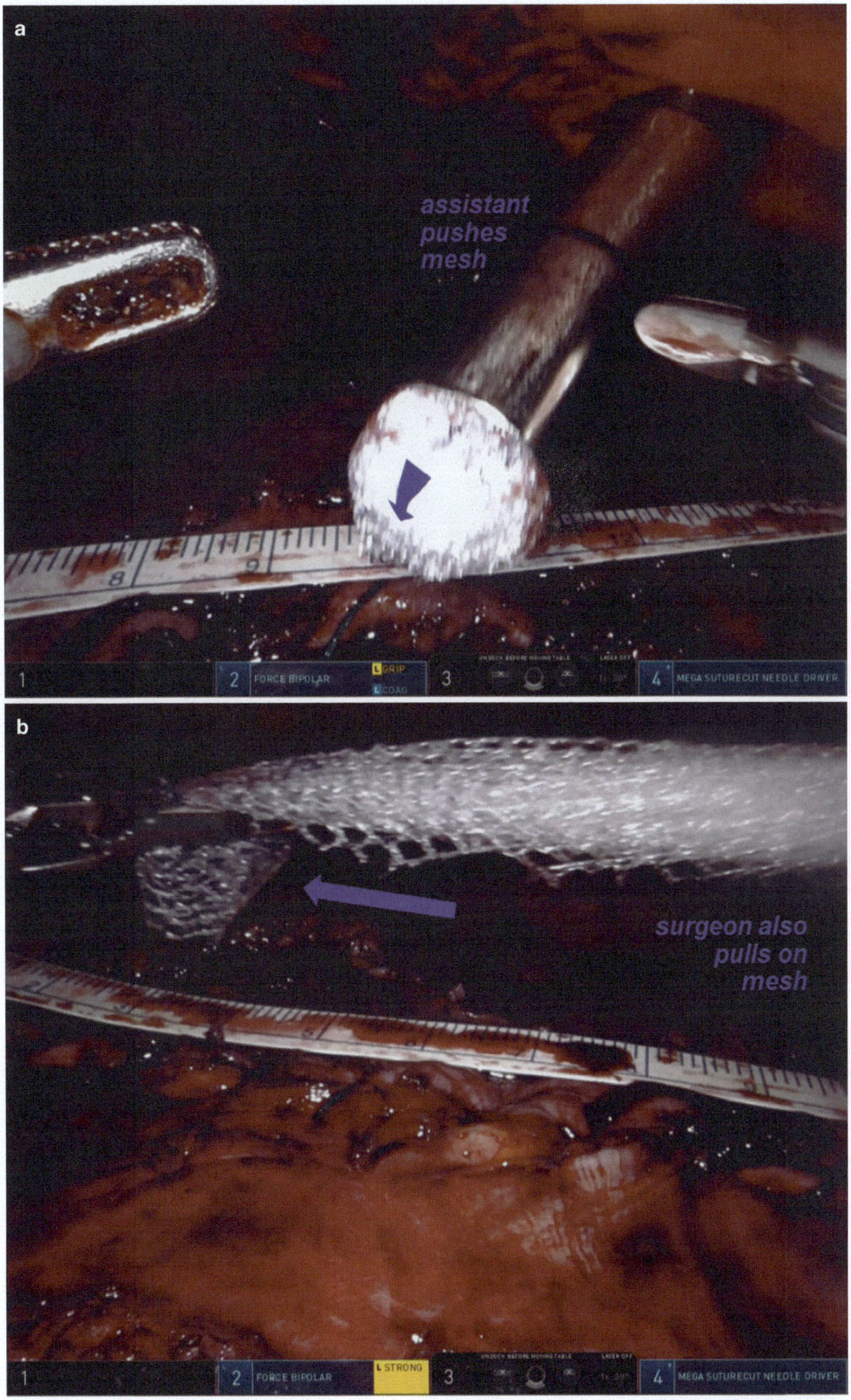


**Fig. 7.29** (**a**) and (**b**) Introduction of the mesh. (**c**) Unfurling the mesh. (**d**) and (**e**) Anchoring the mesh, only if necessary to unfurl and situate it. (**f**) Proper placement of the mesh

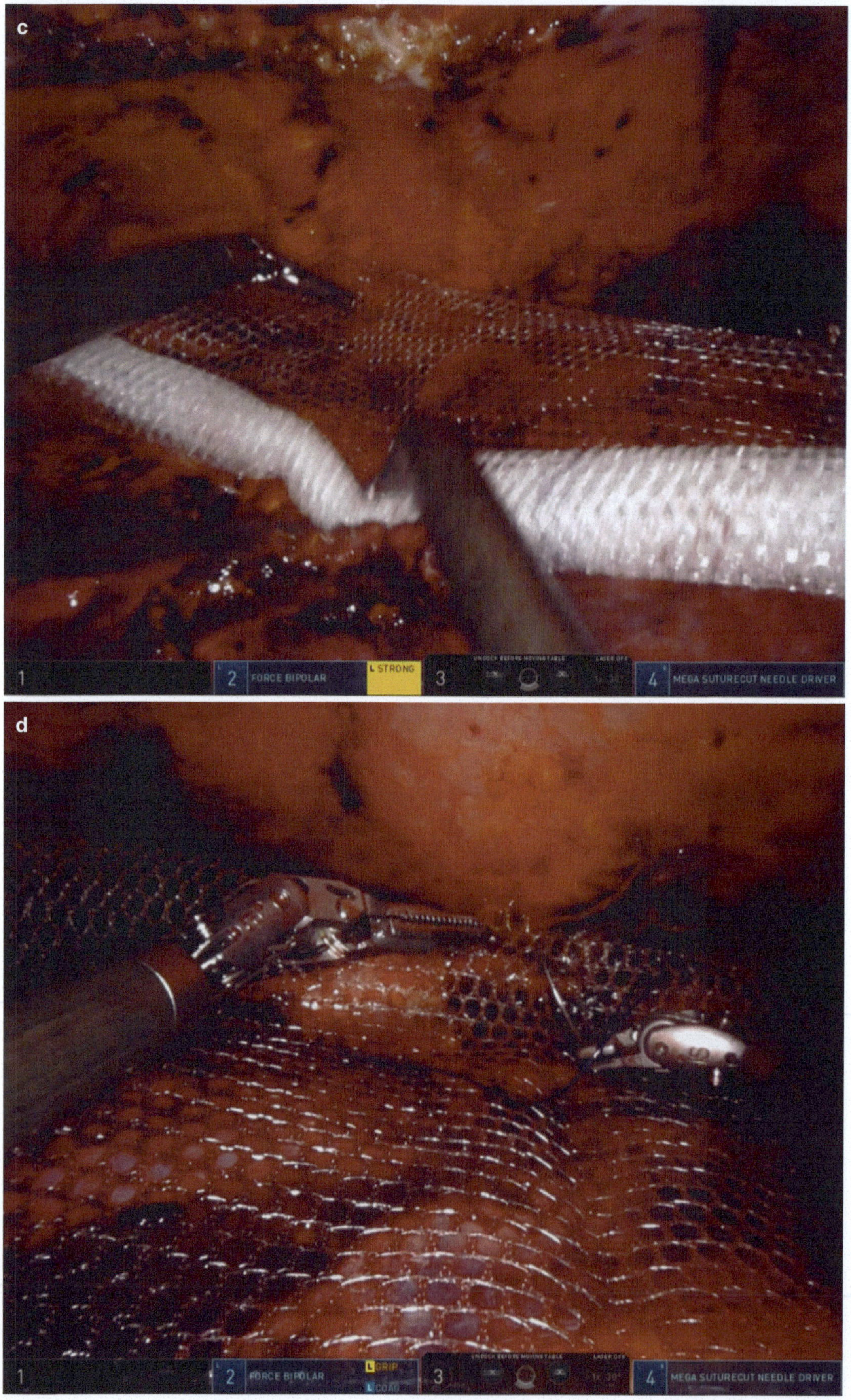


**Fig. 7.29** (continued)

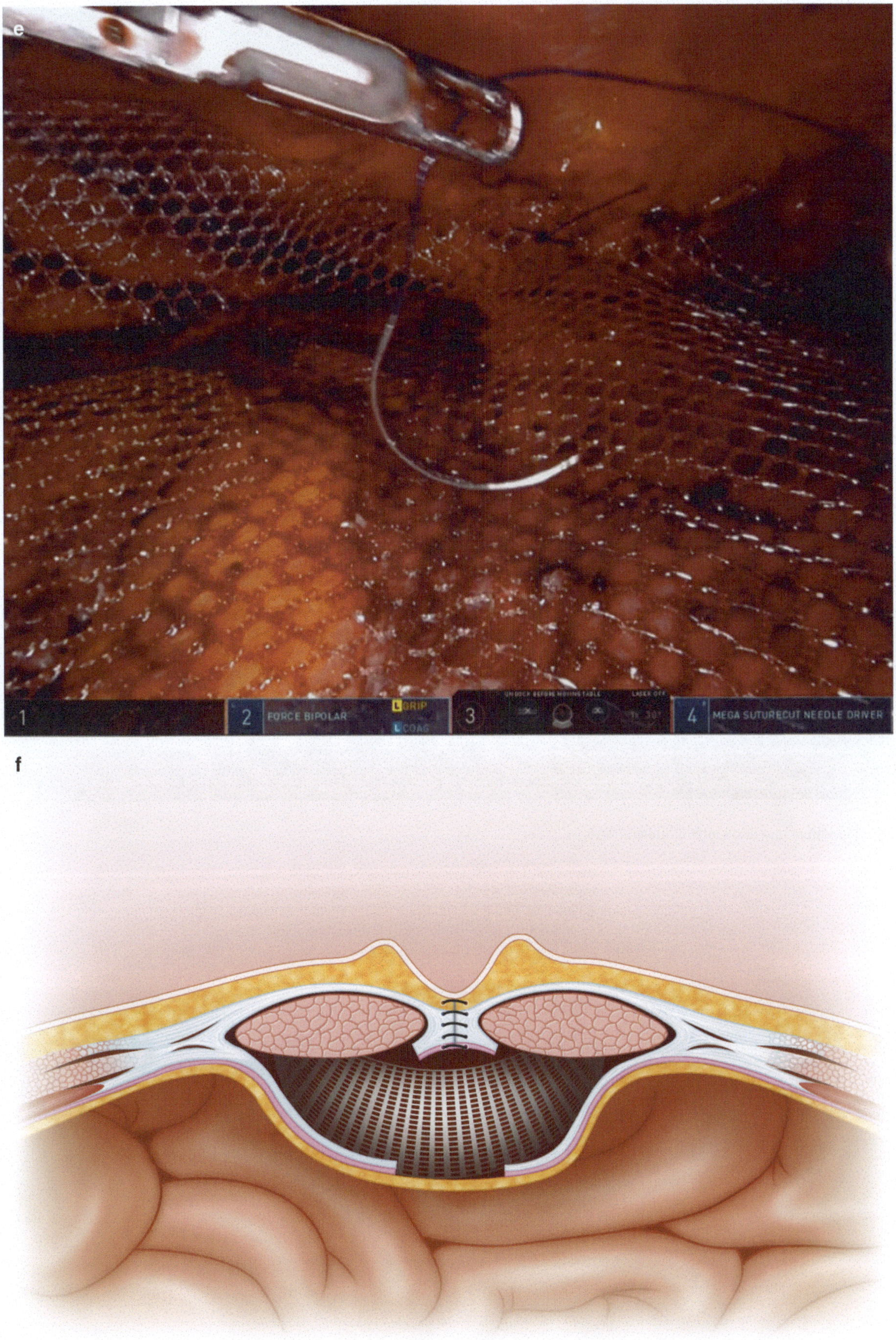


**Fig. 7.29** (continued)

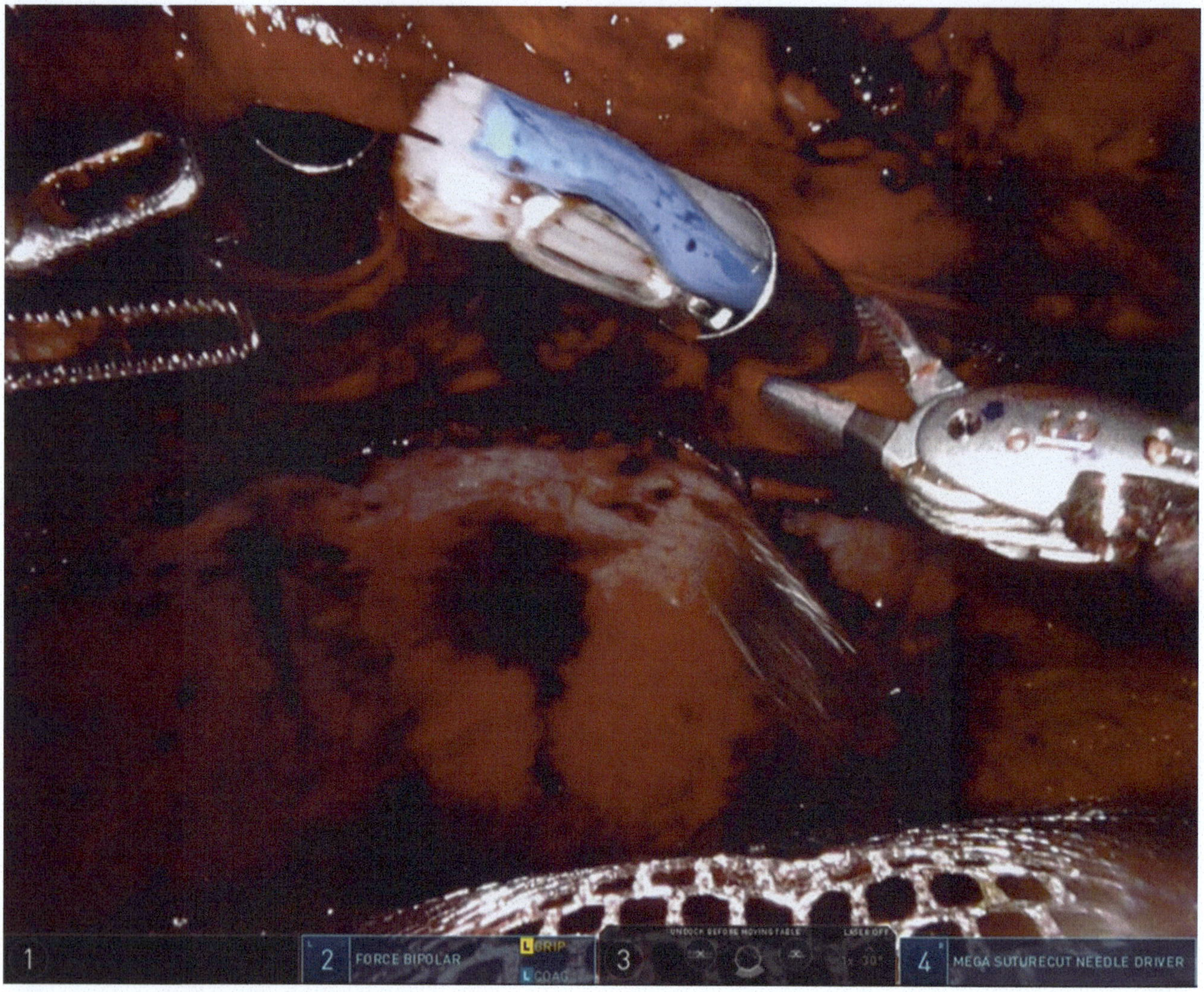


Fig. 7.30 Placement of a drain after a bilateral TAR

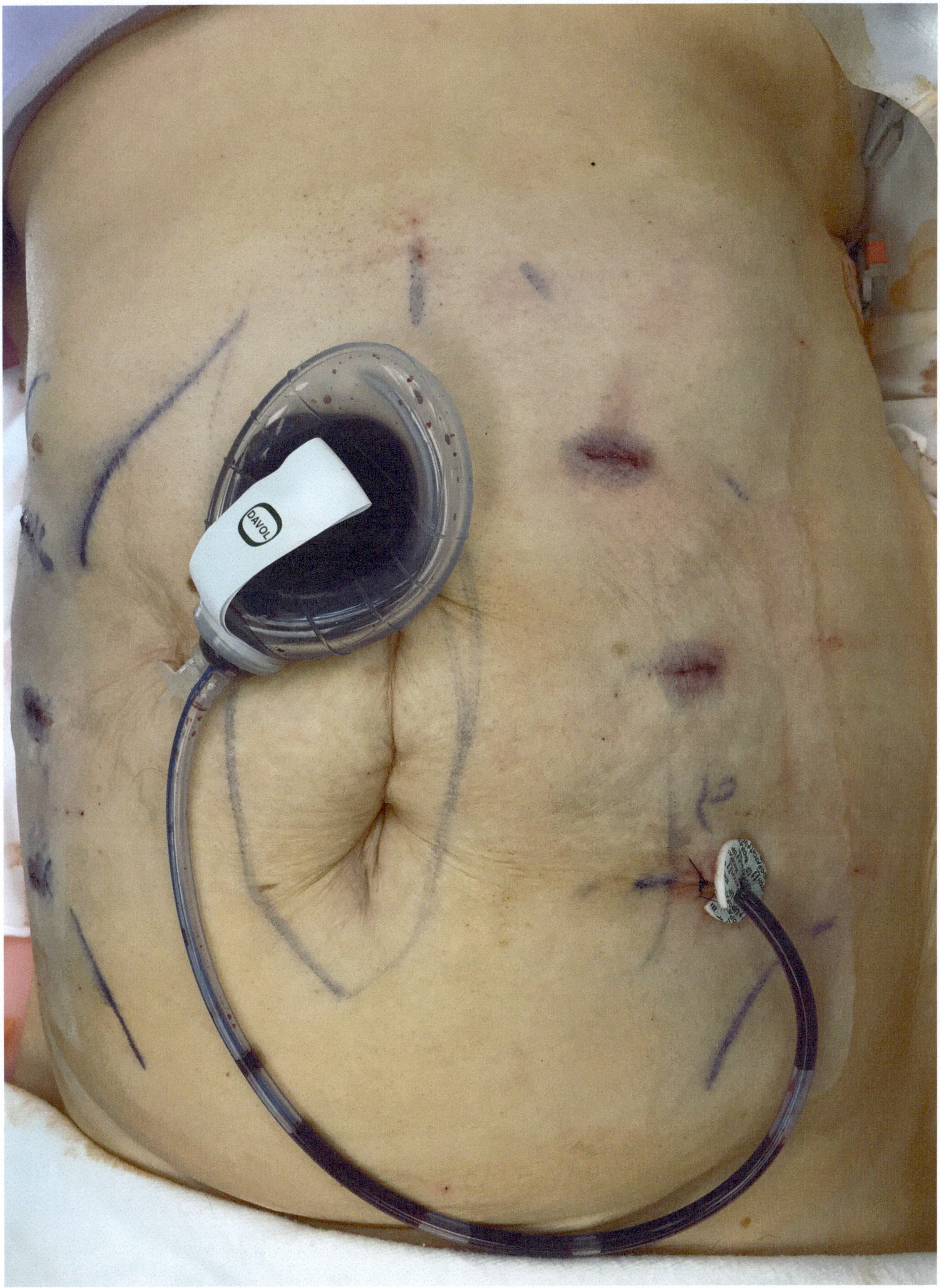


**Fig. 7.31** Skin closure and dressings, with drain

## References

1. Radu VG. Retromuscular approach in ventral hernia repair: endoscopic Rives-Stoppa procedure. Chirurgia. 2019;114:109. https://doi.org/10.21614/chirurgia.114.1.109.
2. Maman D, Greenwald D, Kreniske J, Royston A, Powers S, Bauer J. Modified Rives-Stoppa technique for repair of complex incisional hernias in 59 patients. Ann Plast Surg. 2012;68:190–3. https://doi.org/10.1097/sap.0b013e318212f380.
3. Bauer J, Harris M, Gorfine S, Kreel I. Rives-Stoppa procedure for repair of large incisional hernias: experience with 57 patients. Hernia. 2002;6:120–3. https://doi.org/10.1007/s10029-002-0071-3.
4. Cox TC, Pearl JP, Ritter EM. Rives-Stoppa incisional hernia repair combined with laparoscopic separation of abdominal wall components: a novel approach to complex abdominal wall closure. Hernia. 2010;14:561–7. https://doi.org/10.1007/s10029-010-0704-x.
5. Tastaldi L, Alkhatib H. Incisional hernia repair. Surg Clin North Am. 2018;98:511–35. https://doi.org/10.1016/j.suc.2018.02.006.
6. Warren JA, Love M. Incisional hernia repair. Surg Clin North Am. 2018;98:537–59. https://doi.org/10.1016/j.suc.2018.01.008.

## Suggested Reading

Belyansky I, Reza Zahiri H, Sanford Z, Weltz AS, Park A. Early operative outcomes of endoscopic (eTEP access) robotic-assisted retromuscular abdominal wall hernia repair. Hernia. 2018;22:837–47. https://doi.org/10.1007/s10029-018-1795-z.

Gokcal F, Morrison S, Kudsi OY. Robotic retromuscular ventral hernia repair and transversus abdominis release: short-term outcomes and risk factors associated with perioperative complications. Hernia. 2019;23(2):375–85. https://doi.org/10.1007/s10029-019-01911-1.

Liu R. Dr Rockson Liu [YouTube Channel]. Retrieved from https://www.youtube.com/channel/UCfr51Rf6cQWnZ2dqY7TskxQ/videos.

# Robotic Subcostal Hernia Repair: Totally Extraperitoneal (TEP)

8

Naseem Bou-Ayash, Fahri Gokcal, and Omar Yusef Kudsi

## Introduction

Subcostal hernias are atypical hernias, which may be difficult to repair using traditional methods such as open onlay repair. The difficulty is mainly due to the proximity of the hernia to the costal margin, which limits the space needed for adequate defect closure, mesh fixation, and mesh overlap. Minimally invasive subcostal hernia repair can be achieved with both intraperitoneal and extraperitoneal mesh placement techniques. Although the intraperitoneal onlay mesh (IPOM) technique is commonly adopted for a variety of midline hernias [1], the repair of subcostal hernias may prove challenging with an intraperitoneal approach because of their proximity to vital structures, especially at the stage of mesh fixation.

On the other hand, extraperitoneal methods such as the totally extraperitoneal retromuscular technique (TEP-RM) with transversus abdominis release (TAR) may provide a wide workspace which can comfortably accommodate the mesh, thereby allowing for greater mesh overlap and ultimately improved patient outcomes. Moreover, TEP-RM can eliminate the need for any mesh fixation, because the mesh is to be held in place between the rectus abdominis and posterior sheath. The robotic platform allows for greater precision and control while dissecting the retrorectus space and has been shown to achieve favorable results in TEP-RM repair [2].

## Procedure: Illustrated Steps

Figures 8.1, 8.2, 8.3, 8.4, 8.5, 8.6, 8.7, 8.8, 8.9, 8.10, 8.11, 8.12, 8.13, 8.14, 8.15, 8.16, 8.17, 8.18, 8.19, 8.20, 8.21, 8.22, 8.23, 8.24, 8.25, 8.26, 8.27, 8.28, 8.29, 8.30, 8.31, 8.32, 8.33, 8.34, 8.35, 8.36, 8.37, 8.38, 8.39, 8.40, 8.41, 8.42, 8.43, 8.44, 8.45, 8.46, and 8.47 illustrate the technical aspects of robotic subcostal TEP-RM repair with adjunctive TAR.

N. Bou-Ayash · F. Gokcal
Department of Surgery, Good Samaritan Medical Center, Brockton, MA, USA

O. Y. Kudsi (✉)
Department of Surgery, Good Samaritan Medical Center, Tufts University School of Medicine, Boston, MA, USA


O. Y. Kudsi (ed.), *Robotic Hernia Surgery*, https://doi.org/10.1007/978-3-030-46667-1_8

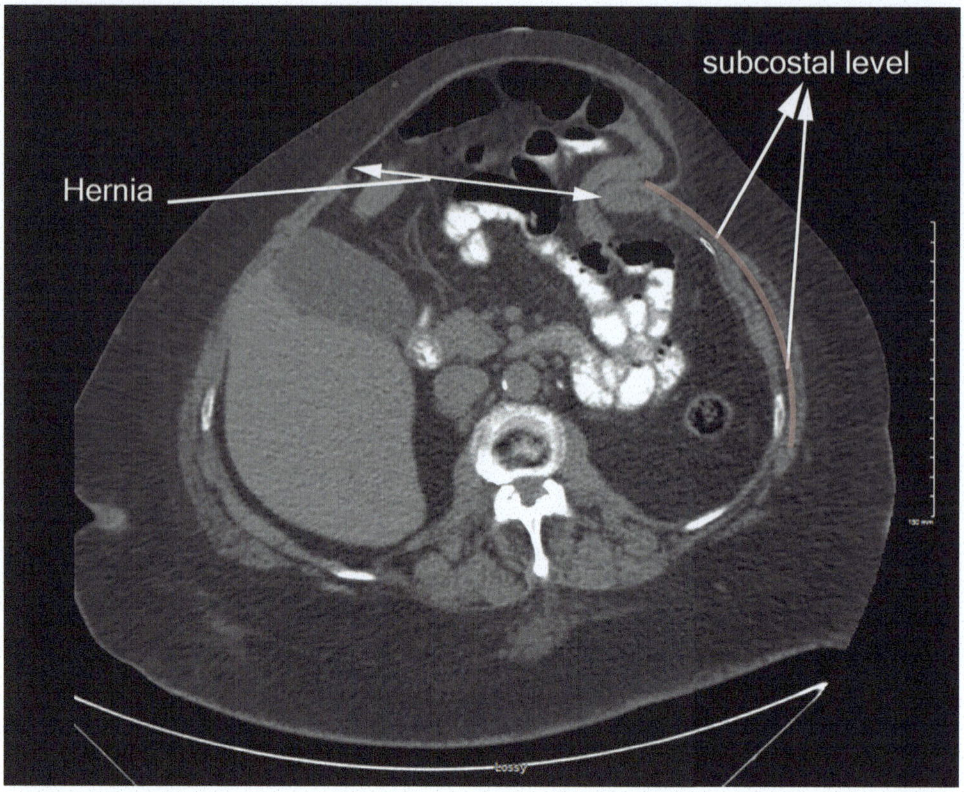


**Fig. 8.1** Computerized tomography (CT) scan (transverse) showing the subcostal hernia traversing the left rectus muscle

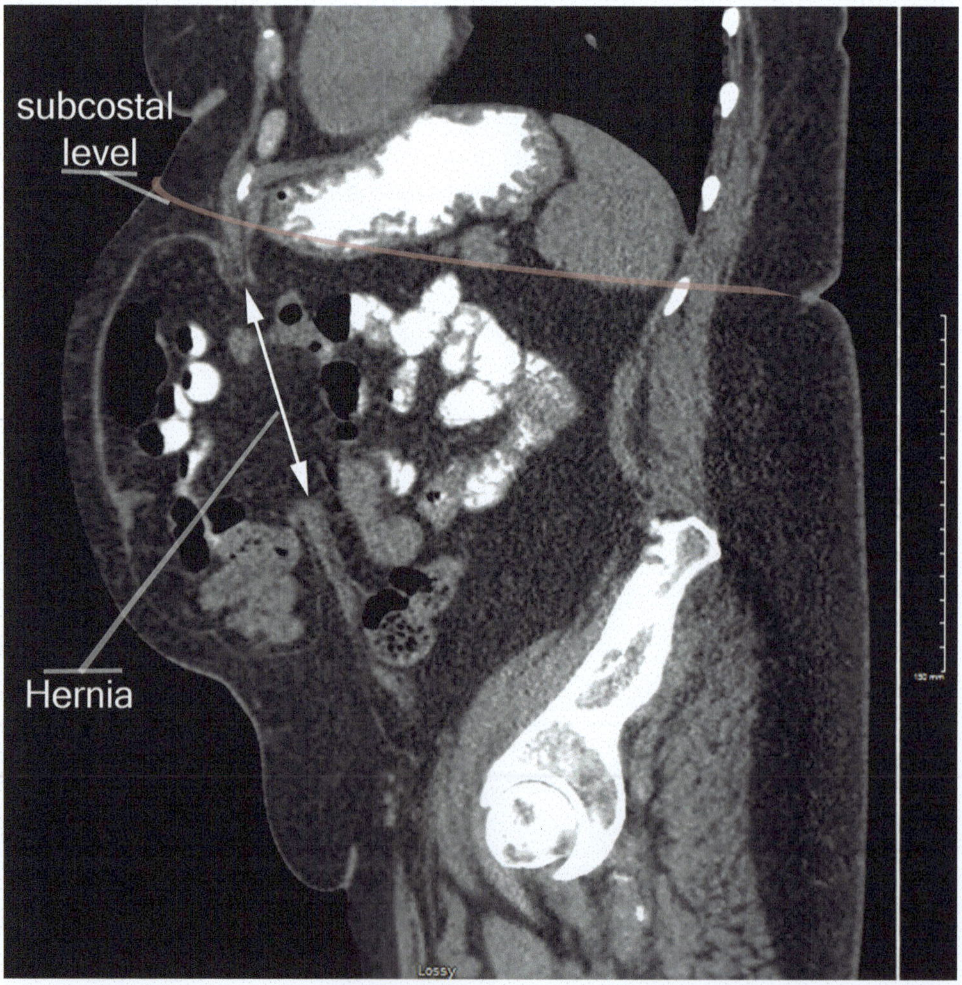


**Fig. 8.2** CT scan (sagittal) showing the bowel-containing large hernia below the costal margin

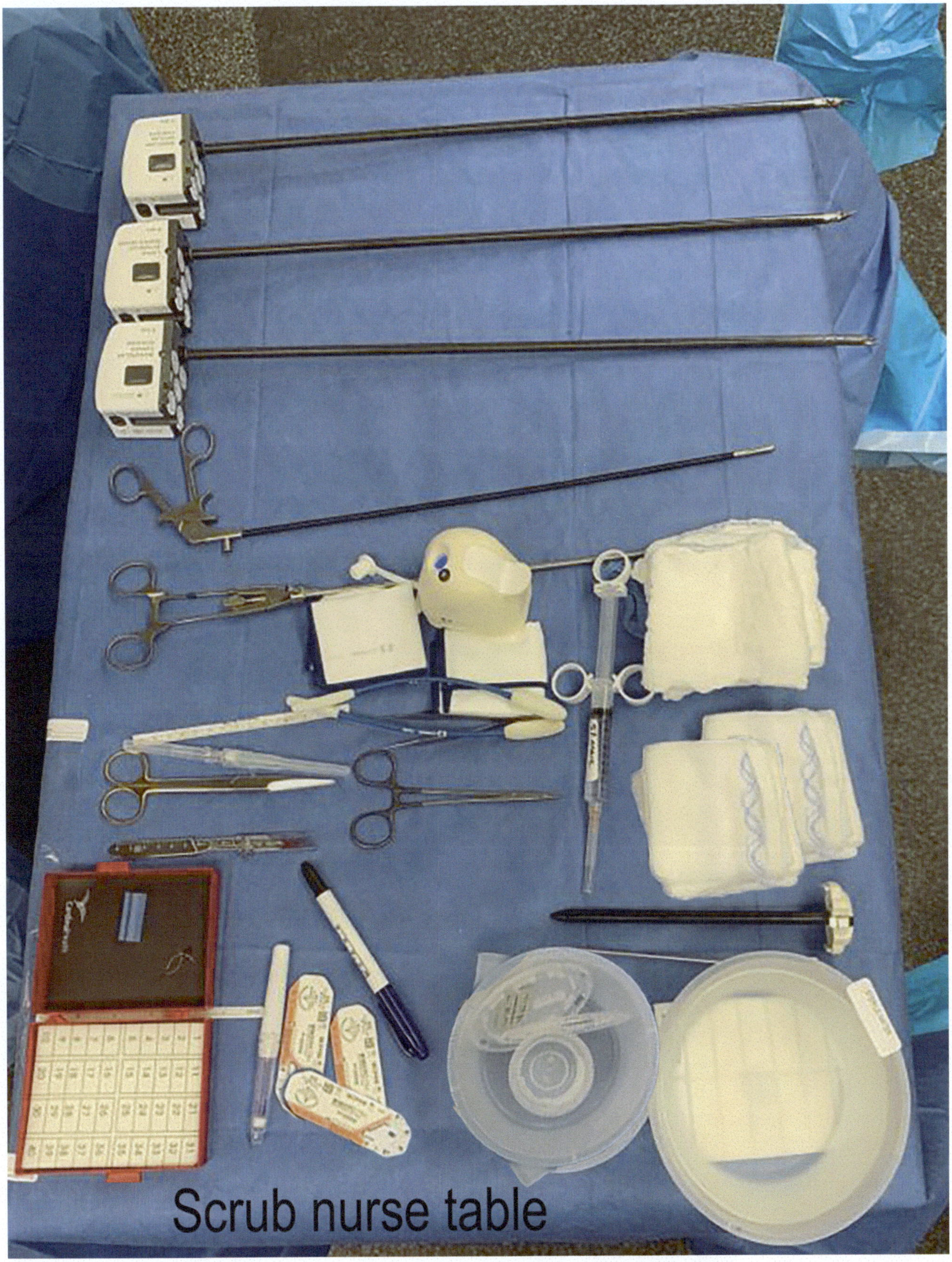


**Fig. 8.3** Scrub nurse table setup with the robotic and open instruments, including monopolar scissors, bipolar fenestrated forceps, and needle driver

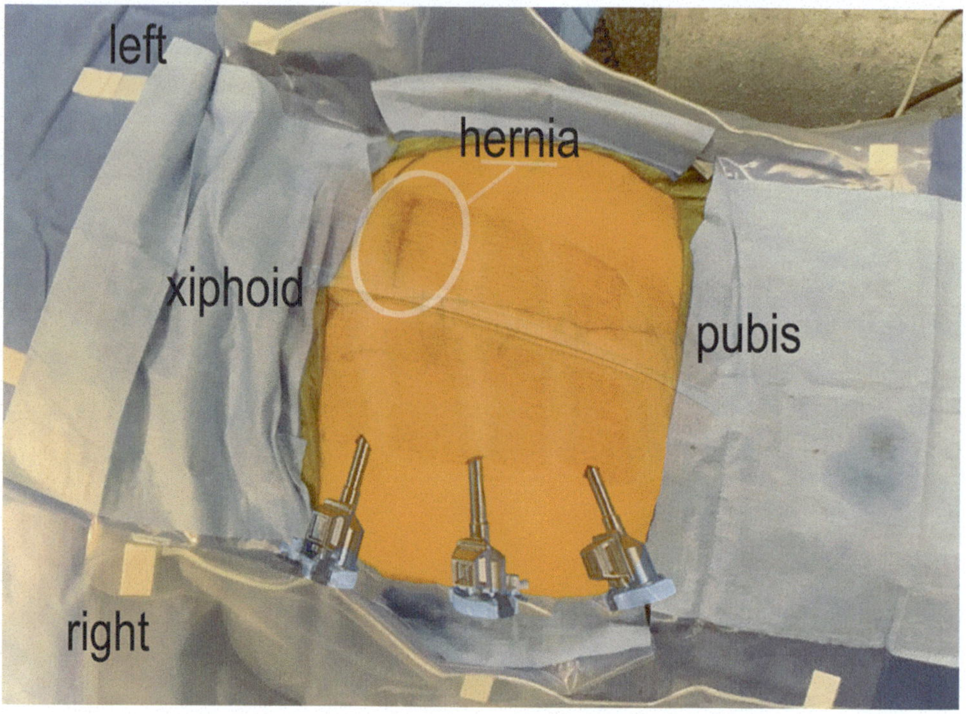


**Fig. 8.4** The hernia area is demarcated, along with the trocar insertion sites

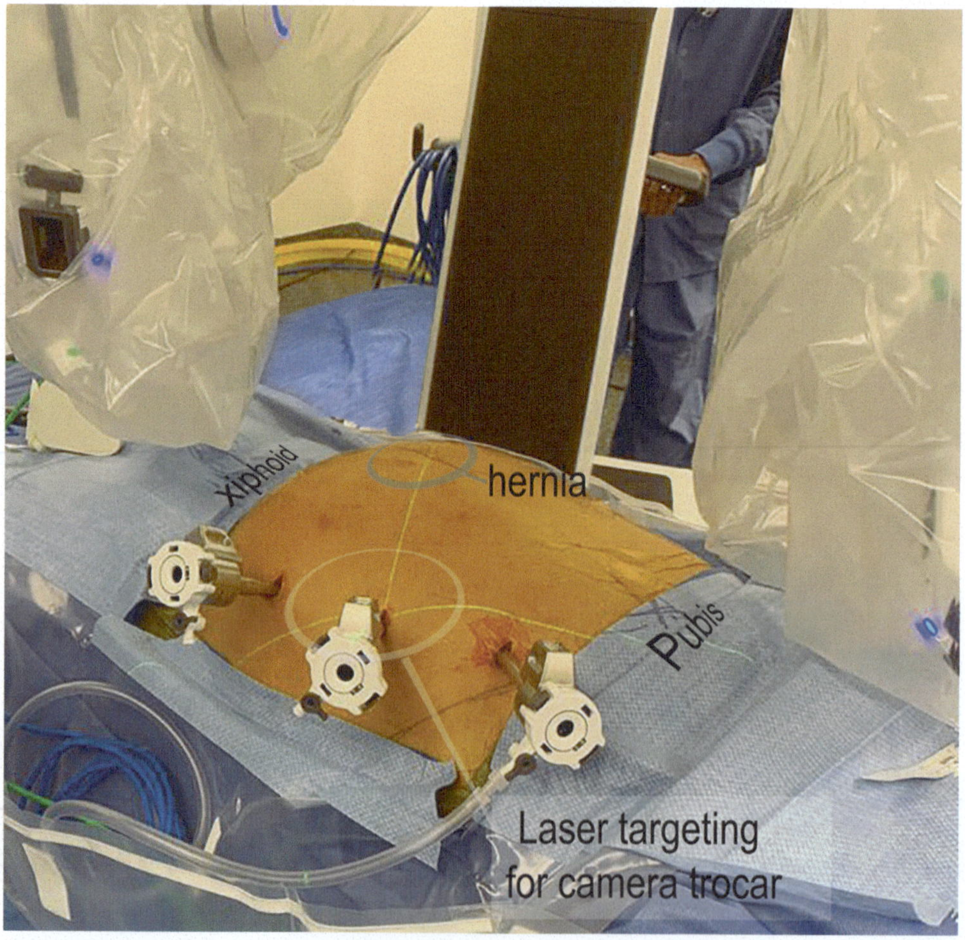


**Fig. 8.5** After totally extraperitoneal (TEP) access is achieved (described in Chap. 3), the patient-side cart of the robot is advanced by an assistant with the guidance of the surgeon. Laser targeting is used to identify the camera trocar insertion point. Once the arms are docked, the surgical target is selected and the system automatically positions the boom to allow for optimal arm configuration

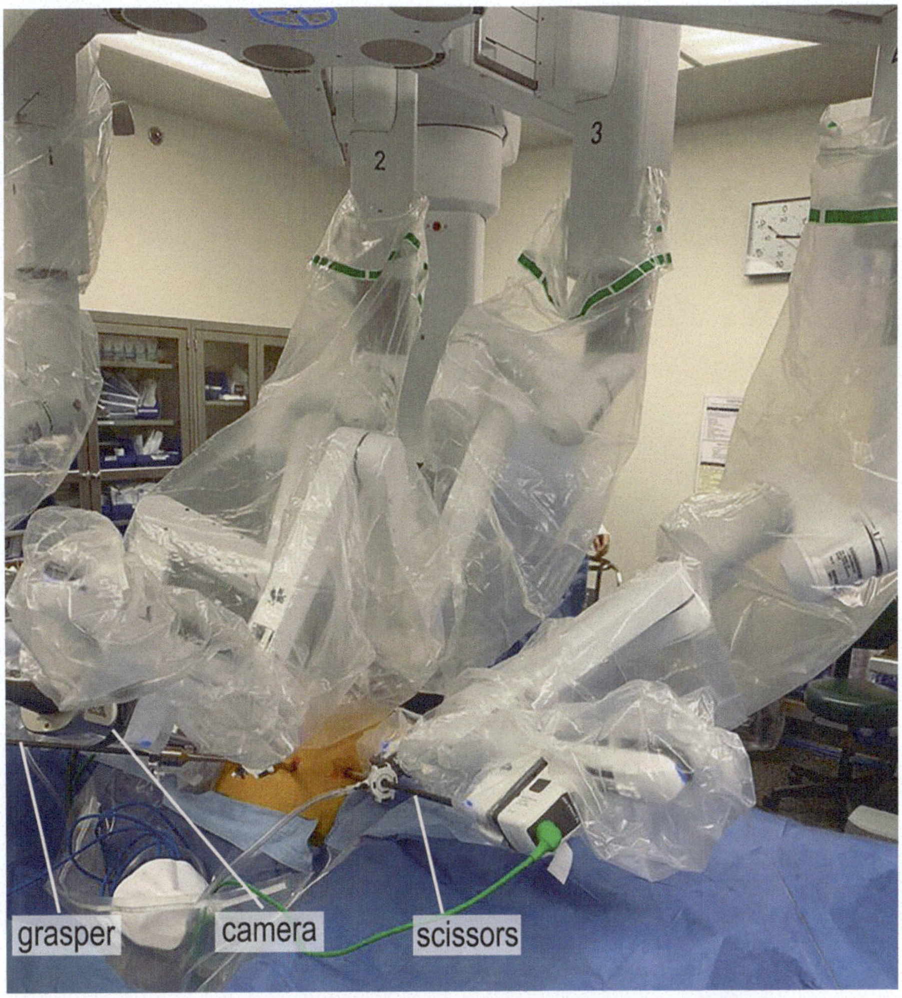


**Fig. 8.6** External view after docking, showing the scissors with the right robotic arm and the grasper with the left robotic arm

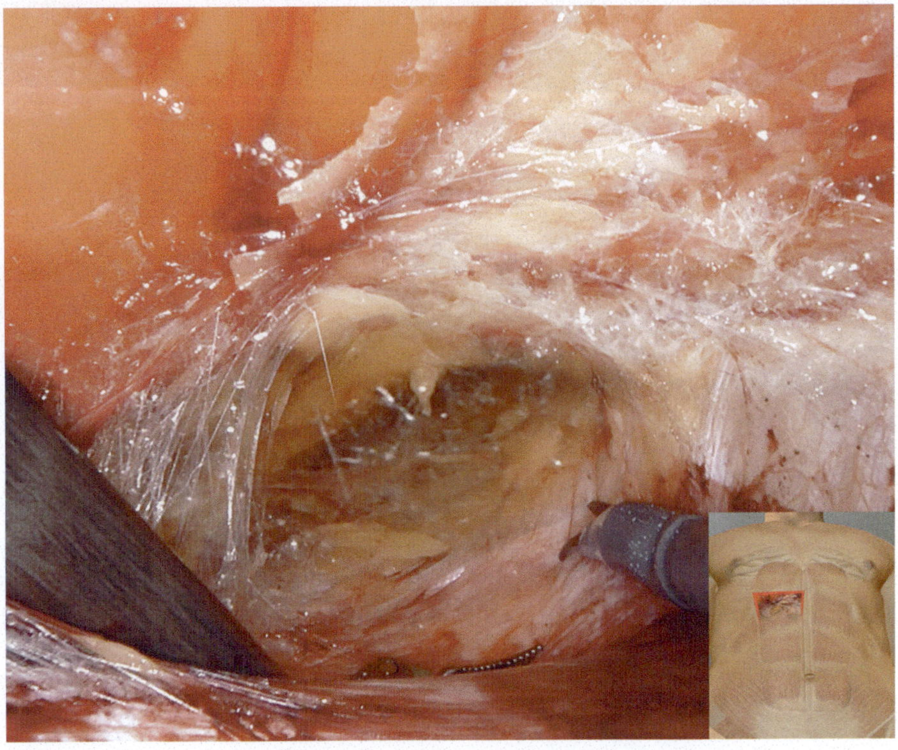

**Fig. 8.7** The right retrorectus space is entered and loose connective tissue is dissected

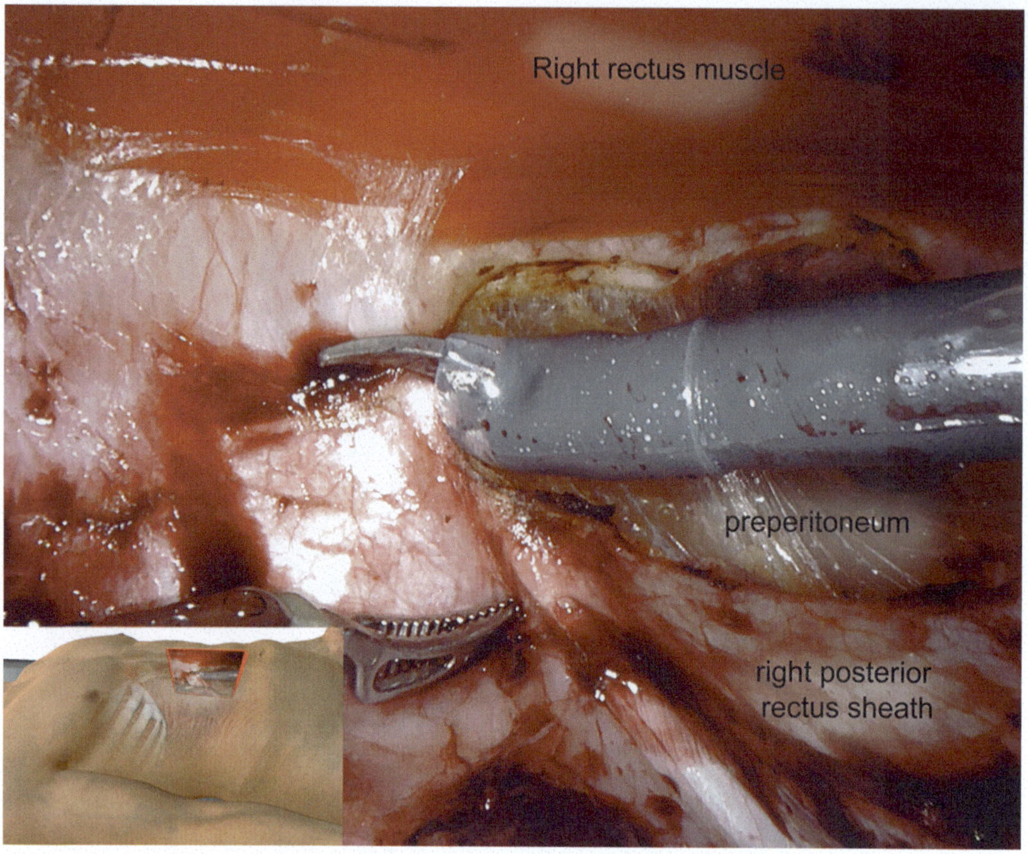


**Fig. 8.8** After ipsilateral retrorectus dissection is performed, the medial aspect of the rectus sheath is divided to enter the preperitoneal space inferior to the linea alba

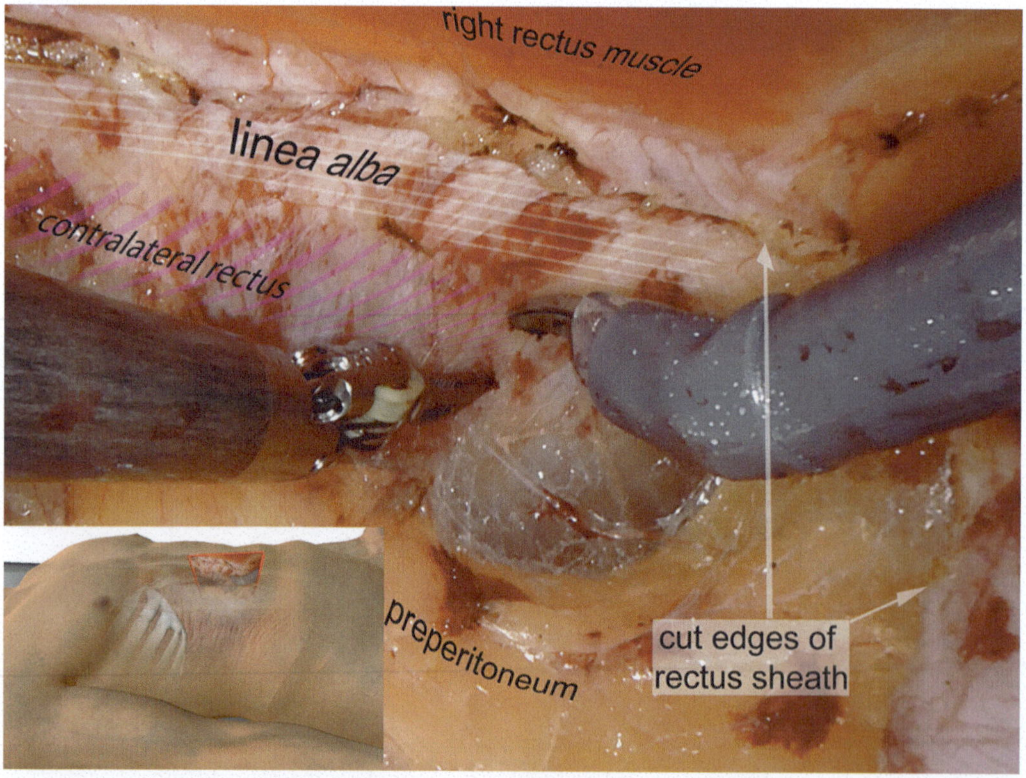


**Fig. 8.9** The medial part of the contralateral posterior rectus sheath is incised to complete crossover

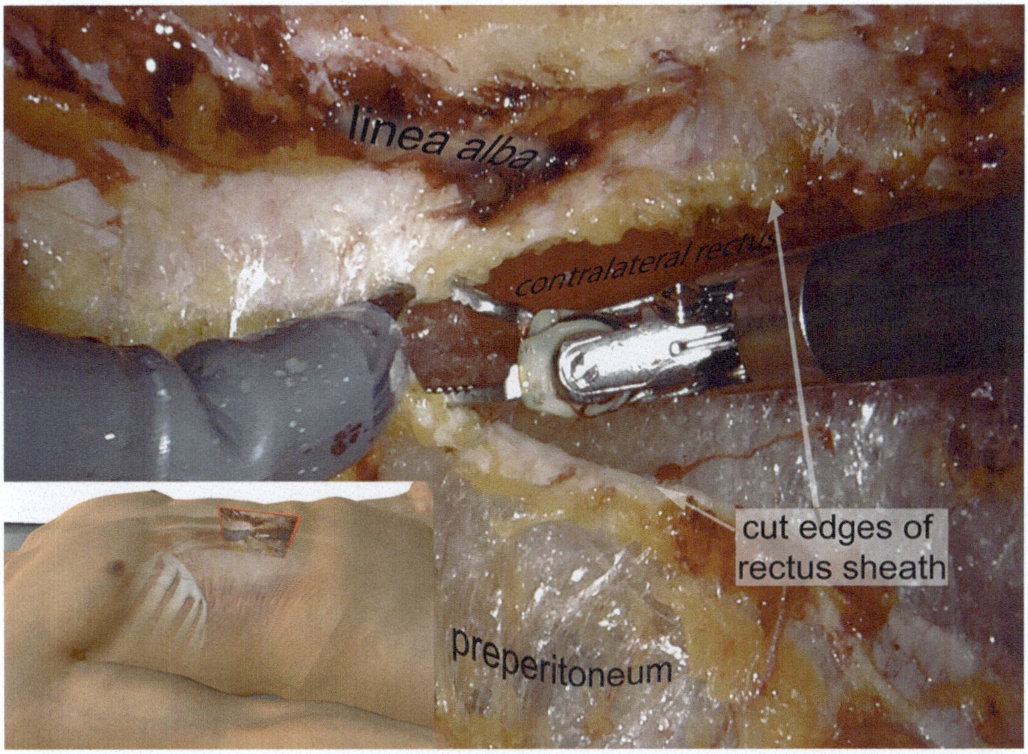


**Fig. 8.10** Contralateral rectus sheath dissection is continued in the cranial direction

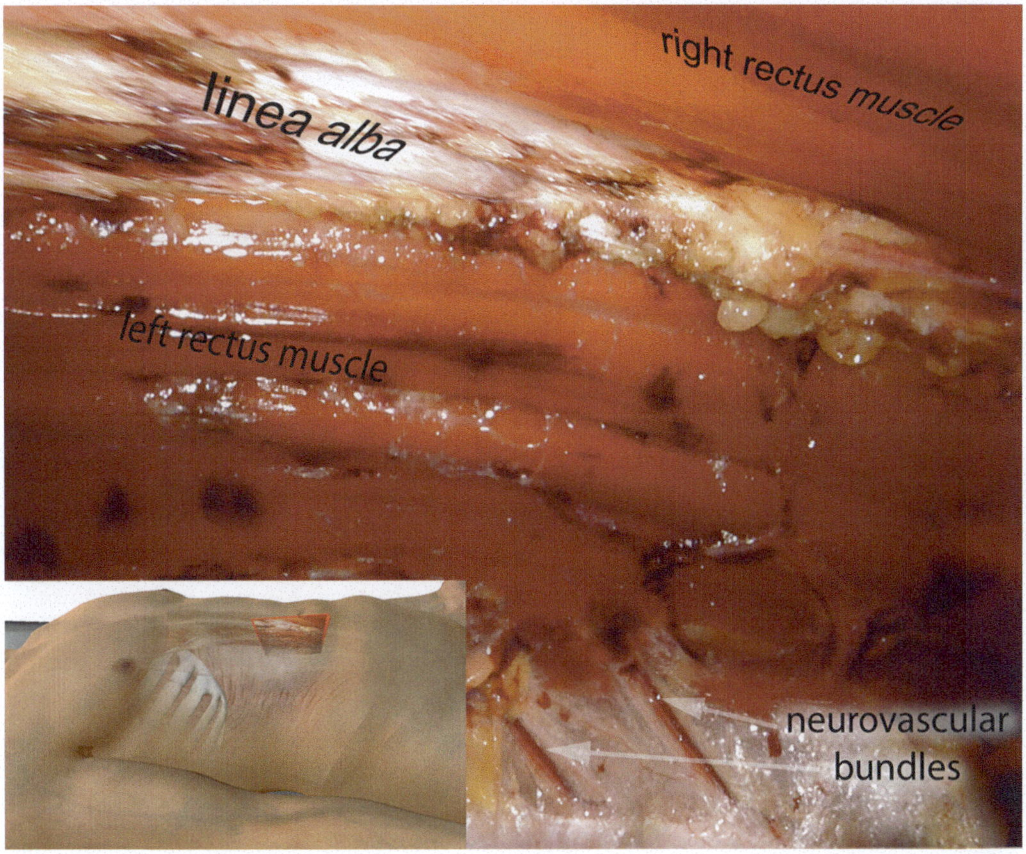


**Fig. 8.11** Throughout dissection, neurovascular bundles are identified and preserved

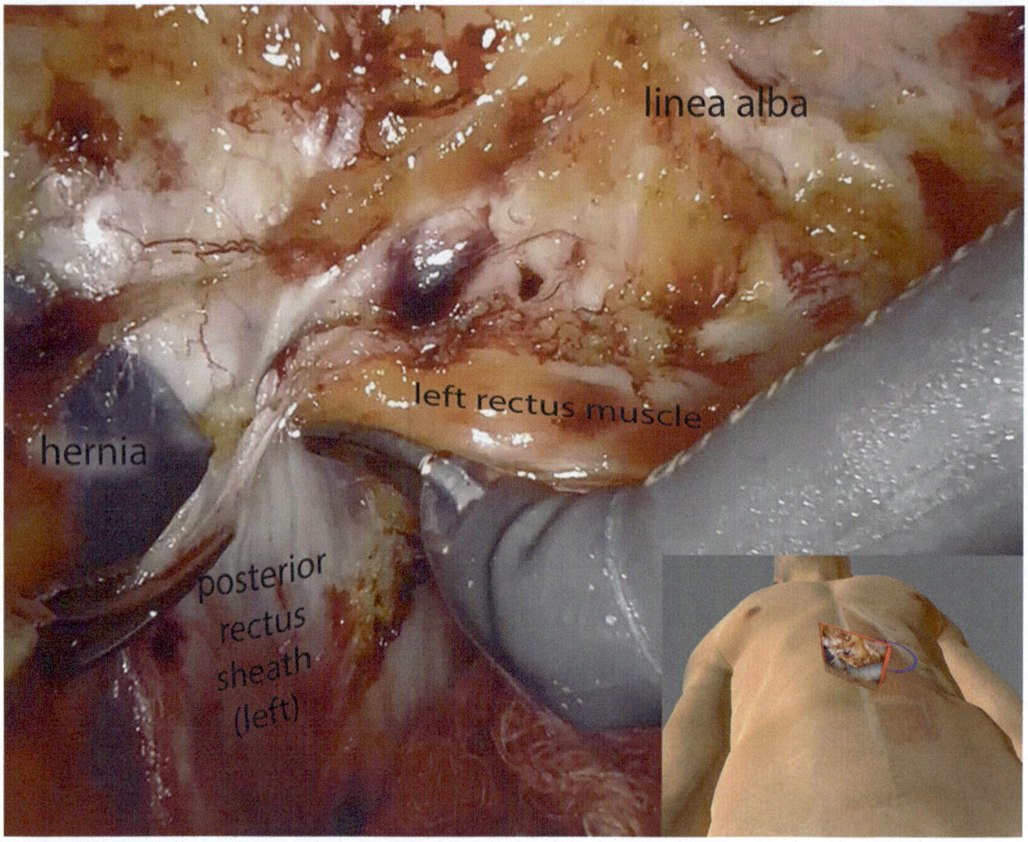


Fig. 8.12 As the dissection proceeds, the hernia site is encountered

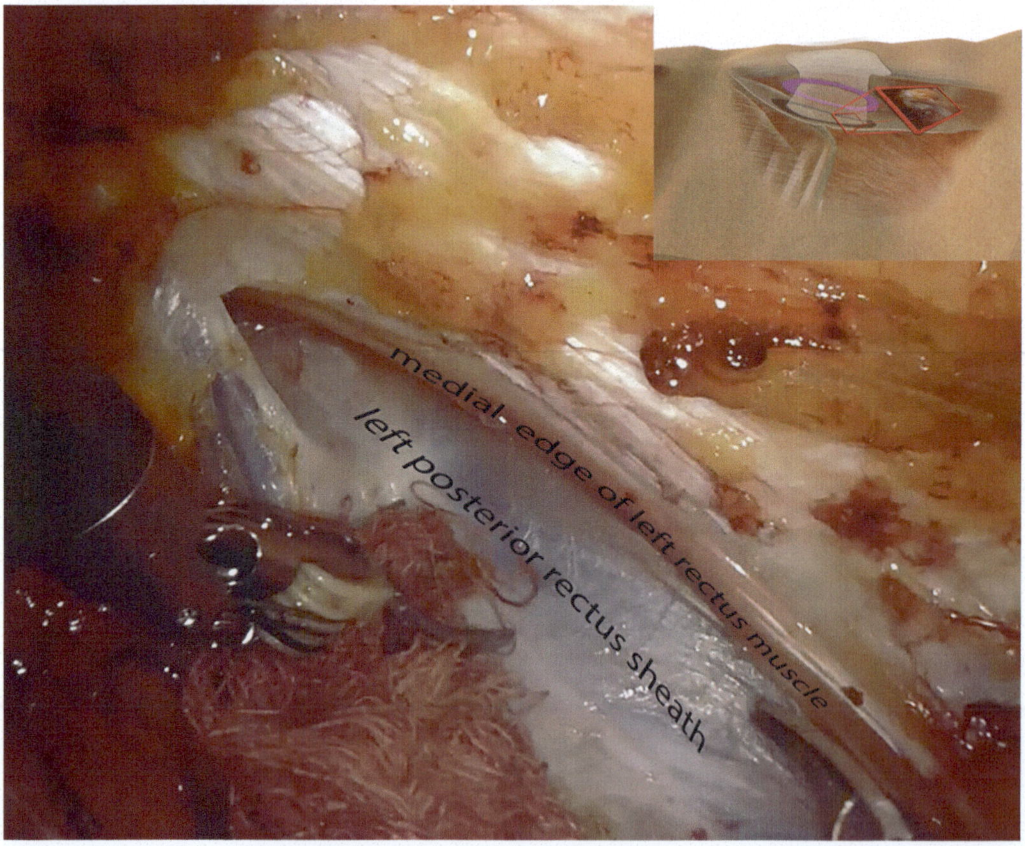


Fig. 8.13 The sub-figure illustration shows the "chef hat" shape of the hernia. Dissection is carried out along the medial aspect of the hernia

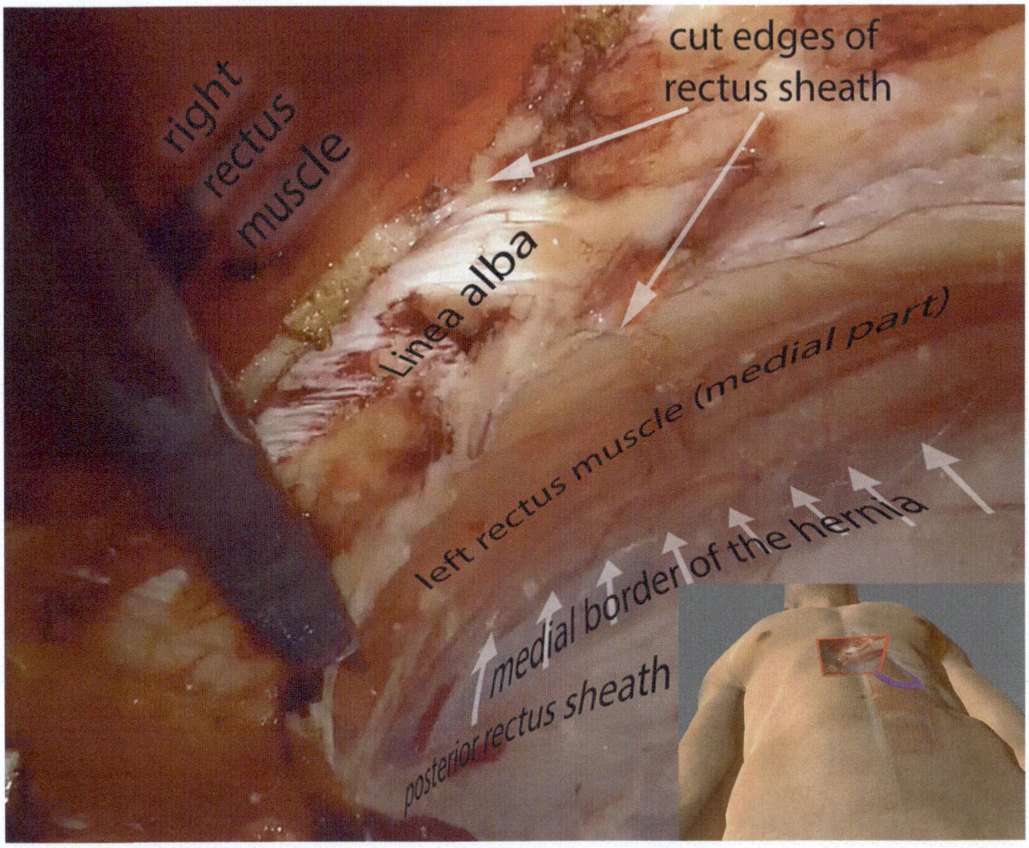


**Fig. 8.14** The hernia sac is identified, bordered by the medial part of the left rectus muscle

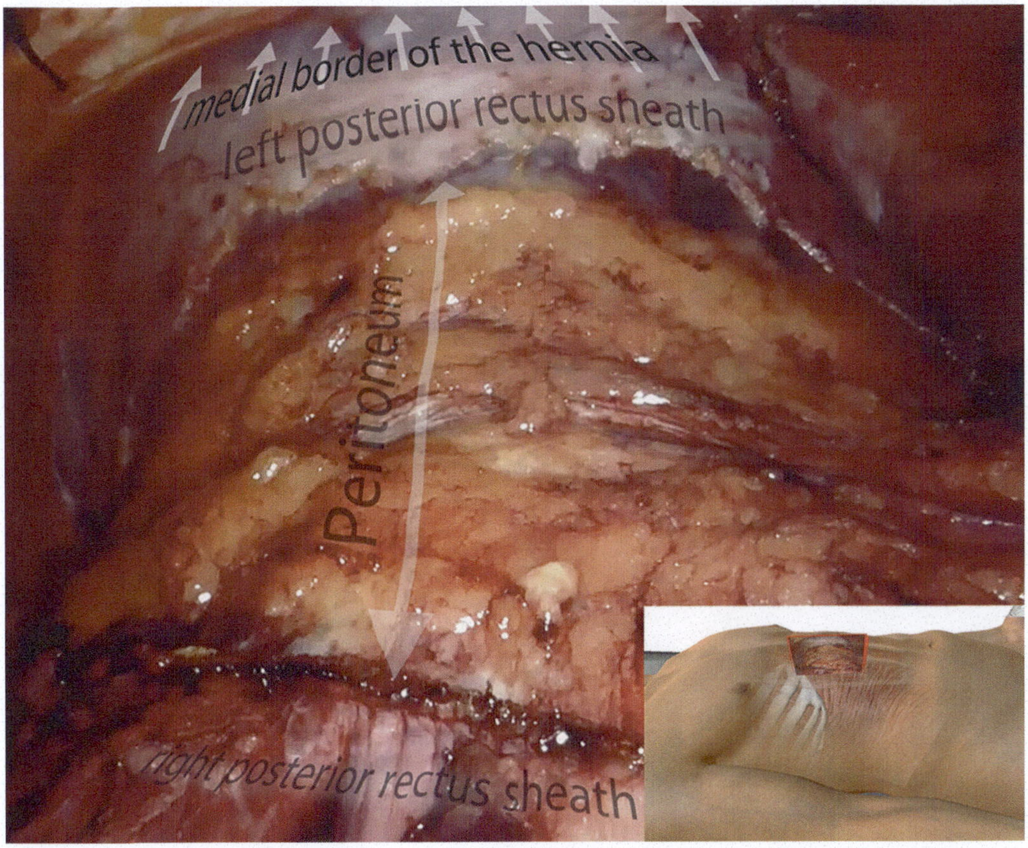


**Fig. 8.15** The right and left medial edges of the posterior rectus sheaths are connected by the peritoneum

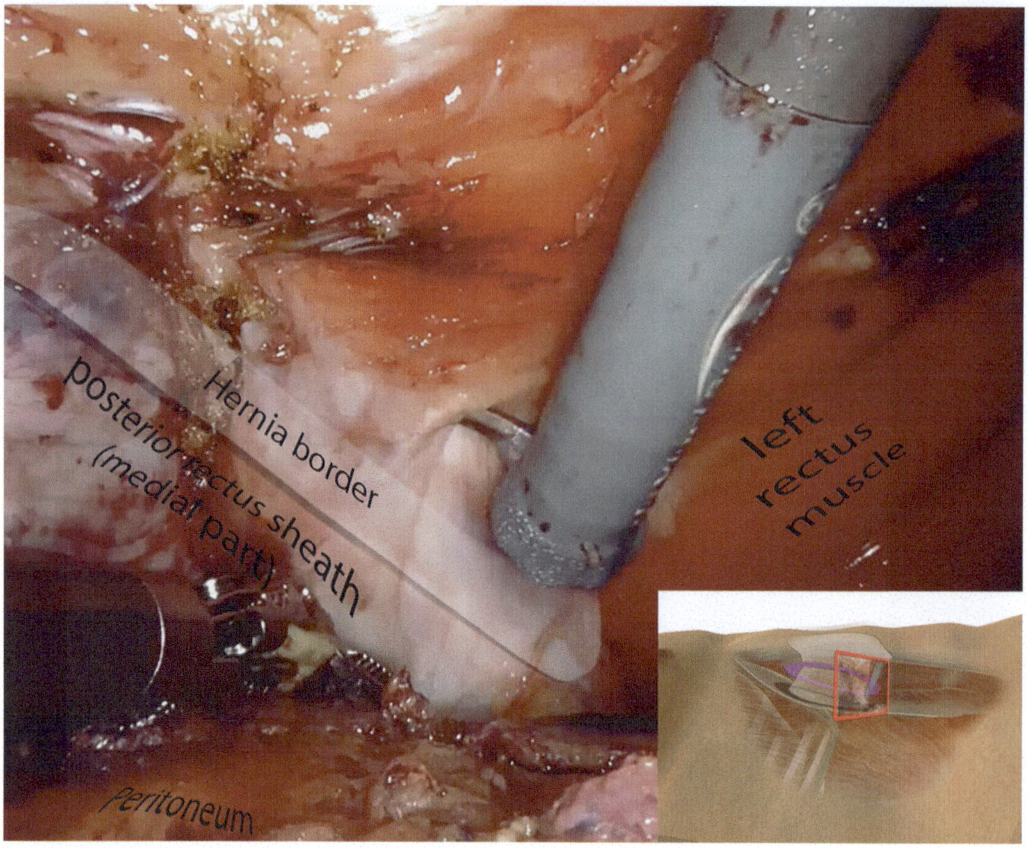


**Fig. 8.16** Circumferential dissection is carried out around the inferior border of the hernia sac

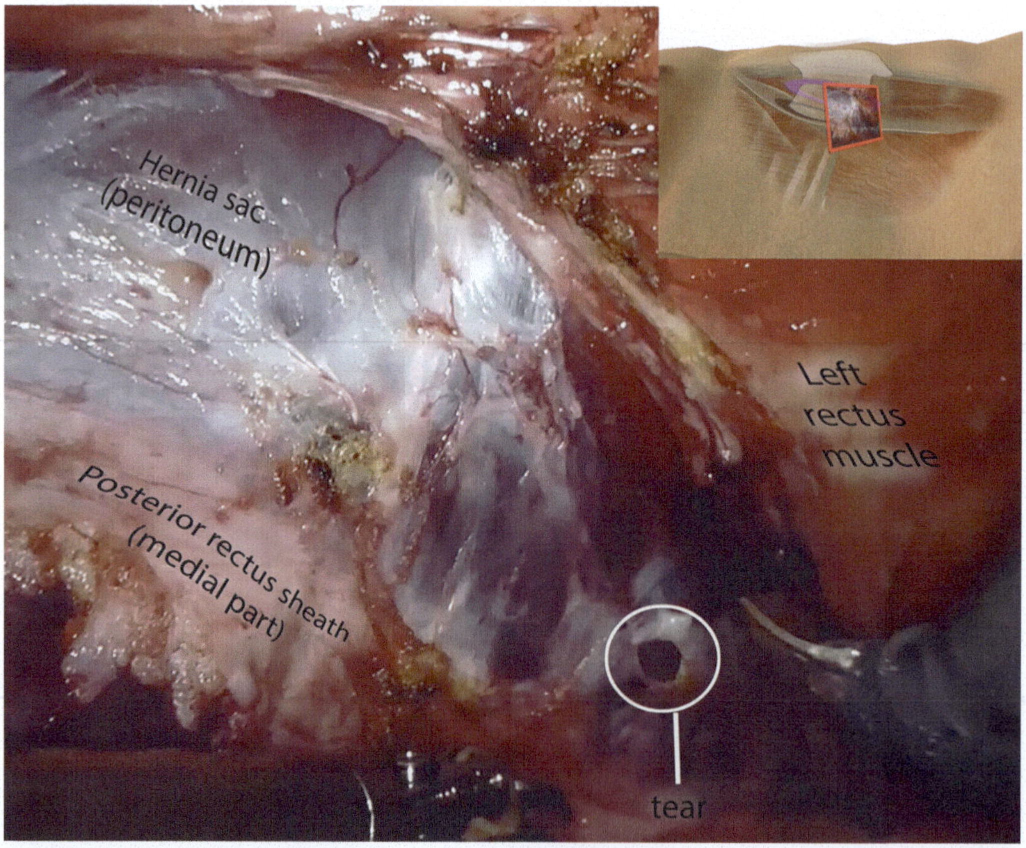


**Fig. 8.17** An inadvertent tear is caused in the peritoneum, which forms the hernia sac

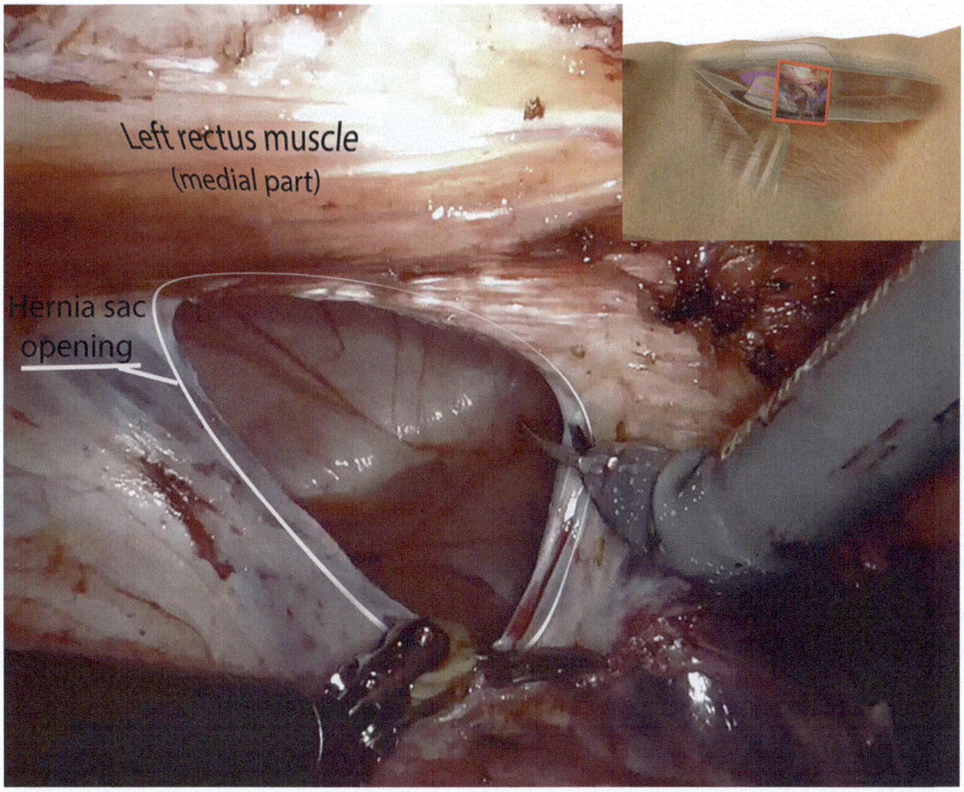


**Fig. 8.18** Because of the hernia shape and the angle of the dissection plane, the decision is made to divide the hernia sac at the level of the hernia neck, instead of performing complete reduction of the hernia sac and its contents

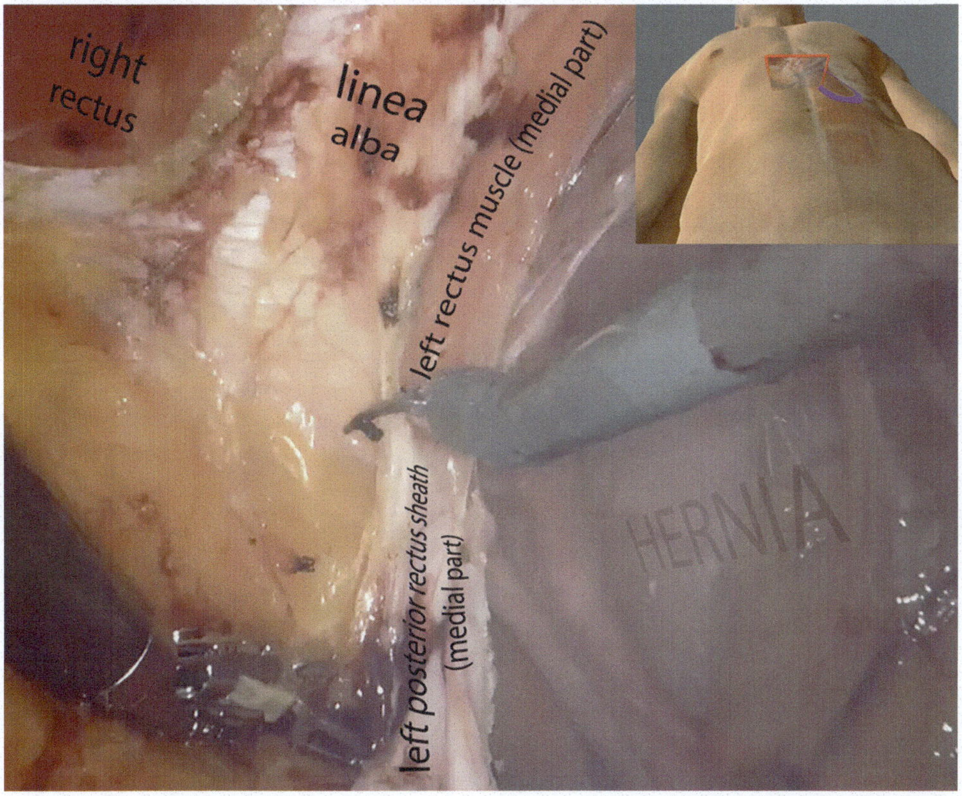


**Fig. 8.19** The hernia sac opening is enlarged by dissecting in the cranial direction, separating the left posterior rectus sheath from the overlying rectus muscle

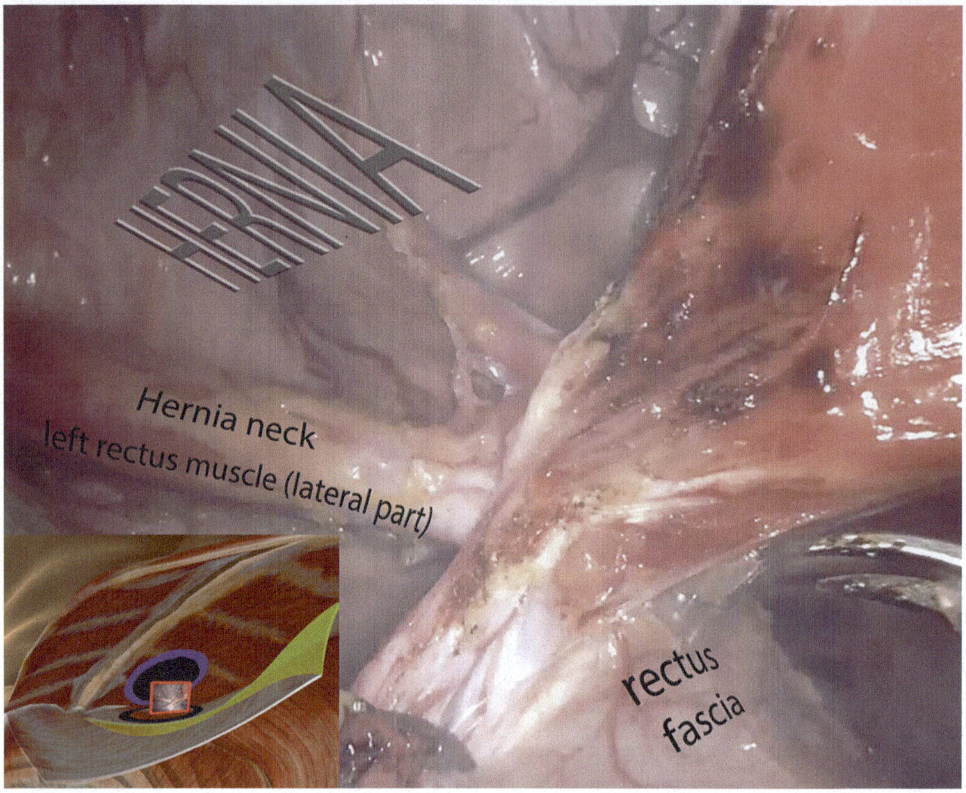


**Fig. 8.20** The hernia neck is bordered by the lateral aspect of the left rectus muscle. The sub-figure illustration shows the camera view from the inside (retromuscular space)

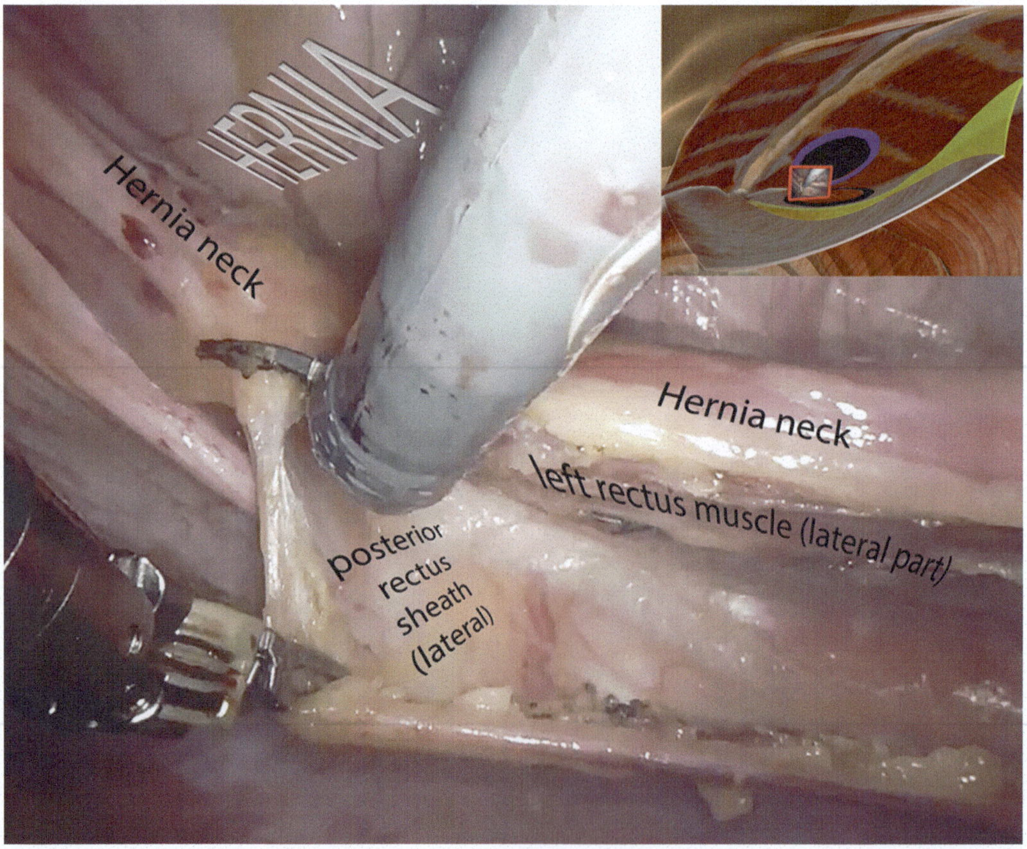


**Fig. 8.21** Circumferential dissection is continued around the superolateral portion of the hernia neck

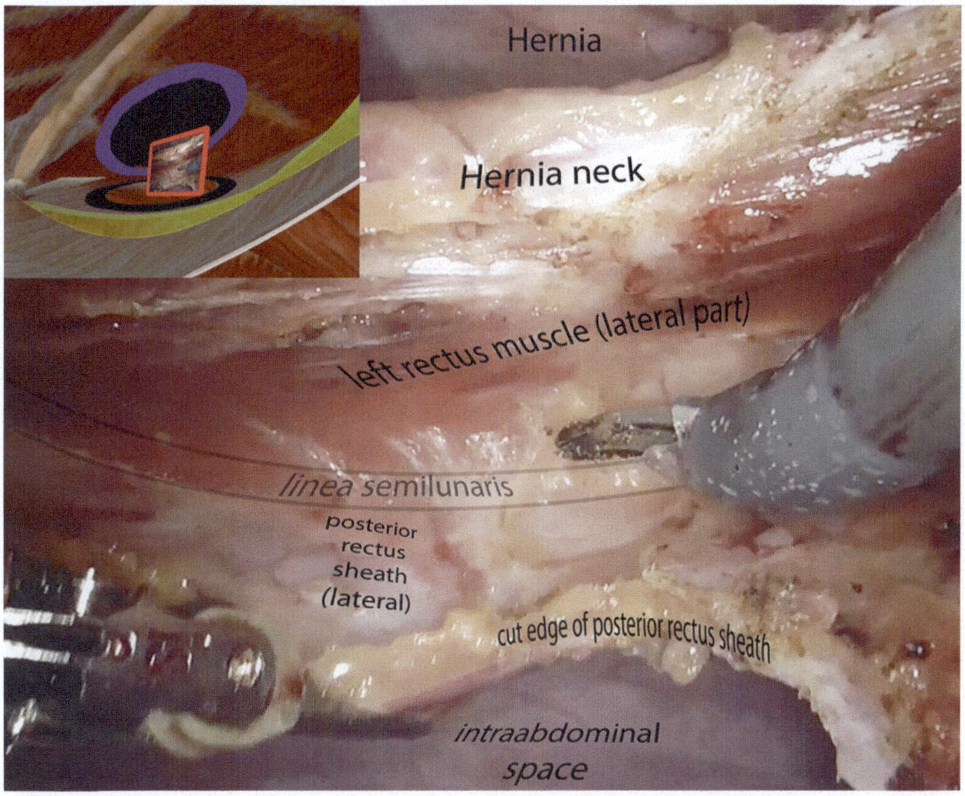


**Fig. 8.22** Dissection of the lateral border of the posterior rectus sheath, where transversus abdominis muscle fibers will be visualized later

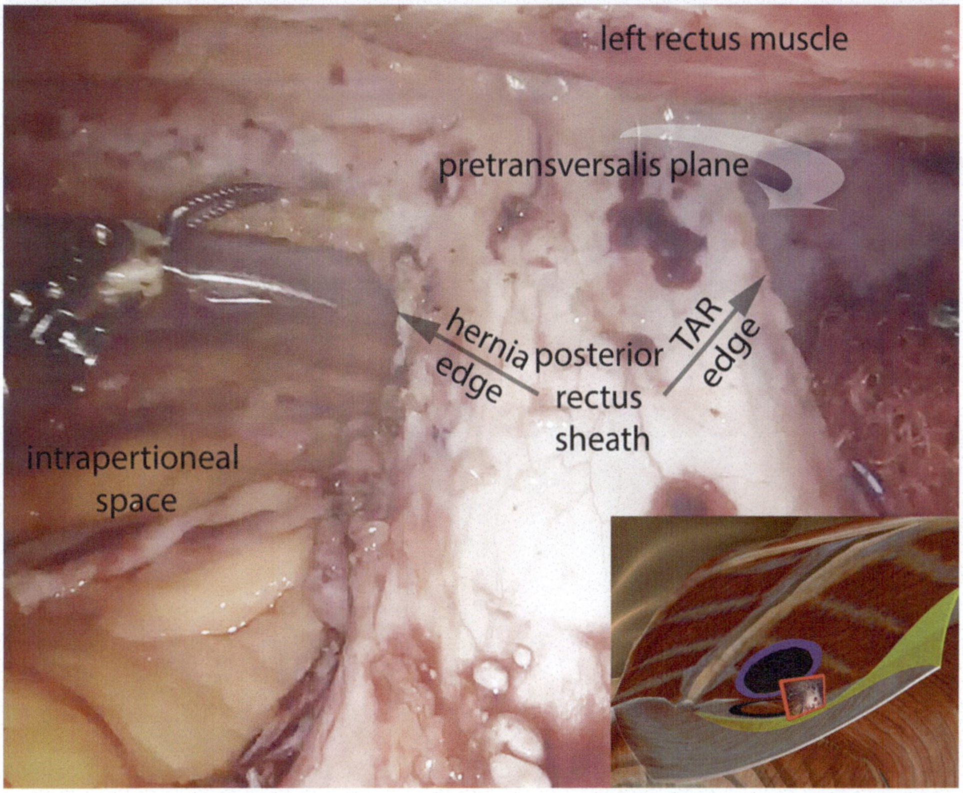


**Fig. 8.23** The lateral part of the posterior rectus sheath is bordered by the hernia medially and the transversus abdominis muscle laterally, where transversus abdominis release (TAR) is performed

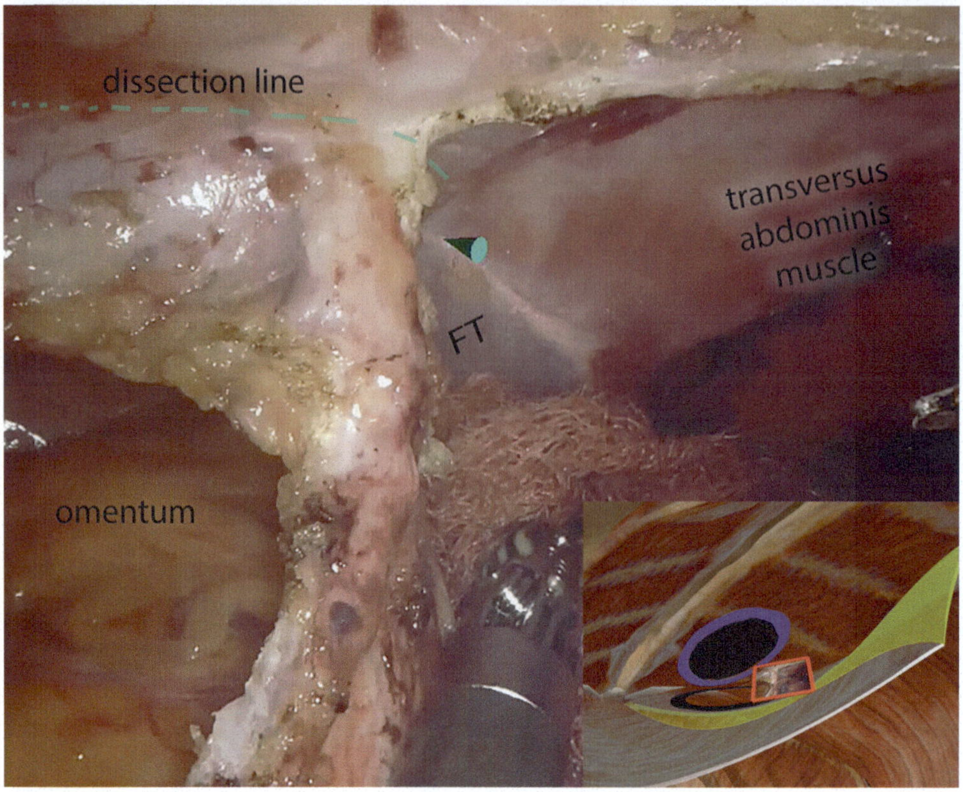


**Fig. 8.24** Transversus abdominis aponeurosis release is continued at the level of the linea semilunaris

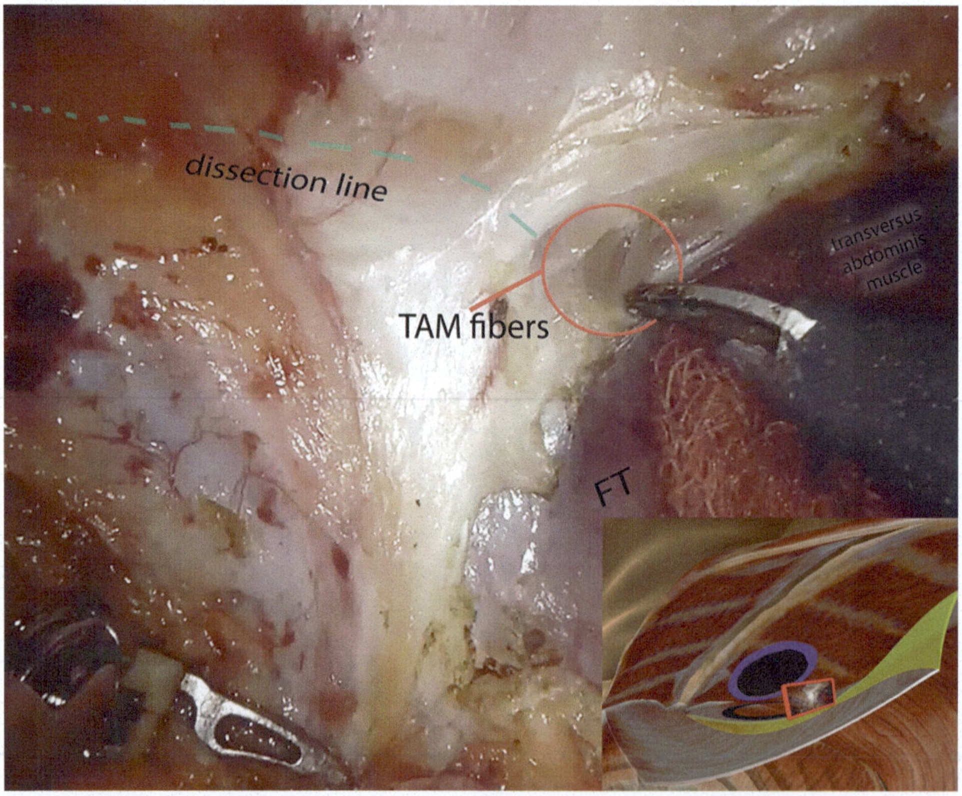


**Fig. 8.25** Identification of the transversus abdominis muscle fibers superiorly, where TAR is to be continued. FT fascia transversalis, TAM transversus abdominis muscle

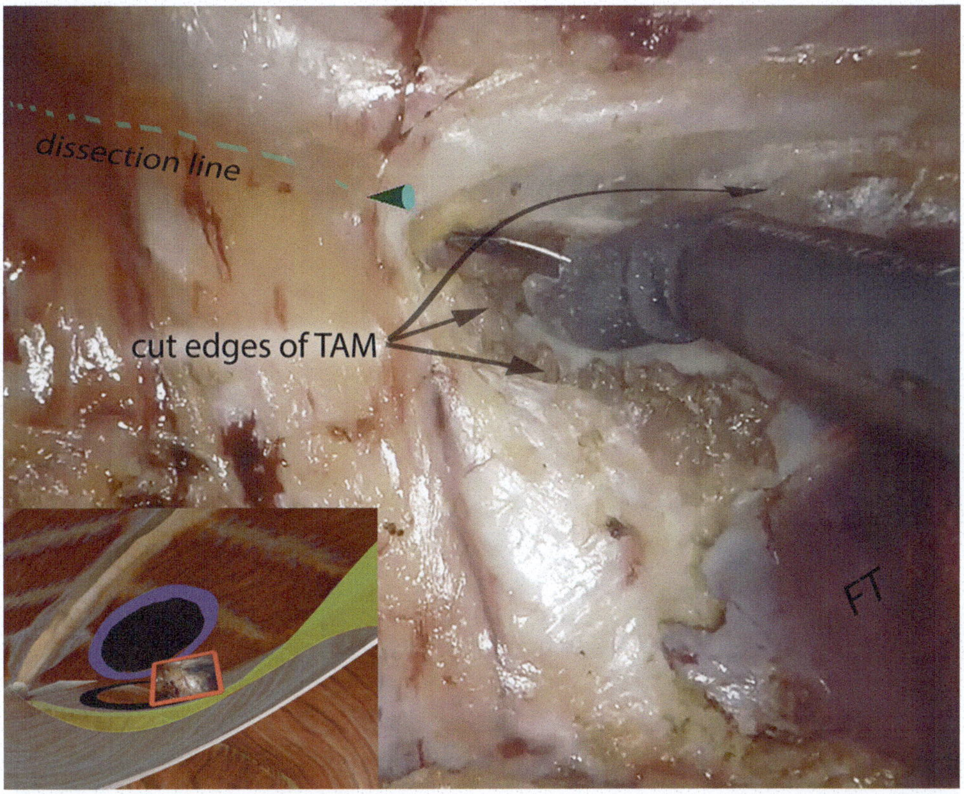


**Fig. 8.26** Proceeding with TAR superiorly. FT fascia transversalis

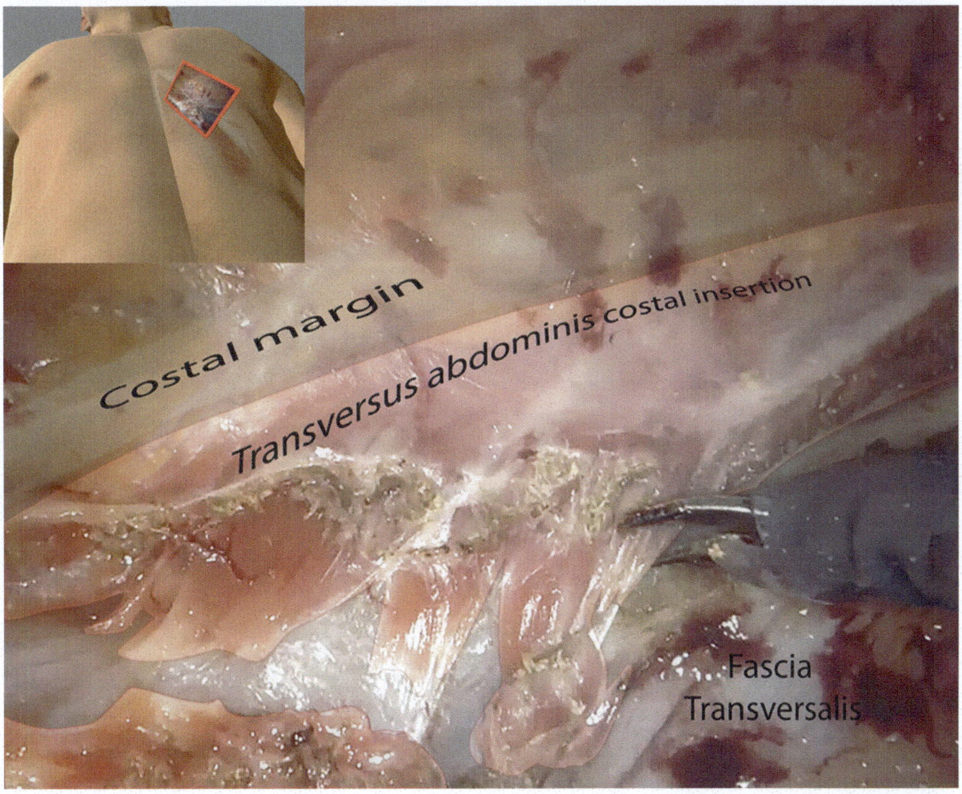


**Fig. 8.27** The separated transversus abdominis muscle fibers are shown below the costal margin

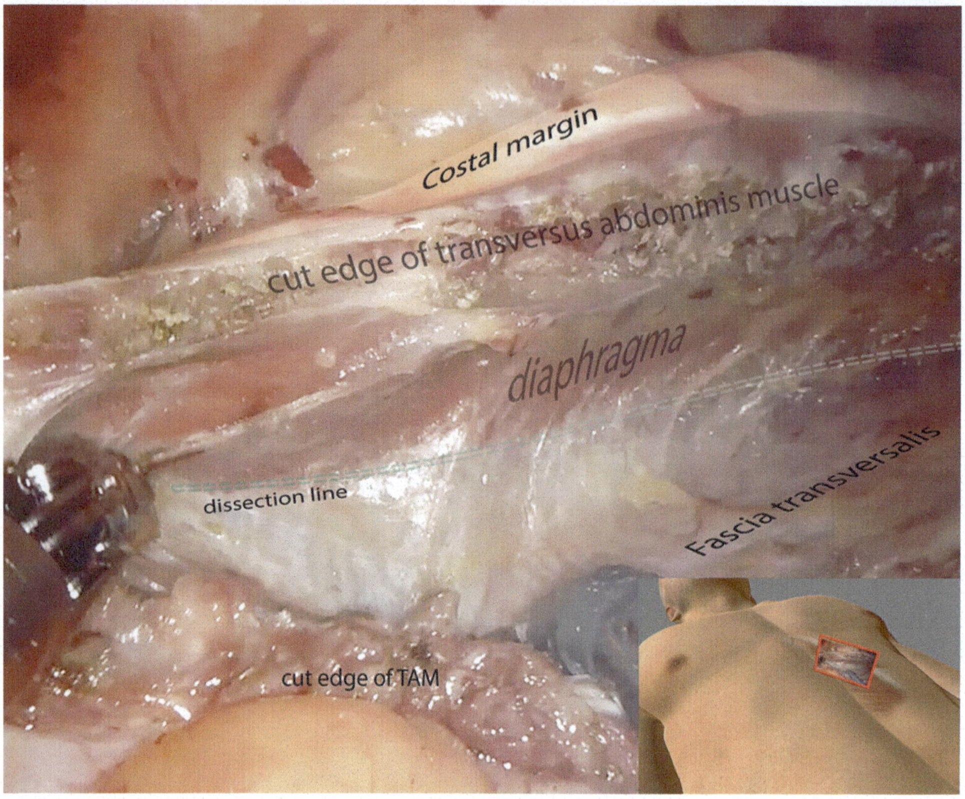


**Fig. 8.28** As TAR is continued medially, the diaphragm can be visualized just under the costal margin, where the transversus abdominis muscle inserts

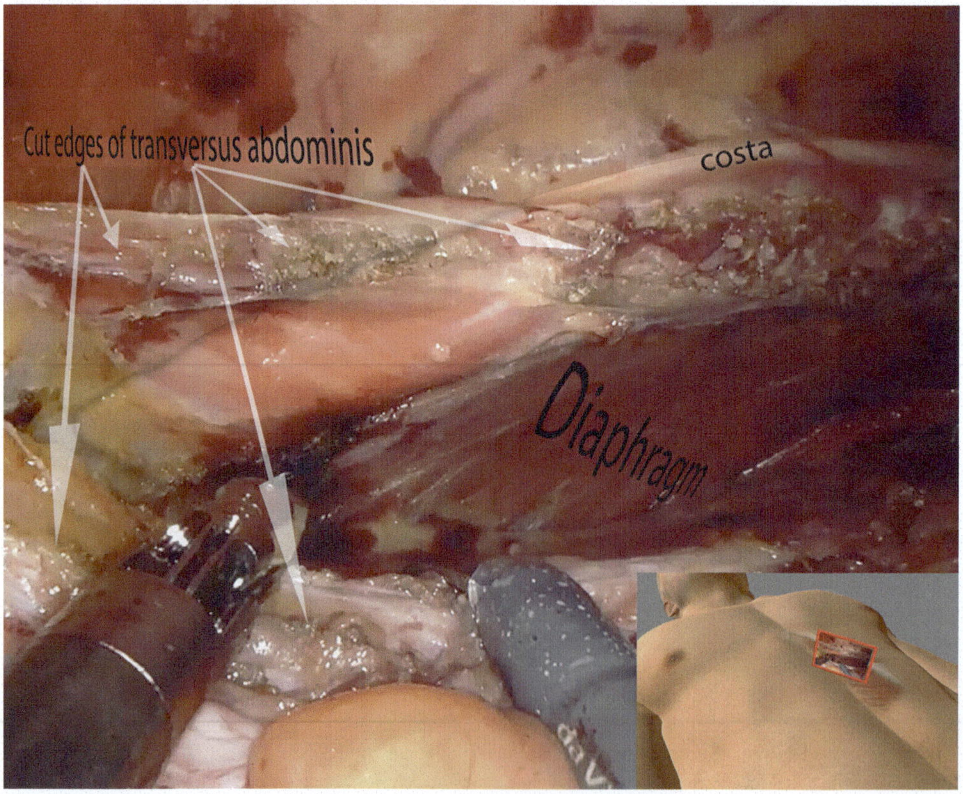


**Fig. 8.29** The diaphragm is then exposed by separating it from the underlying fascia transversalis

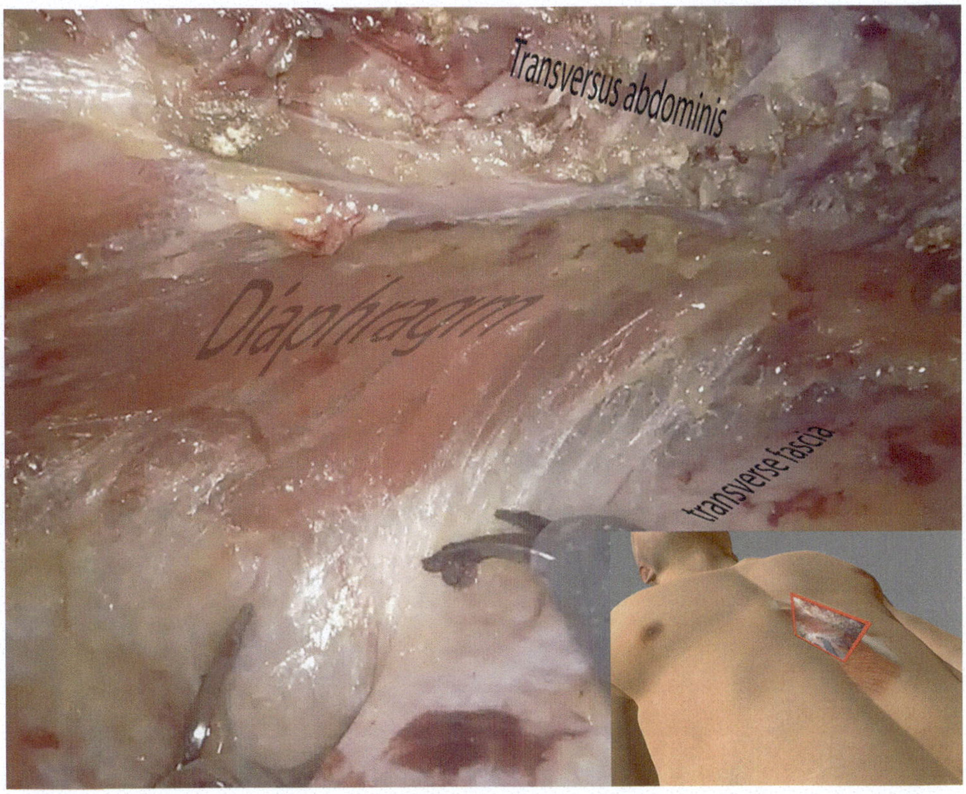


**Fig. 8.30** Dissection is continued superiorly. Gentle pressure along the posterior layer may help identify the dissection plane

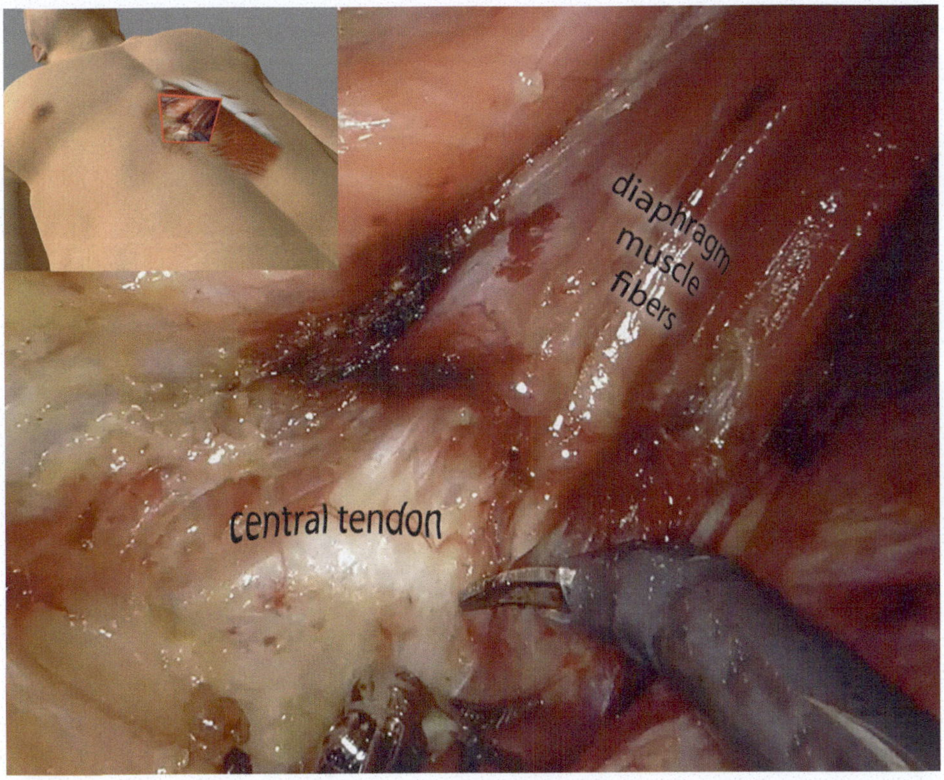


**Fig. 8.31** The dissection continues until the central tendon is reached

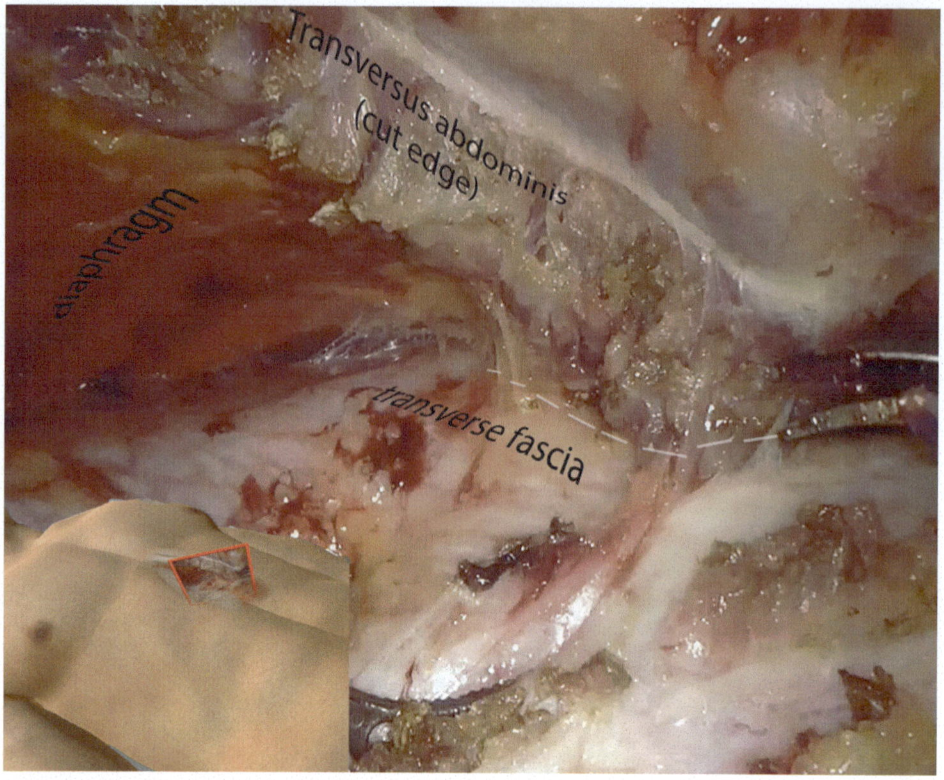


Fig. 8.32 Separation of the transverse fascia from the diaphragm is continued laterally

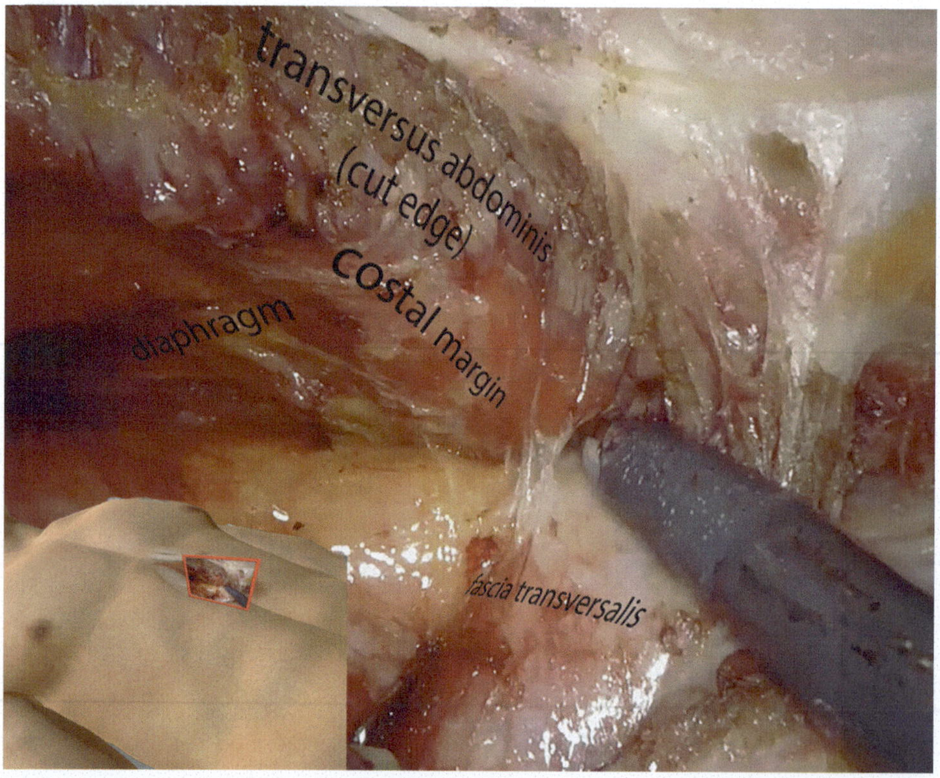


Fig. 8.33 The dissection continues towards the lateral costal margin, where the diaphragm and transversus abdominis meet

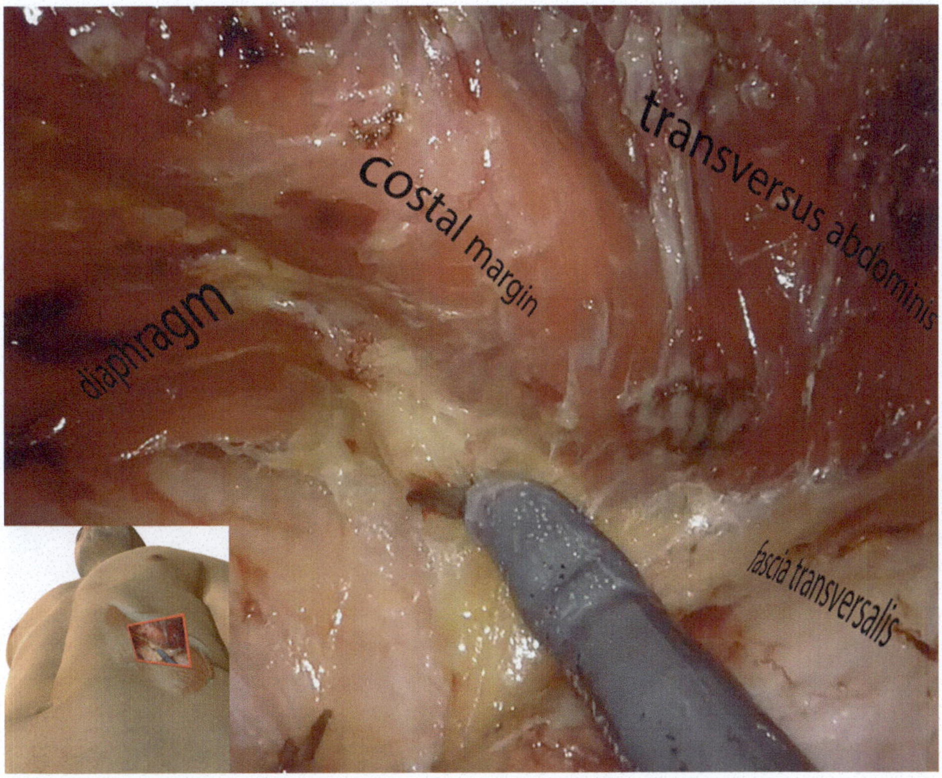


Fig. 8.34 Dissection is continued laterally

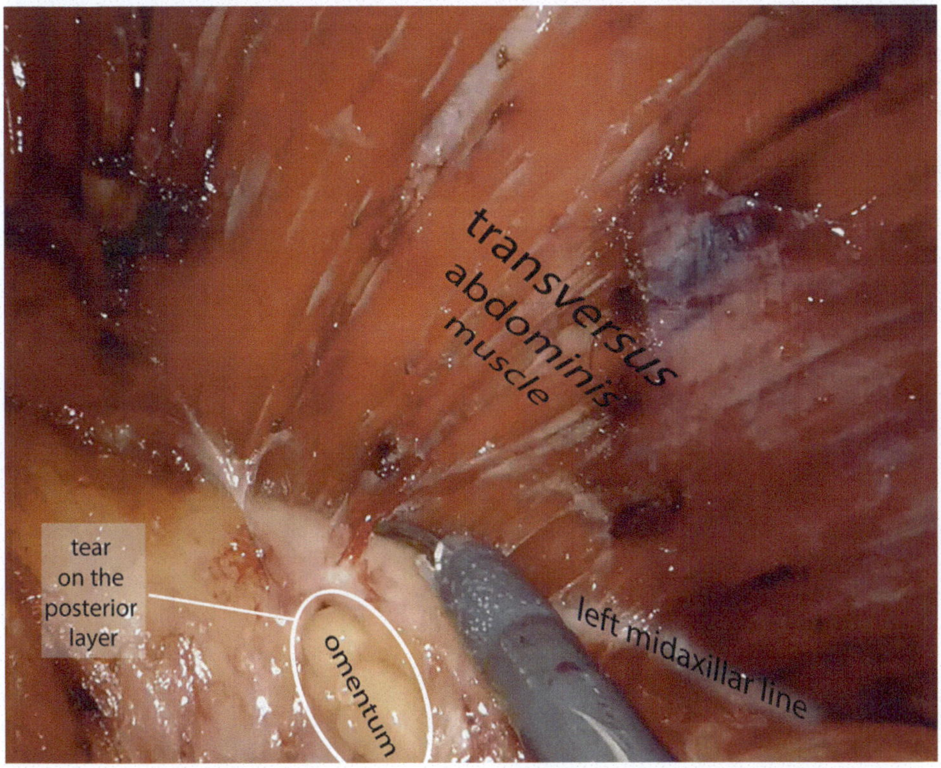


Fig. 8.35 An inadvertent tear is noticed in the posterior fascia, through which a small portion of the omentum protrudes

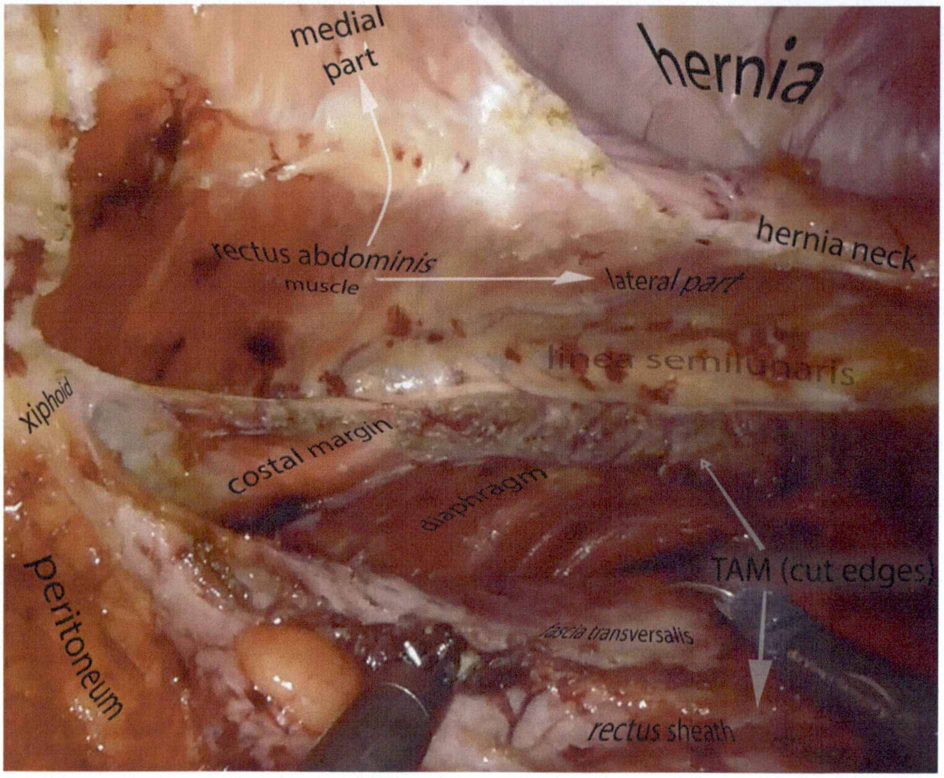


**Fig. 8.36** View of the hernia site, showing all its anatomical borders

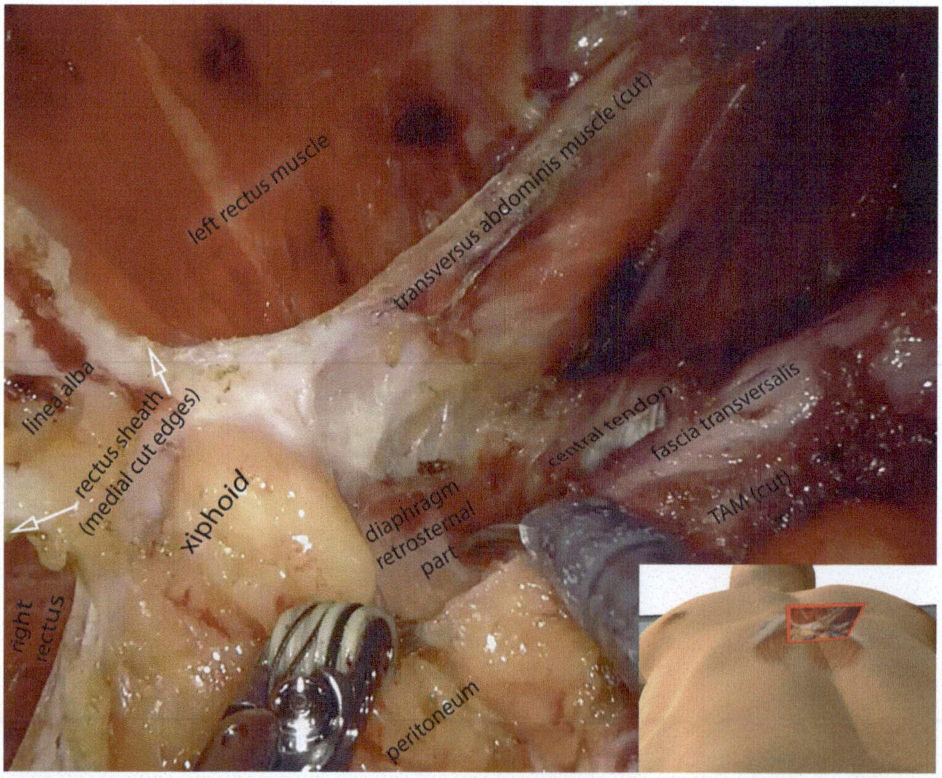


**Fig. 8.37** Dissection is continued medially, at the retrosternal aspect of the diaphragm

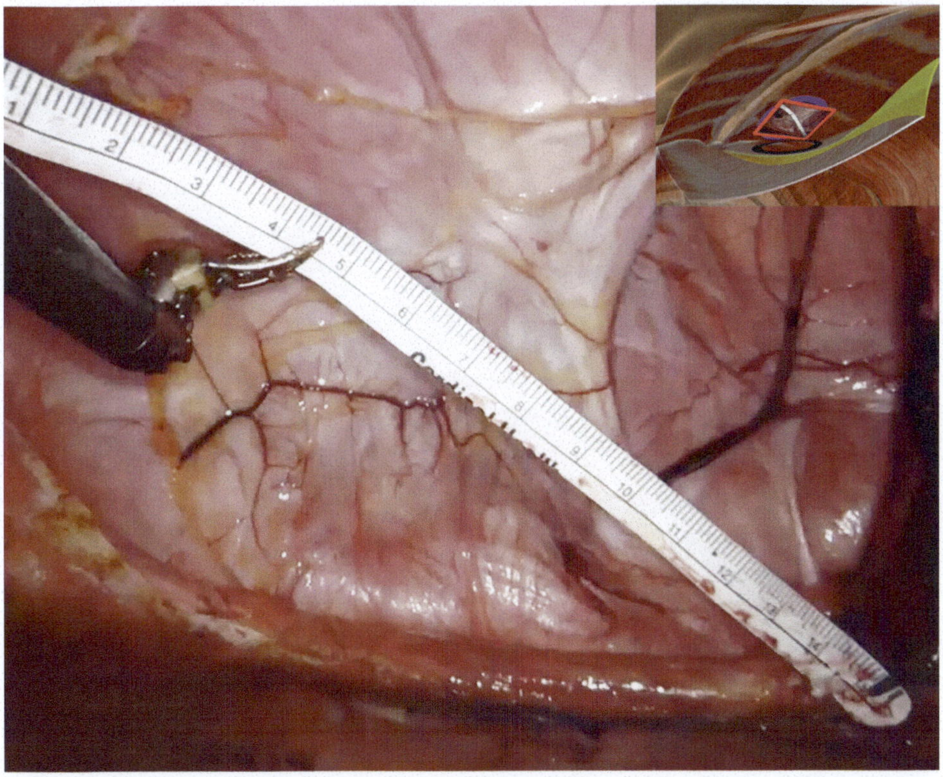

Fig. 8.38 After the necessary dissection is completed, the hernia defect is measured

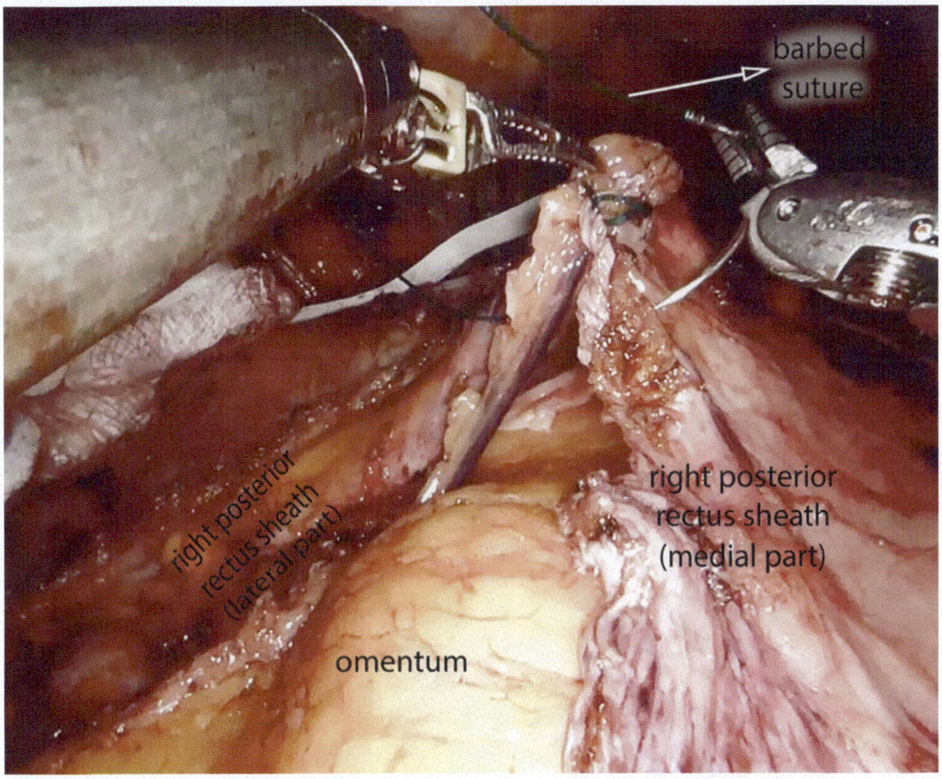


Fig. 8.39 A barbed suture is used to approximate the edges of the posterior rectus sheath (hernia opening)

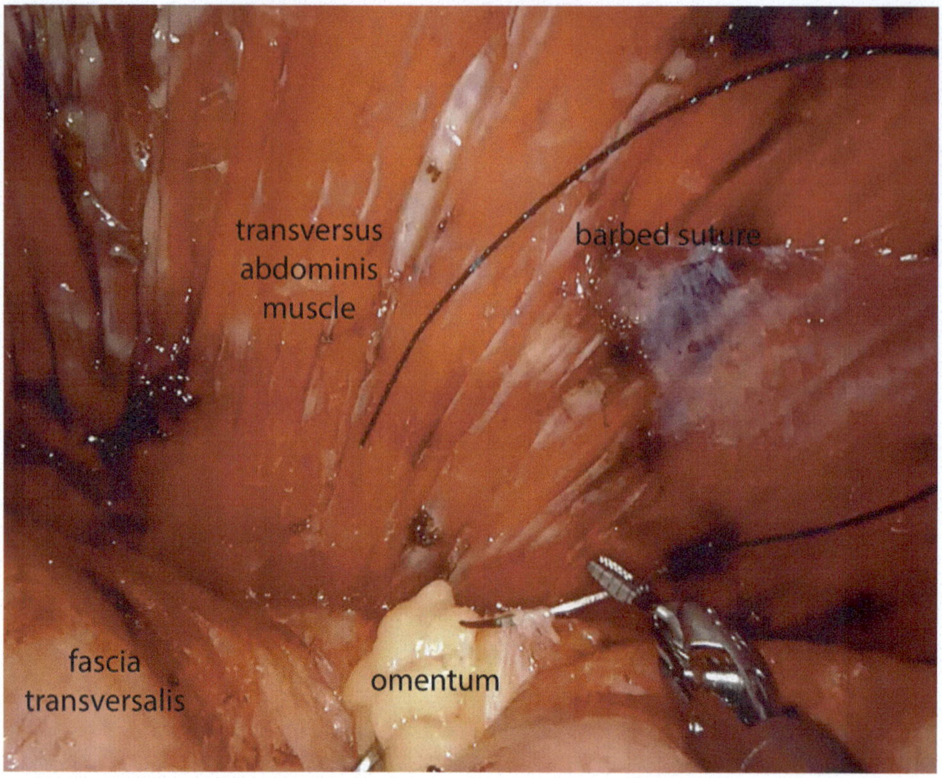


Fig. 8.40 Another barbed suture is used to close the peritoneal tear mentioned in Fig. 8.35, after reducing the herniated omentum

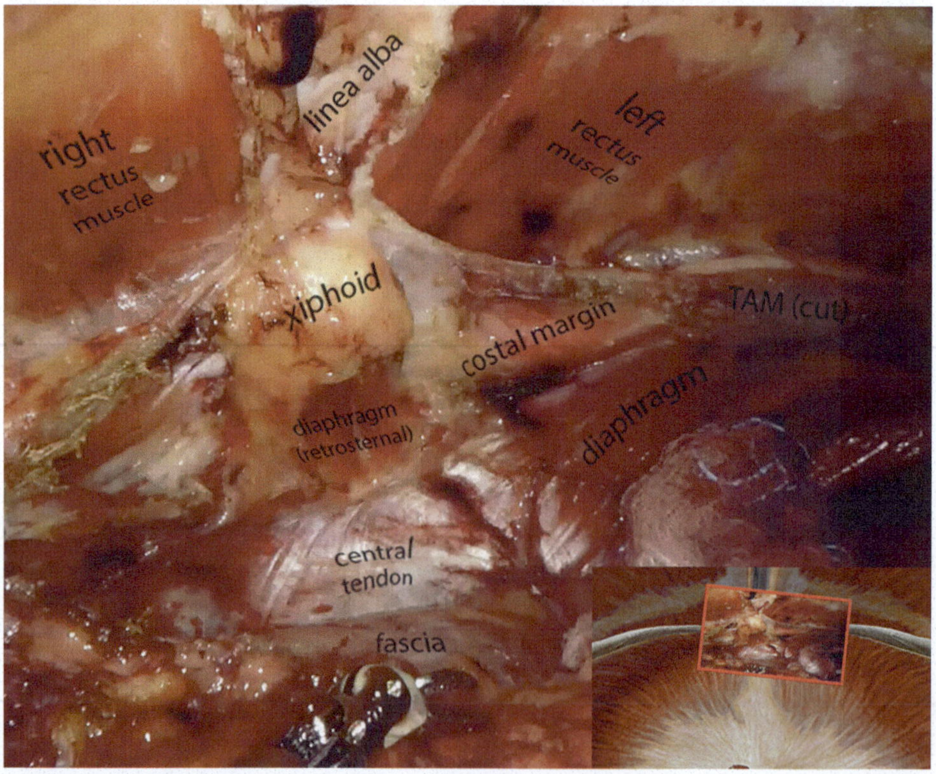


Fig. 8.41 Inferior view of the subxiphoid region and diaphragm

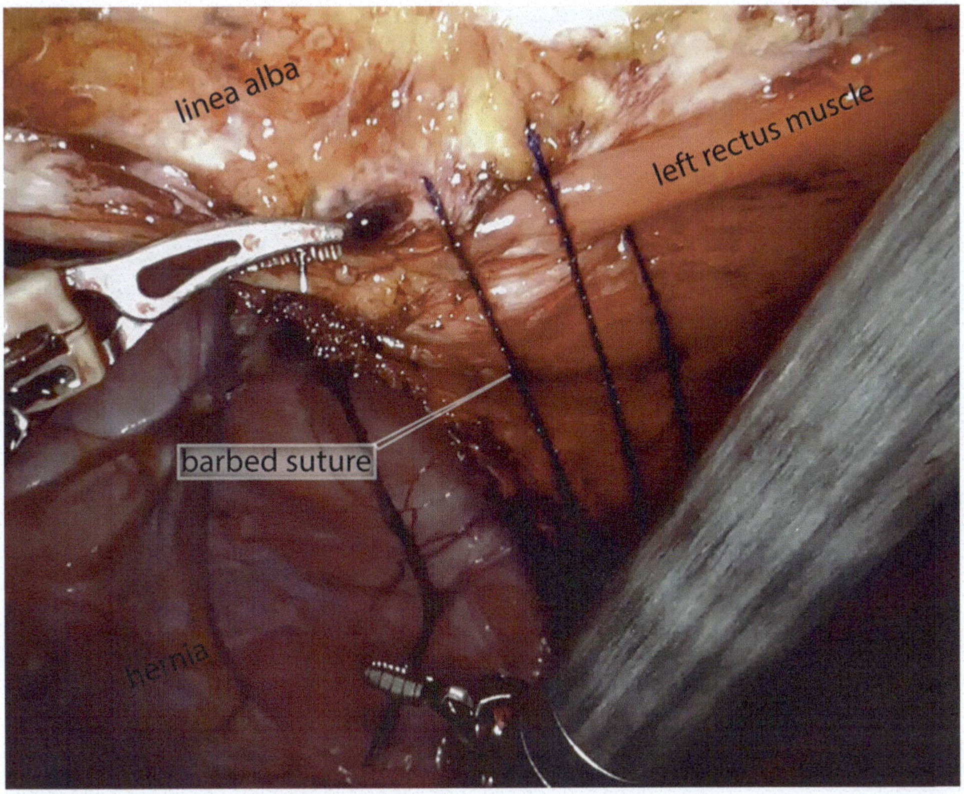


Fig. 8.42 Closure of the hernia defect; suturing in the caudocranial direction

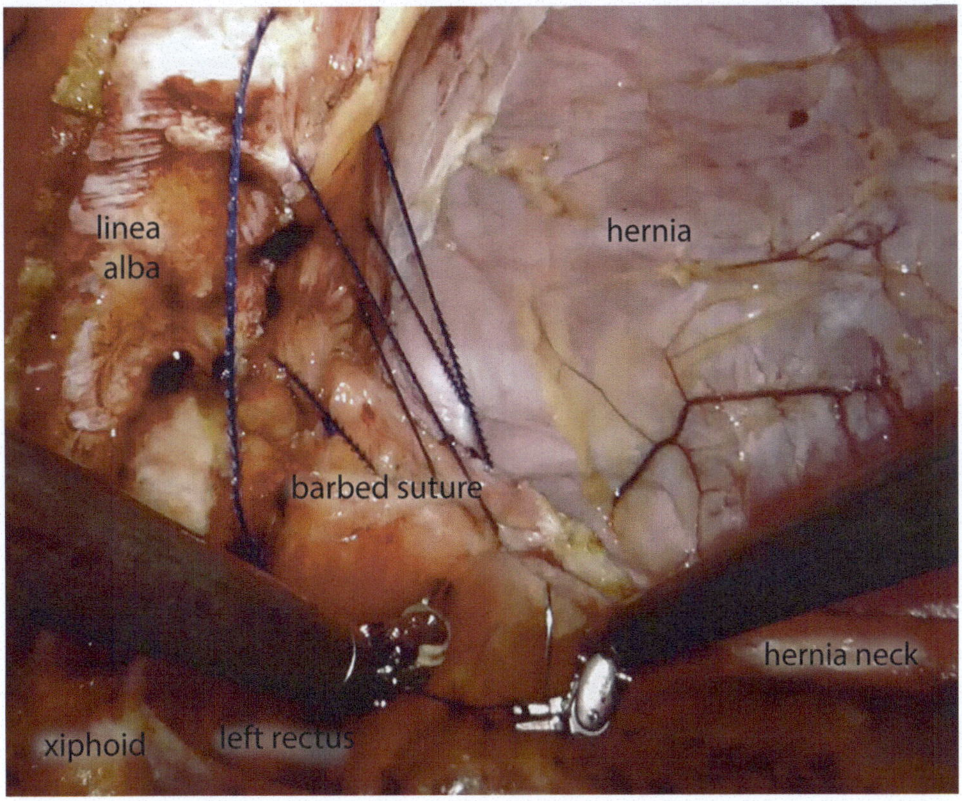


Fig. 8.43 Closure of the hernia defect; suturing in the craniocaudal direction

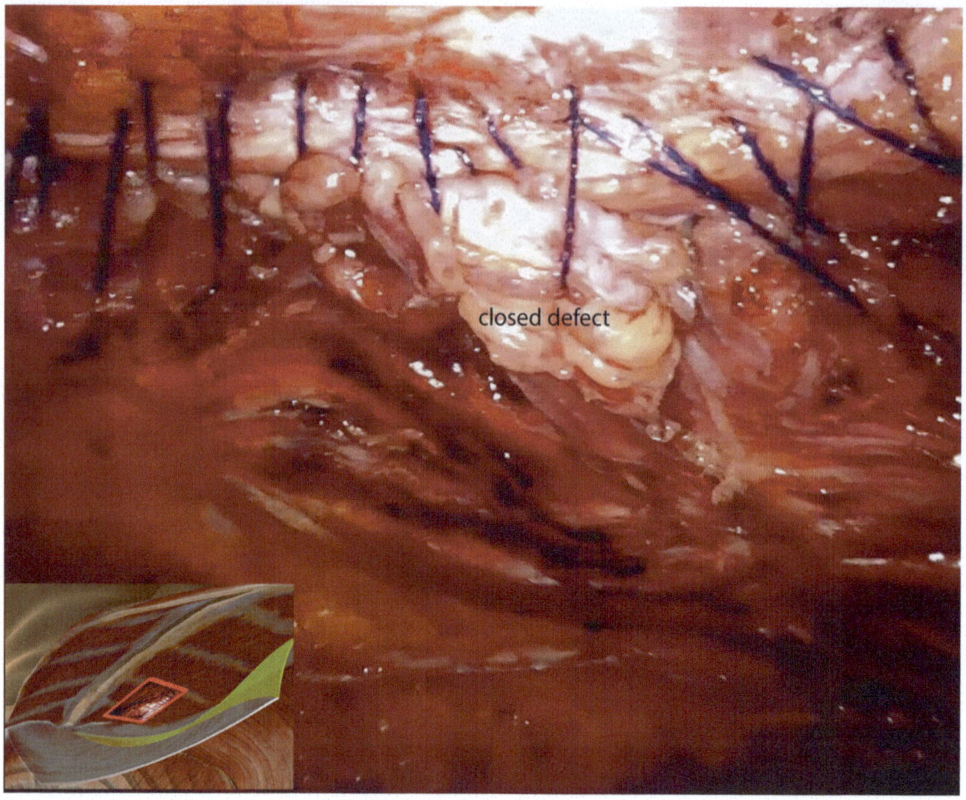


Fig. 8.44 After sutures have been placed along the hernia neck, the defect is closed

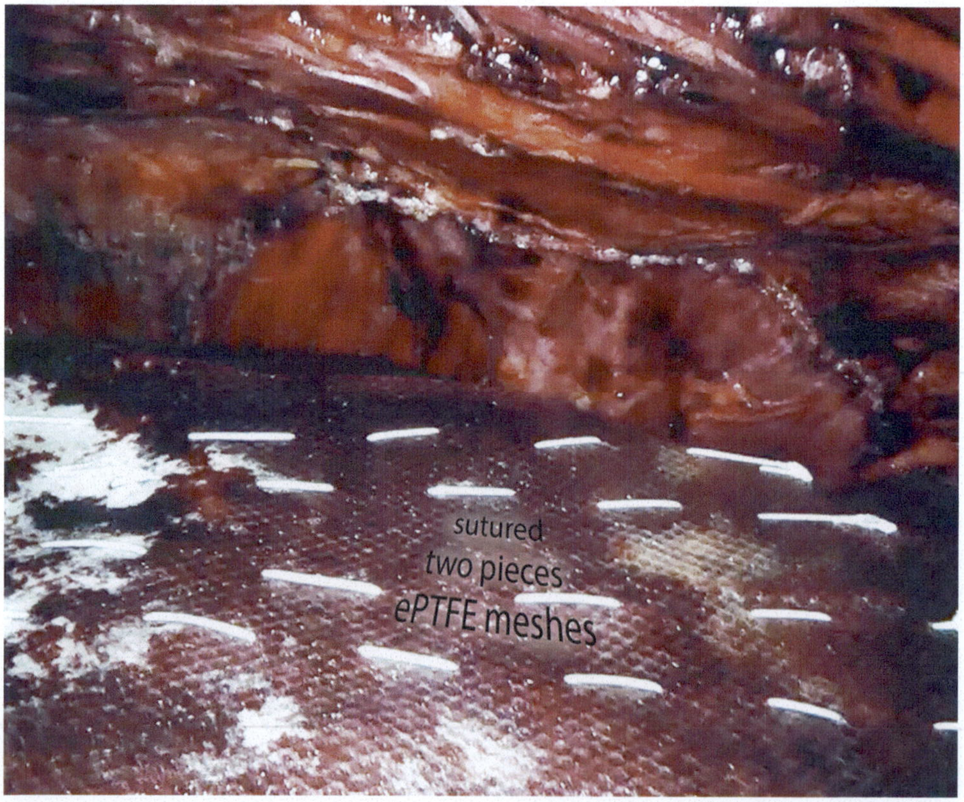


Fig. 8.45 Two pieces of expanded polytetrafluoroethylene (ePTFE) mesh are sutured together to adequately reinforce the repair

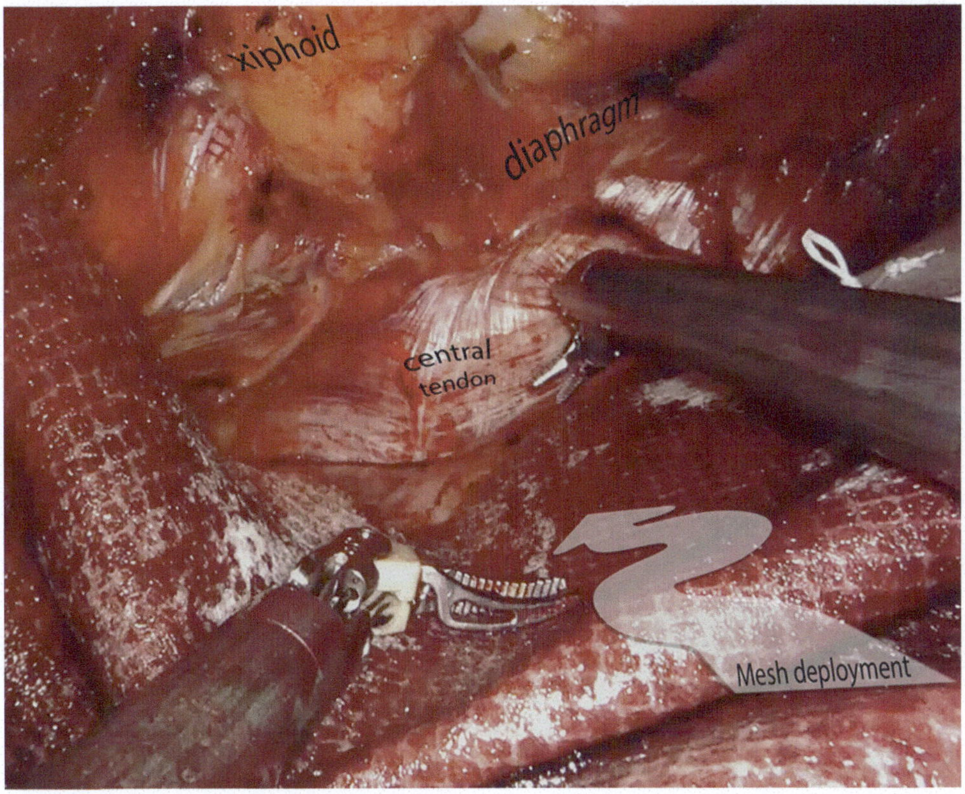


**Fig. 8.46** The mesh is deployed to cover all edges of the surgical plane

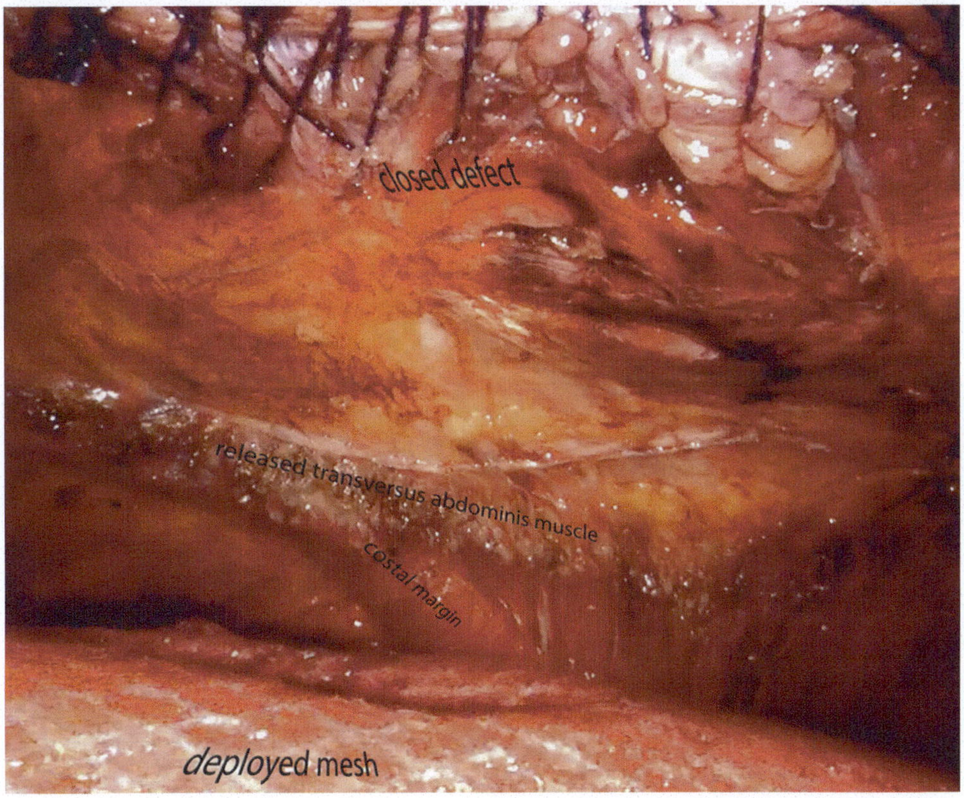


**Fig. 8.47** Final view of the deployed mesh with the overlying closed defect

## References

1. Moreno-Egea A, Carrillo-Alcaraz A. Management of non-midline incisional hernia by the laparoscopic approach: results of a long-term follow-up prospective study. Surg Endosc. 2012;26:1069–78. https://doi.org/10.1007/s00464-011-2001-x.
2. Kudsi OY, Gokcal F, Chang K. Robotic intraperitoneal onlay versus totally extraperitoneal (TEP) retromuscular mesh ventral hernia repair: a propensity score matching analysis of short-term outcomes. Am J Surg. 2020:pii: S0002-9610(20)30004-0. https://doi.org/10.1016/j.amjsurg.2020.01.003. [Epub ahead of print].

# Robotic Hybrid Lateral Incisional Hernia Repair: Totally Extraperitoneal (TEP)

9

Naseem Bou-Ayash, Fahri Gokcal, and Omar Yusef Kudsi

## Introduction

Lateral incisional hernias have been defined by the European Hernia Society (EHS) as those arising lateral to the linea semilunaris, below the subcostal region and above the iliac region [1]. These incisional hernias often occur after previous operations, especially those that involve injury to intercostal nerves. Subsequent laxity of the lateral abdominal wall layers due to denervation increases the risk of an incisional hernia.

Although these hernias have traditionally been repaired with the open approach, the previously compromised and thin lateral abdominal wall layers are difficult to identify and manipulate to ensure adequate mesh placement and fixation. This approach may further disrupt posterior layer integrity and ultimately complicate its approximation. The robotic platform, with the delicate dissection it provides, is better able to address these challenges. When both open and robotic approaches are combined into the hybrid technique, surgeons gain the advantage of robotic precise dissection and the time-efficient defect closure afforded by open surgery. The hybrid technique has been shown to offer operative times similar to those of the open approach [2–4].

## Procedure: Illustrated Steps

Figures 9.1, 9.2, 9.3, 9.4, 9.5, 9.6, 9.7, 9.8, 9.9, 9.10, 9.11, 9.12, 9.13, 9.14, 9.15, 9.16, 9.17, 9.18, 9.19, 9.20, 9.21, 9.22, 9.23, 9.24, 9.25, 9.26, 9.27, 9.28, 9.29, 9.30, 9.31, 9.32, 9.33, 9.34, 9.35, 9.36, and 9.37 illustrate the technical aspects of hybrid robotic totally extraperitoneal (TEP) retromuscular repair of a large lateral incisional hernia with transversus abdominis release (TAR).

N. Bou-Ayash · F. Gokcal
Department of Surgery, Good Samaritan Medical Center, Brockton, MA, USA

O. Y. Kudsi (✉)
Department of Surgery, Good Samaritan Medical Center, Tufts University School of Medicine, Boston, MA, USA


O. Y. Kudsi (ed.), *Robotic Hernia Surgery*, https://doi.org/10.1007/978-3-030-46667-1_9

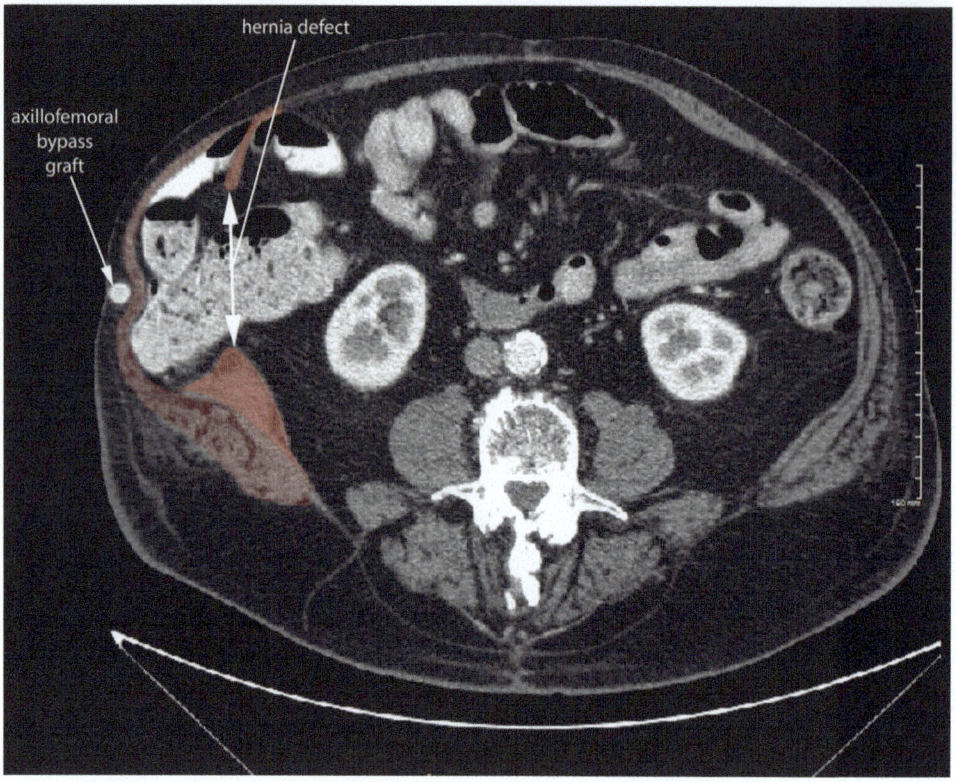


**Fig. 9.1** CT scan (transverse) showing the highlighted right-sided incisional hernia containing colon

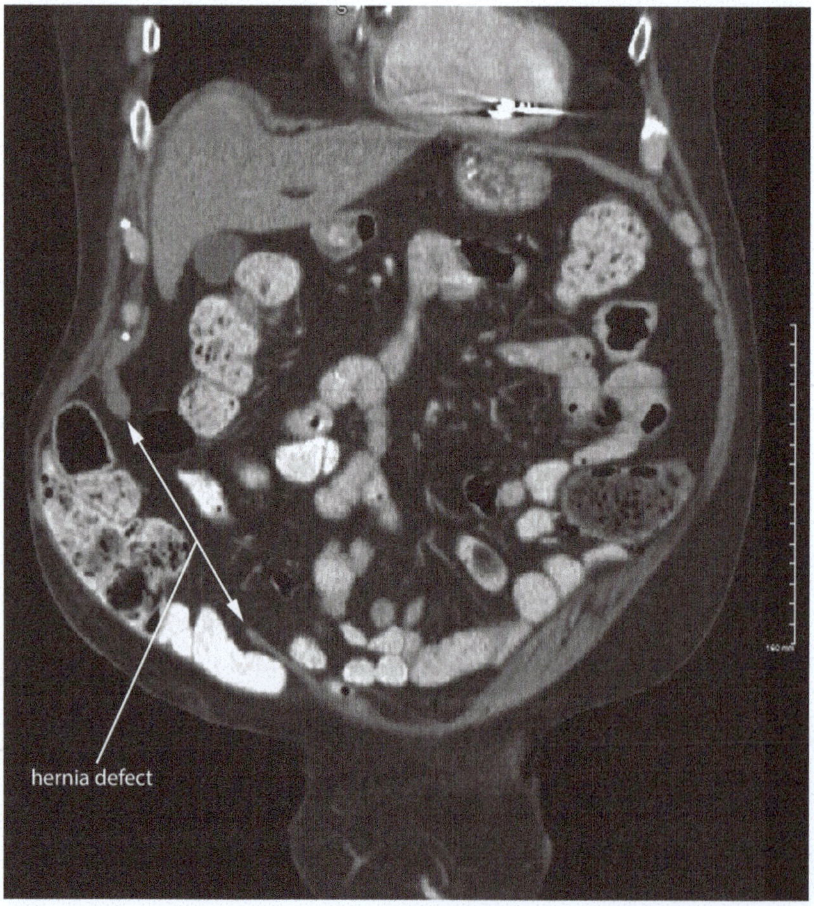


**Fig. 9.2** CT scan (coronal) showing the incisional hernia

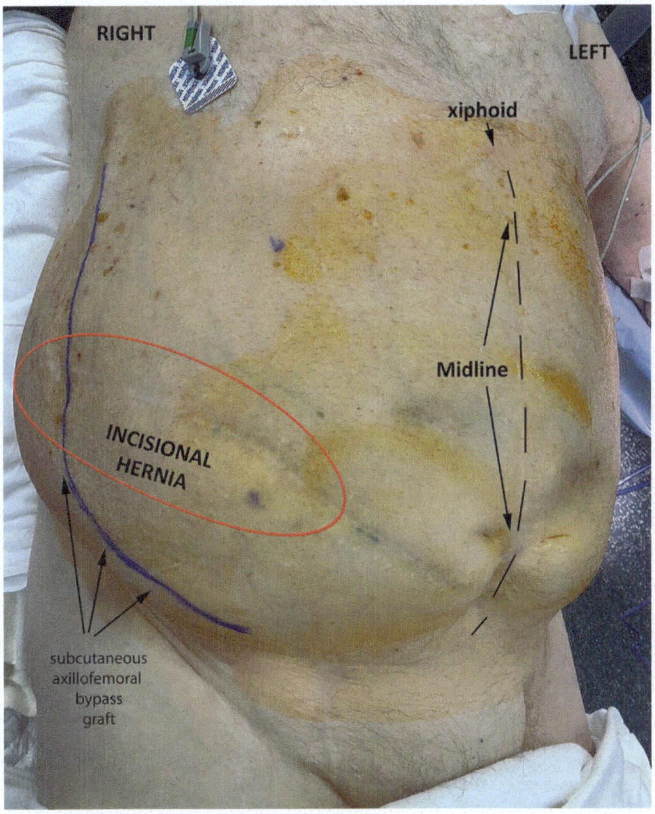


Fig. 9.3 The patient is placed in the semi–lateral decubitus position. An external view of the incisional hernia is shown, with the hernia side being raised with the help of a beanbag. Skin overlying the previous subcutaneous axillofemoral bypass graft is marked

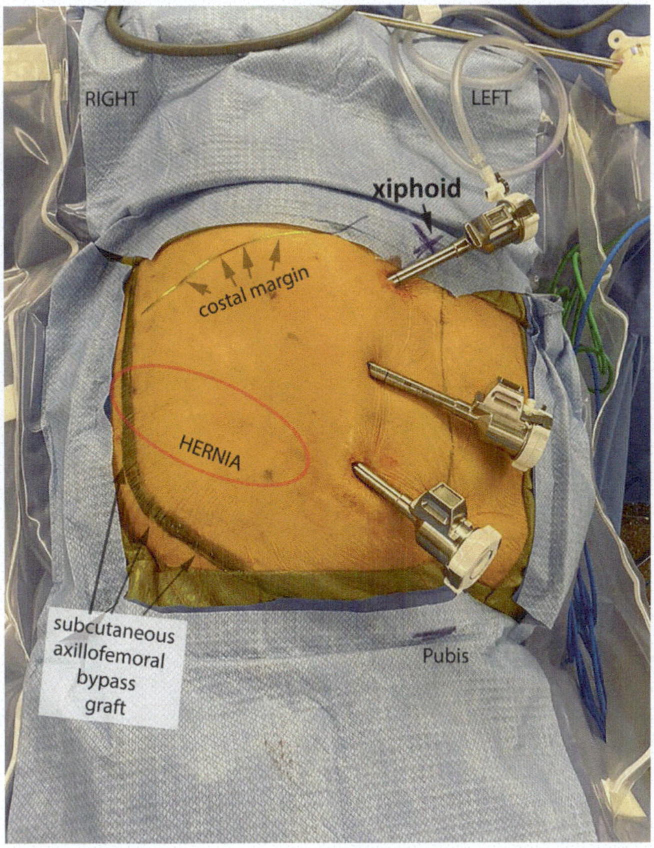


Fig. 9.4 After sterile draping of the surgical site, three trocars are inserted using totally extraperitoneal (TEP) access (described in Chap. 3)

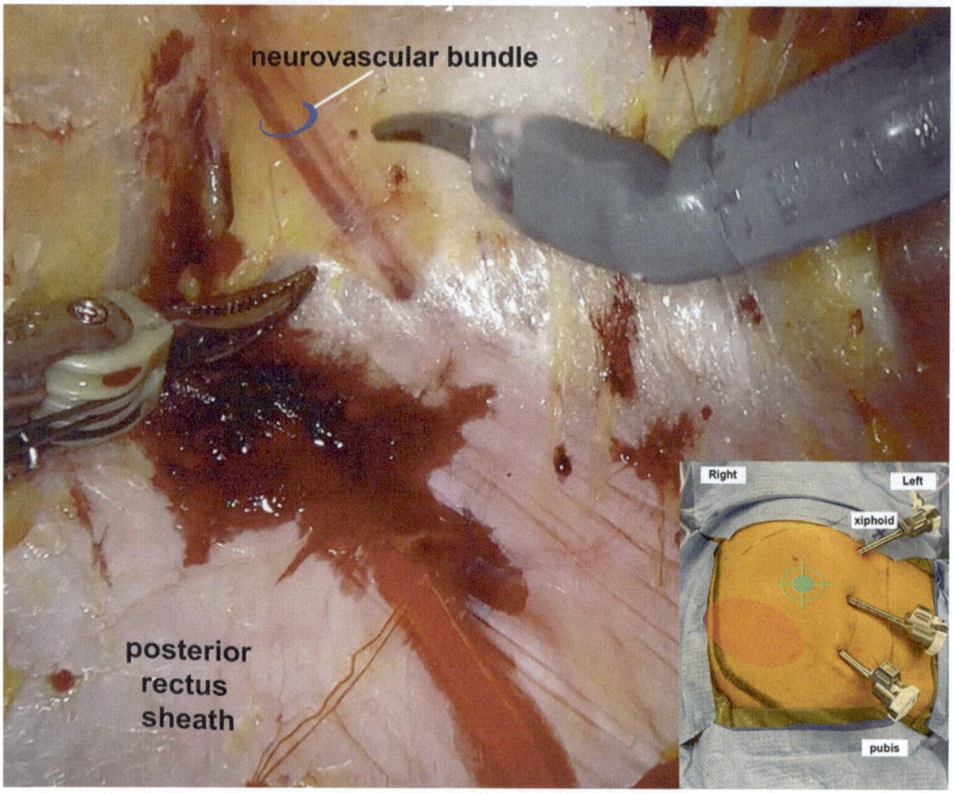


**Fig. 9.5** Ipsilateral retrorectus dissection is performed, and neurovascular bundles on the lateral abdominal wall are identified and preserved. The sub-figure shows trocar positions, captured image, and hernia location

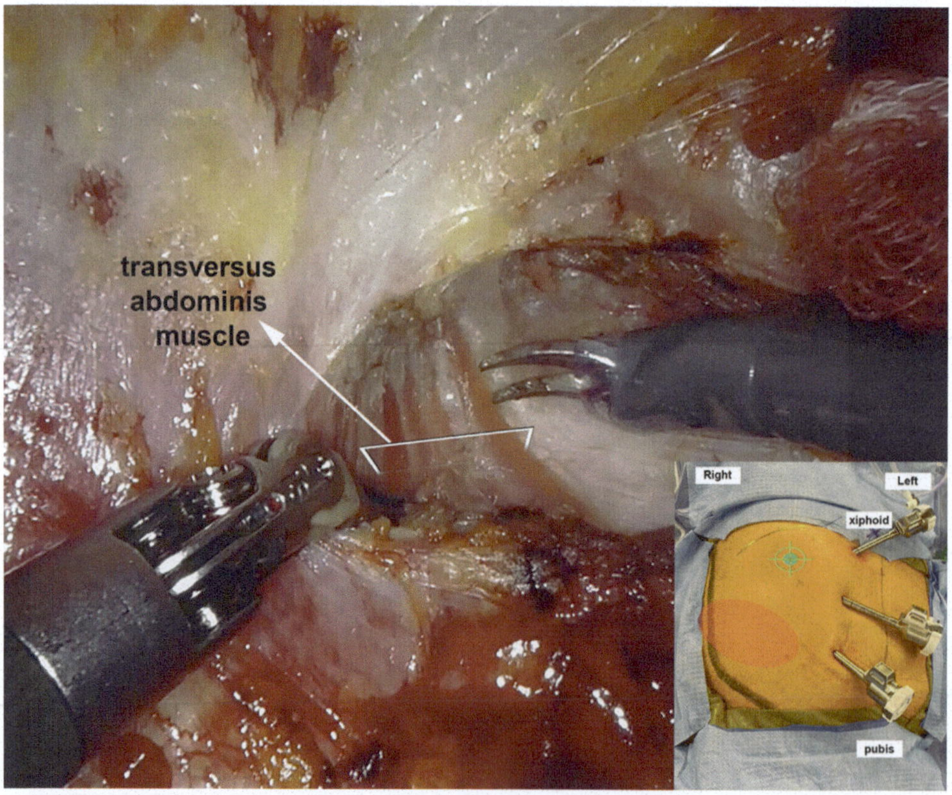


**Fig. 9.6** Ipsilateral transversus abdominis release (TAR) is initiated, proceeding in the caudal direction

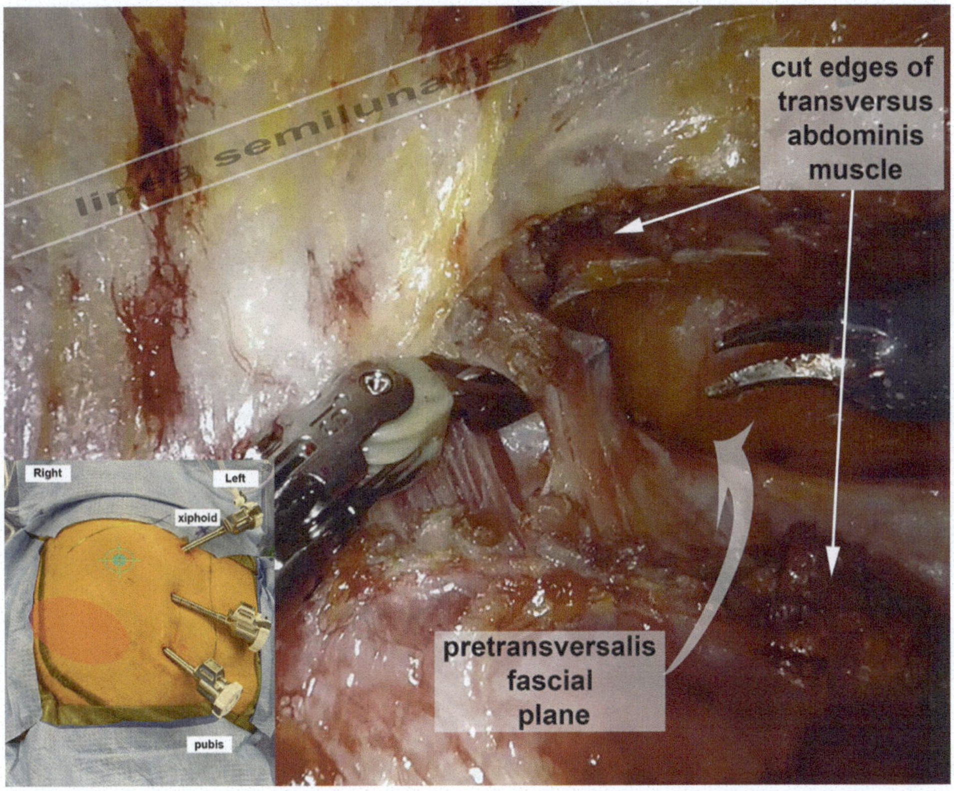


**Fig. 9.7** Continuation of TAR

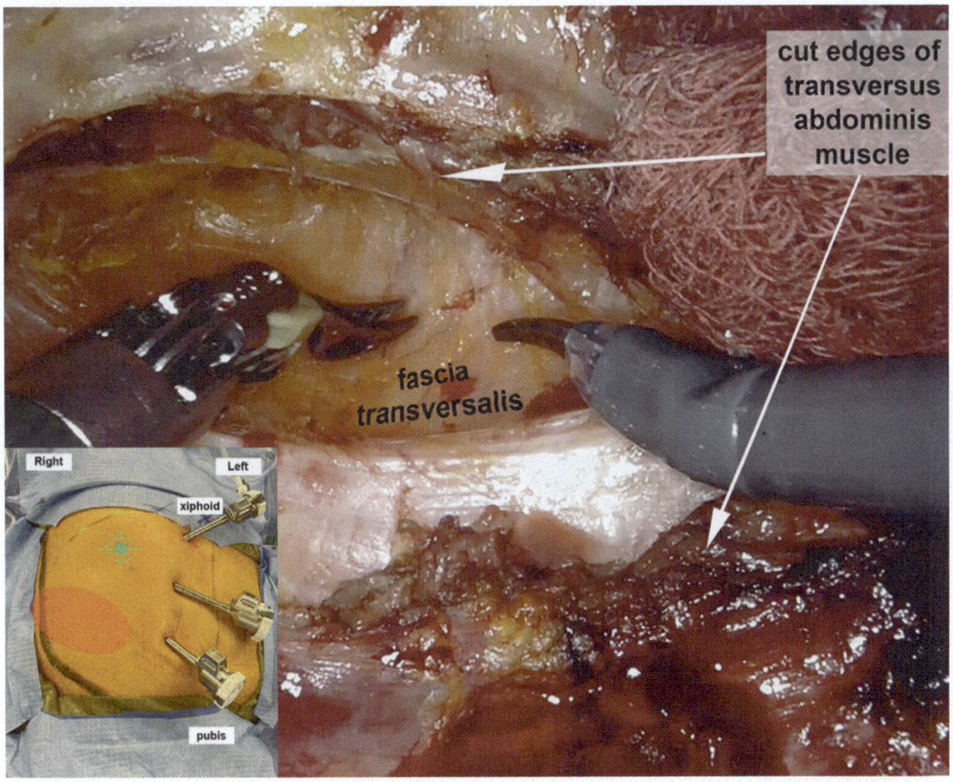


**Fig. 9.8** As TAR is performed, the fascia transversalis and peritoneum are visualized

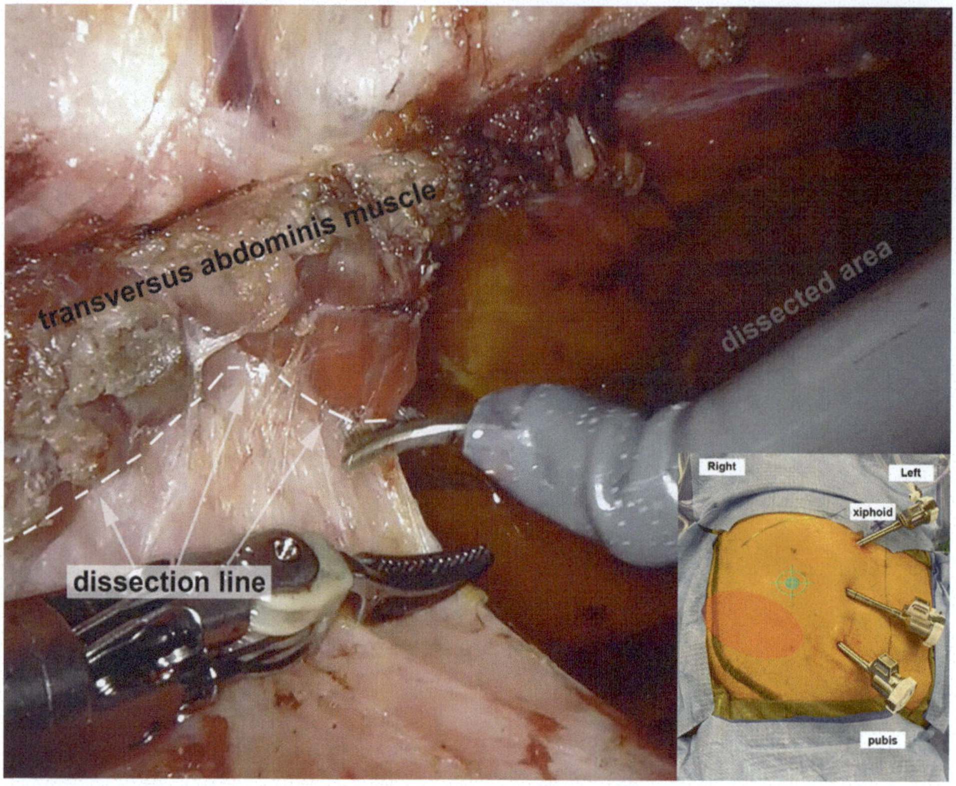


**Fig. 9.9** The dissection line is revealed using traction against the fascia transversalis

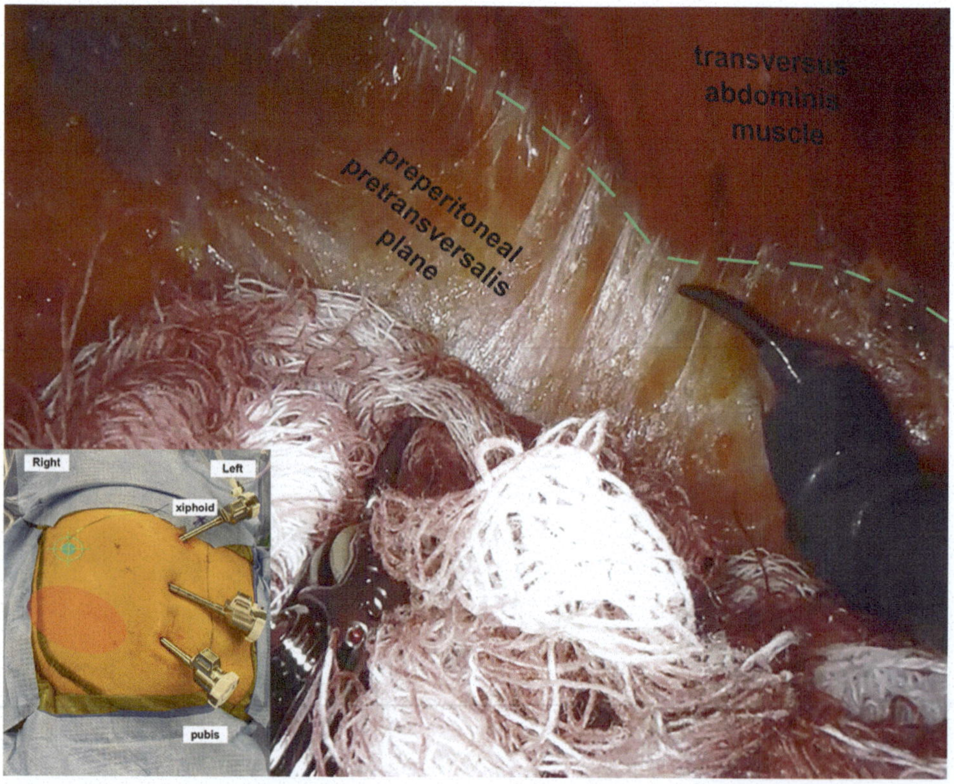


**Fig. 9.10** Lateral dissection towards the anterior axillary line

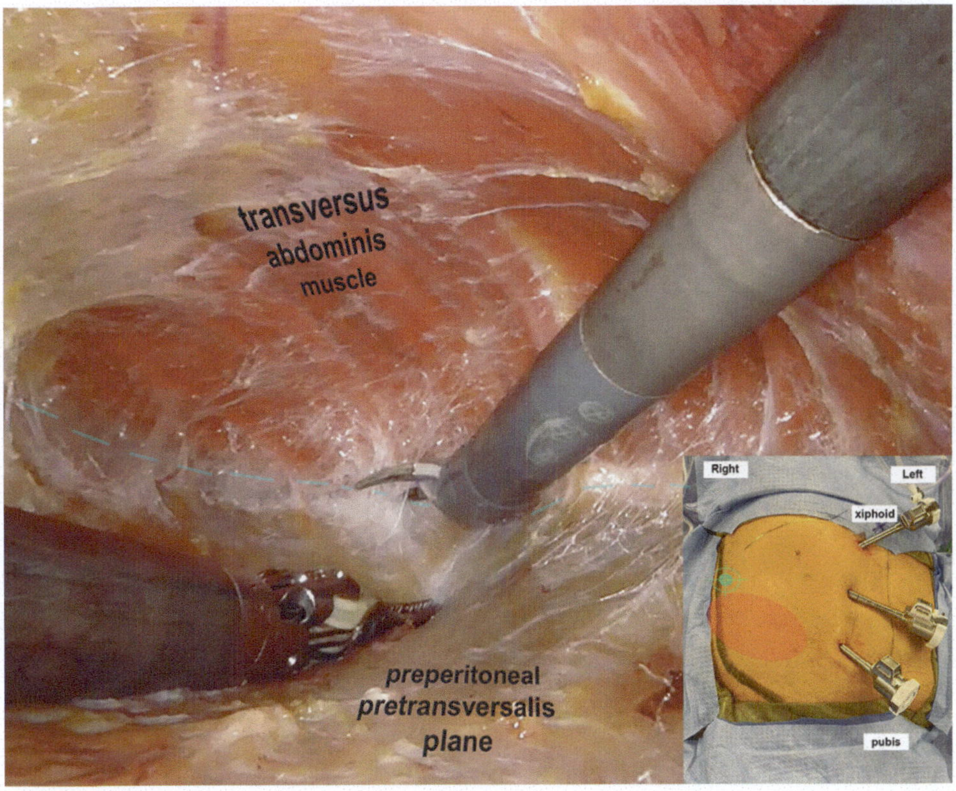


**Fig. 9.11** Lateral dissection towards the mid-axillary line

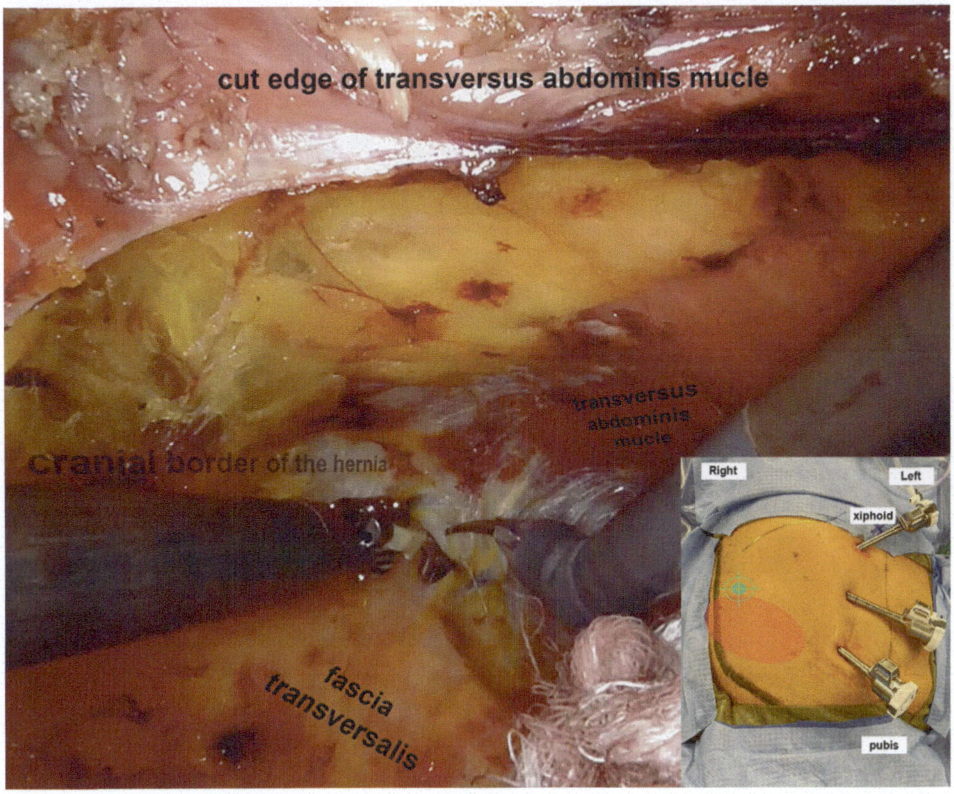


**Fig. 9.12** The dissection is carried out towards the cranial border of the hernia

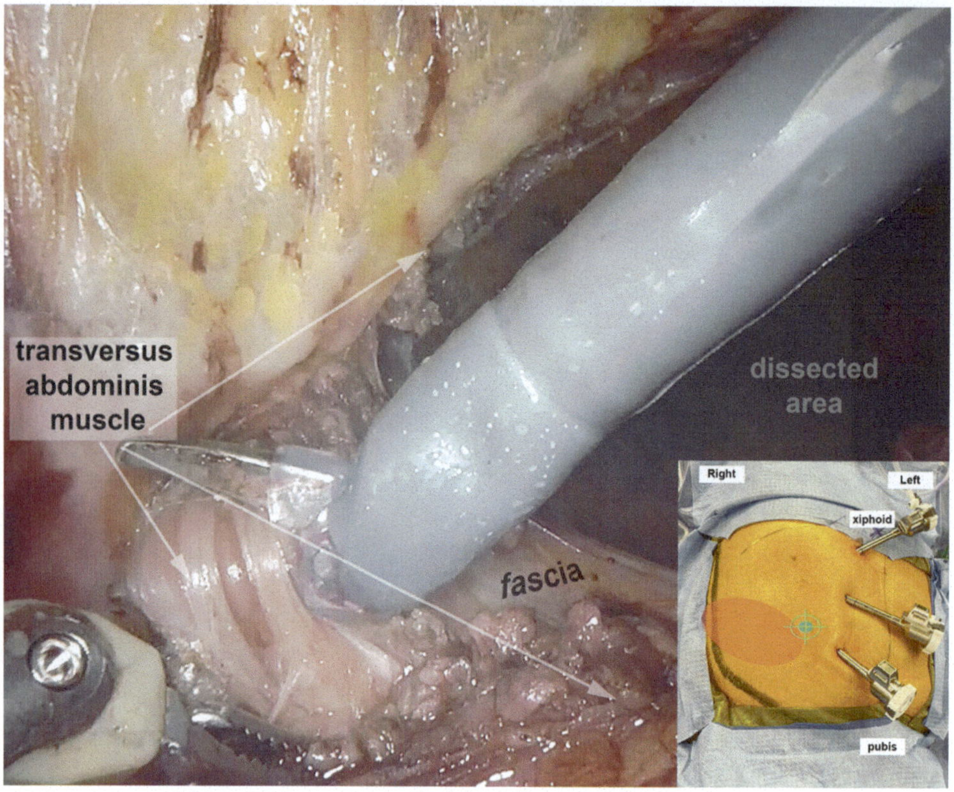


Fig. 9.13 Circumferential dissection around the hernia facilitates the upcoming hernia reduction. TAR is continued

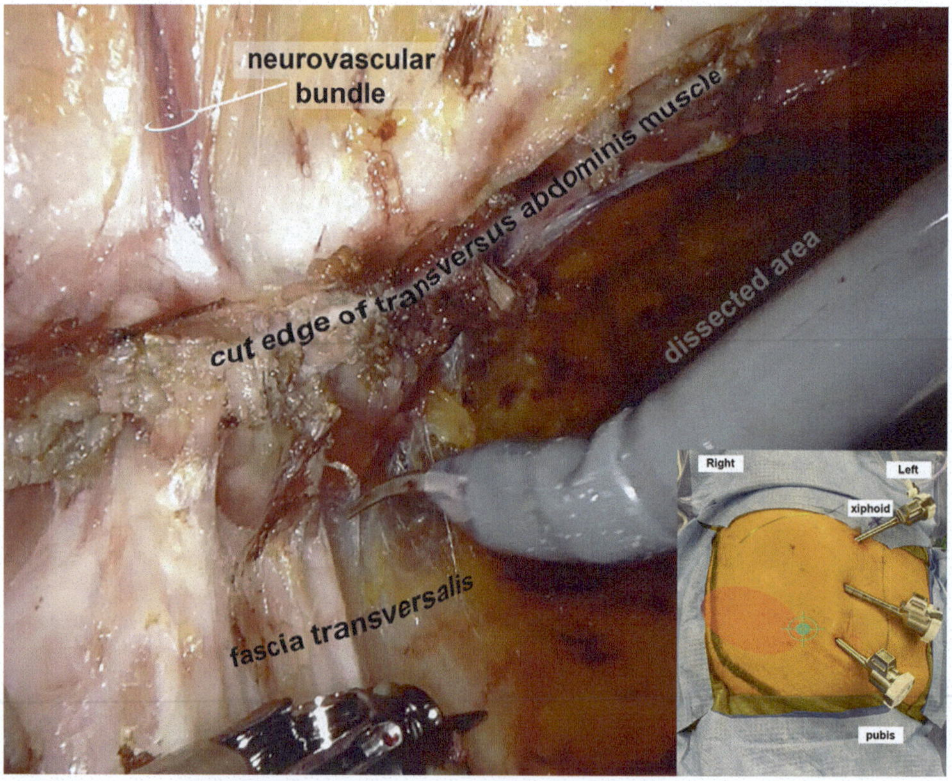


Fig. 9.14 Retromuscular dissection is continued around the hernia

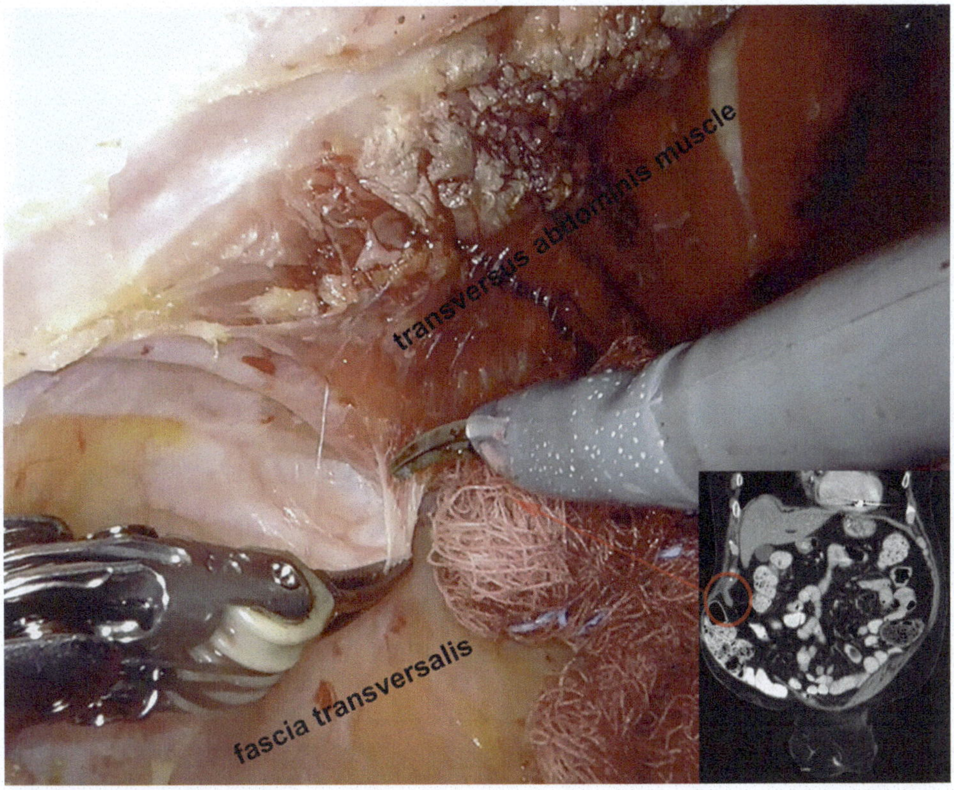


**Fig. 9.15** Traction against the fascia transversalis prevents inadvertent breach of the hernia sac

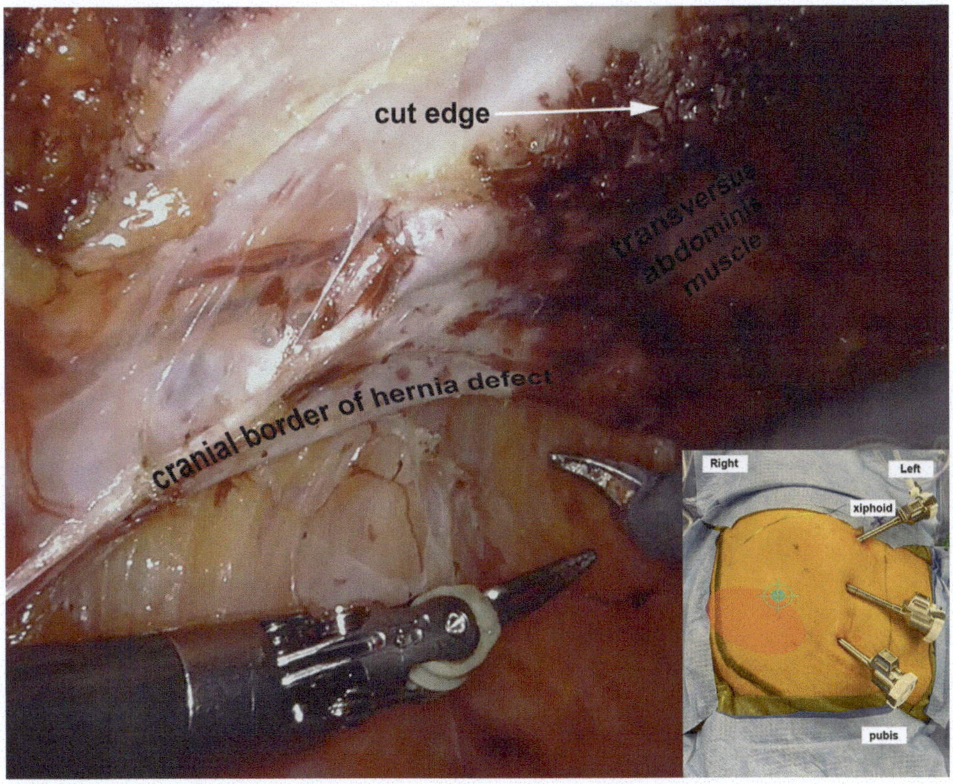


**Fig. 9.16** To isolate the hernia sac without any peritoneal tear, circumferential dissection is of utmost importance

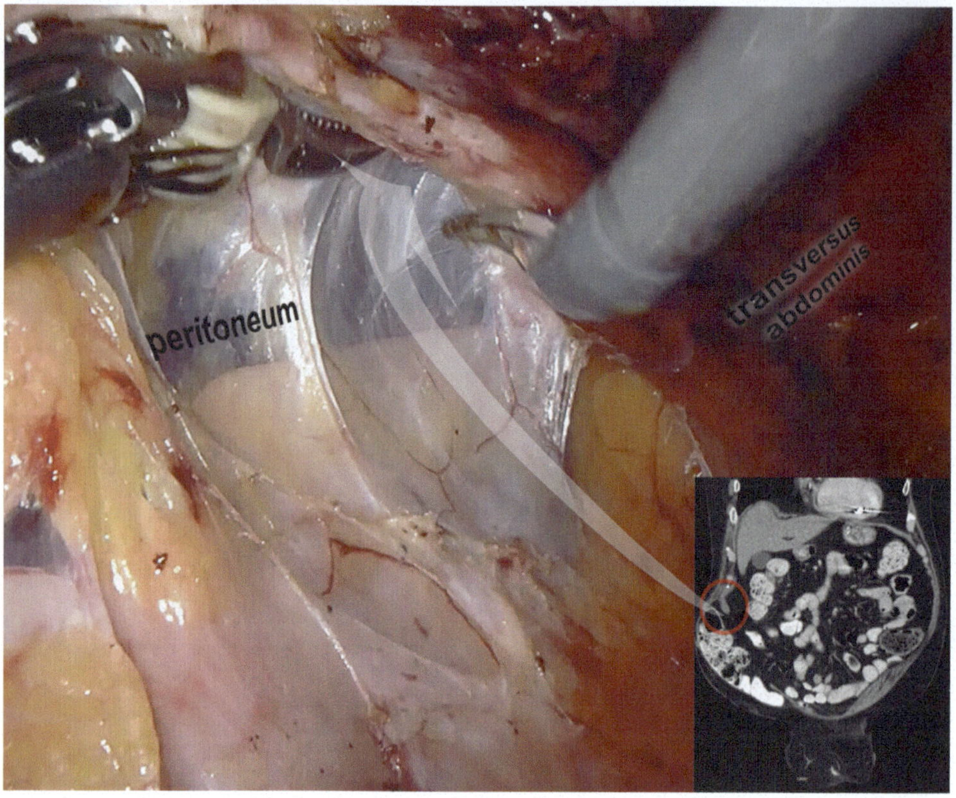


Fig. 9.17 The cranial spherical border of the hernia sac is blocked by the transversus abdominis muscle, which prevents hernia reduction at this point

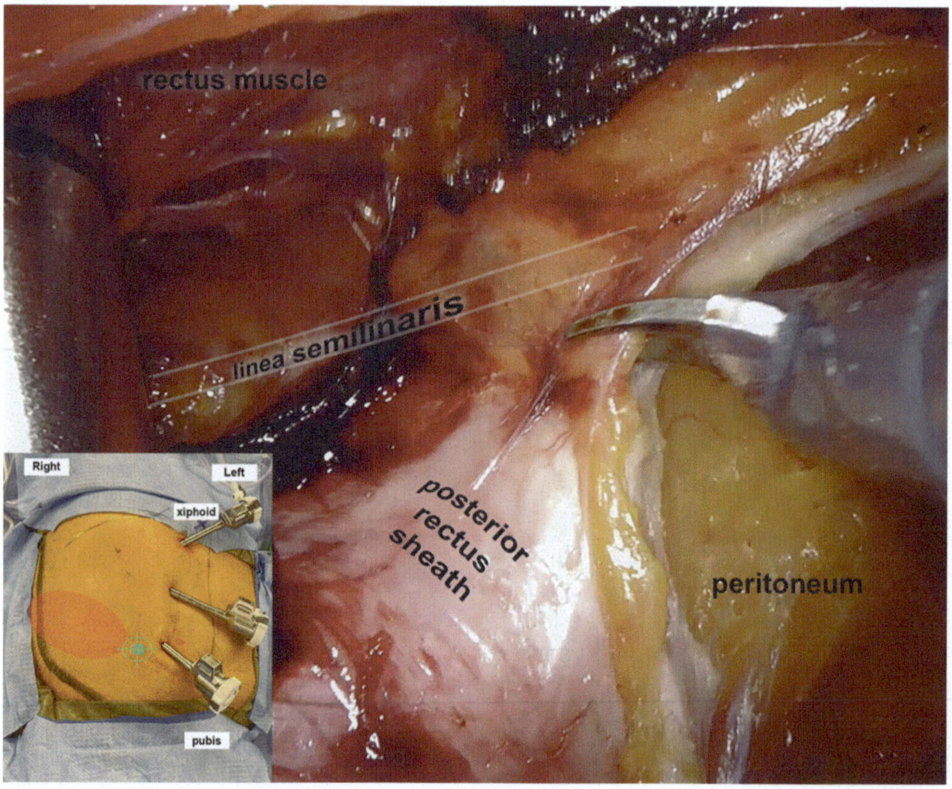


Fig. 9.18 At this level, the lateral border of the posterior rectus sheath does not contain transversus abdominis muscle fibers. Dissection is continued in the cranio-caudal direction

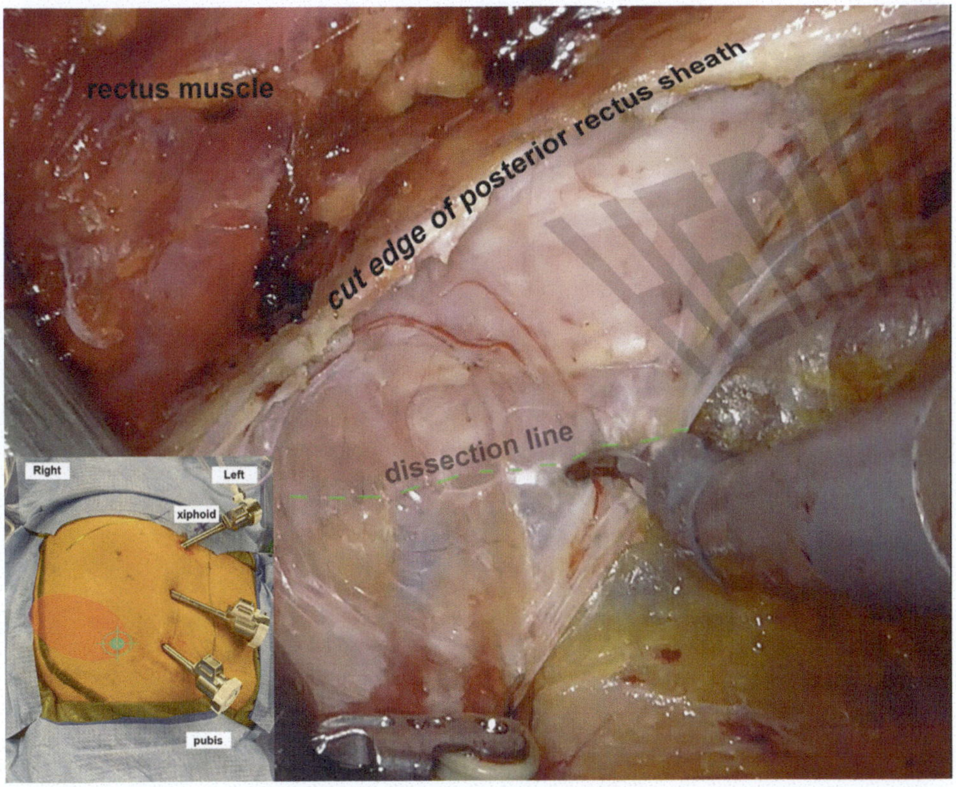


**Fig. 9.19** The hernia sac is stripped from the pseudosac, which consists of oblique muscles

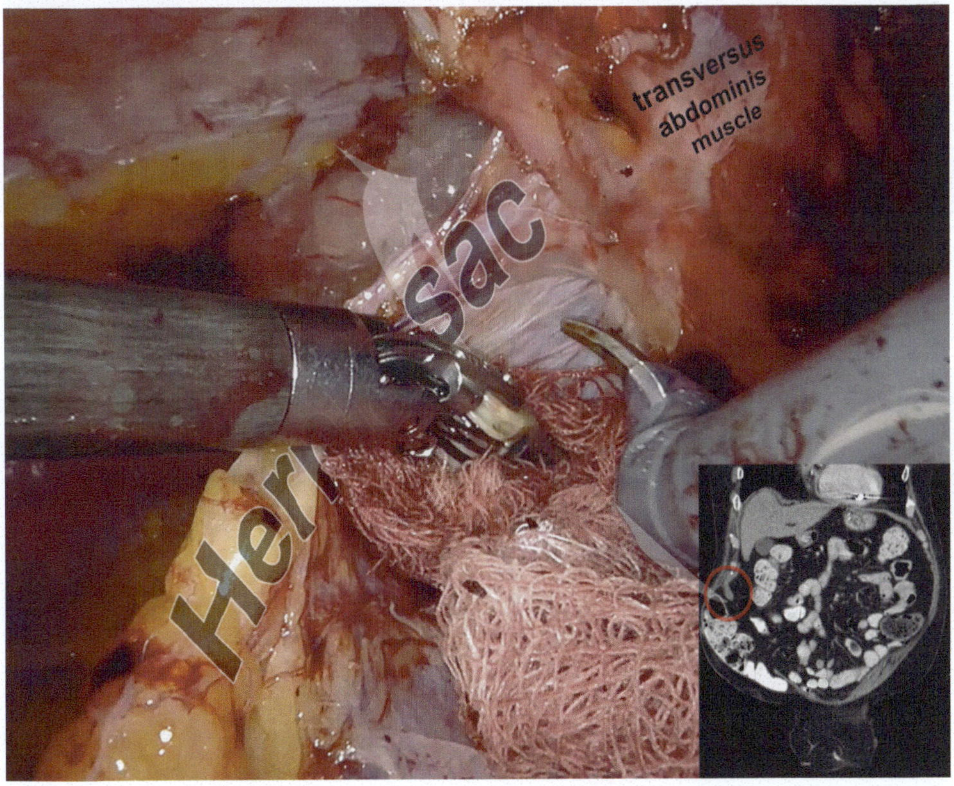


**Fig. 9.20** After the inferior portion of the hernia sac is separated from the pseudosac, the cranial hernia border is revisited

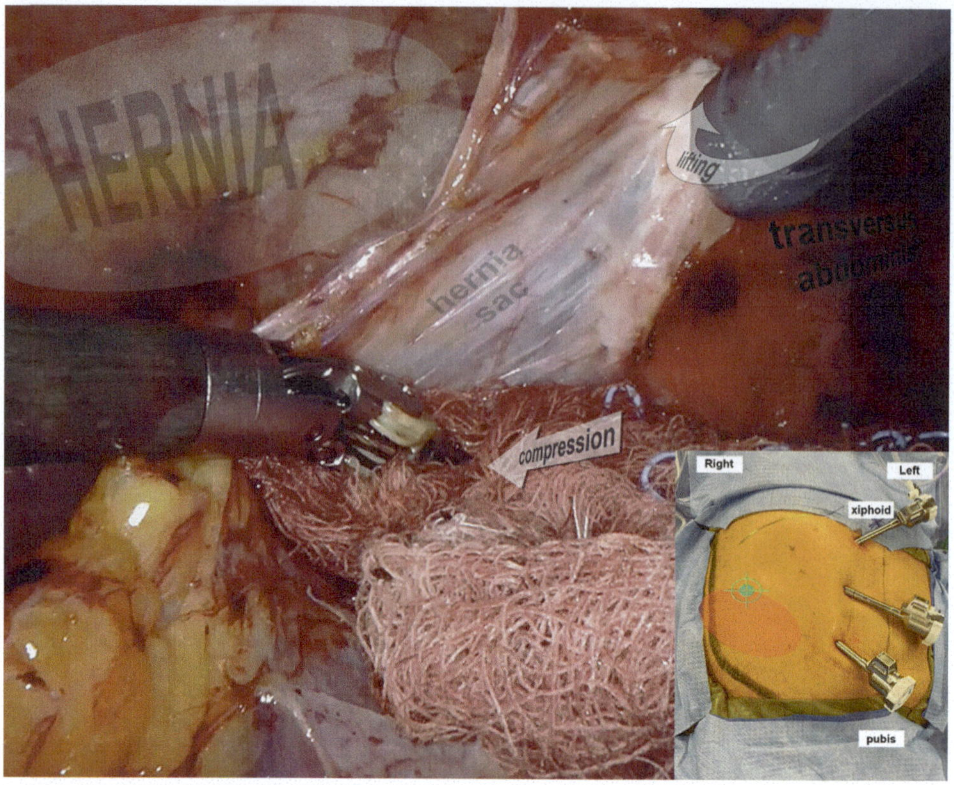


Fig. 9.21 Simultaneous lateral pressure along the hernia sac and traction against the transversus abdominis helps avoid tearing of the hernia sac

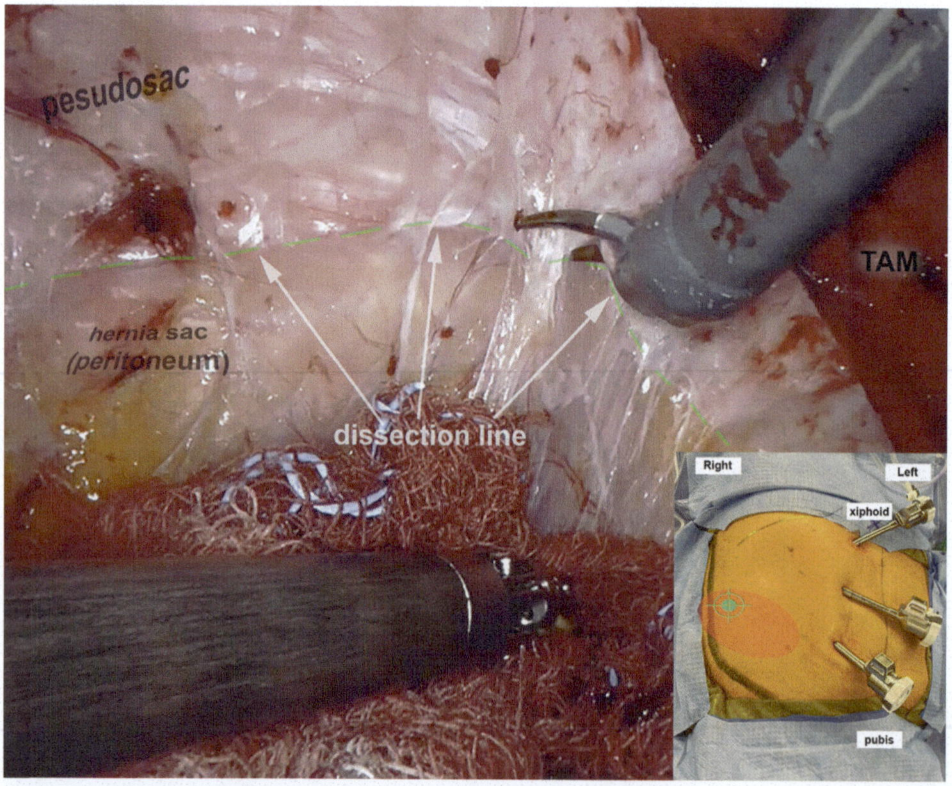


Fig. 9.22 Lateral dissection is continued to free the hernia sac from the pseudosac. The transversus abdominis muscle (TAM) is visualized cranially

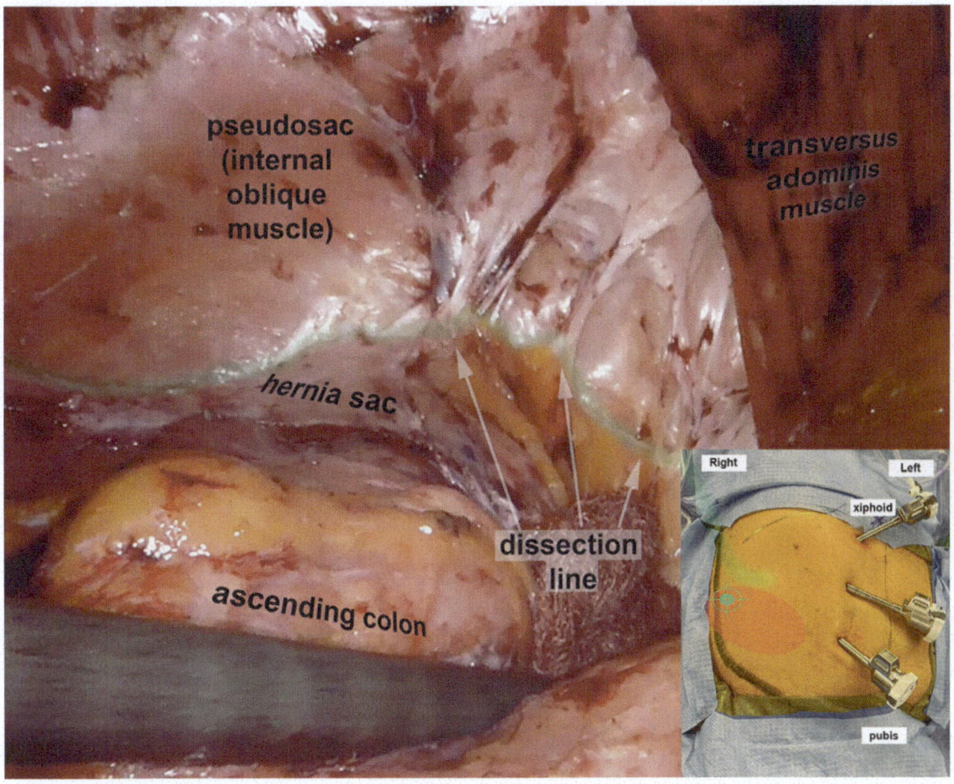


Fig. 9.23 Continuation of lateral dissection

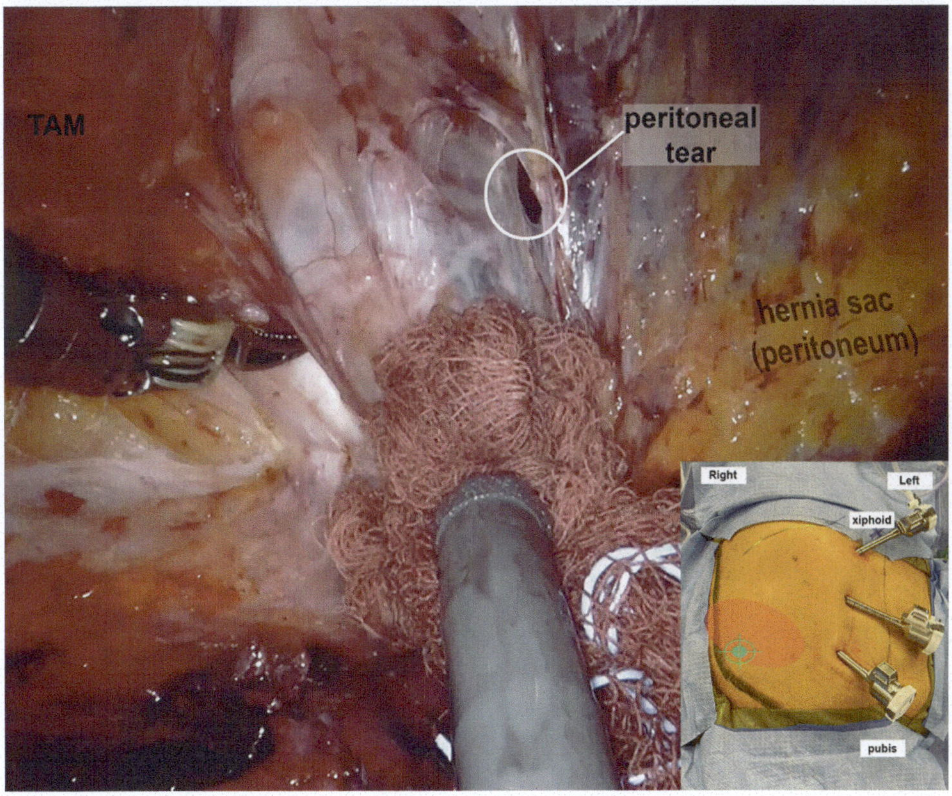


Fig. 9.24 Dissection is continued along the inferior border of the hernia. The transversus abdominis muscle (TAM) is visualized inferiorly

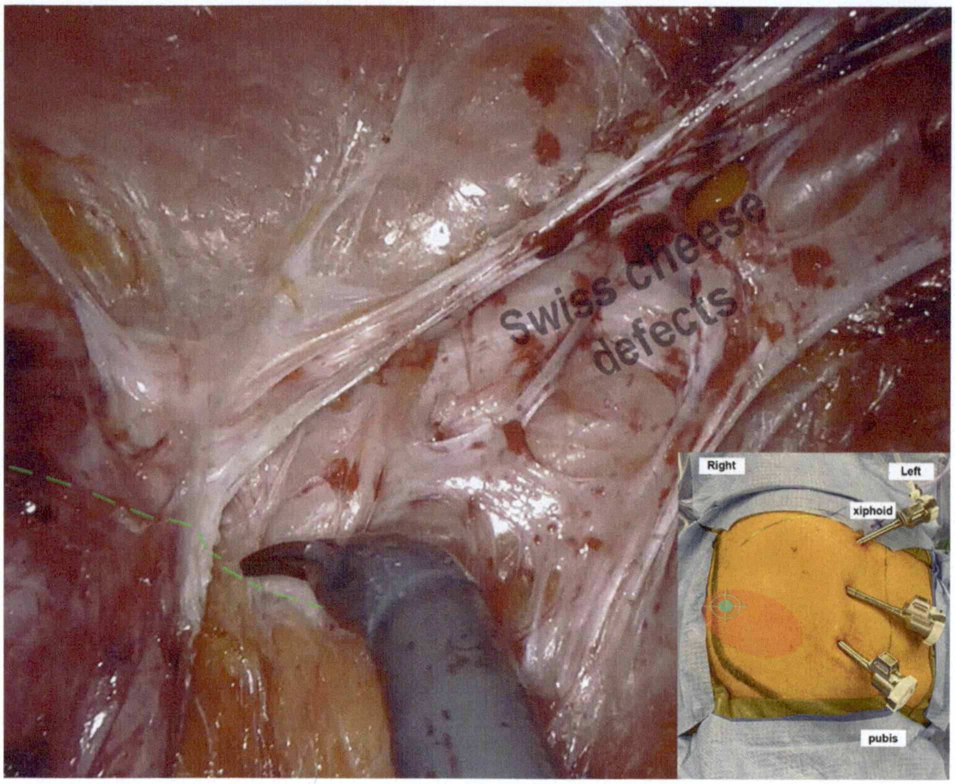


Fig. 9.25 Hernia sac reduction is continued; small "swiss-cheese" defects are revealed

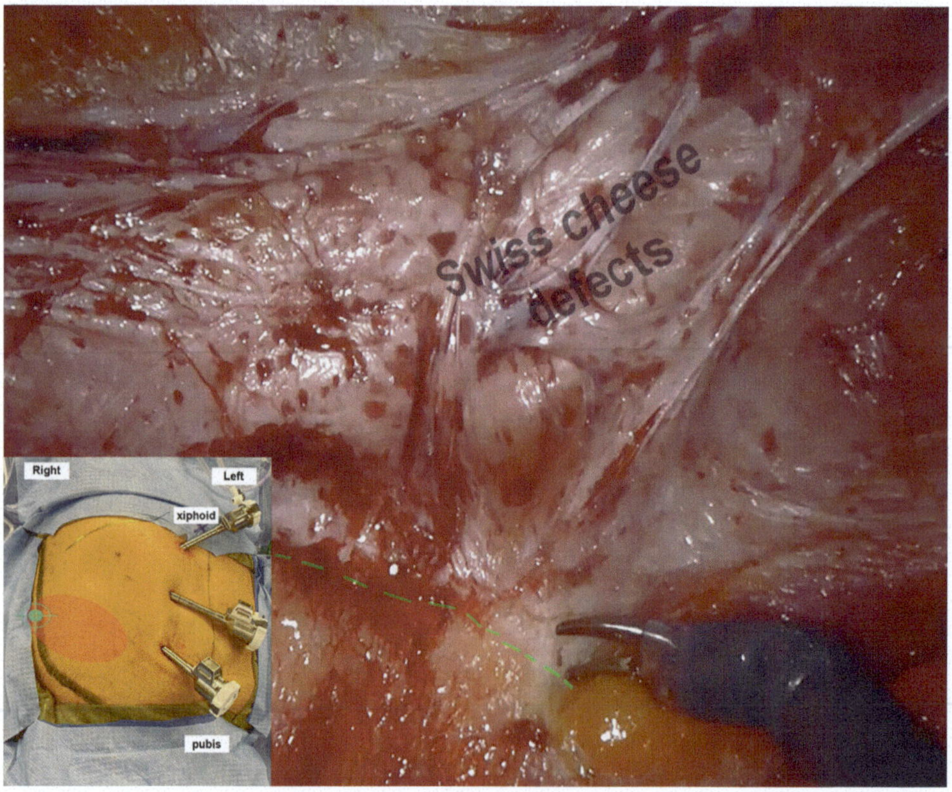


Fig. 9.26 The dissection is continued laterally towards the posterior axillary line

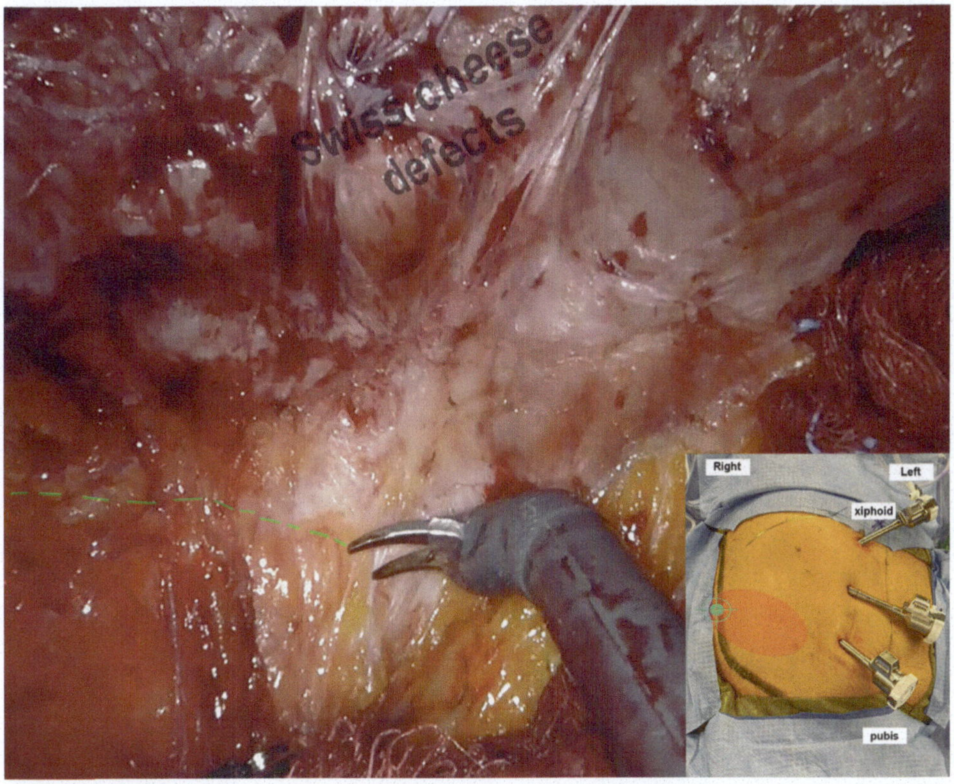


Fig. 9.27 Continuation of lateral dissection

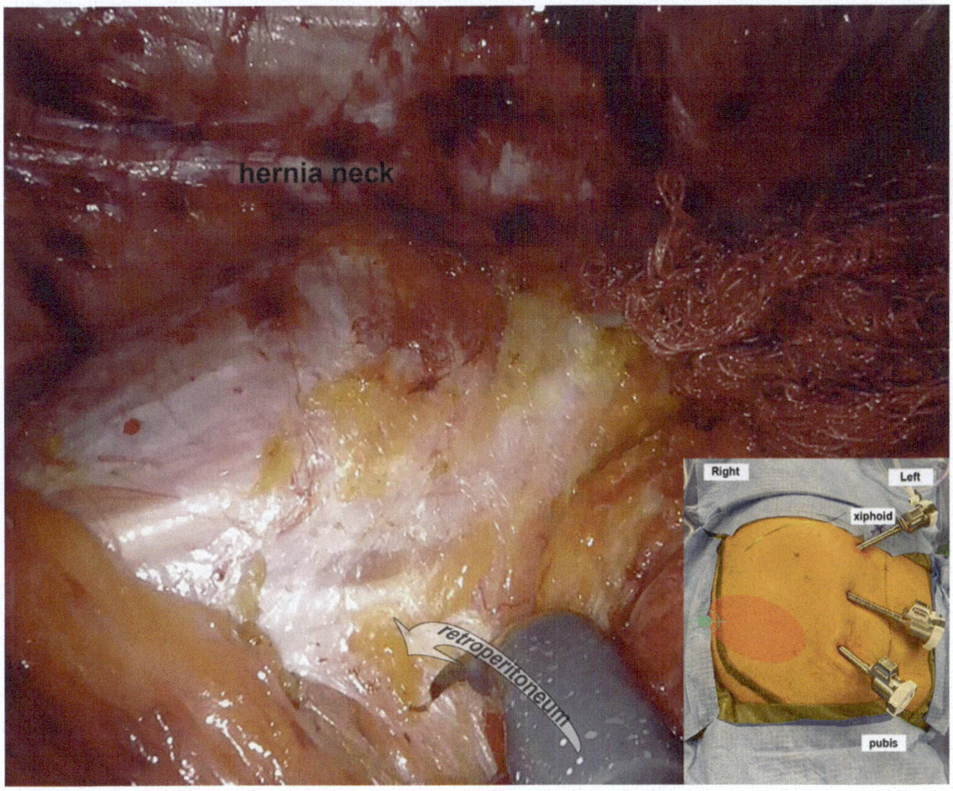


Fig. 9.28 The retroperitoneum is revealed

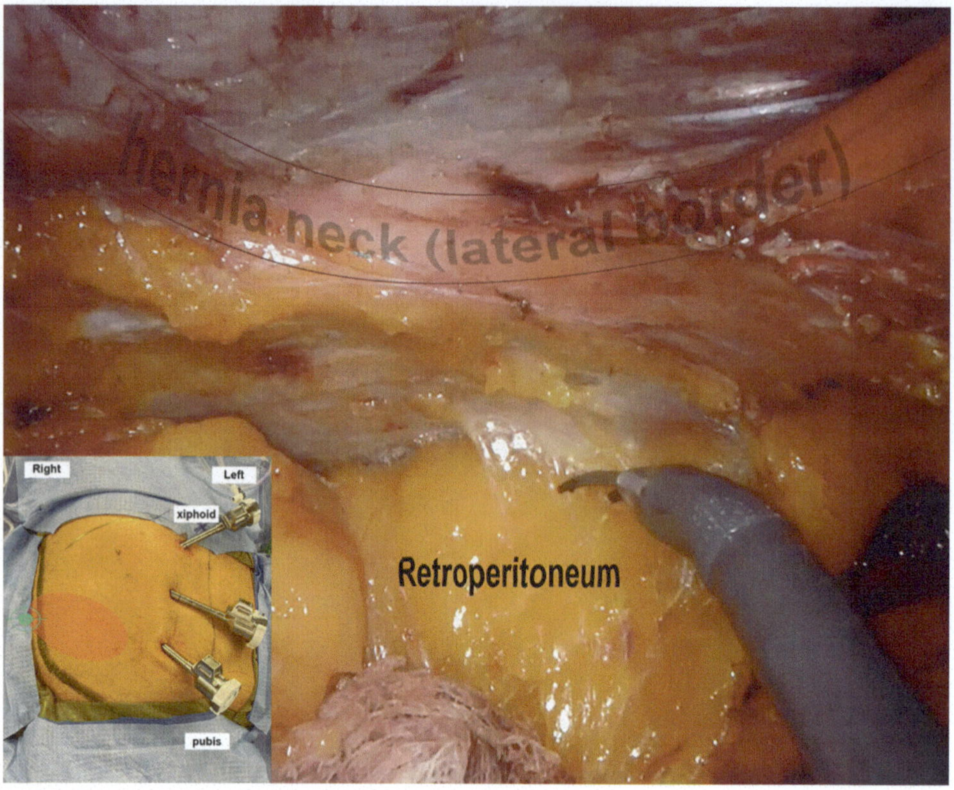


Fig. 9.29 The lateral border of the hernia neck is shown, along with retroperitoneal fatty tissue

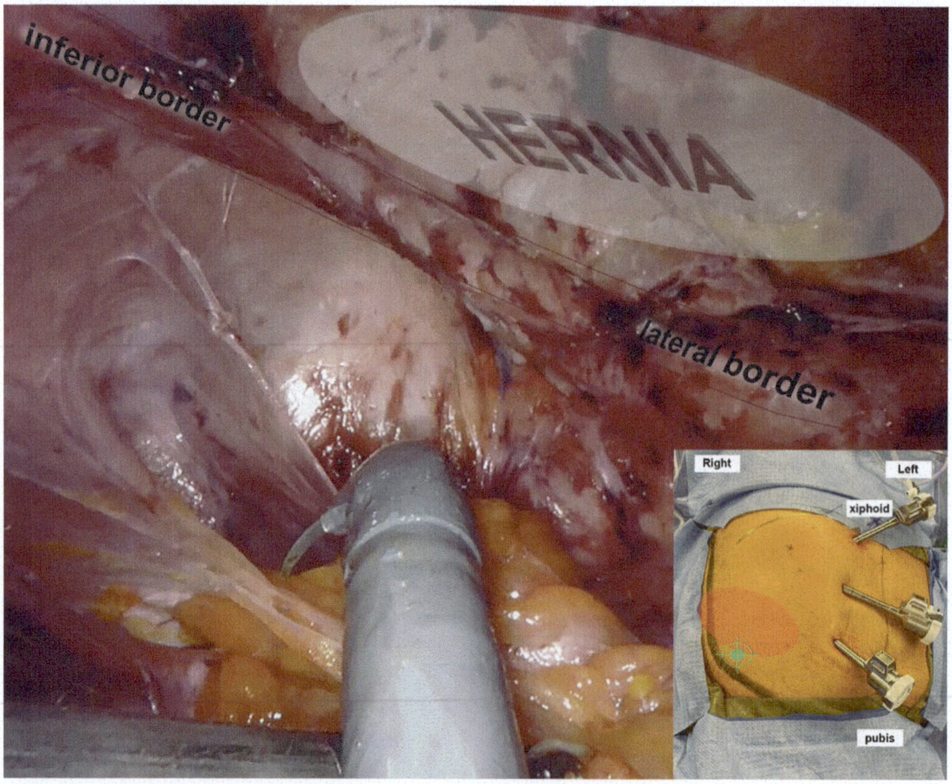


Fig. 9.30 Hernia reduction is continued at the inferior border of the hernia neck

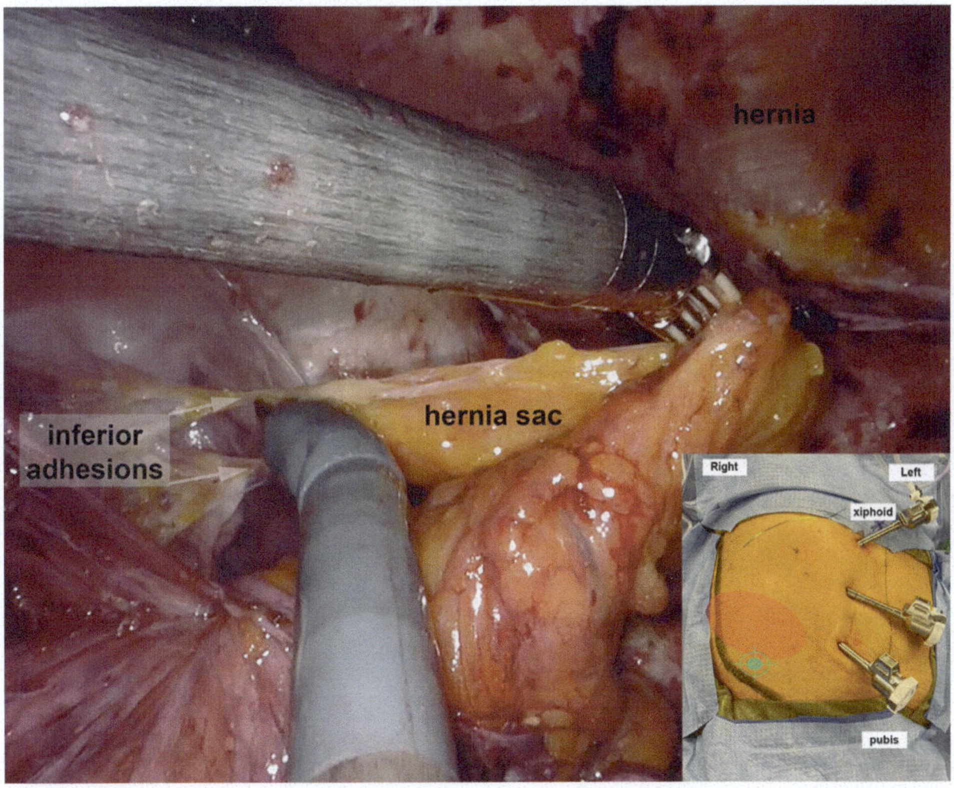


Fig. 9.31 Adhesions are transected to complete hernia sac reduction

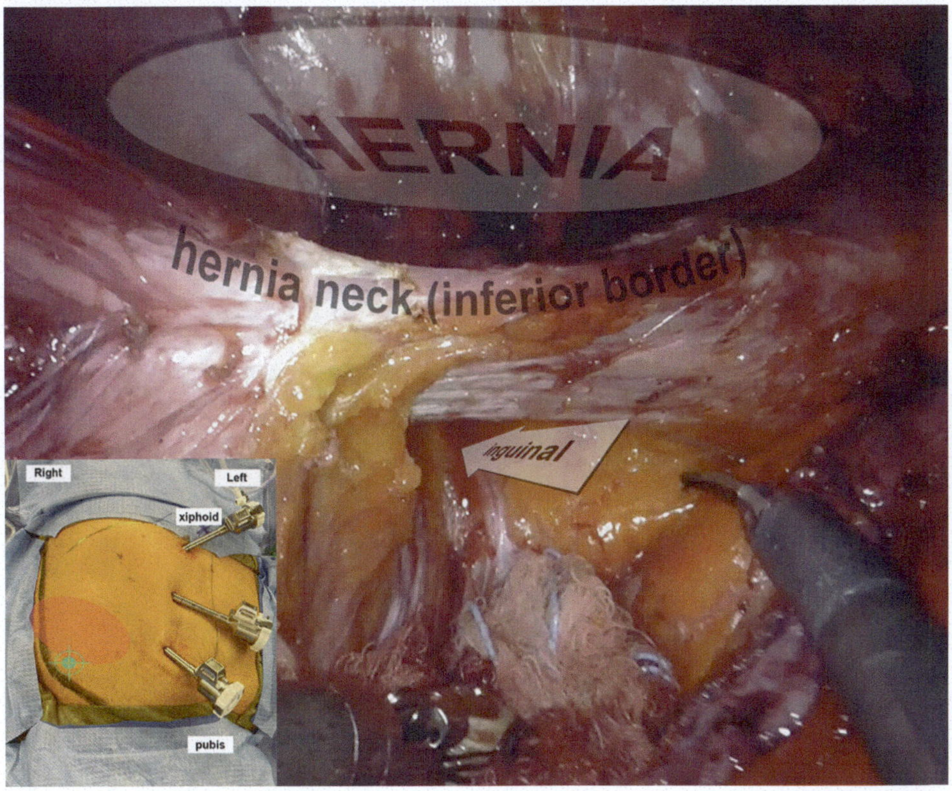


Fig. 9.32 The inguinal region is revealed below the inferior border of the hernia neck

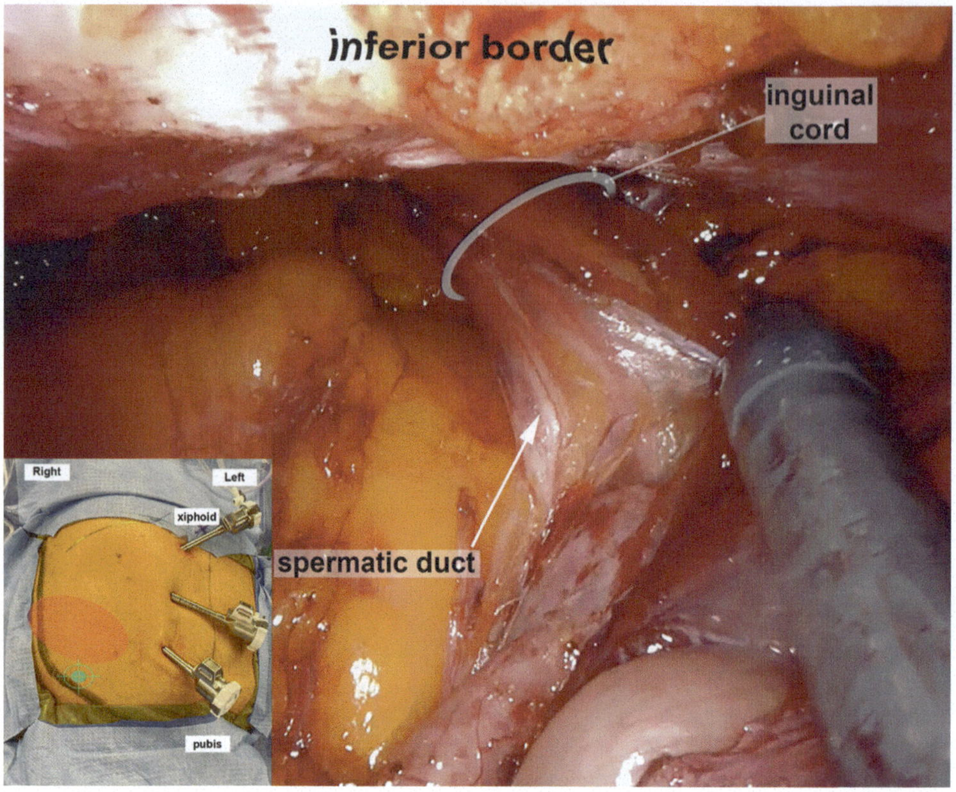


**Fig. 9.33** A closer look at the inguinal cord and its elements

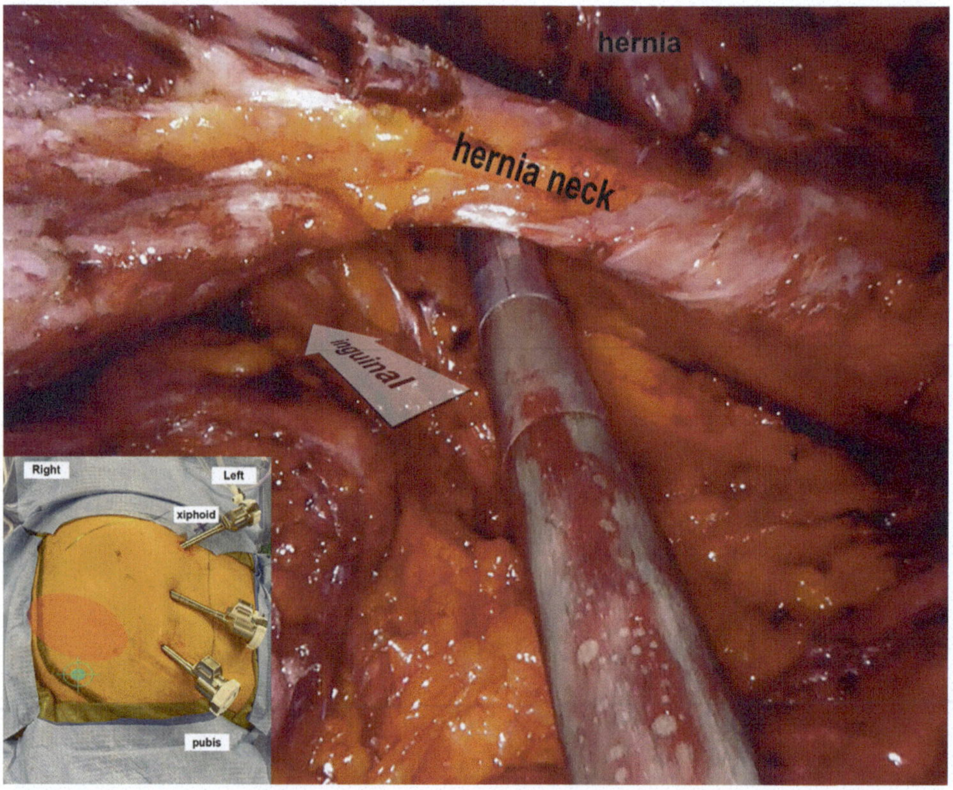


**Fig. 9.34** Inferior view of the dissected area

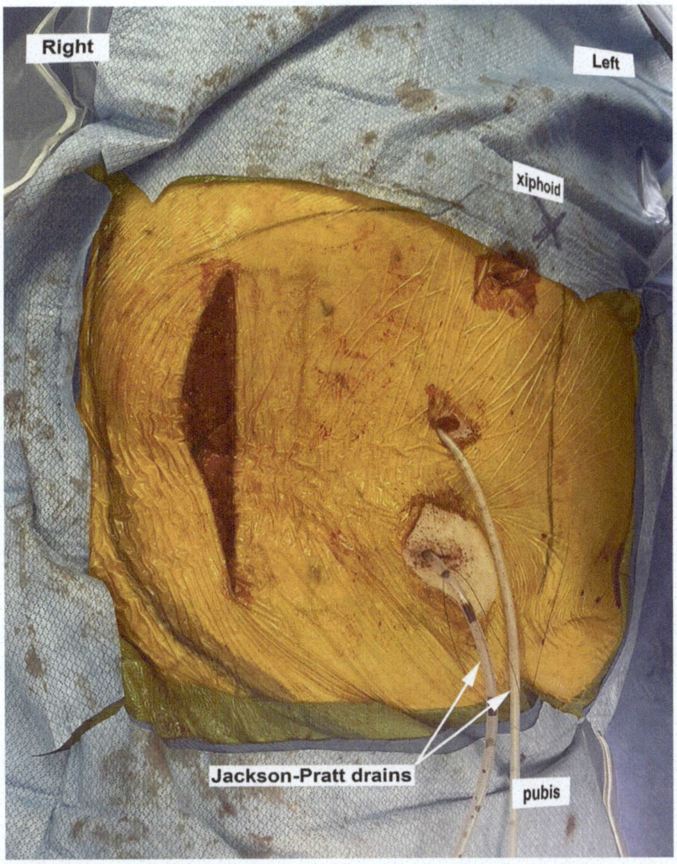


**Fig. 9.35** Transition to the open approach of the hybrid technique. Two pieces of expanded polytetrafluoroethylene (ePTFE) mesh are sewn together and deployed into the dissected area. The anterior defect is closed using barbed sutures. The trocars are then removed, and two Jackson-Pratt drains are placed

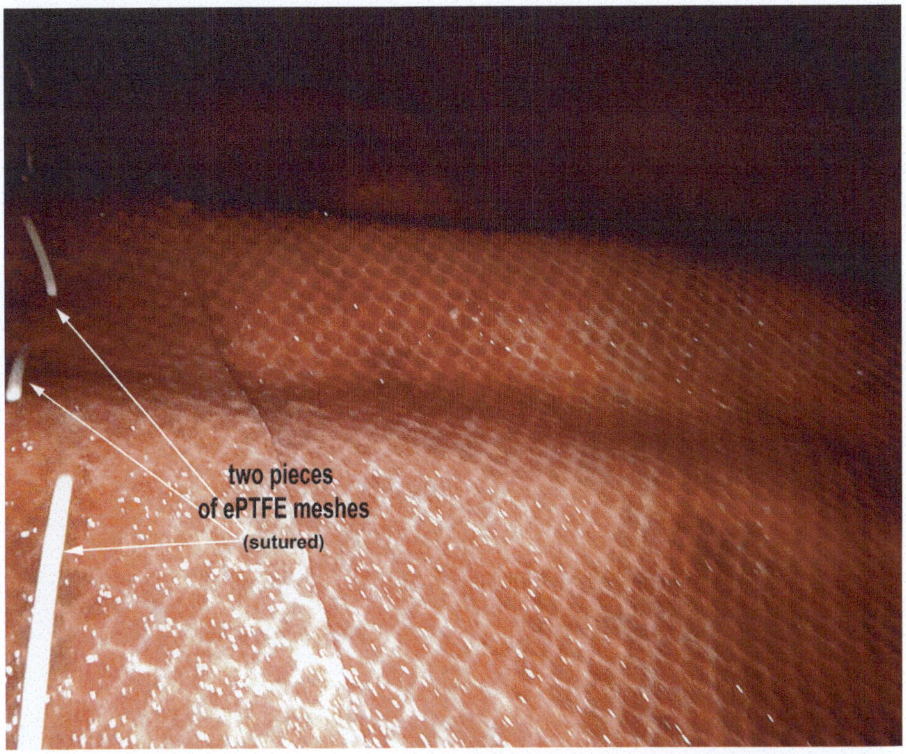


**Fig. 9.36** Laparoscopic view of the ePTFE mesh, obtained to ensure that the mesh is deployed without folding or wrinkles. Skin and trocar incisions are closed using absorbable sutures

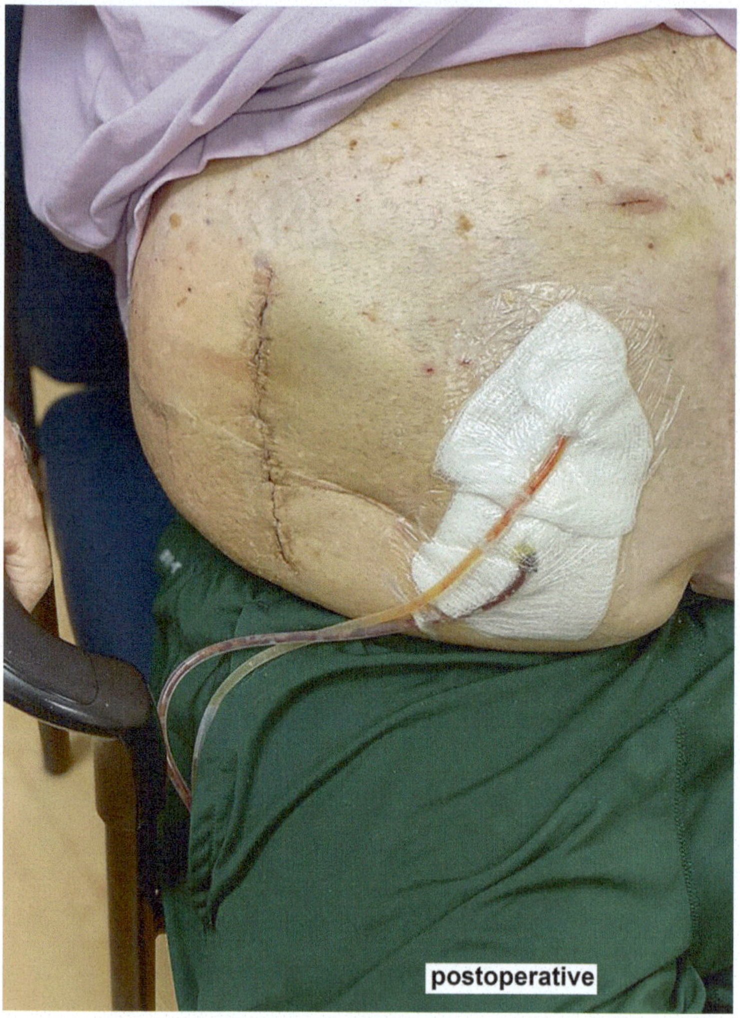


Fig. 9.37 Postoperative results after 1 week

## References


1. Muysoms FE, Miserez M, Berrevoet F, Campanelli G, Champault GG, Chelala E, et al. Classification of primary and incisional abdominal wall hernias. Hernia. 2009;13:407–14. https://doi.org/10.1007/s10029-009-0518-x.
2. Halka JT, Vasyluk A, Demare A, Iacco A, Janczyk R. Hybrid robotic-assisted transversus abdominis release versus open transversus abdominis release: a comparison of short-term outcomes. Hernia. 2019;23:37–42. https://doi.org/10.1007/s10029-018-1858-1.
3. Halka JT, Vasyluk A, DeMare AM, Janczyk RJ, Iacco AA. Robotic and hybrid robotic transversus abdominis release may be performed with low length of stay and wound morbidity. Am J Surg. 2018;215:462–5. https://doi.org/10.1016/j.amjsurg.2017.10.053.
4. Kulaçoðlu H, Özer M. Hybrid repair for secondary lumbar hernias: Three cases with different etiologies. Laparosc Endosc Surg Sci. 2018;25(4):149–156. https://doi.org/10.14744/less.2018.22932.

# Robotic Flank Hernia Repair: Totally Extraperitoneal (TEP)

# 10

Rockson Liu, Azure Adkins, and Sora Ely

## Introduction

Flank or lumbar hernias are located in the lumbar region, the borders of which are the posterior border of the external oblique laterally, the 12th rib superiorly, the erector spinae muscle medially, and the iliac crest inferiorly. About 80% of flank hernias are due to trauma or surgery. Operations that commonly use a flank incision include nephrectomy, adrenalectomy, liver resection, and abdominal aortic aneurysm (AAA) repair. Hernias form in this area postoperatively because of nerve damage causing muscle atrophy, muscle/tendon avulsion, or weakness of the aponeurosis. There are also primary lumbar hernias, which can be congenital or spontaneous.

Symptoms of flank hernias are a palpable posterolateral mass that often reduces on recumbency and enlarges with straining. Hernias in this location have a low risk of incarceration, as they are usually wide-necked.

## Procedure: Illustrated Steps

In the case illustrated in this chapter (Figs. 10.1, 10.2, 10.3, 10.4, 10.5, 10.6, 10.7, 10.8, 10.9, 10.10, 10.11, 10.12, 10.13, 10.14, 10.15, 10.16, 10.17, 10.18, 10.19, 10.20, 10.21, 10.22, 10.23, 10.24, 10.25, 10.26, 10.27, and 10.28), the patient is a 66-year-old man with a history of a right nephrectomy, two renal transplants, and previous hernia repairs, who presented with an enlarging, symptomatic right flank hernia. Because of the extensive abdominal surgical history, we elected to perform an extended totally extraperitoneal (eTEP) hernia operation, in order to stay outside of the abdominal cavity. This technique requires mid transverse abdominis release (TAR) in order to continue to develop the preperitoneal space lateral to the retrorectus space. By performing this operation, we are able to stay out of the abdominal cavity and place the mesh against well-vascularized muscle, which is very important in this patient because he is immunocompromised, owing to the need to take long-term immunosuppressive medications.

The hernia width was 15 cm and the length was 8 cm. A macroporous polyester mesh that measured 30 cm wide and 20 cm long was placed in the retromuscular space and secured with multiple sutures. The patient was discharged home on the second postoperative day and has been doing well postoperatively.

R. Liu (✉) · A. Adkins
Alta Bates Summit Medical Center, Epic Care, Oakland, CA, USA

S. Ely
Department of General Surgery, University of California San Francisco East Bay, Highland Hospital, Oakland, CA, USA


O. Y. Kudsi (ed.), *Robotic Hernia Surgery*, https://doi.org/10.1007/978-3-030-46667-1_10

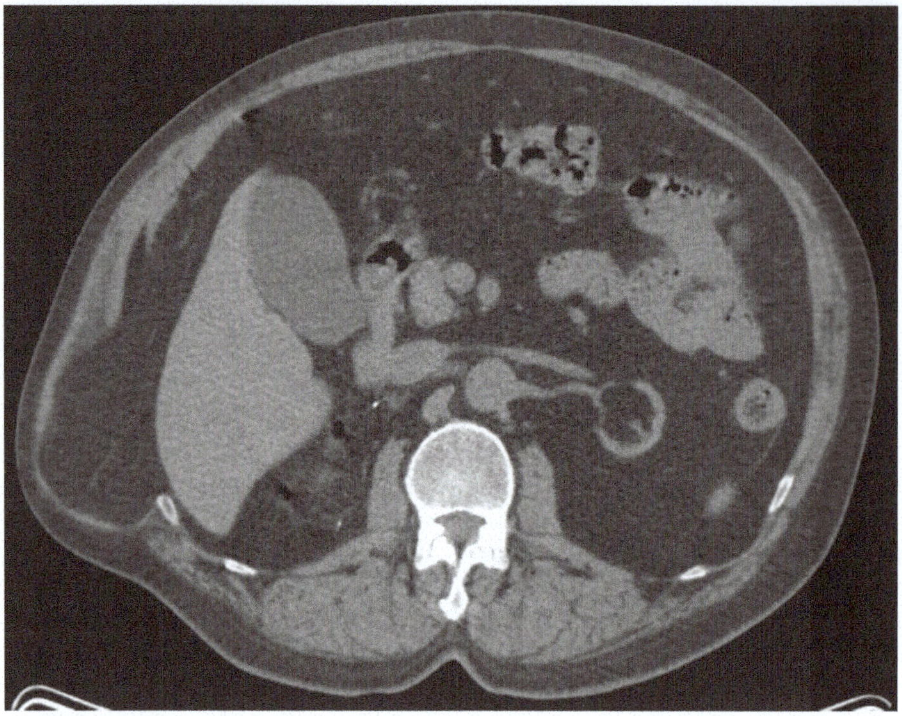

**Fig. 10.1** CT imaging of right flank hernia: axial view

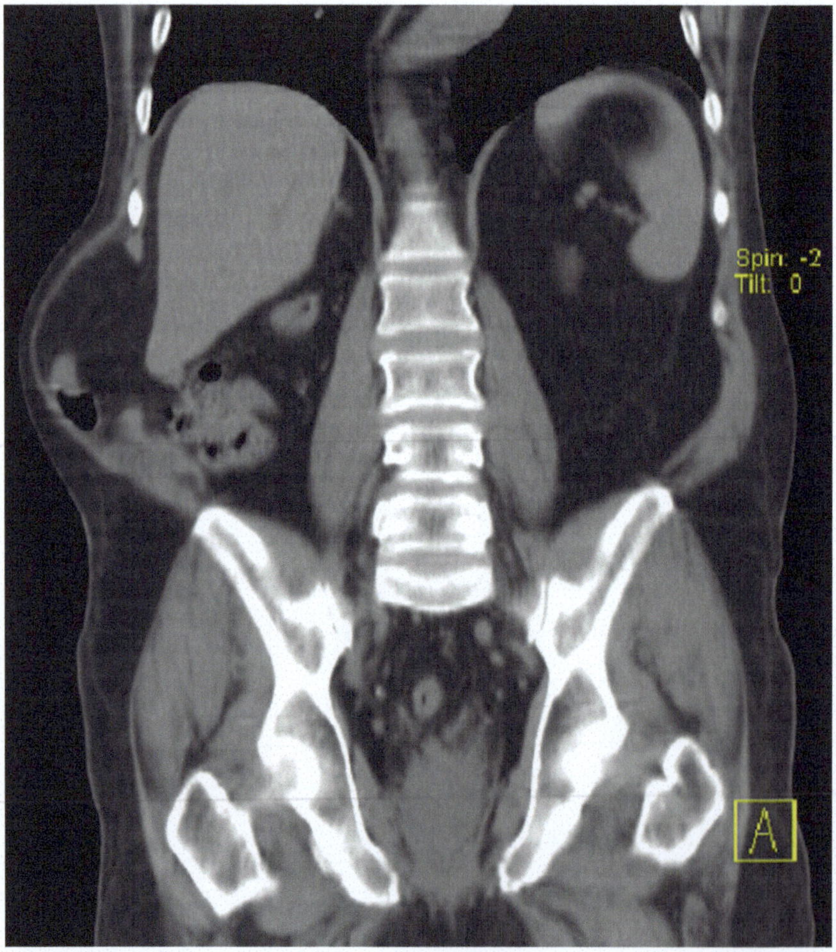


**Fig. 10.2** CT imaging of right flank hernia: coronal view

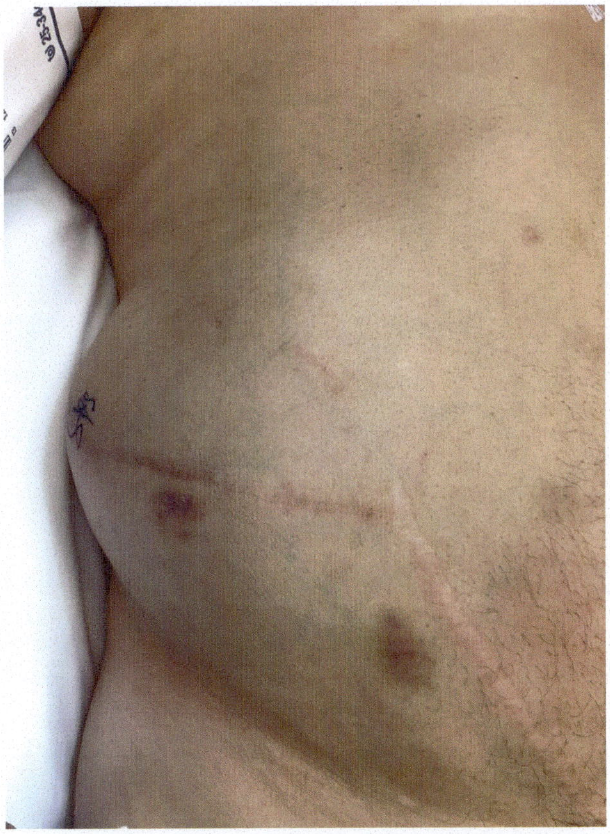

Fig. 10.3 Preoperative photo of hernia

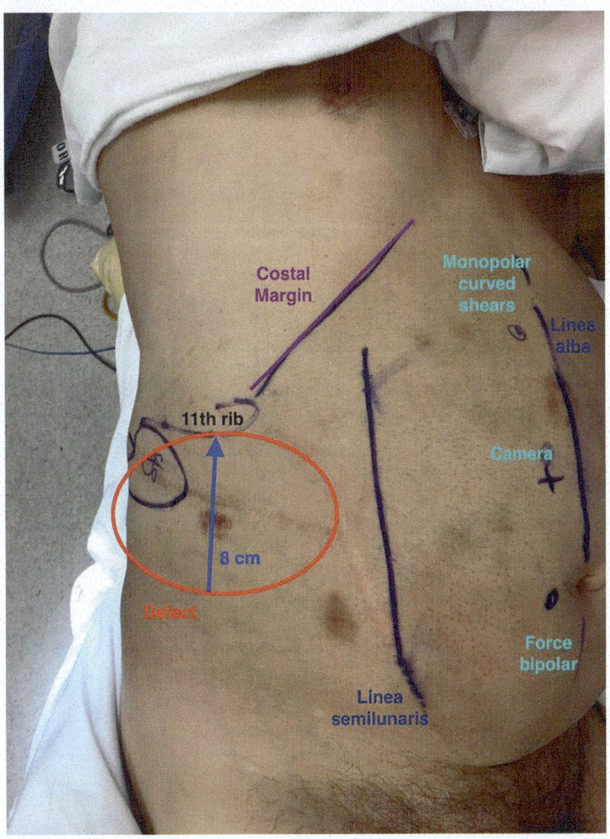


Fig. 10.4 Annotated preoperative photo with anatomy marked. This photo shows the right hernia in addition to the relevant surgical anatomy. The port placement and instruments used in each port are also marked

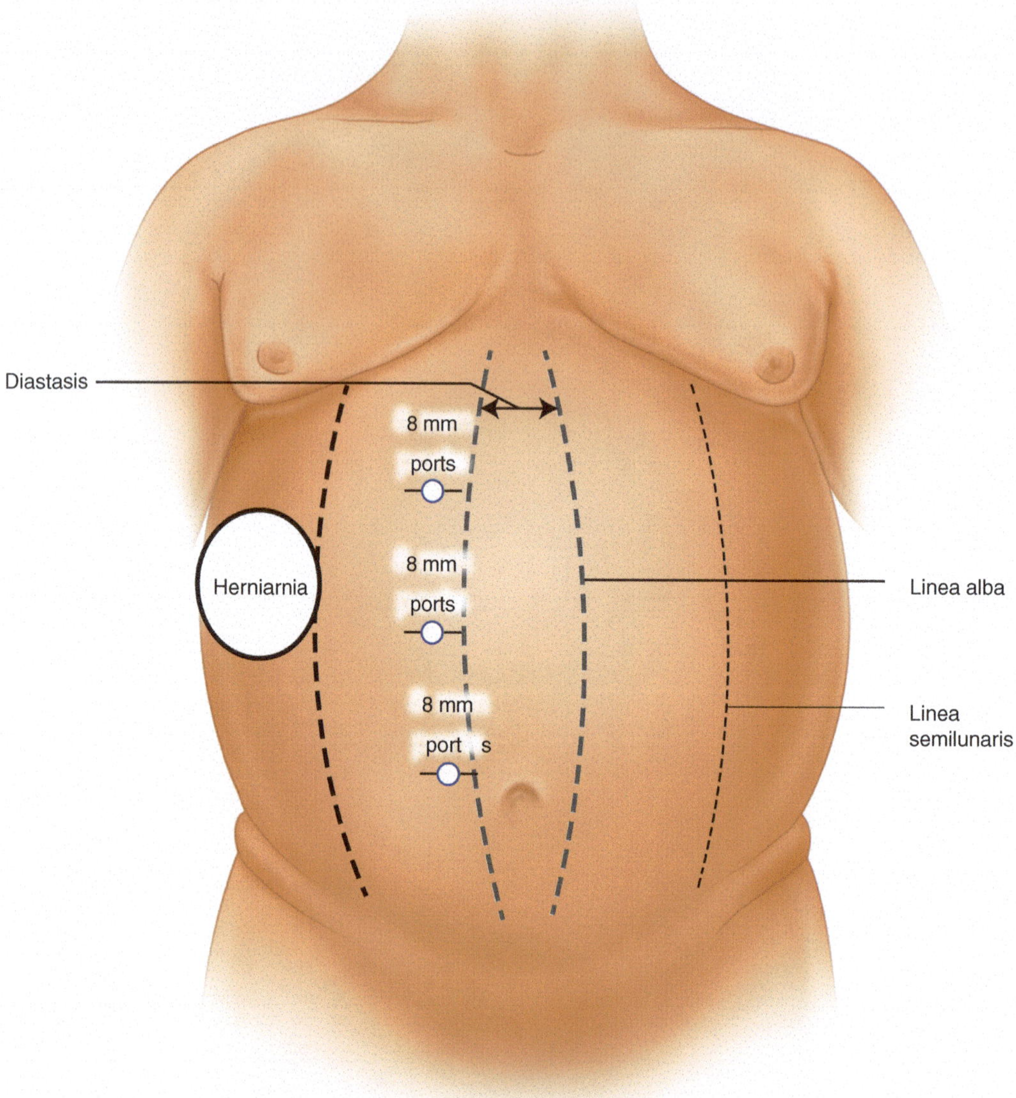


**Fig. 10.5** Port placement at right rectus

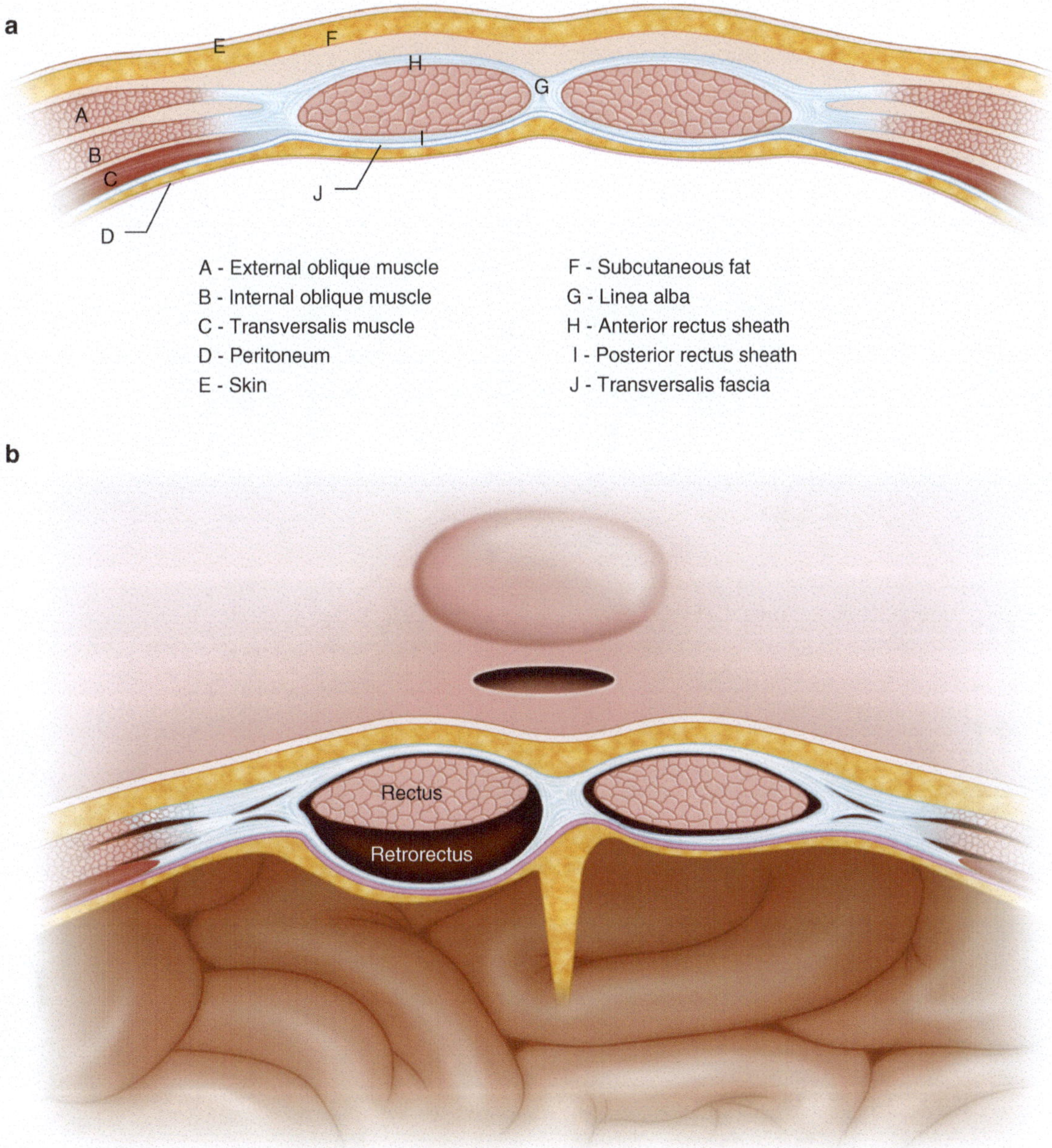


**Fig. 10.6** (**a**) Illustration of anatomy. (**b**) Port placement

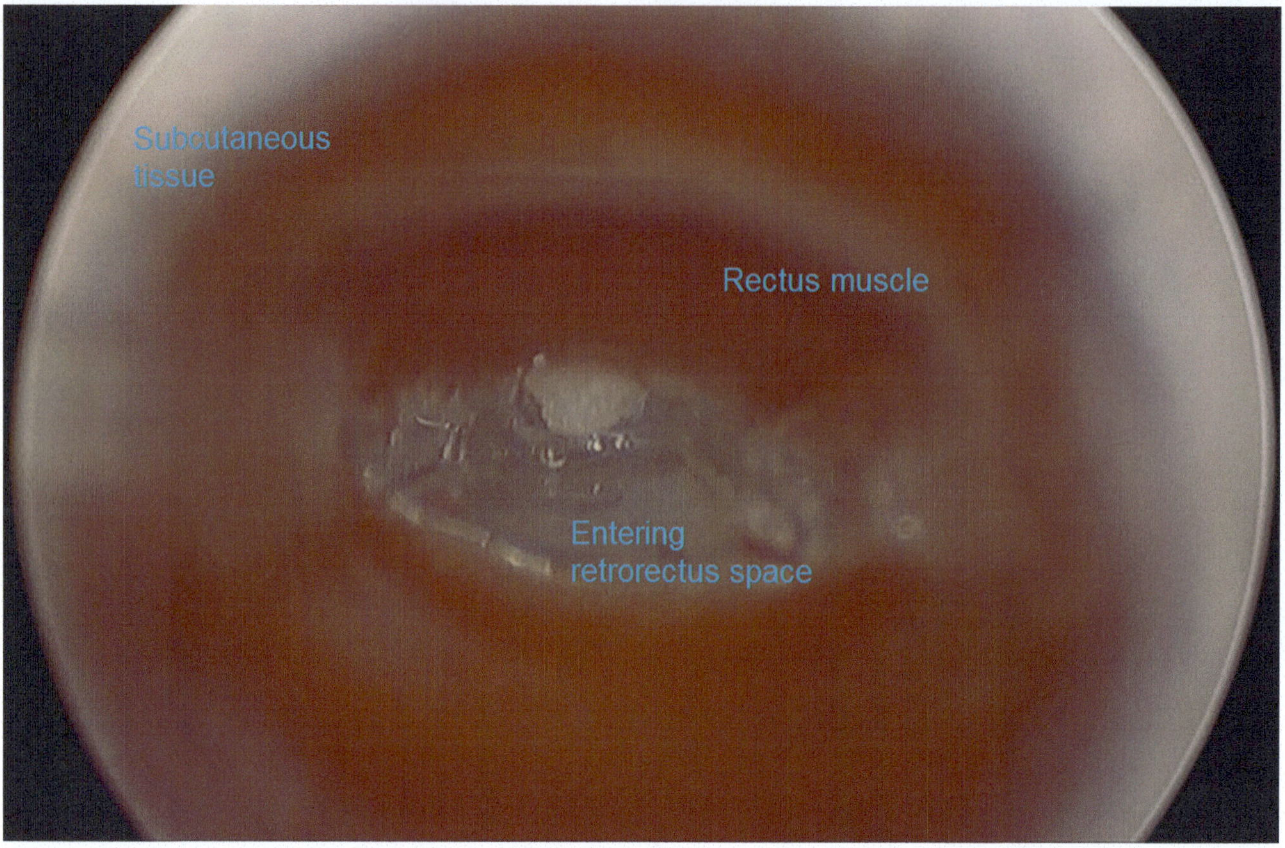


**Fig. 10.7** Laparoscopic entry under direct visualization utilizing 5-mm optical Applied Medical Kii Fios trocar. Subcutaneous tissue, the anterior rectus sheath, and then rectus muscle were dissected with the trocar and $CO_2$ insufflated 15 mmHg

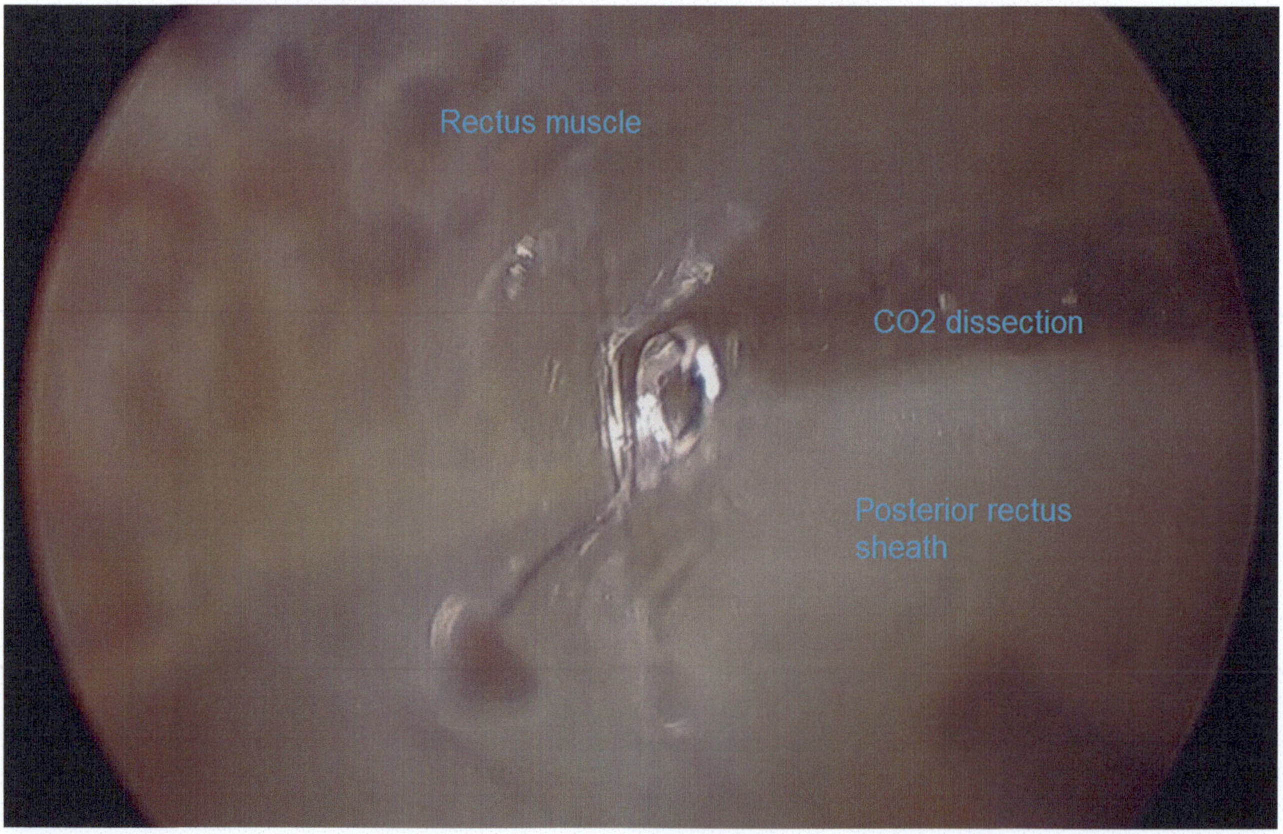


**Fig. 10.8** $CO_2$ dissection in the retrorectus space, utilizing the trocar

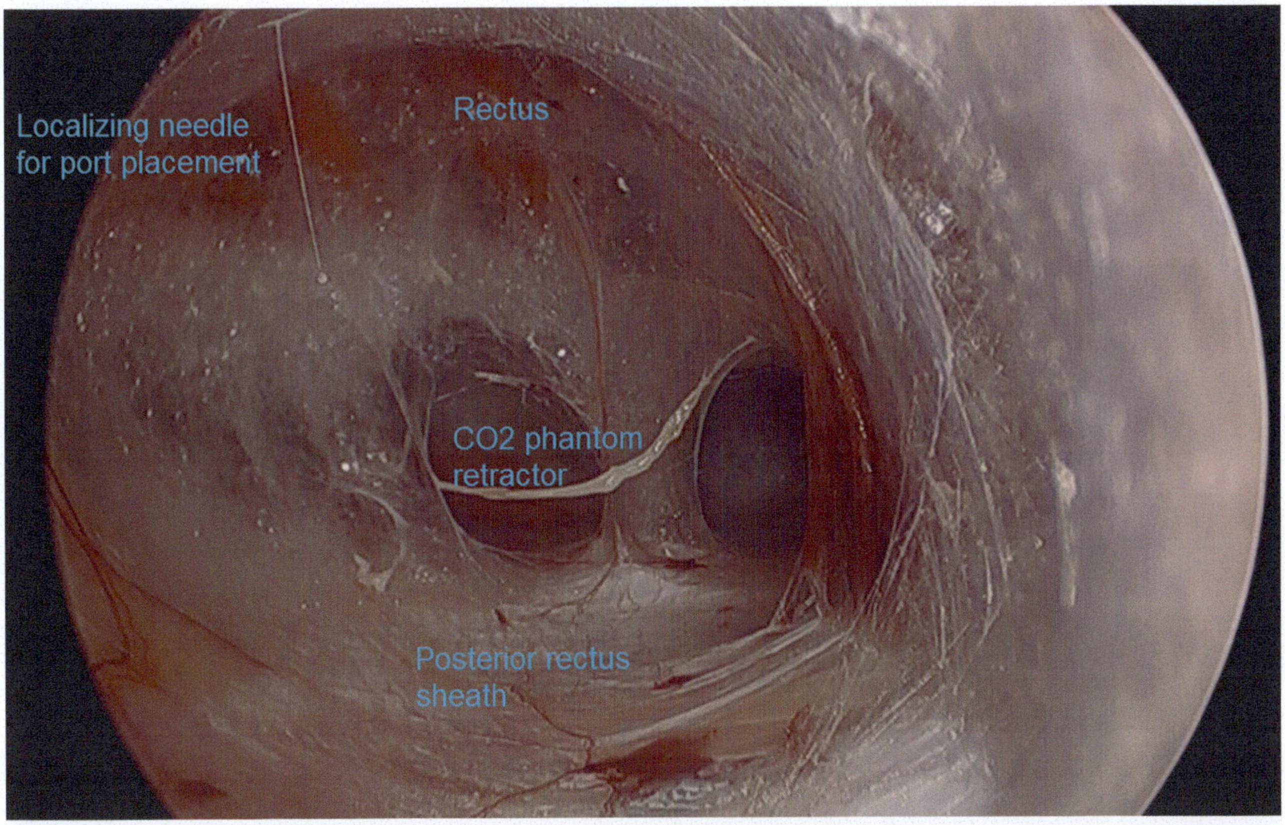


**Fig. 10.9** Port placement using contained $CO_2$ as a phantom retractor with visualization of caudal dissection created to have space for placement of the second and third trocars (6 cm distance between ports), with finder needle used to identify the preferred tract

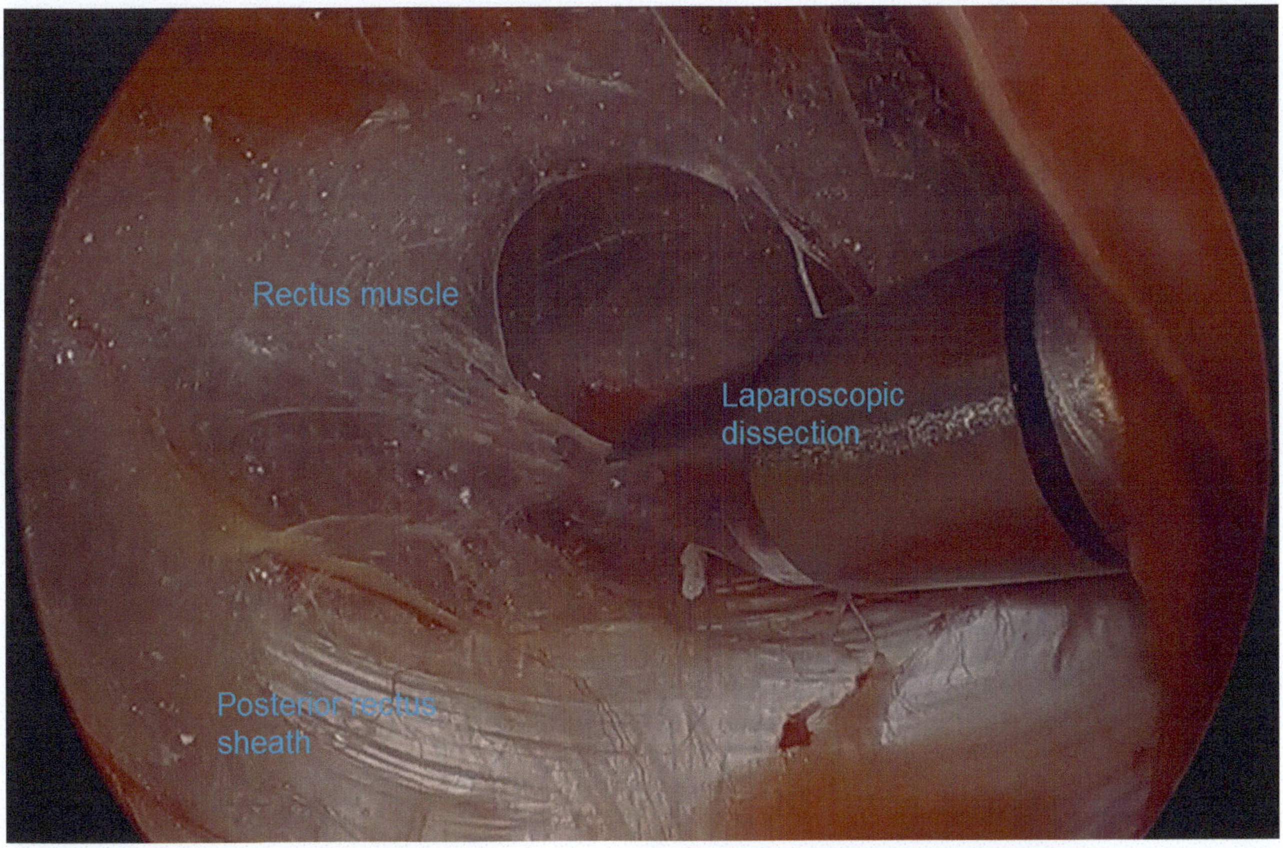


**Fig. 10.10** Laparoscopic dissection cranially with a monopolar Maryland dissector to create space for robotic instrument insertion

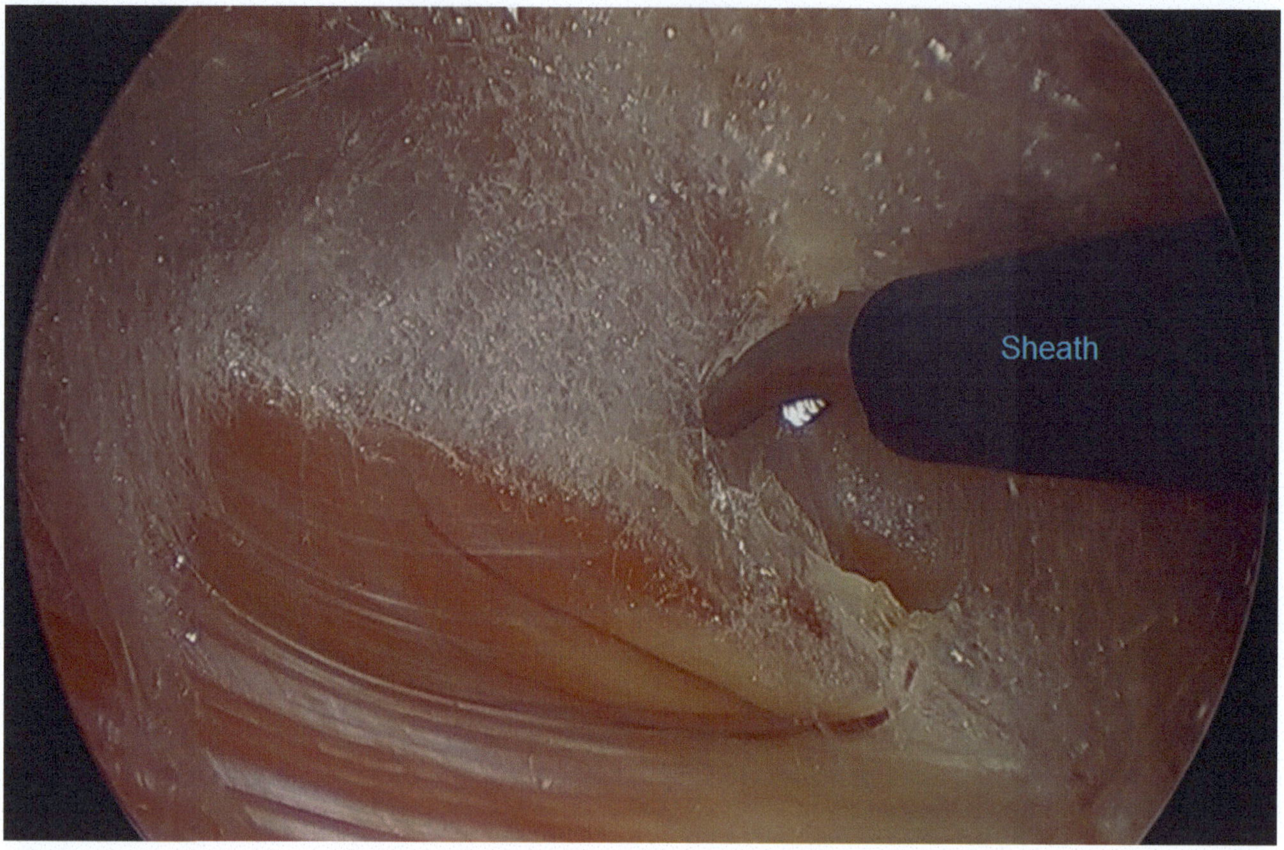


**Fig. 10.11** Utilization of sheath for Maryland dissector to avoid arcing on the metal robot port in this small space

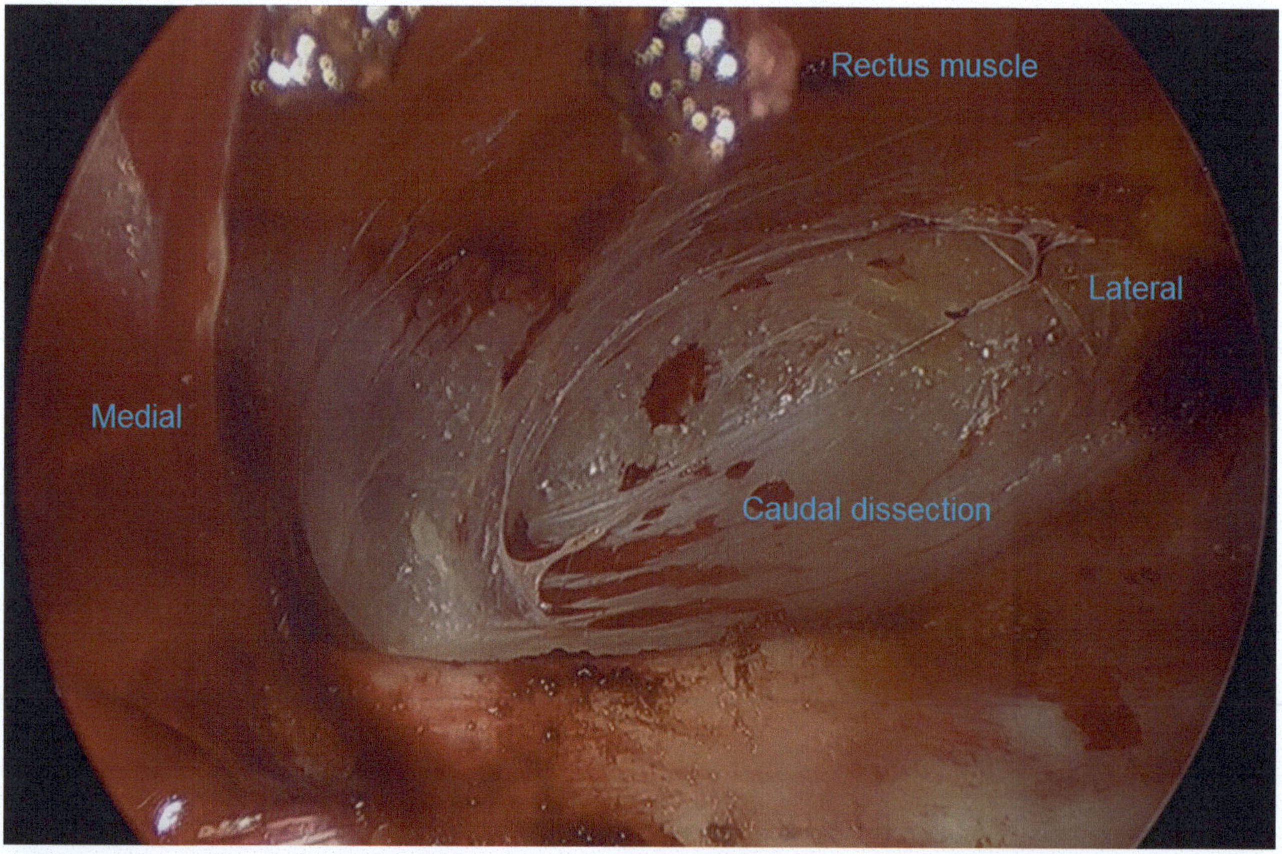


**Fig. 10.12** Dissected retrorectus space

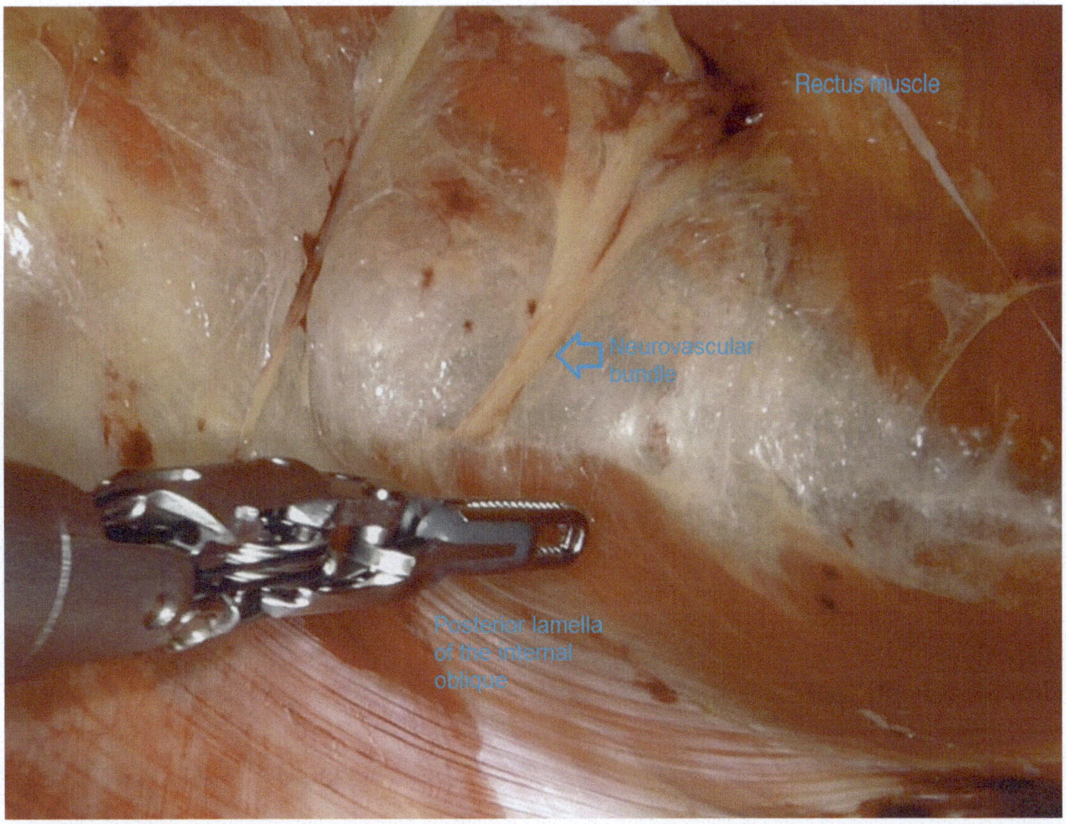


**Fig. 10.13** Lateral right rectus space with visible neurovascular bundle and posterior sheath with posterior lamella of the internal oblique muscle. (The robot is now docked and monopolar and bipolar scissors are in use)

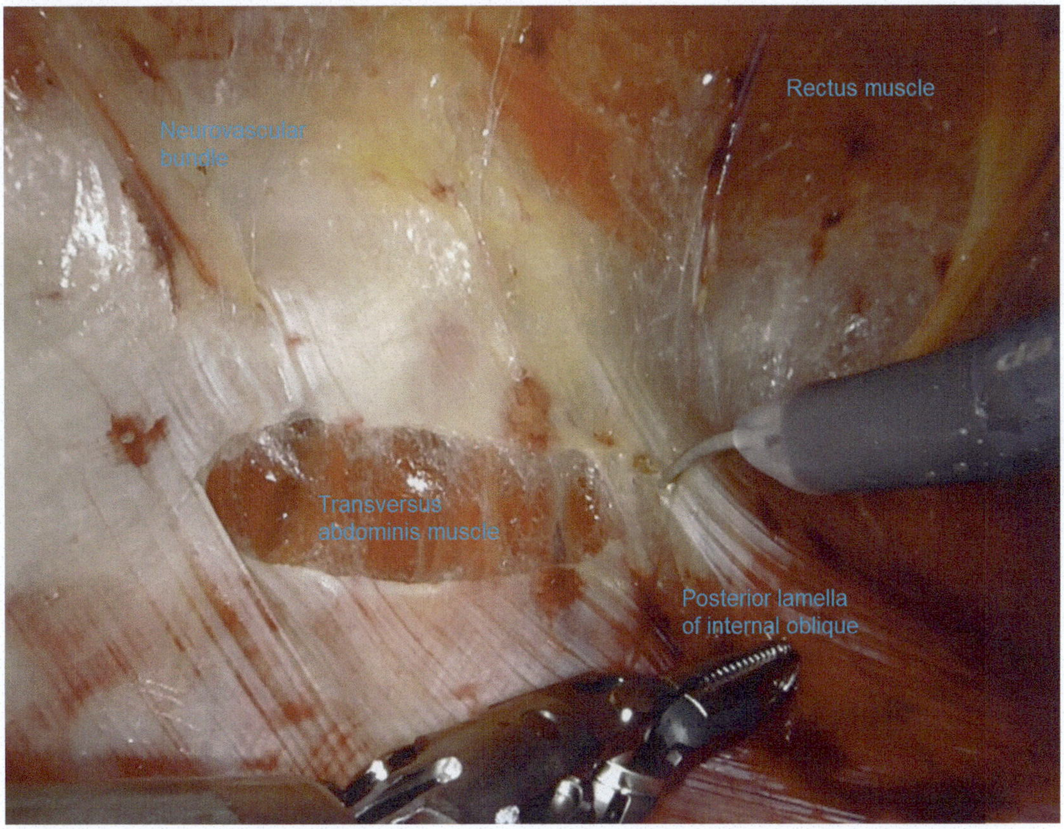


**Fig. 10.14** Opening the posterior lamella of the internal oblique muscle to access the transversus abdominis muscle

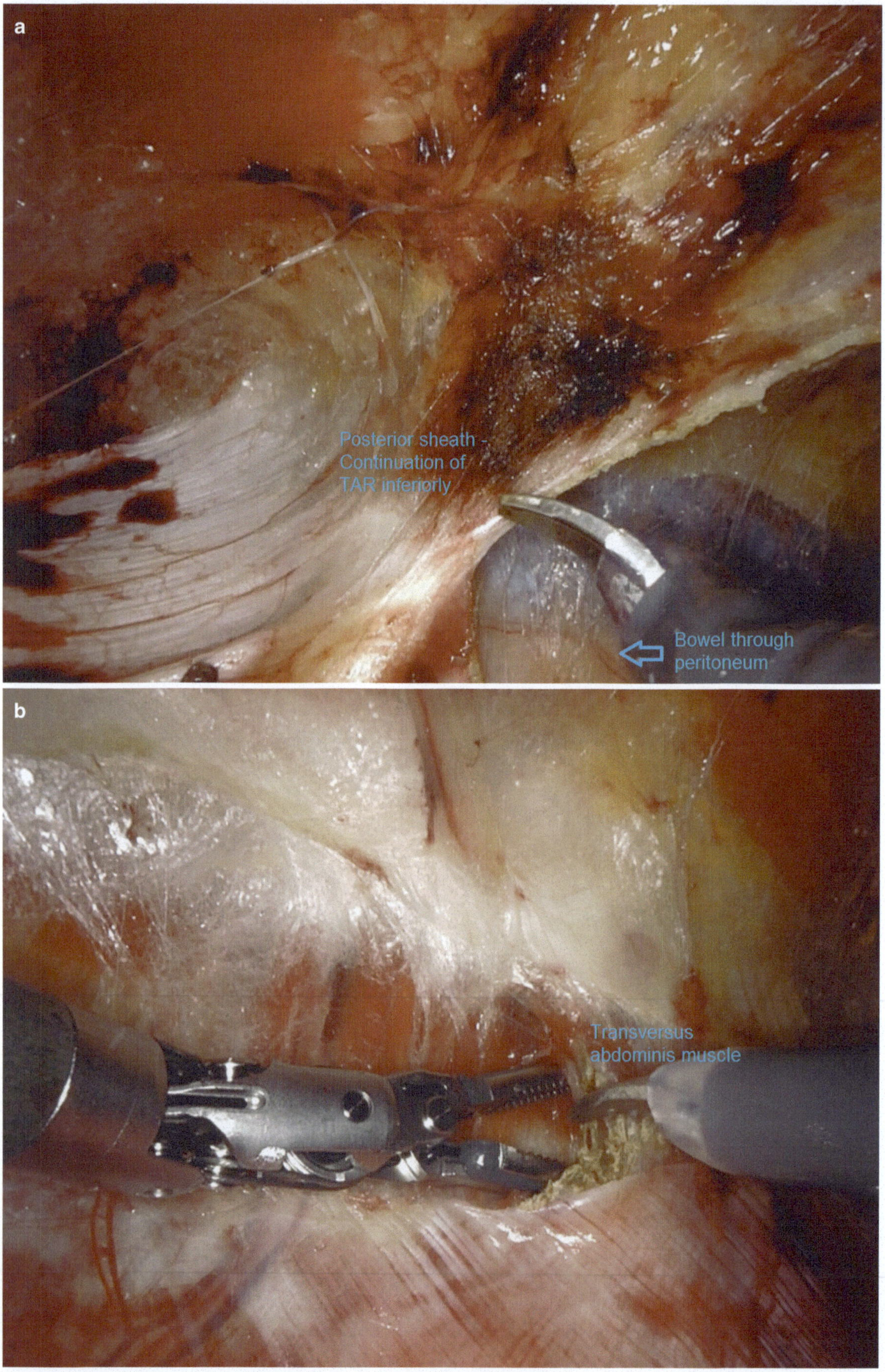


**Fig. 10.15** (**a**–**d**) Transversus abdominis release (TAR)

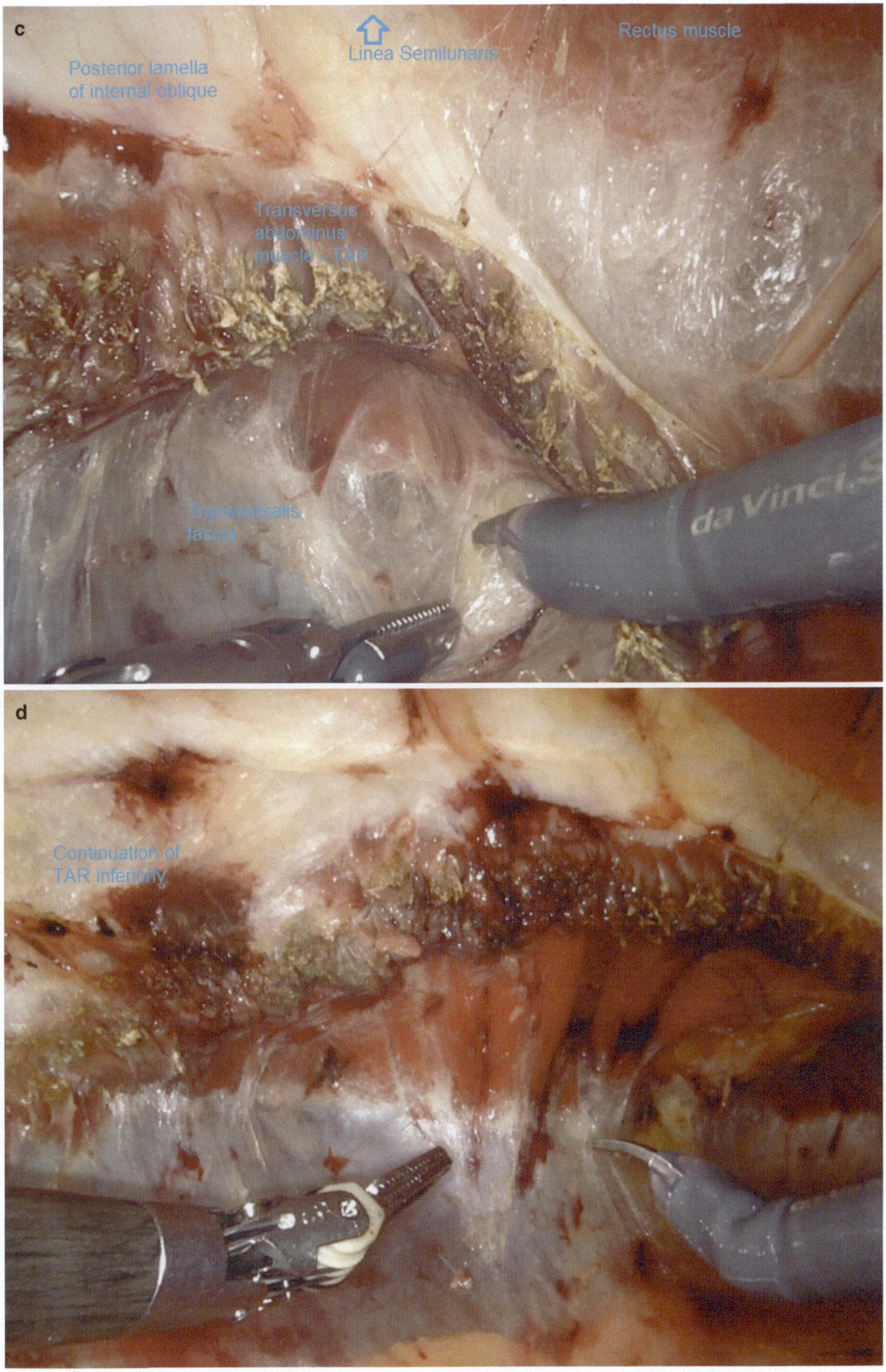


**Fig. 10.15** (continued)

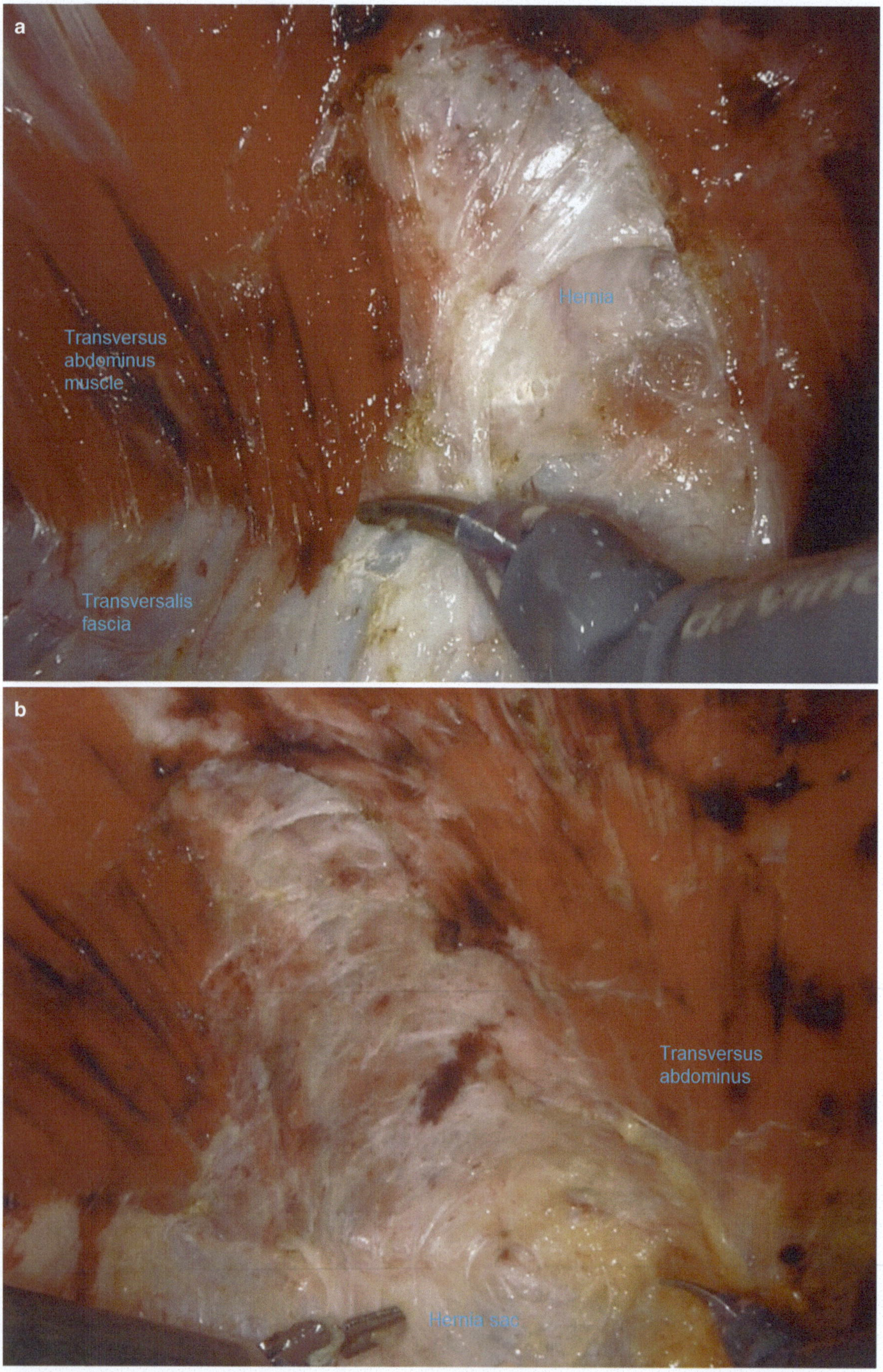


**Fig. 10.16** (**a**) and (**b**) Medial portion of right flank hernia defect

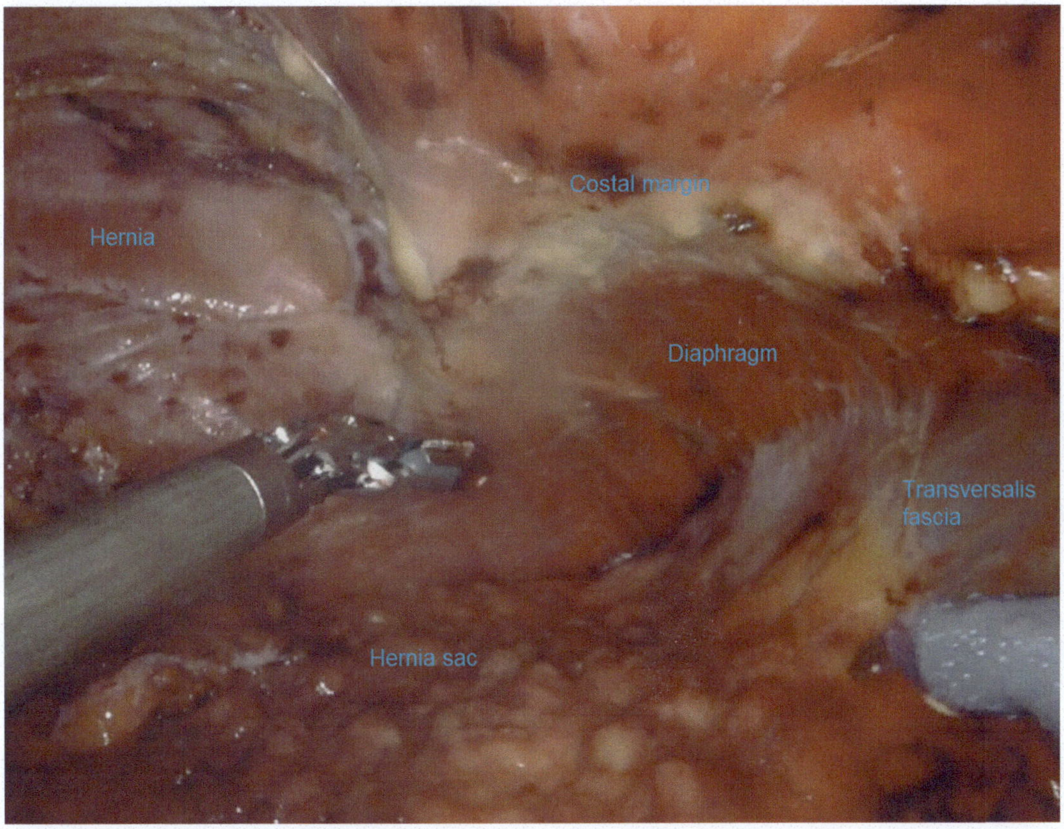


**Fig. 10.17** Cranial dissection with visible diaphragm and rib

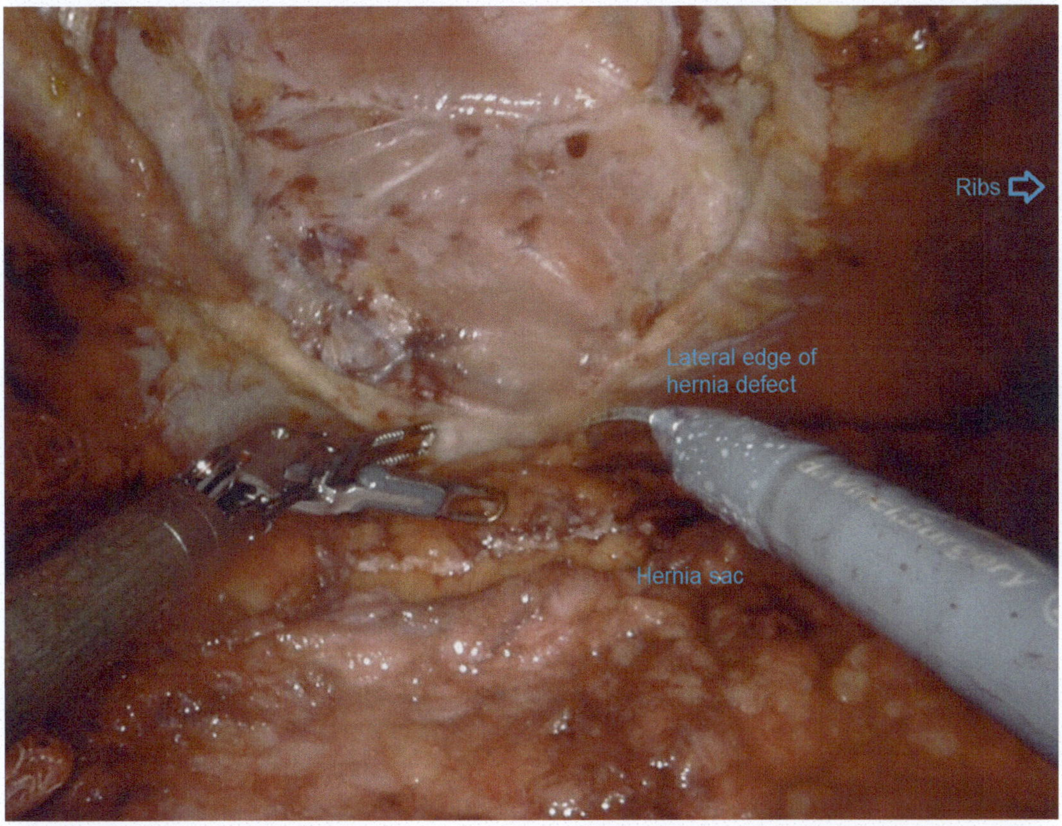


**Fig. 10.18** Posterolateral dissection of hernia defect

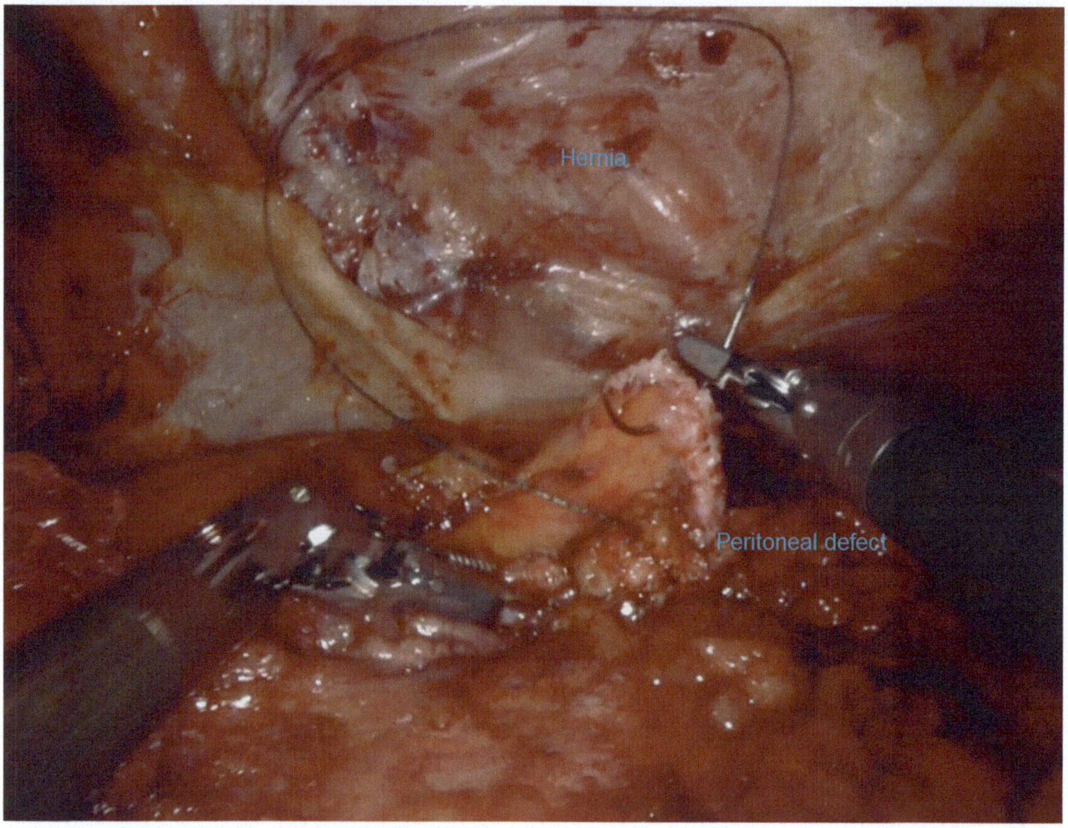


Fig. 10.19 Closure of peritoneal hole utilizing 3-0 barbed suture (v-loc)

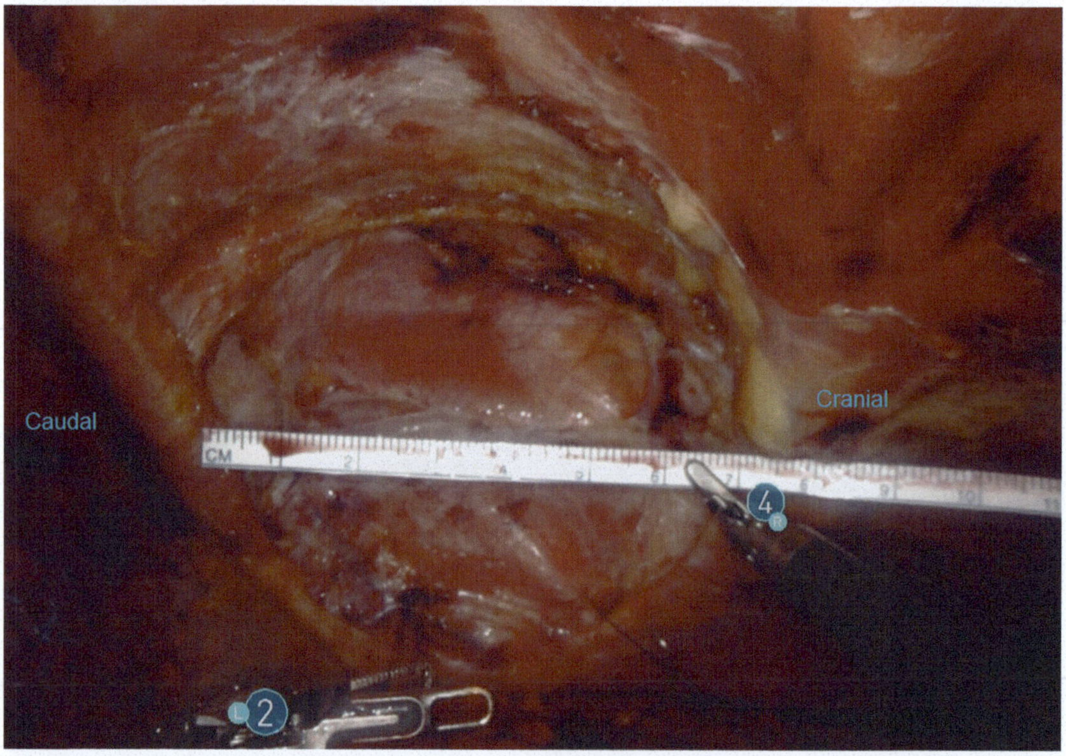


Fig. 10.20 Measuring cranial-caudal width of defect

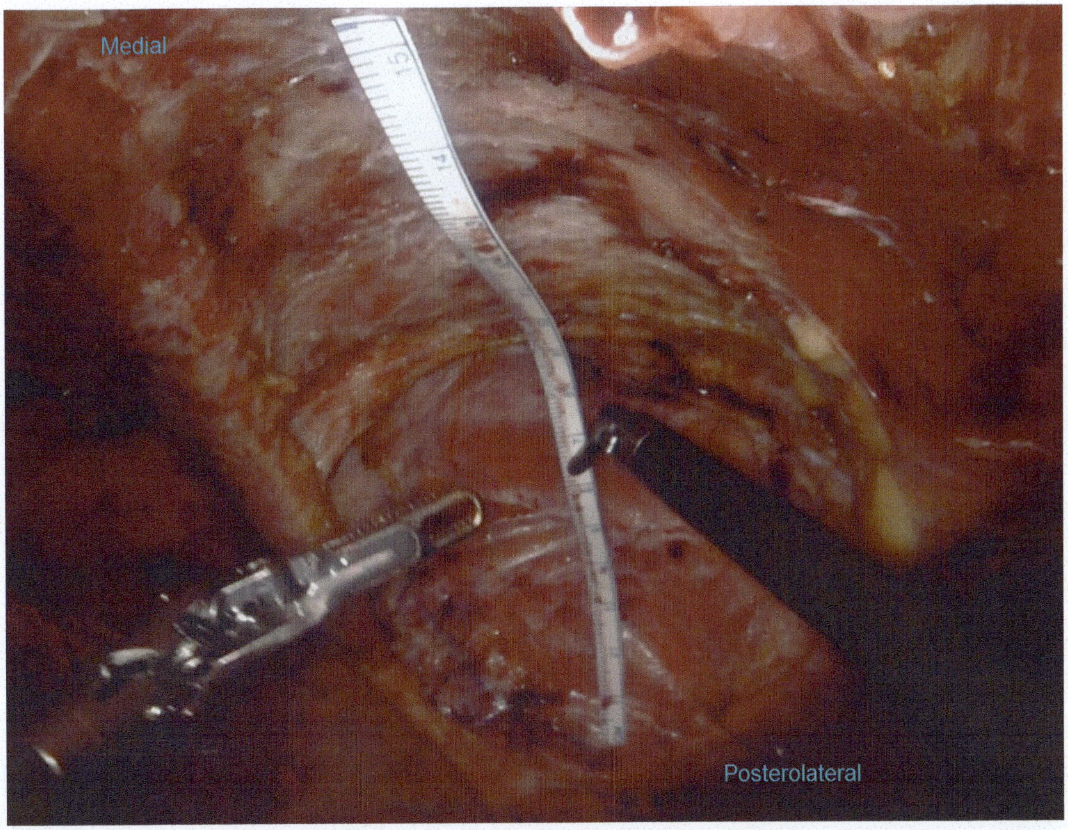


Fig. 10.21 Measuring medial-posterolateral length of defect

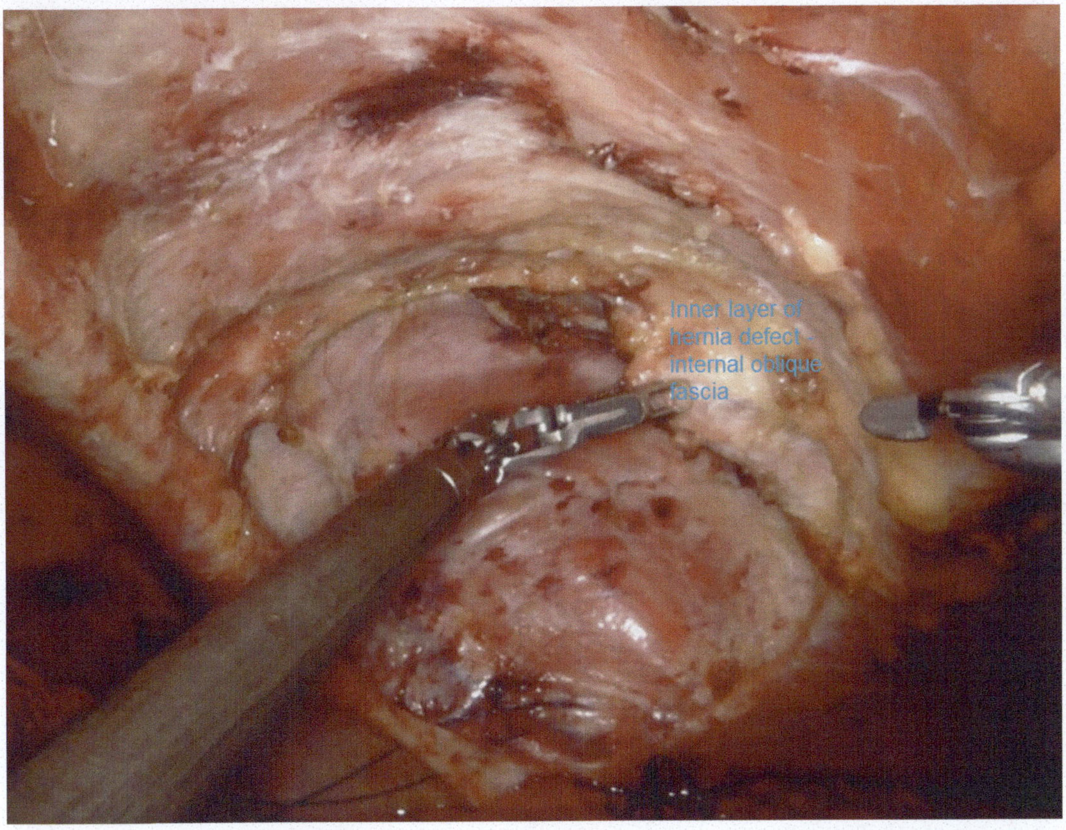


Fig. 10.22 Assessing layers of the defect

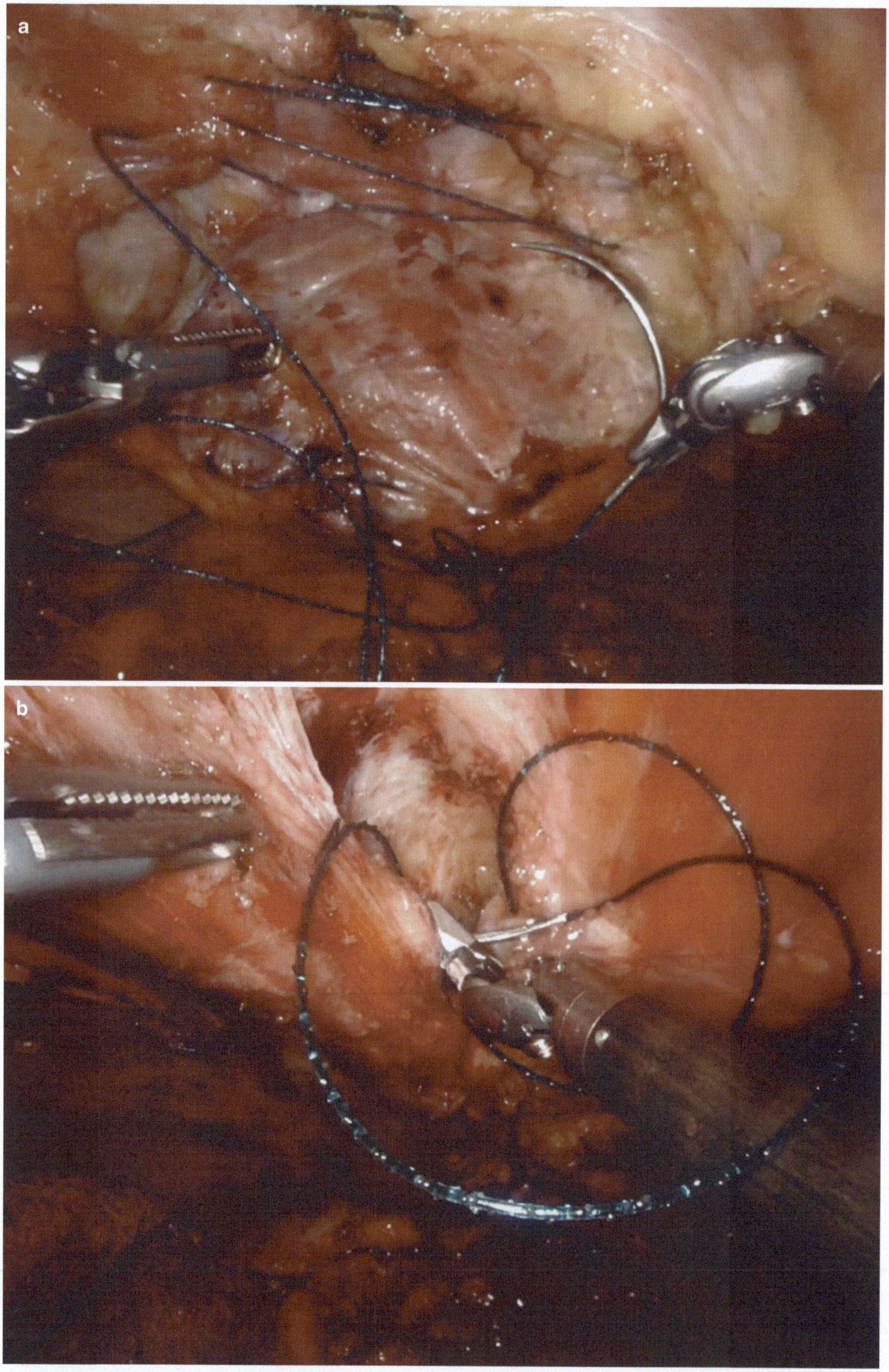

**Fig. 10.23** (**a**) and (**b**) Multilayer closure of oblique muscle and fascia utilizing 180-day absorbable v-loc

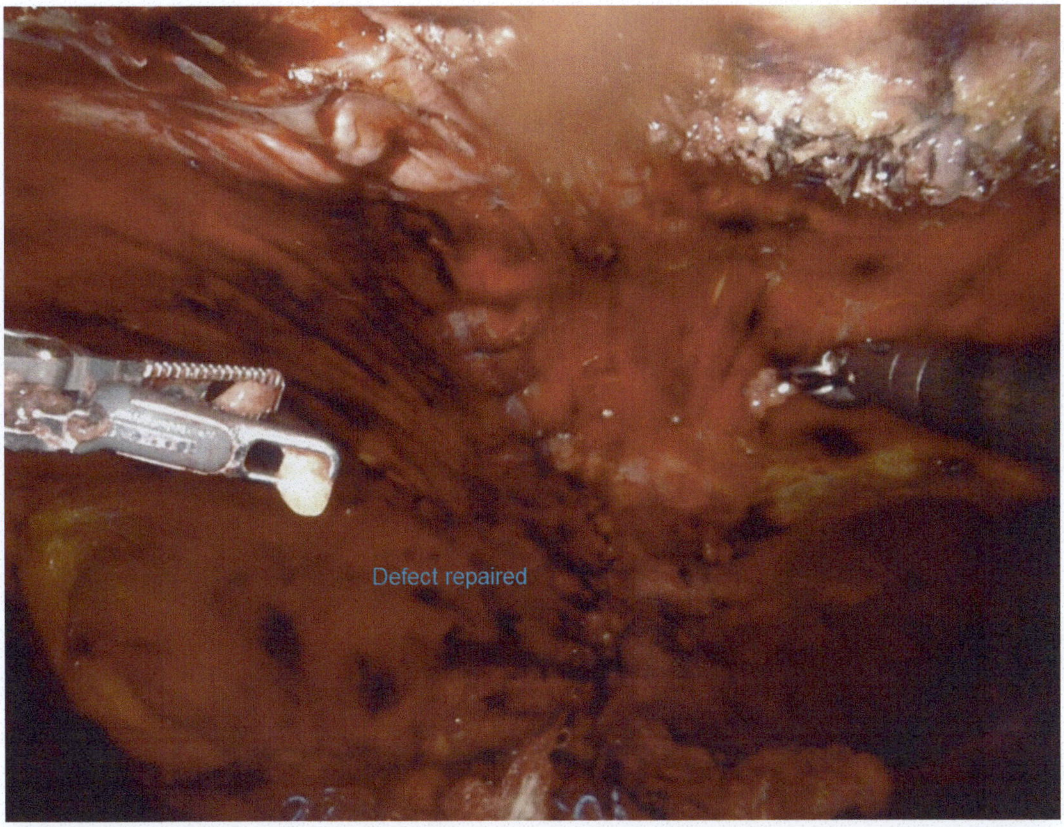


**Fig. 10.24** Approximation of transversus abdominis

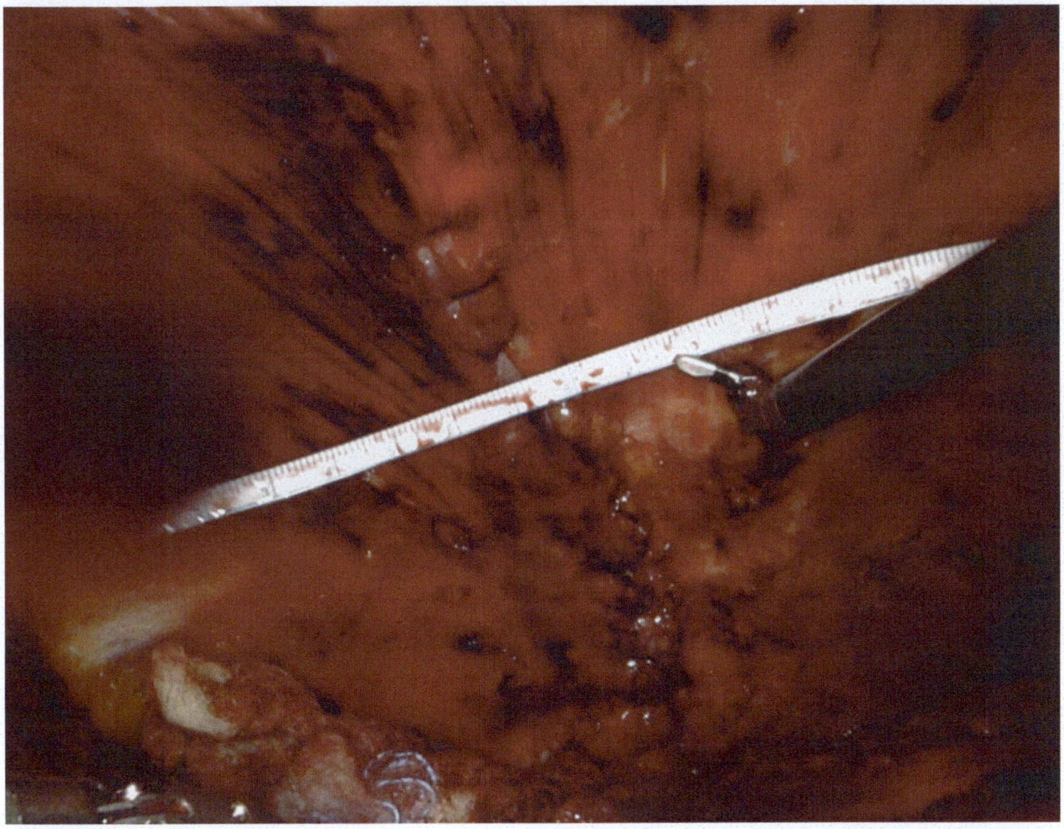

**Fig. 10.25** Measuring space for mesh

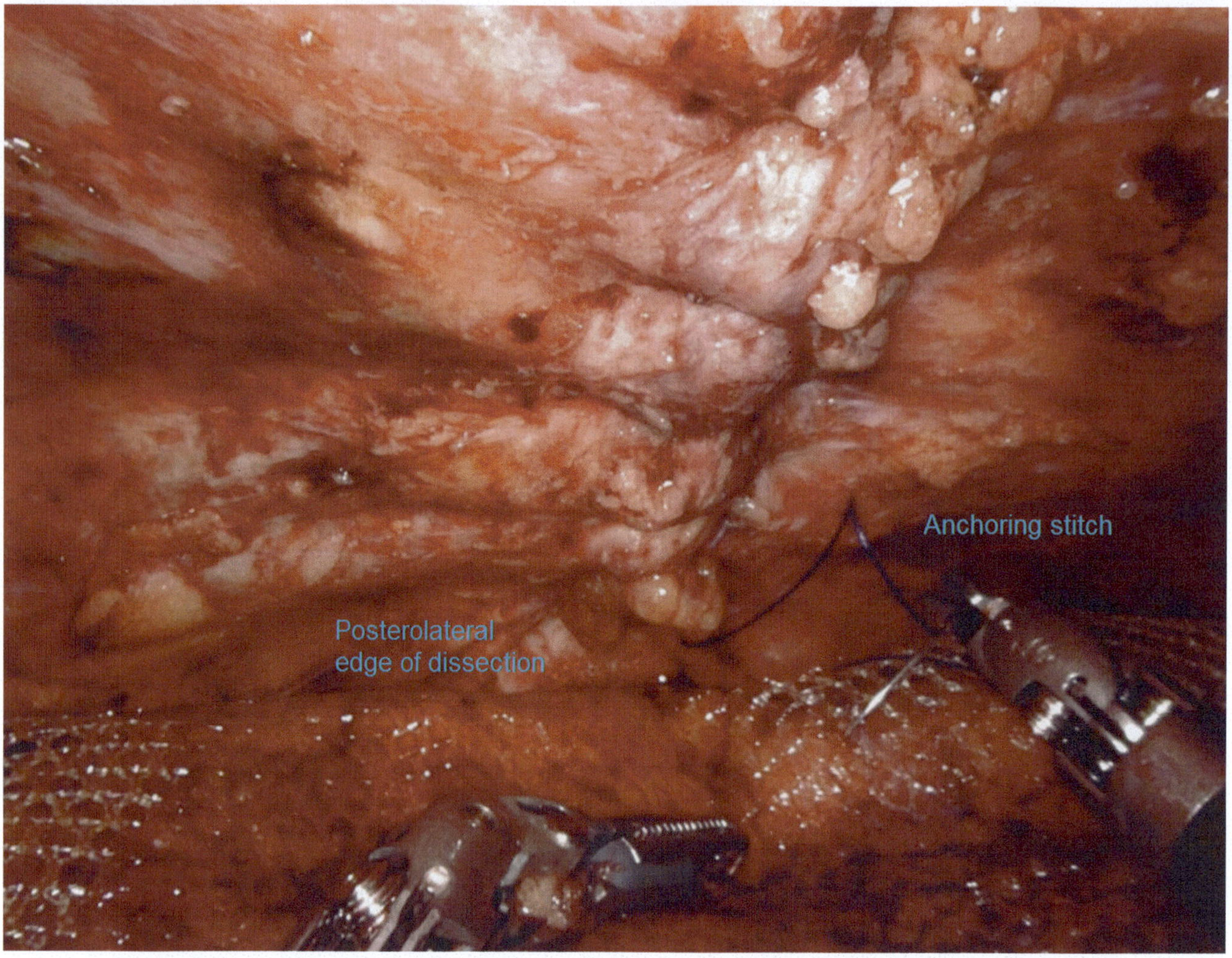


**Fig. 10.26** Placement of mesh in posterolateral space with mesh cut to size; the mesh is anchored with 3-0 Vicryl suture

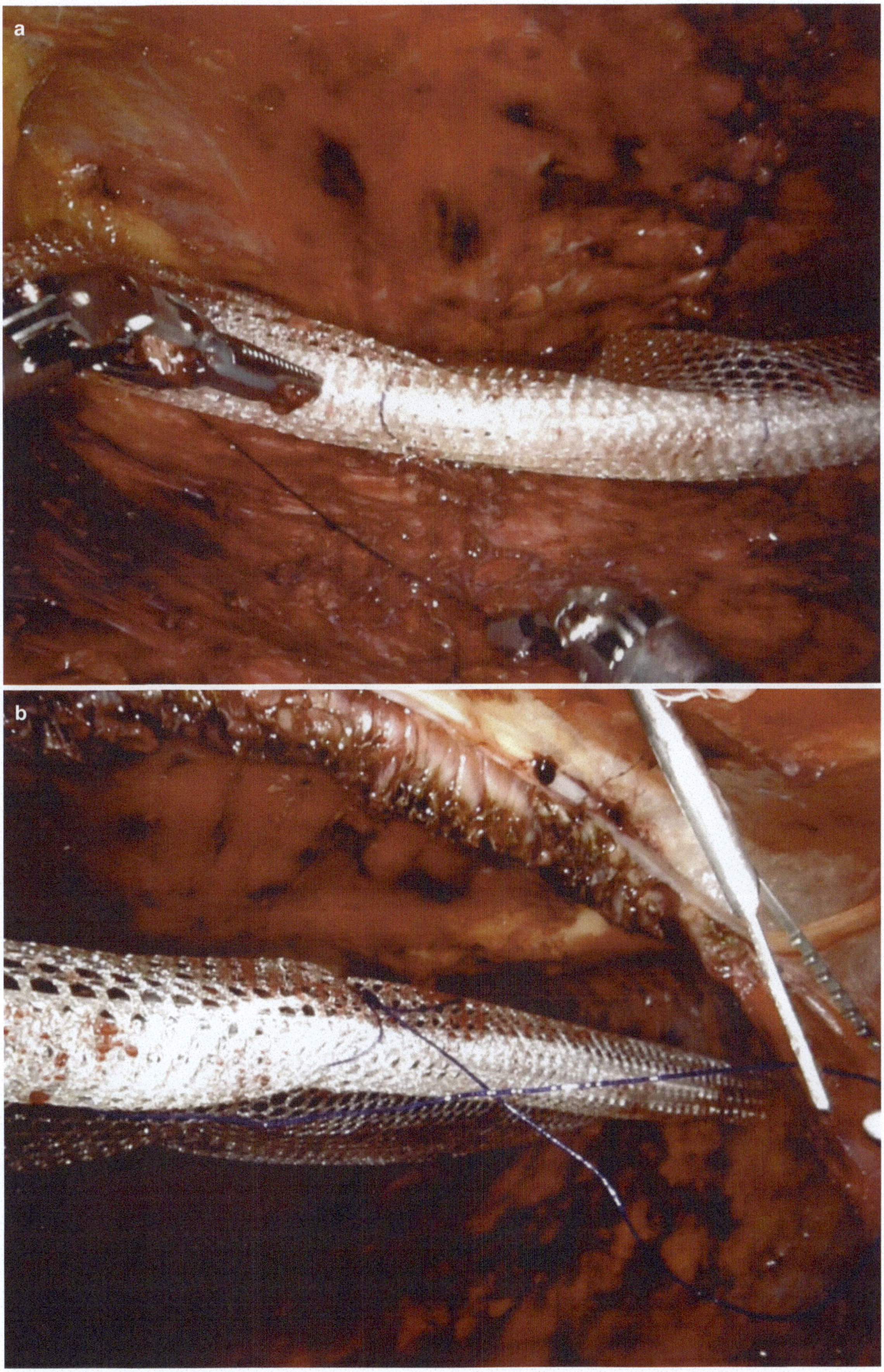


**Fig. 10.27** (**a–c**) Placement of mesh on the "ceiling" utilizing temporary suspension sutures to facilitate mesh fixation

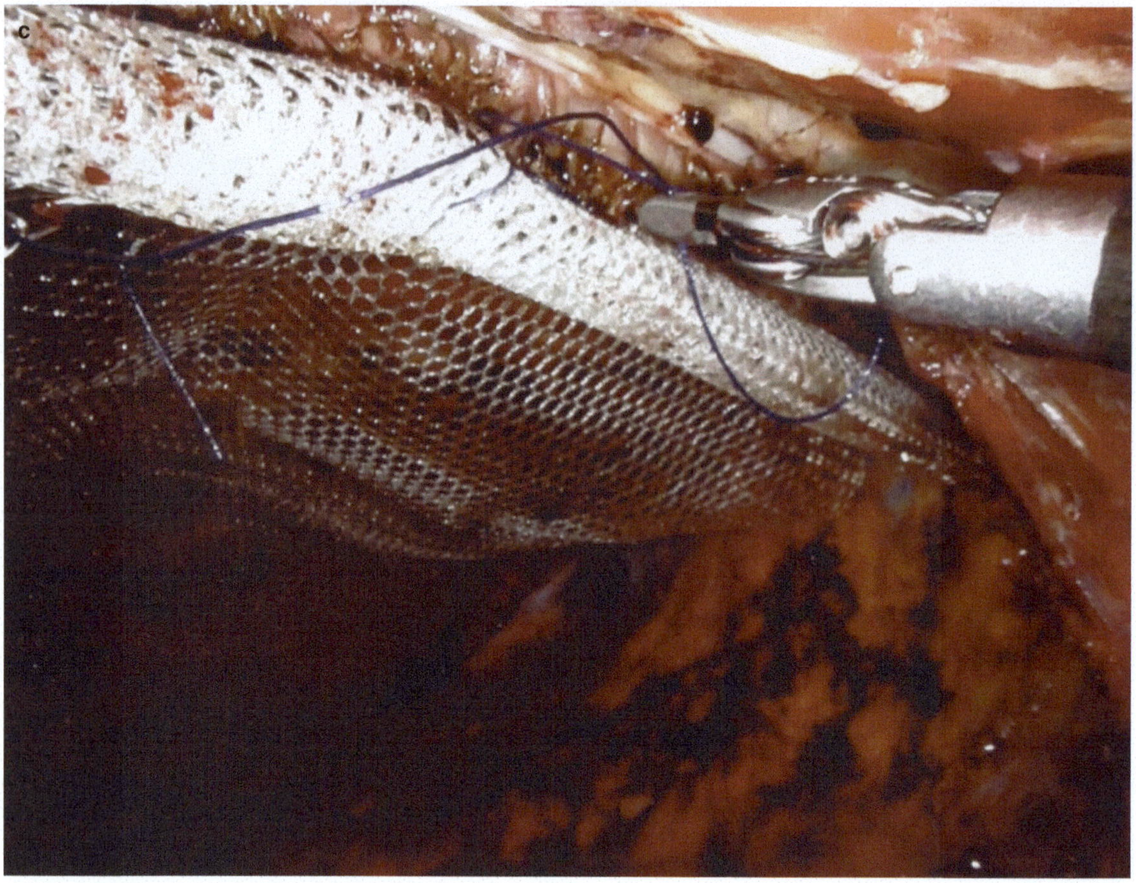


Fig. 10.27 (continued)

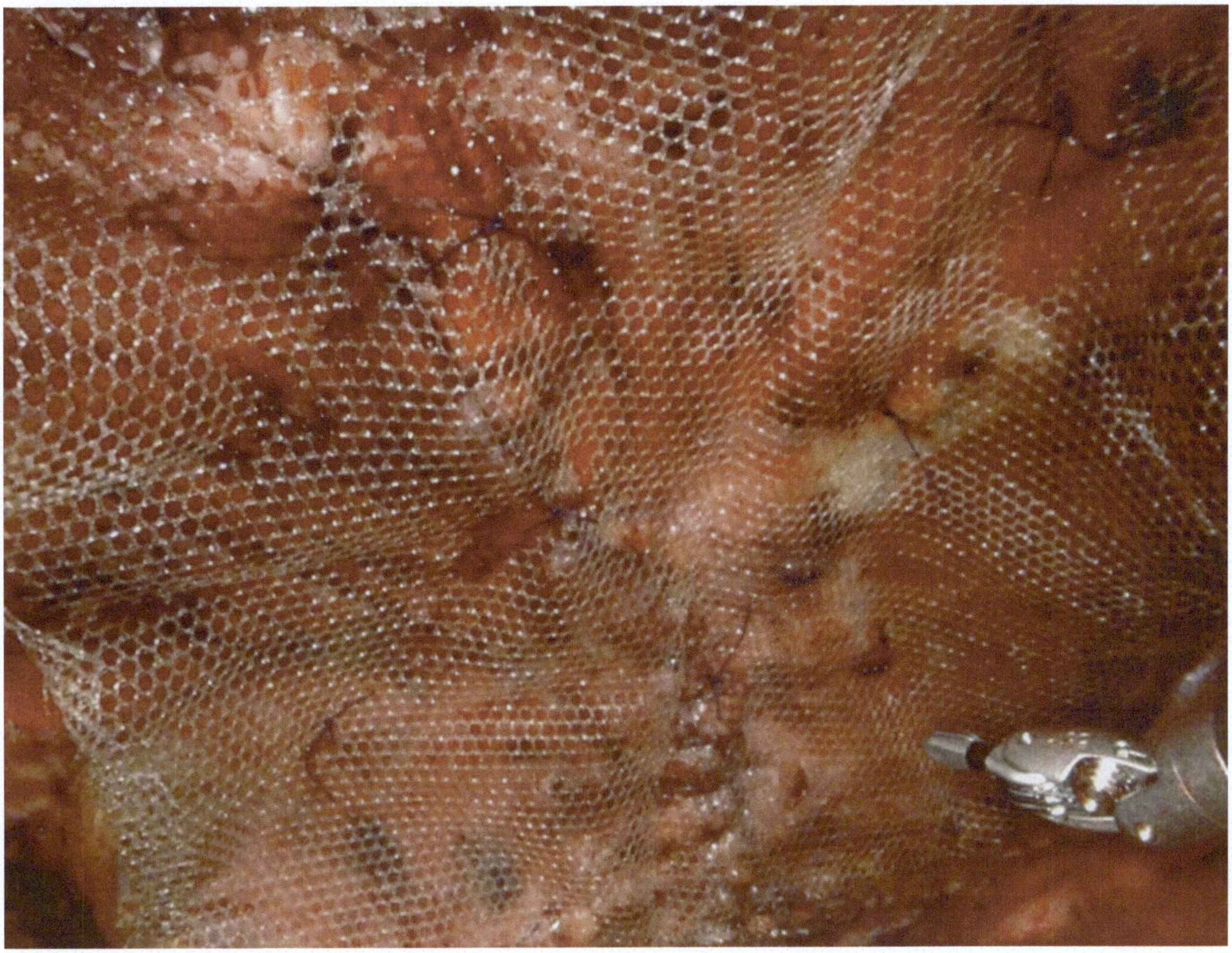

Fig. 10.28 Final mesh placement

## Suggested Reading


Akinduro OO, Jones F, Turner J, Cason F, Clark C. Rare case of a strangulated intercostal flank hernia following open nephrectomy: a case report and review of literature. Int J Surg Case Rep. 2015;17:143–5. https://doi.org/10.1016/j.ijscr.2015.11.015.

Dakin GF, Kendrick ML. Challenging hernia locations: flank hernias. In: Jacob BP, Ramshaw B, editors. The SAGES manual of hernia repair. New York: Springer; 2013. p. 531–40.

Salameh JR, Salloum EJ. Lumbar incisional hernias: diagnostic and management dilemma. JSLS. 2004;8:391–4.

# Robotic Parastomal Hernia Repair: Modified Retromuscular Sugarbaker

# 11

David J. Morrell, Jeffrey A. Blatnik, and Eric M. Pauli

## Introduction

Parastomal hernias remain technically challenging to repair and continue to have high rates of recurrence and high rates of surgical site occurrences. A variety of operative repairs have been proposed to manage parastomal hernias—each with its own constellation of benefits and clear drawbacks. Repair method is generally selected based on the characteristics of the hernia, the patient comorbidities, and the skill and training level of the surgeon. Methods differ in a variety of ways: open *vs.* minimally invasive operation, stoma left in situ *vs.* stoma relocation, primary repair *vs.* mesh-based repair, permanent synthetic *vs.* biologic *vs.* bioabsorbable mesh, uncut *vs.* keyhole *vs.* cruciate mesh configuration, and underlay *vs.* sublay *vs.* onlay mesh positioning. The need to repair a concomitant midline hernia and the need to include myofascial releases to afford the repair are additional considerations.

We recently described a method of parastomal hernia repair utilizing a transversus abdominis release, bowel transposition to within the pre-peritoneal pocket, and retromuscular mesh reinforcement (as described in the Suggested Reading by Pauli et al.). This so-called Pauli parastomal hernia repair (PPHR) represents a modified retromuscular Sugarbaker technique. The advantages of the method include the ability to leave the stoma in situ and the ability to repair large midline and/or parastomal hernias without the need to cut the mesh, thus avoiding an area of weakness into which most recurrent parastomal hernias occur. Additionally, retromuscular mesh positioning has a myriad of well-described advantages.

## Procedure: Illustrated Steps

Figures 11.1, 11.2, 11.3, 11.4, 11.5, 11.6, 11.7, 11.8, 11.9, 11.10, 11.11, 11.12, 11.13, 11.14, 11.15, 11.16, 11.17, 11.18, 11.19, 11.20, 11.21, 11.22, 11.23, 11.24, 11.25, 11.26, 11.27, 11.28, 11.29, 11.30, 11.31, 11.32, 11.33, and 11.34 illustrate details of the technical steps in the robotic-assisted approach to PPHR. This chapter focuses on repairs requiring only a unilateral posterior rectus sheath and transversus abdominis release to achieve wide retromuscular mesh reinforcement—a technique employed in the setting of an isolated parastomal hernia with no midline component. The steps necessary to perform the contralateral myofascial release are identical to those outlined in Chap. 6. Despite the slight variation in requirements for a unilateral versus bilateral component separation, the underlying principle of both versions of the operation remain the same: wide retromuscular mesh reinforcement of all hernia defects.

D. J. Morrell
Department of Surgery, Penn State Health Milton S. Hershey Medical Center, Hershey, PA, USA

J. A. Blatnik
Department of Surgery, Section of Minimally Invasive Surgery, Washington University School of Medicine, St. Louis, MO, USA

E. M. Pauli (✉)
Department of Surgery, Division of Minimally Invasive and Bariatric Surgery, Penn State Health Milton S. Hershey Medical Center, Hershey, PA, USA
e-mail: epauli@pennstatehealth.psu.edu


O. Y. Kudsi (ed.), *Robotic Hernia Surgery*, https://doi.org/10.1007/978-3-030-46667-1_11

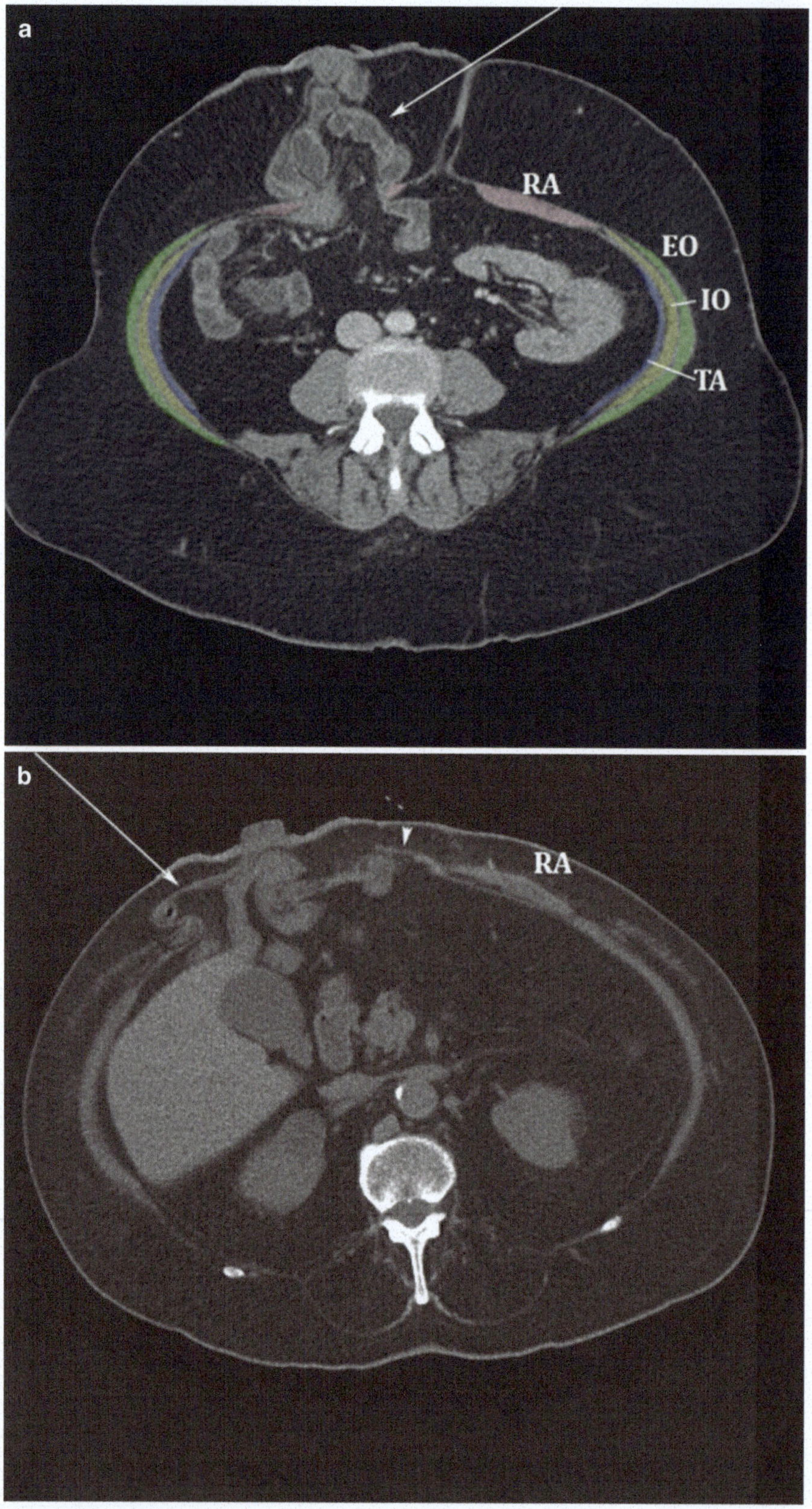


**Fig. 11.1** Preoperative CT images demonstrating typical parastomal hernia appearance in two patients with no prior history of component separation. (**a**) In this CT image, the patient has an end ileostomy with a small parastomal hernia (*arrow*) containing loops of non-obstructed small bowel immediately proximal to the ostomy. (**b**) In this CT image, the patient has an end ileostomy with a midline incisional hernia (*arrowhead*) in addition to a small parastomal hernia (*arrow*) containing a non-obstructed loop of small bowel. This patient would require bilateral posterior component separations to allow for wide mesh overlap of the parastomal and midline hernia defects. EO external oblique, IO internal oblique, RA rectus abdominis, TA transversus abdominis

a

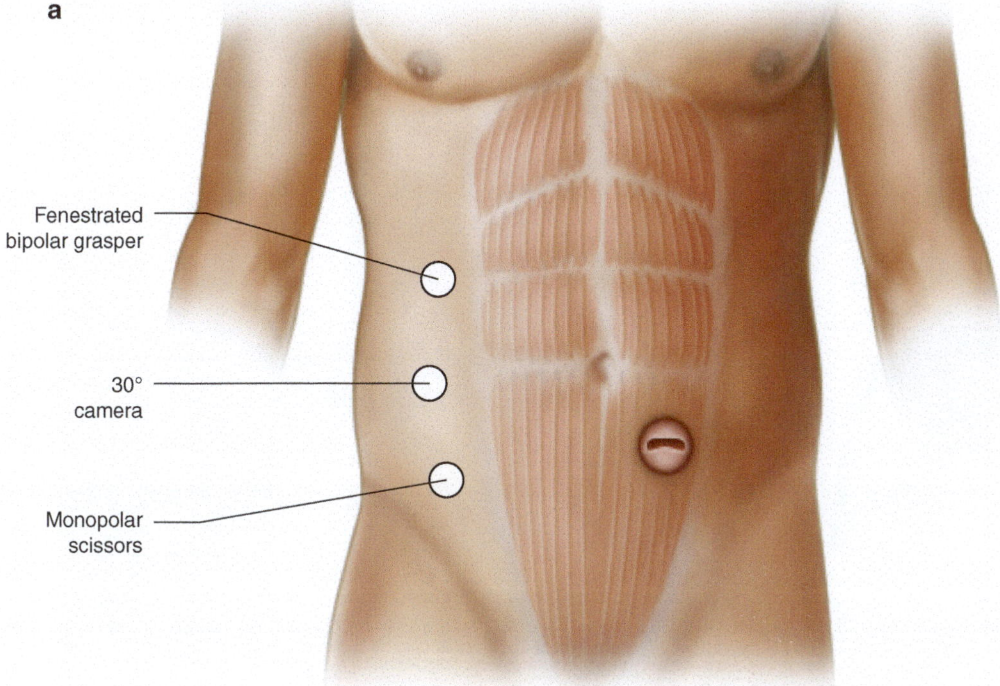


b

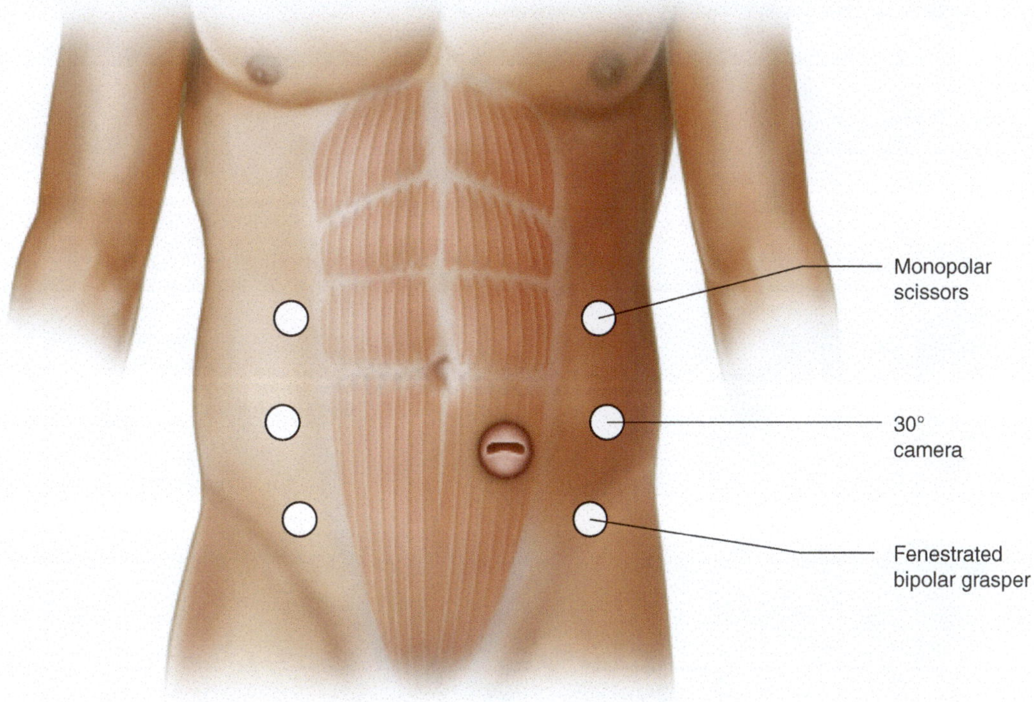


**Fig. 11.2** The location of port sites for the procedure. (**a**) Port placement when a unilateral component separation is planned. (**b**) Port placement when a bilateral component separation is planned to permit repair of concomitant midline or contralateral defects. The ports contralateral to the ostomy site are placed first, to perform the component separation ipsilateral to the ostomy site prior to proceeding to the contralateral component separation, at which point new ports are placed adjacent to the ostomy

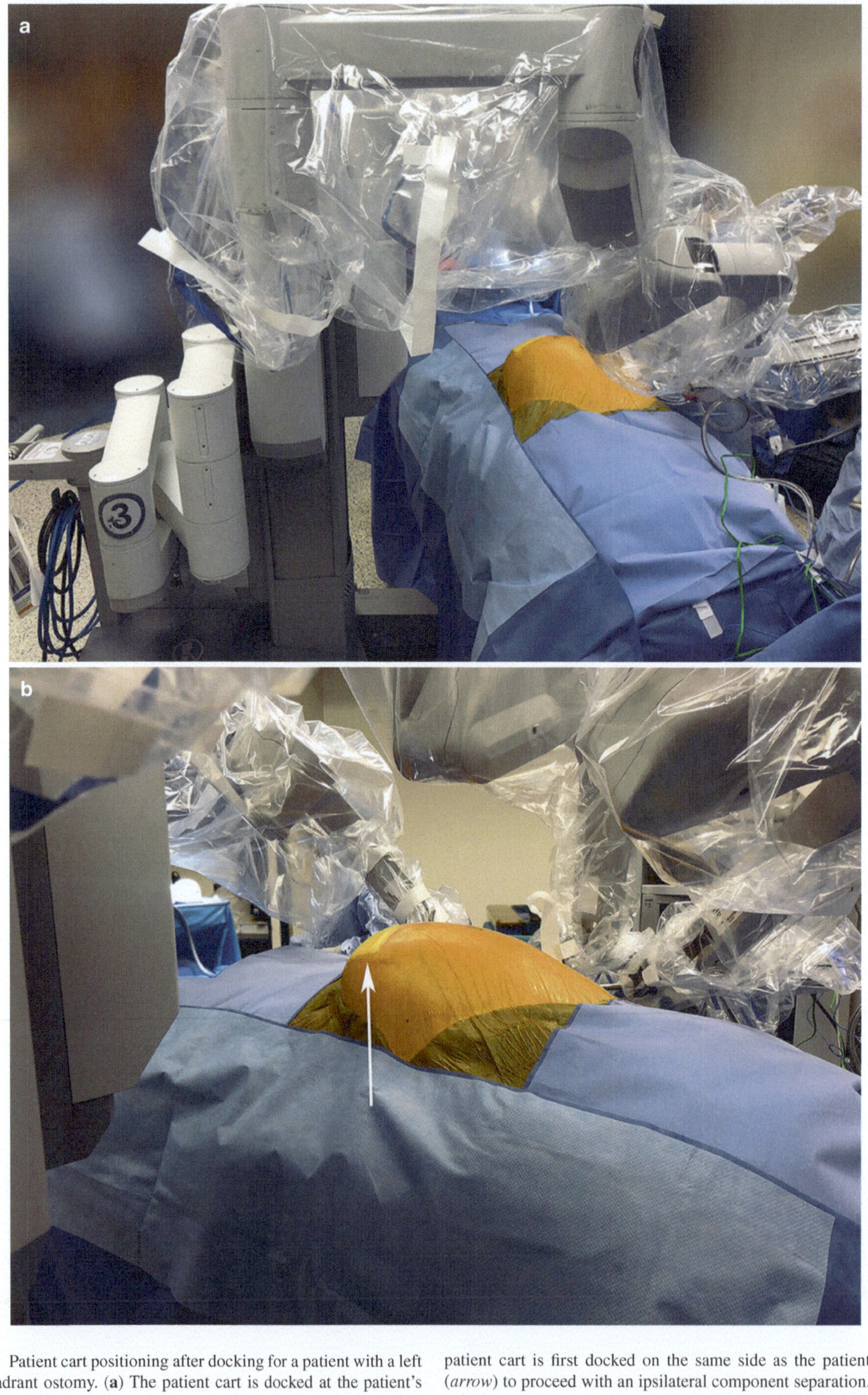


**Fig. 11.3** Patient cart positioning after docking for a patient with a left lower quadrant ostomy. (**a**) The patient cart is docked at the patient's side opposite from the desired working ports, with the center column over the patient's hip. For the da Vinci® Xi or Si system (Intuitive Surgical, Sunnyvale, CA), the third working arm is docked. (**b**) The patient cart is first docked on the same side as the patient's ostomy (*arrow*) to proceed with an ipsilateral component separation. (**c**) When a bilateral component separation is performed, the patient cart is undocked after completing the ipsilateral component separation and moved to the opposite side of the patient

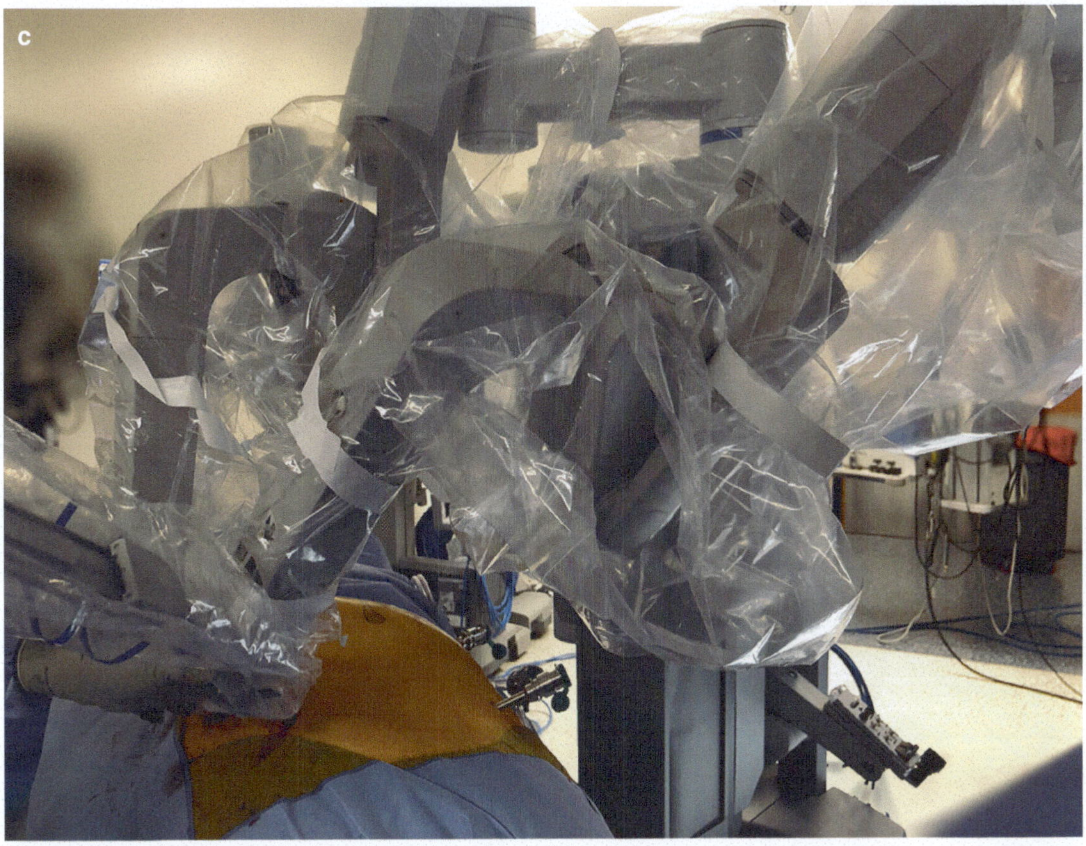


Fig. 11.3 (continued)

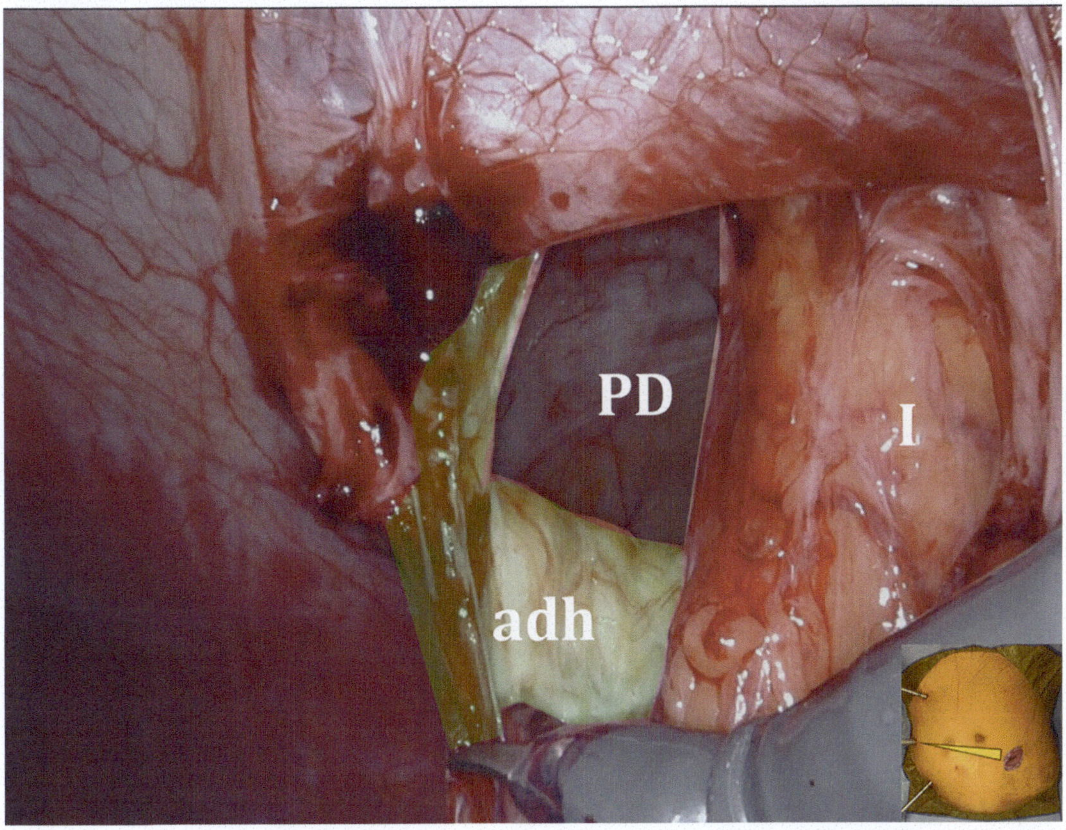


Fig. 11.4 After entering the abdominal cavity, lysis of visceral adhesions (adh) to the anterior abdominal wall and pelvis is undertaken. The hernia contents are reduced and the ostomy is left in situ. The *inset image* demonstrates the direction of the camera. I ileostomy, PD parastomal defect

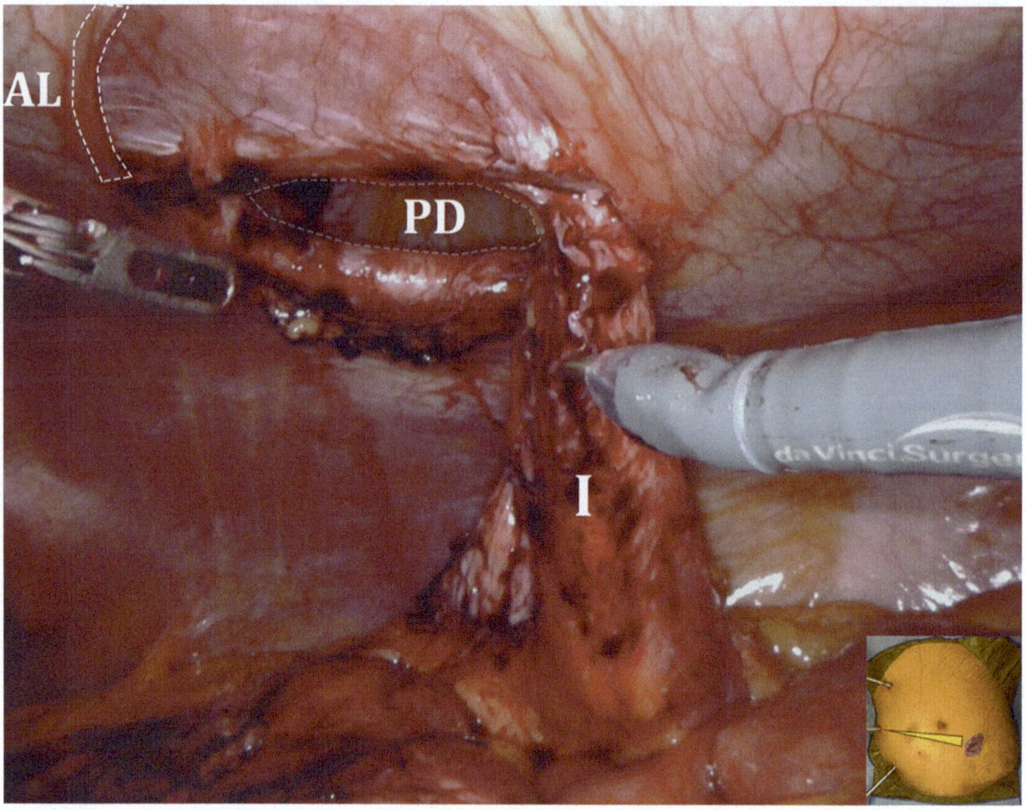


Fig. 11.5 View of the parastomal defect around the ostomy after completion of lysis of adhesions and reduction of parastomal hernia content. AL arcuate line

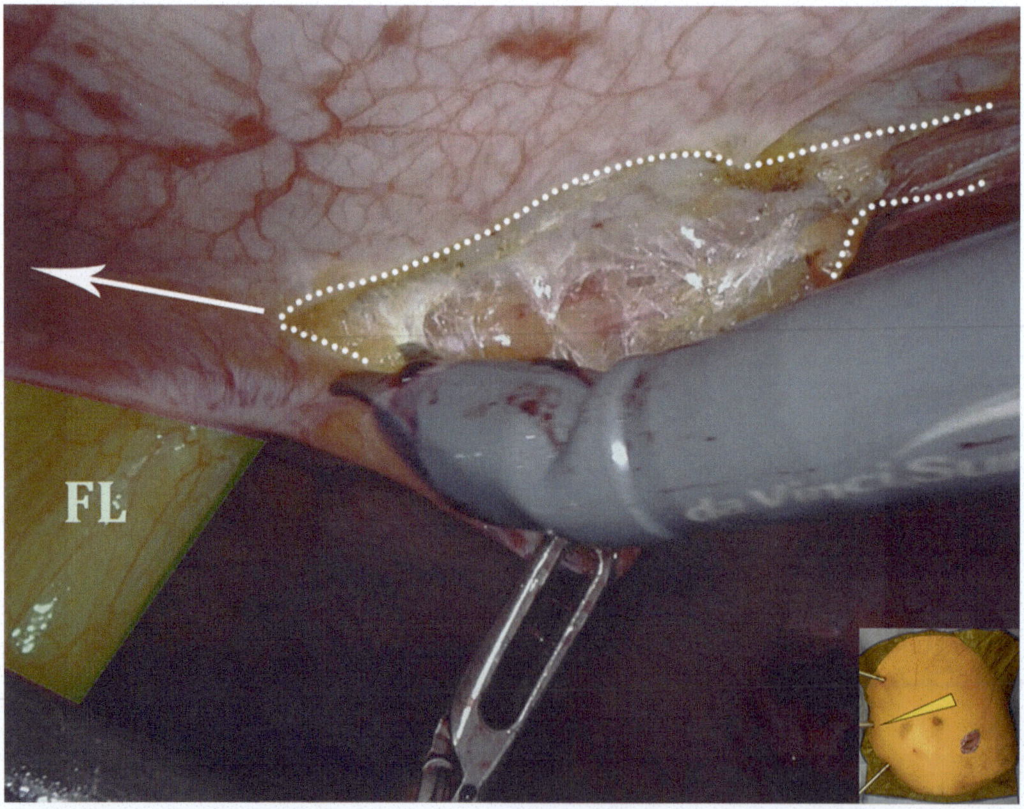


Fig. 11.6 The peritoneum is incised and dissected to uncover the posterior rectus sheath and linea alba. The *dotted line* represents the cut edges of peritoneum, and the *arrow* indicates the planned trajectory of the incision. FL falciform ligament

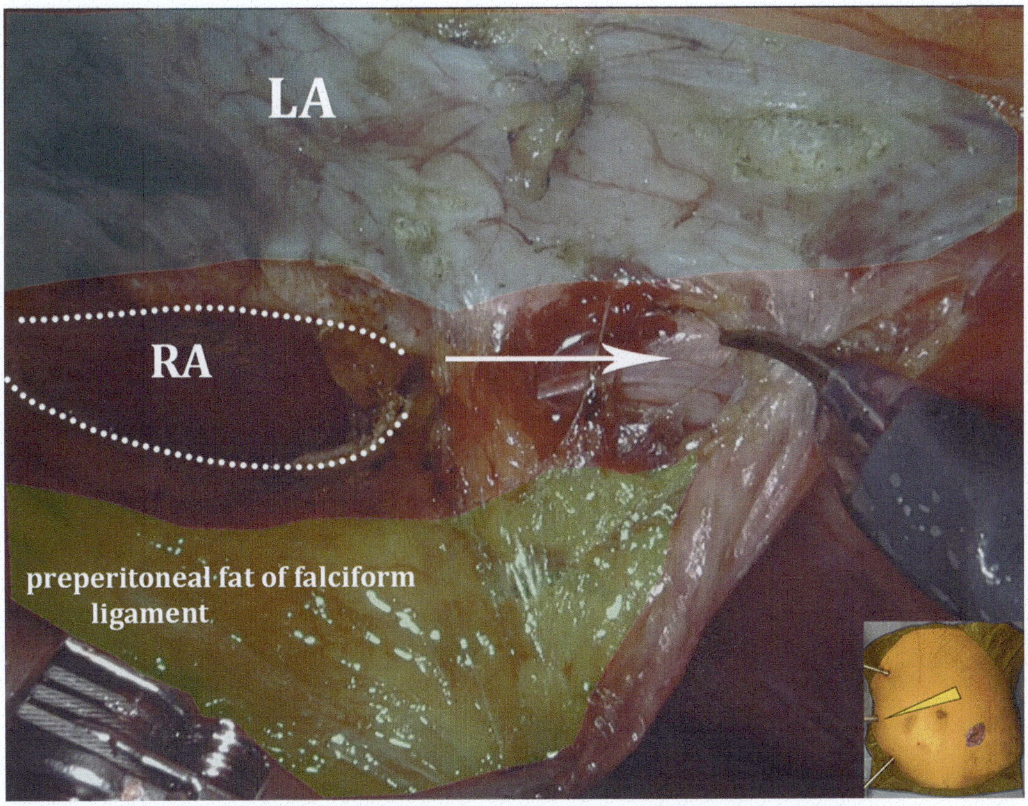


**Fig. 11.7** The posterior rectus sheath is incised approximately 0.5 cm lateral to the linea alba (LA) and the incision is extended across the full length of the rectus muscle. The *dotted line* represents the cut edges of the posterior rectus sheath, and the *arrow* indicates the planned trajectory of the incision

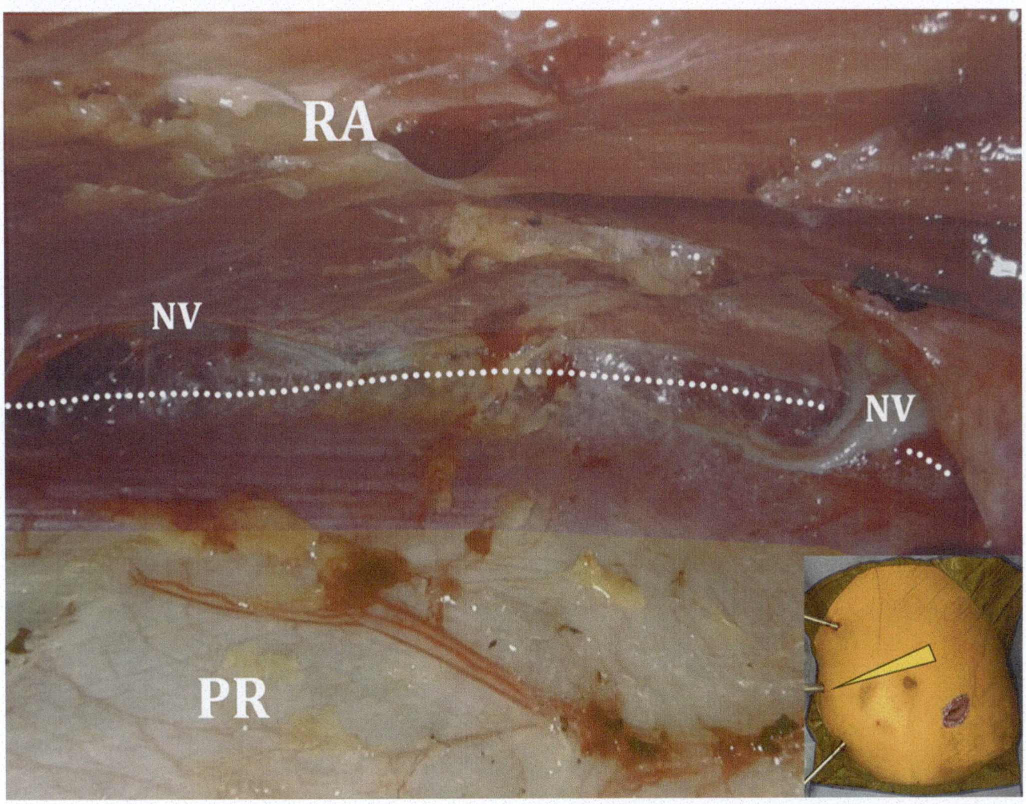


**Fig. 11.8** The retrorectus plane is developed laterally by separating the posterior rectus sheath from the rectus abdominis muscle. This plane continues laterally to the linea semilunaris (*dotted line*), where care should be taken to identify and preserve the neurovascular bundles (NV) entering the rectus itself. PR posterior rectus sheath

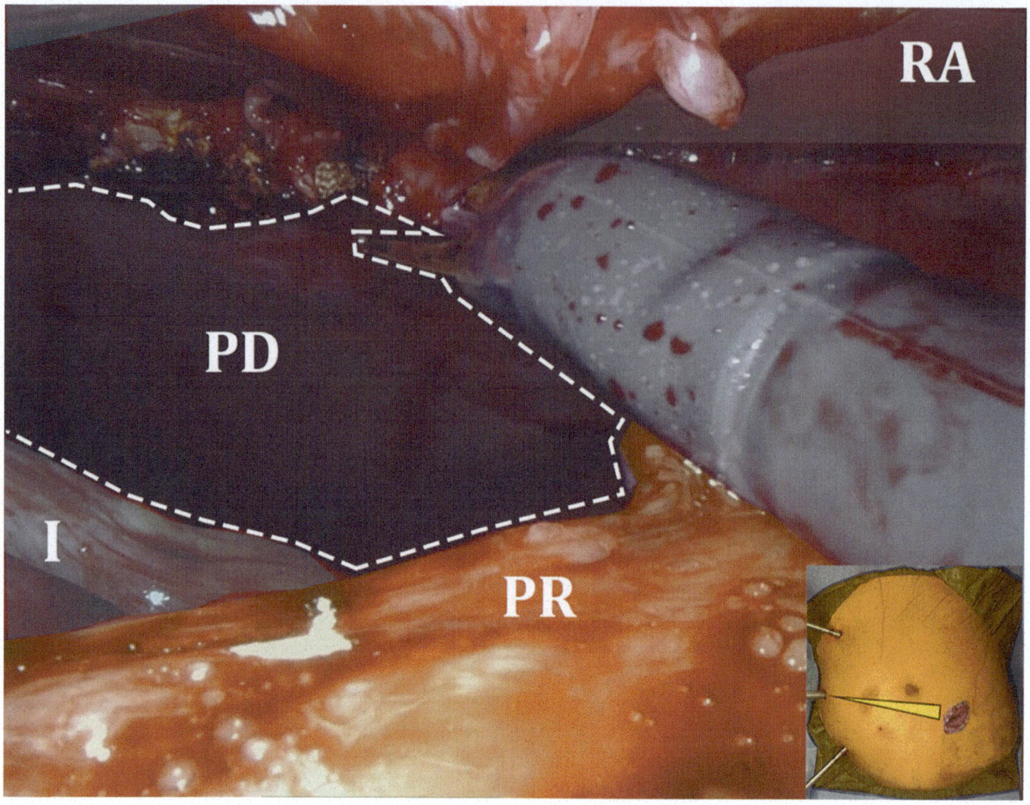


**Fig. 11.9** At the level of the ostomy, care is taken to not injure the bowel while extending the posterior rectus dissection around the ostomy. There is intrinsically a parastomal defect in the posterior rectus sheath, where the stoma and hernia content traversed through the rectus abdominis

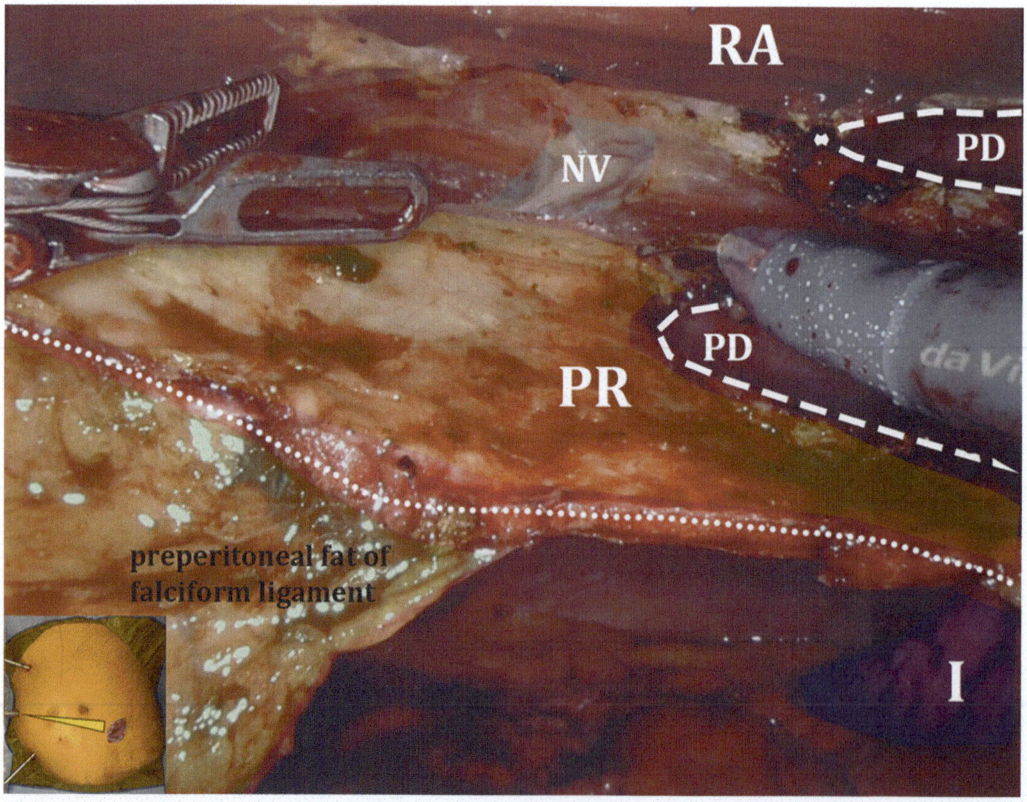


**Fig. 11.10** After completion of the posterior rectus sheath release, the preserved neurovascular bundles supplying the rectus abdominis can easily be identified. In this image, the parastomal defect in the rectus abdominis and posterior rectus sheath can both be seen with the ostomy traversing. The *dotted line* represents the medial cut edge of the posterior rectus sheath

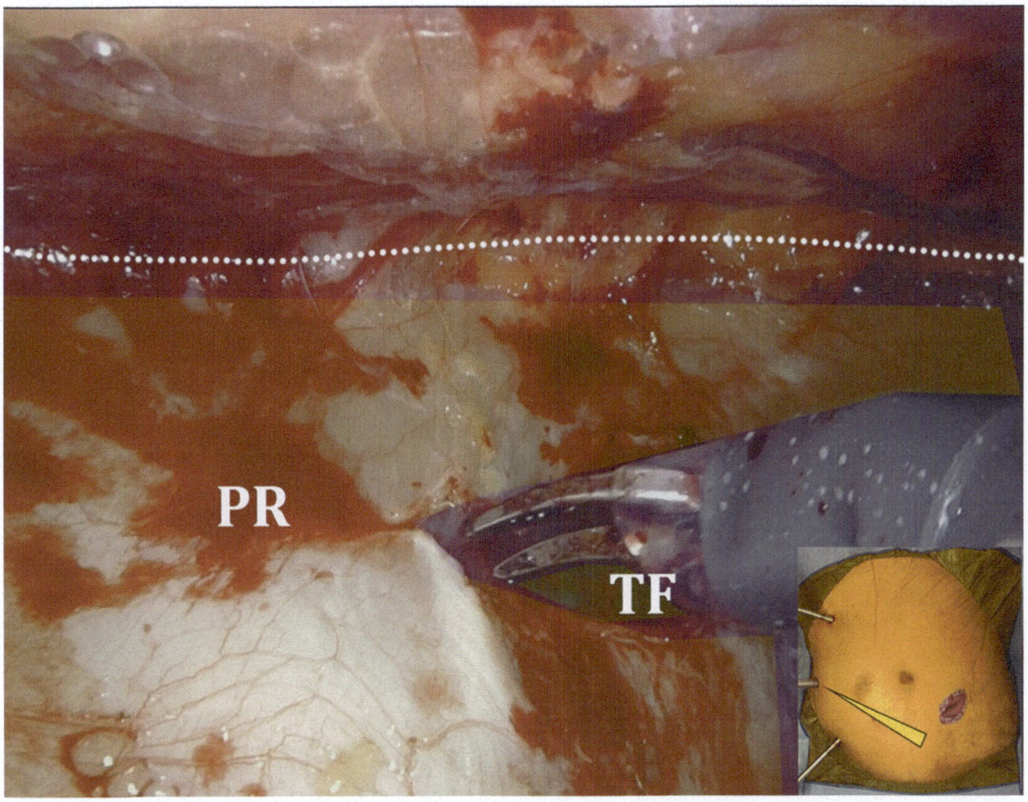


**Fig. 11.11** Just medial to the linea semilunaris (*dotted line*), a transversus abdominis release (TAR) is performed by incising into the posterior rectus sheath. In the lower abdomen, seen here, this "bottom up" TAR approach exposes the underlying transversalis fascia (TF) and peritoneum

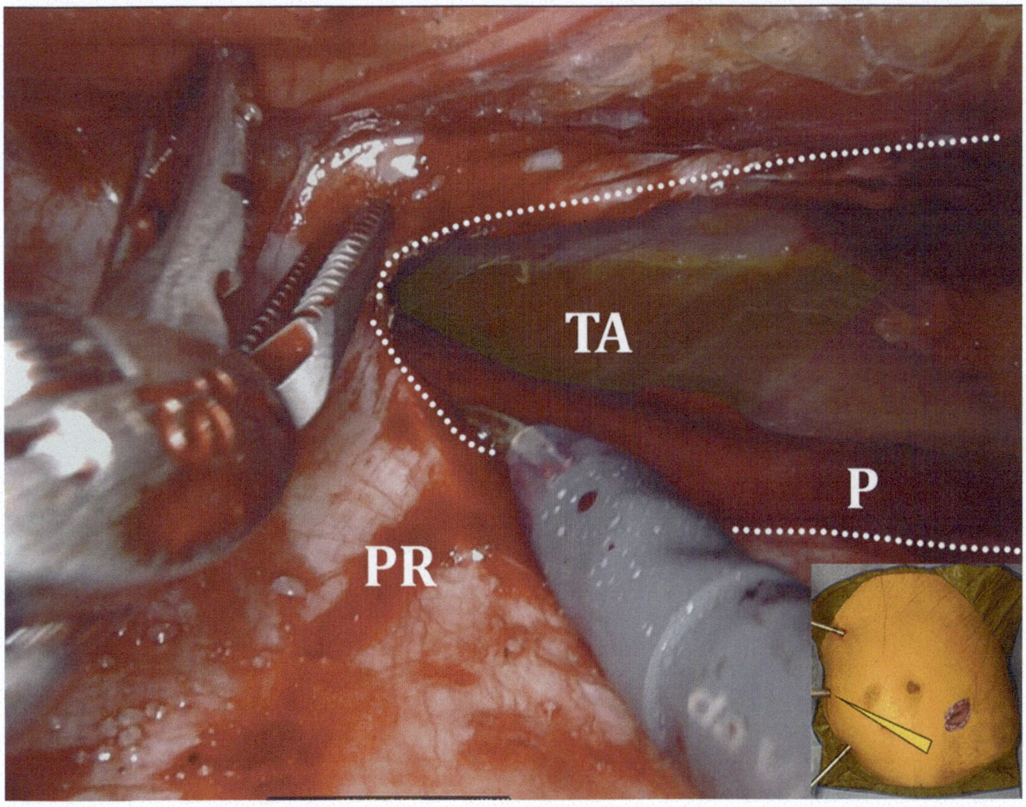


**Fig. 11.12** The dissection is extended laterally from the cut edge of the TAR (*dotted line*) in either the pre-peritoneal or pre-transversalis plane. In this particular case, the peritoneum (P) has been taken off the transversalis fascia that remains on the posterior surface of the transversus abdominis (TA)

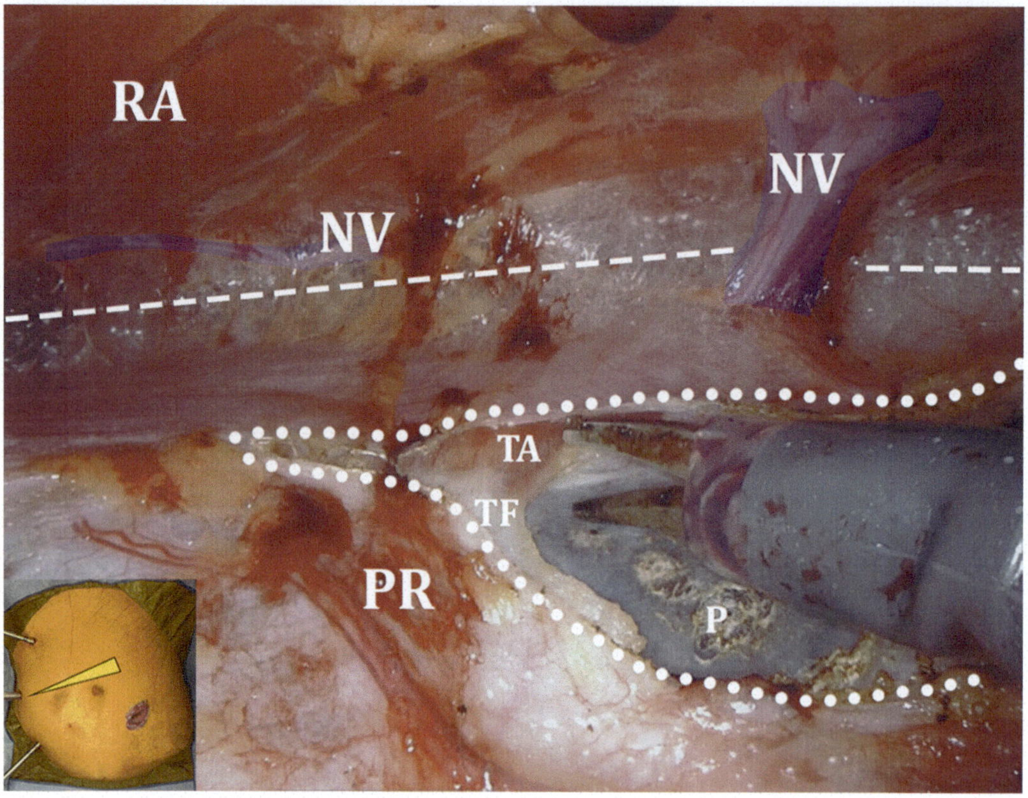


**Fig. 11.13** As the TAR is continued cranially into the upper abdomen, the posterior lamella of the internal oblique is incised, revealing the uncut transversus abdominis and transversalis fascia. The *dashed line* represents the linea semilunaris, and the *dotted line* shows the cut edges of the posterior lamella

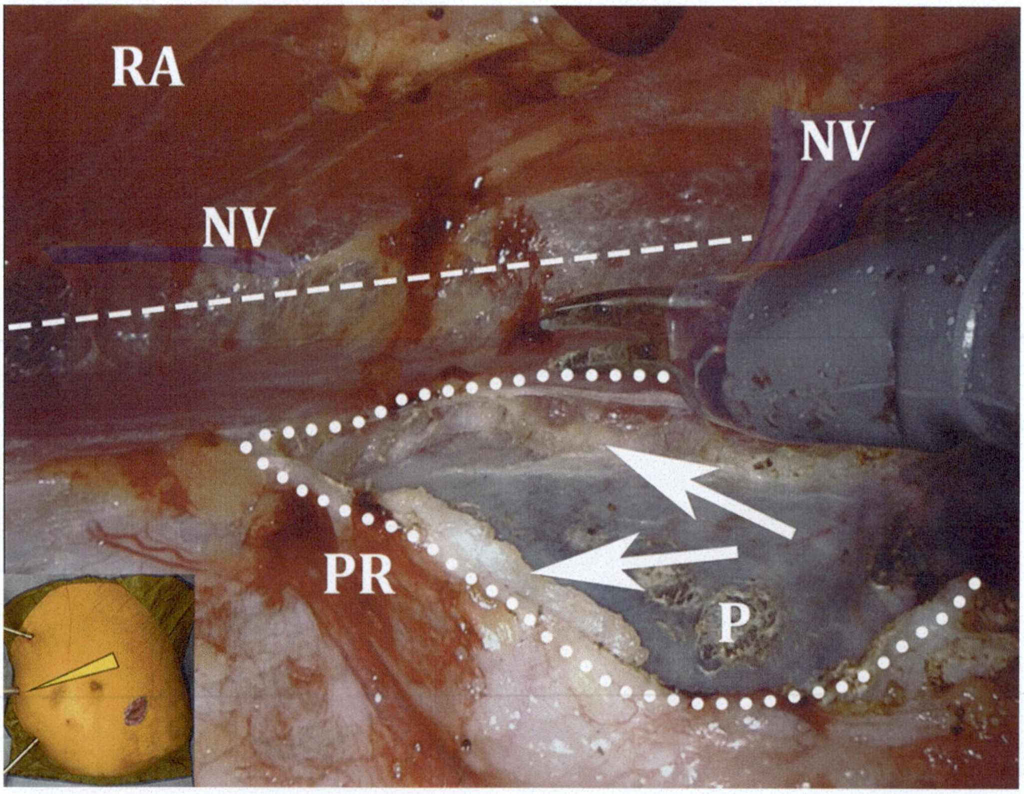


**Fig. 11.14** After incising the posterior lamella of the internal oblique, the fibers of the transversus abdominis are cut to complete the TAR. The *arrows* indicate the cut edges of the transversus abdominis. The *dashed line* represents the linea semilunaris, and the *dotted line* shows the cut edges of the posterior lamella

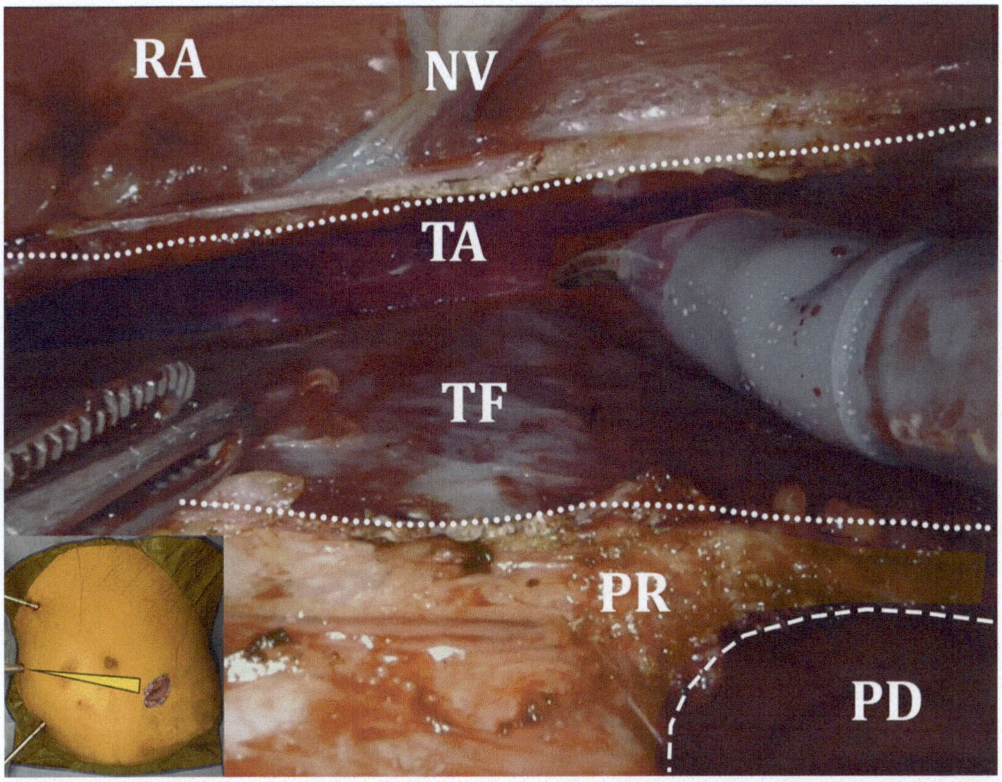


**Fig. 11.15** Following division of the transversus abdominis muscle fibers, dissection lateral to the rectus abdominis can occur in the pre-peritoneal or pre-transversalis plane. In this case, the transversalis fascia is being taken off the transversus abdominis muscle belly, and the parastomal defect in the posterior rectus sheath can be seen. The *dotted lines* show the medial and lateral cut edges of the transversus abdominis. The *dashed line* shows the boundaries of the parastomal defect

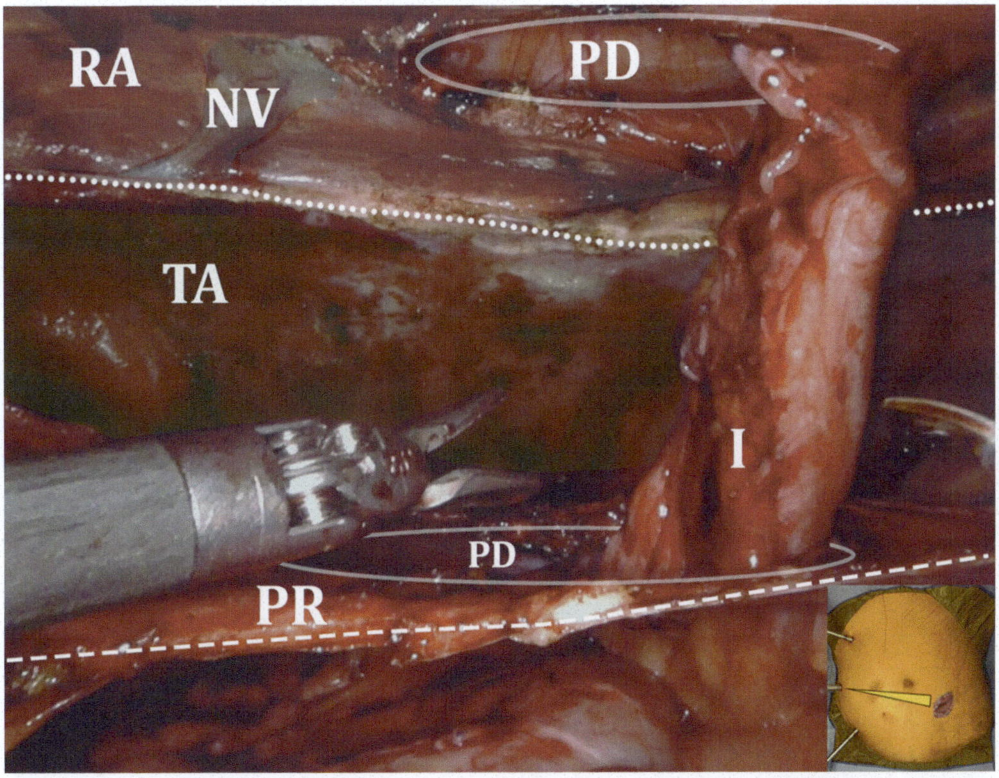


**Fig. 11.16** View of completed transversus abdominis release. The rectus abdominis and transversus abdominis muscles with intact neurovascular bundles remain up; the posterior rectus sheath in continuity with the pre-peritoneal or pre-transversalis plane remain down. The ostomy can be seen traversing the parastomal defect in both the rectus muscle and the posterior rectus sheath. The *dotted line* represents the lateral cut edge of the transversus abdominis, and the *dashed line* is the cut edge the of posterior rectus sheath

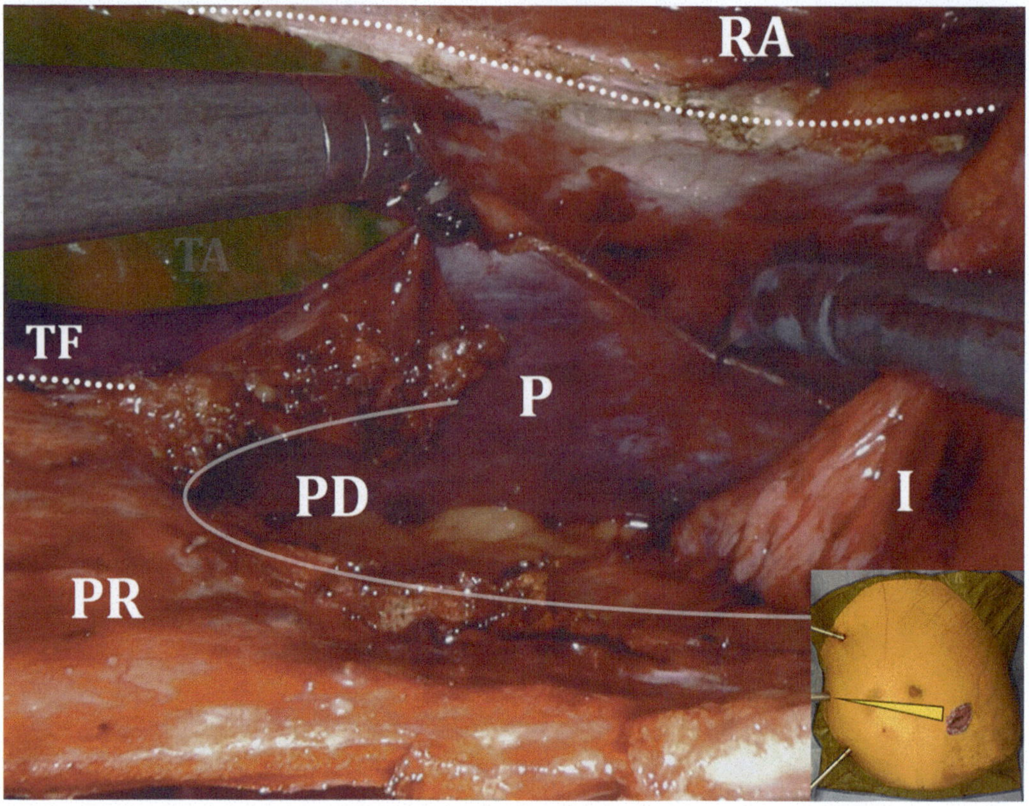


Fig. 11.17 The parastomal defect in the posterior rectus sheath is cut, intentionally extending the defect laterally through the peritoneum and transversalis fascia, which comprise the posterior layer lateral to the rectus abdominis. The *dotted lines* represent the cut edges of the transversus abdominis

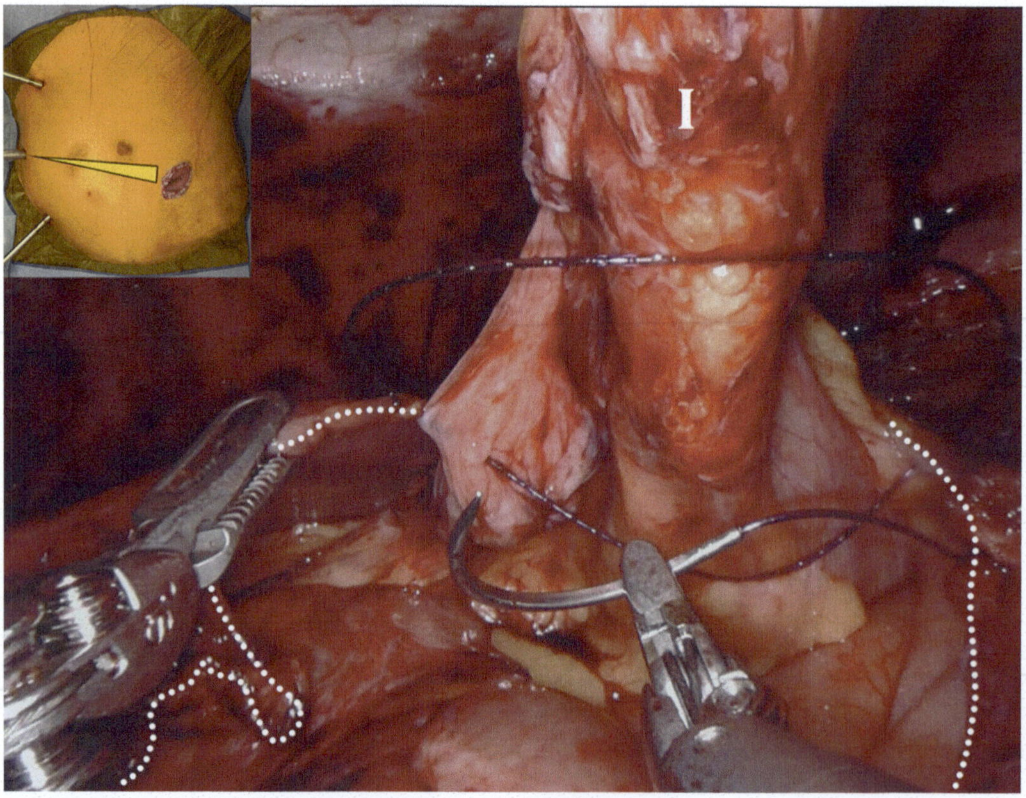


Fig. 11.18 The transversalis fascia and peritoneum are closed with suture in a lateral to medial fashion. This lateralizes the ostomy within the retromuscular space and closes the posterior defect created by the parastomal hernia. The *dotted line* illustrates the cut edges of the lateral extension of the parastomal defect

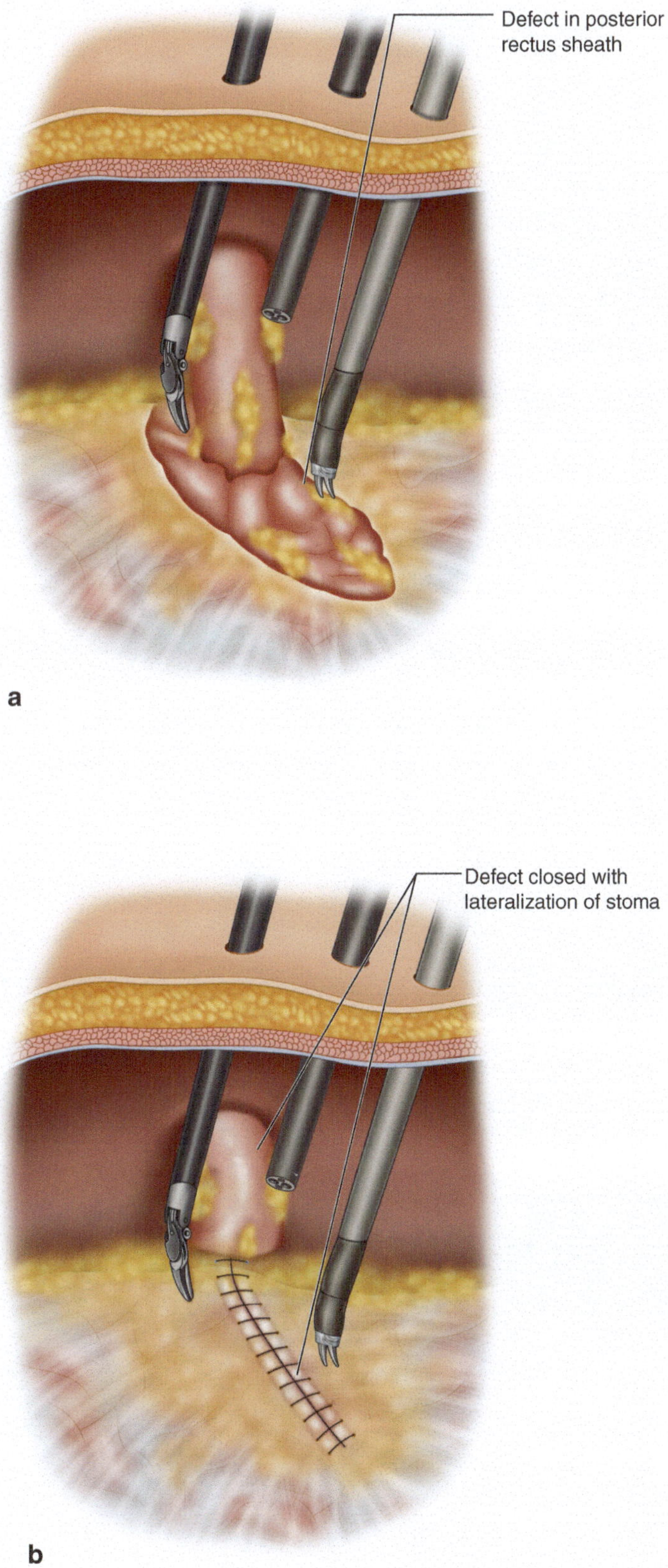


**Fig. 11.19** Maneuvers used to lateralize the bowel into the retromuscular space. (**a**) The defect in the posterior rectus sheath is first extended laterally. (**b**) After extending the defect, it is closed from lateral to medial, with the final proximal ostomy location lateralized

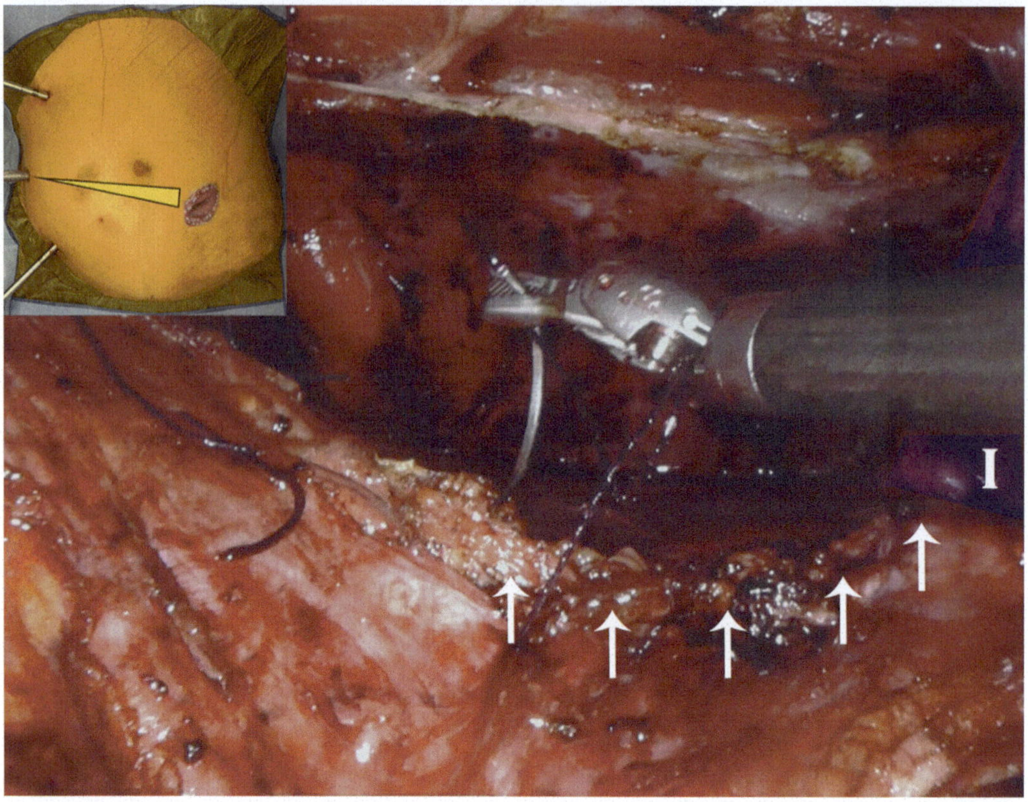


**Fig. 11.20** Completed closure of the posterior parastomal defect demonstrates an intact suture line (*arrows*) extending away from the ostomy

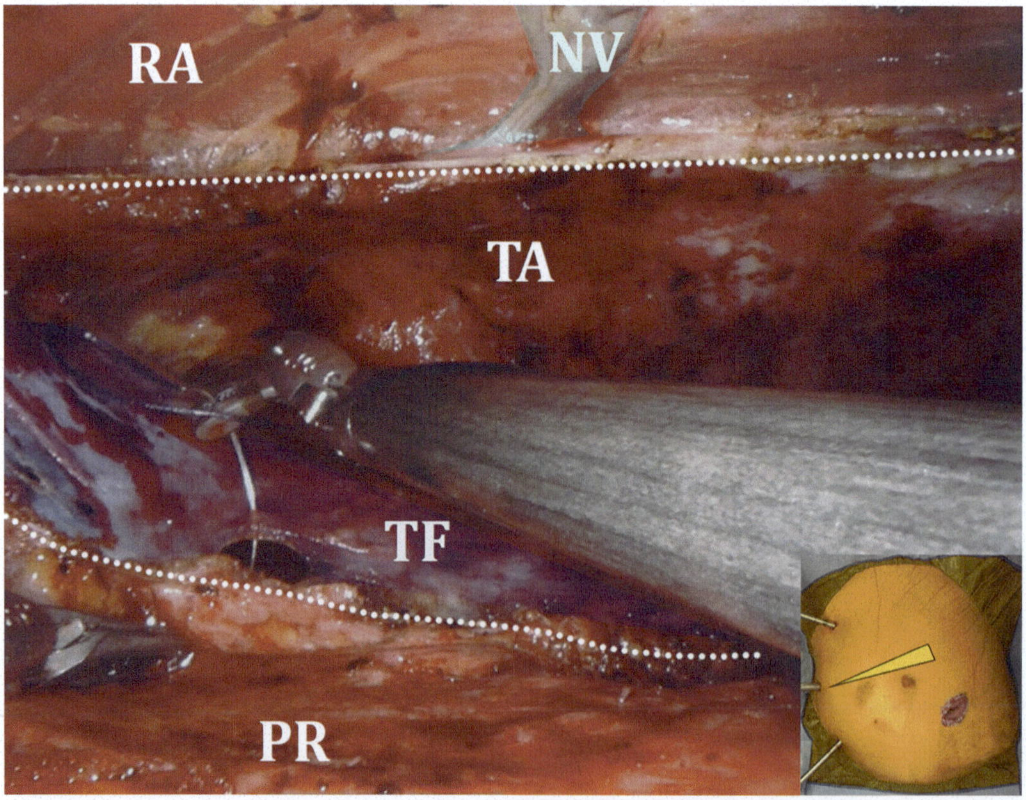


**Fig. 11.21** Additional defects in the posterior rectus sheath or transversalis fascia/peritoneum created during dissection are closed to prevent intraparietal hernia formation. The *dotted lines* represent the cut edge of the transversus abdominis

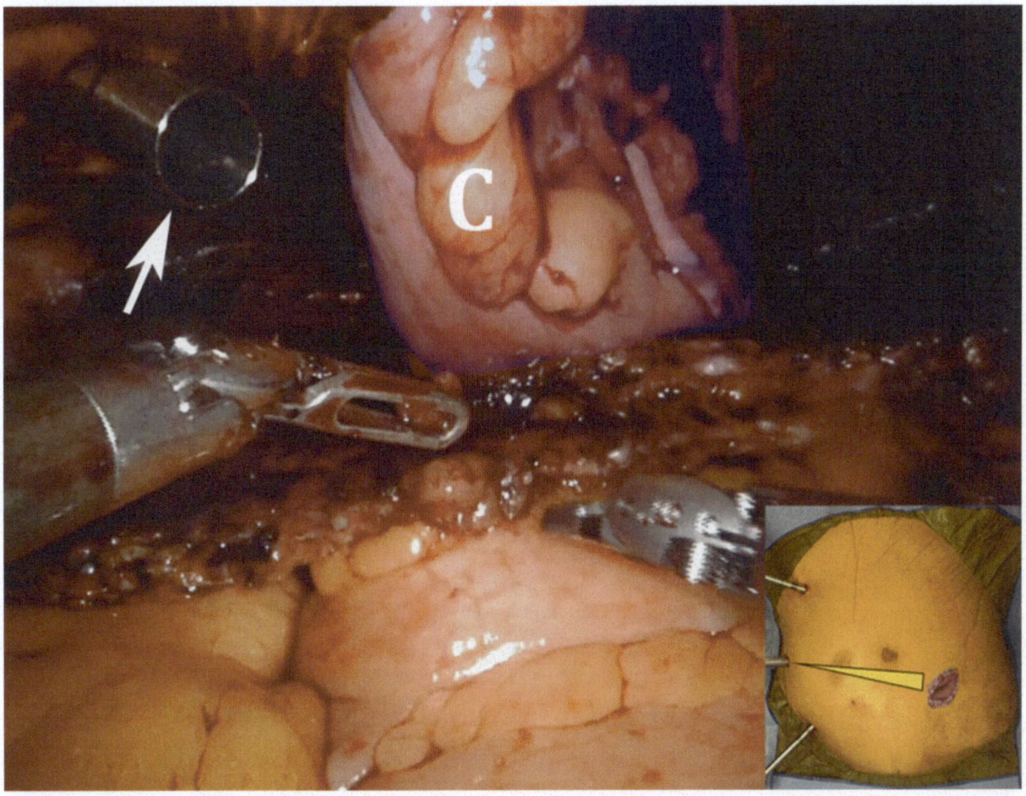


**Fig. 11.22** In patients with midline defects, three contralateral robotic ports (*arrow*) are placed under direct visualization. They are positioned around the stoma to avoid injury and maximize contralateral dissection capabilities. Contralateral posterior rectus sheath release (as shown in Figs. 11.7 and 11.8) and transversus abdominis release (Figs. 11.11, 11.12, 11.13, and 11.14) are performed to allow wide mesh reinforcement of the midline defect. C colostomy

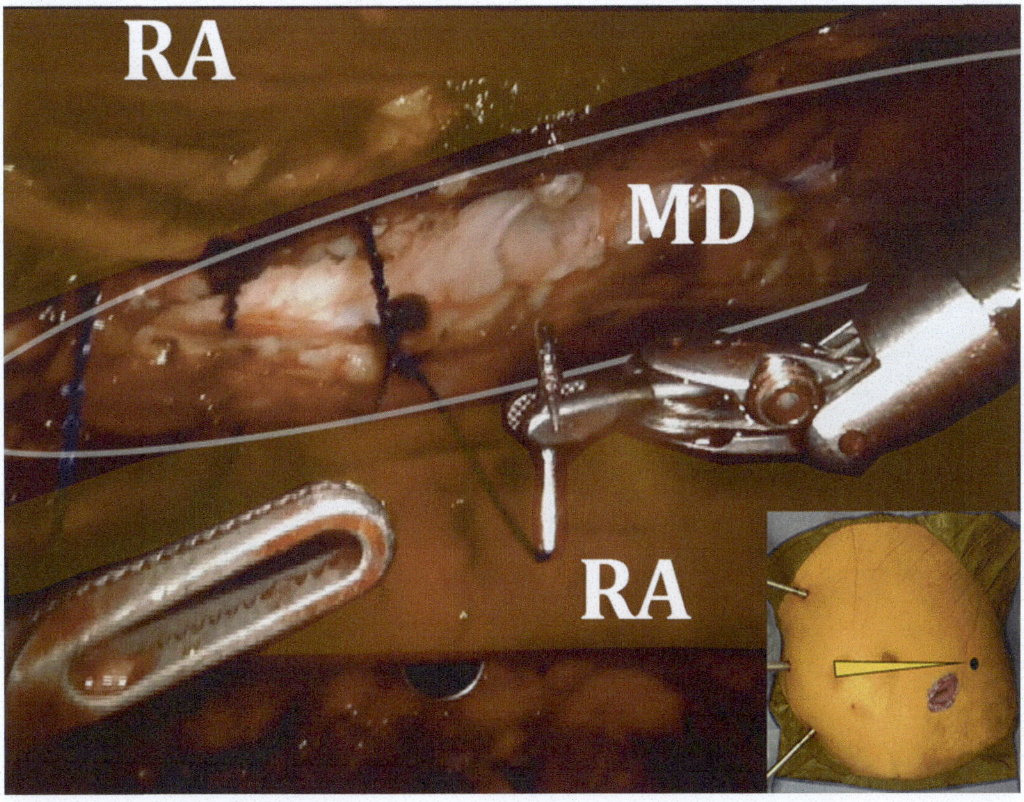


**Fig. 11.23** In patients with midline defects (MD), the anterior fascia is closed to recreate the linea alba between the rectus abdominis muscles. This closure can be performed at a reduced abdominal insufflation pressure (8–10 mmHg)

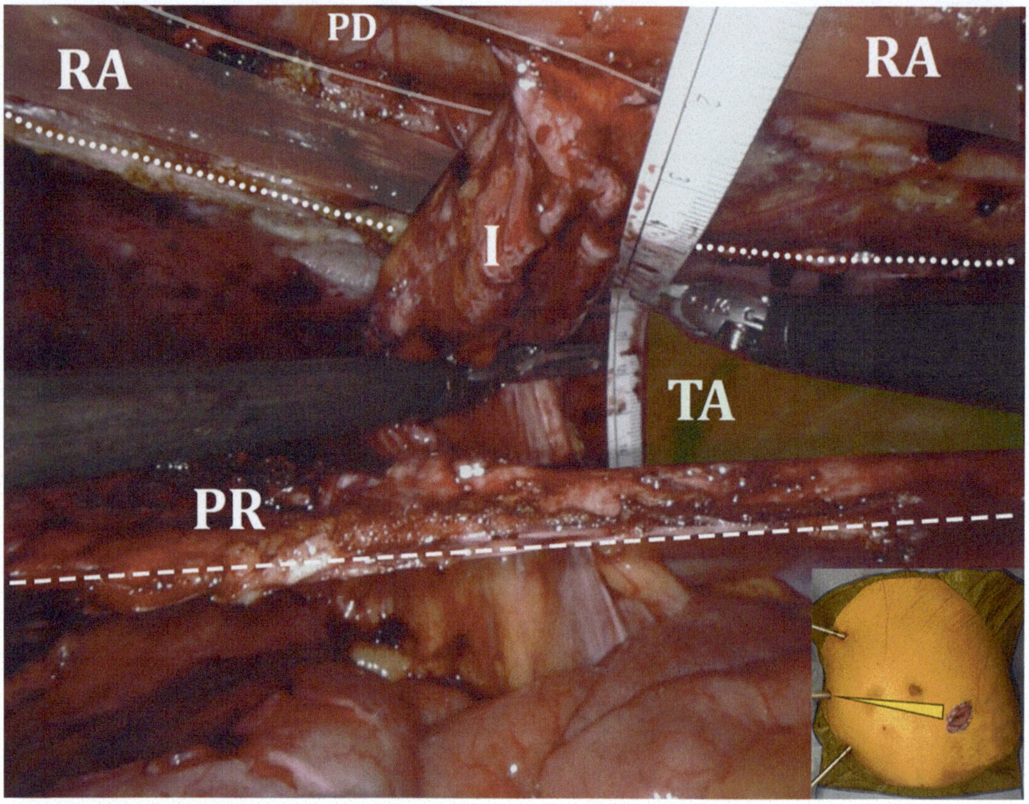


**Fig. 11.24** Complete view of the large retromuscular pocket. The ileostomy can be seen traversing the parastomal defect through the rectus abdominis muscle. A ruler is used to determine the mesh size needed to fill the retromuscular pocket. The *dotted line* represents the cut edge of the transversus abdominis; the *dashed line* shows the cut edge of the posterior rectus sheath

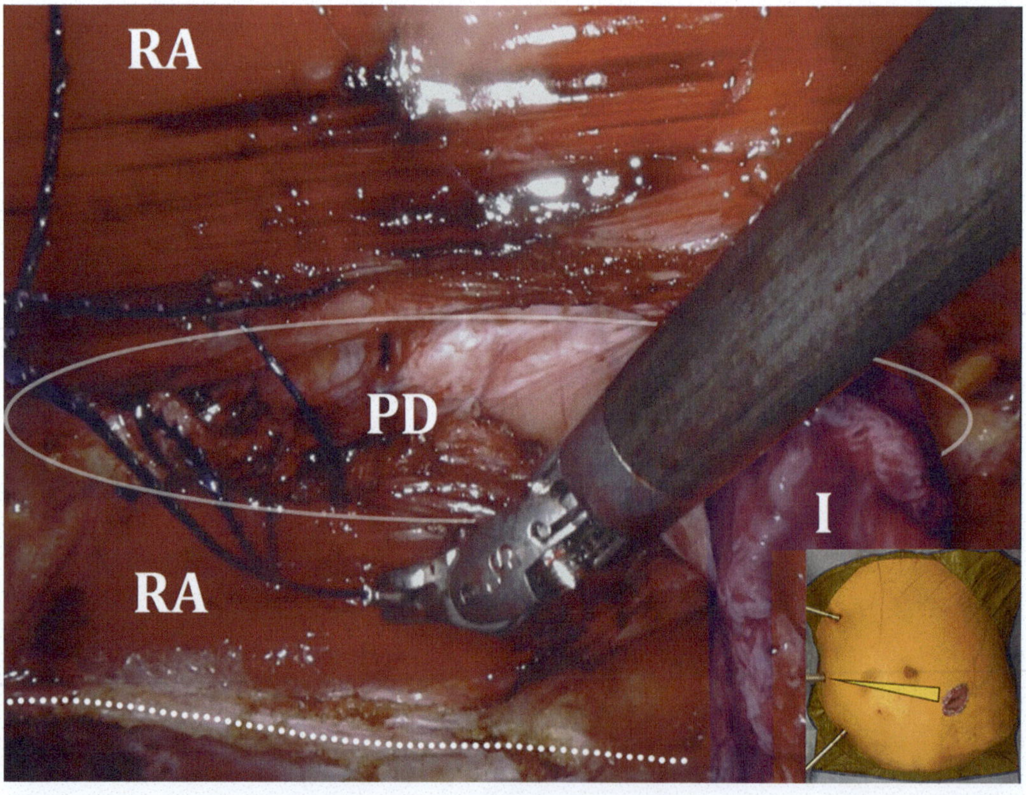


**Fig. 11.25** The anterior parastomal defect is primarily closed by suturing the external oblique aponeurosis to reapproximate the lateral and medial portions of the rectus abdominis around the ostomy. The *dotted line* represents the cut edge of the transversus abdominis

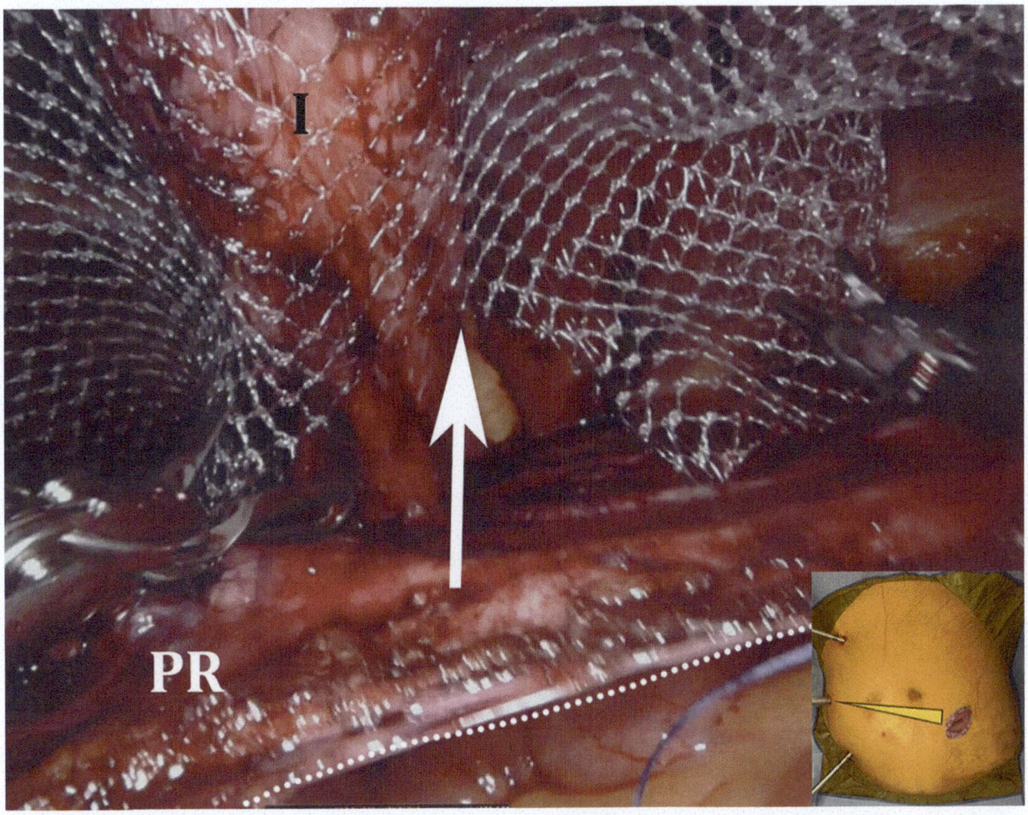


**Fig. 11.26** An uncoated, reduced-weight, macroporous polypropylene mesh is introduced into the retromuscular space. If desired, a slit is made in the mesh (*arrow*) to allow for lateral extension of the mesh beyond where the ostomy enters the retromuscular space. Alternatively, the uncut mesh edge can be positioned at this same location. The *dotted line* indicates the cut edge of the posterior rectus sheath

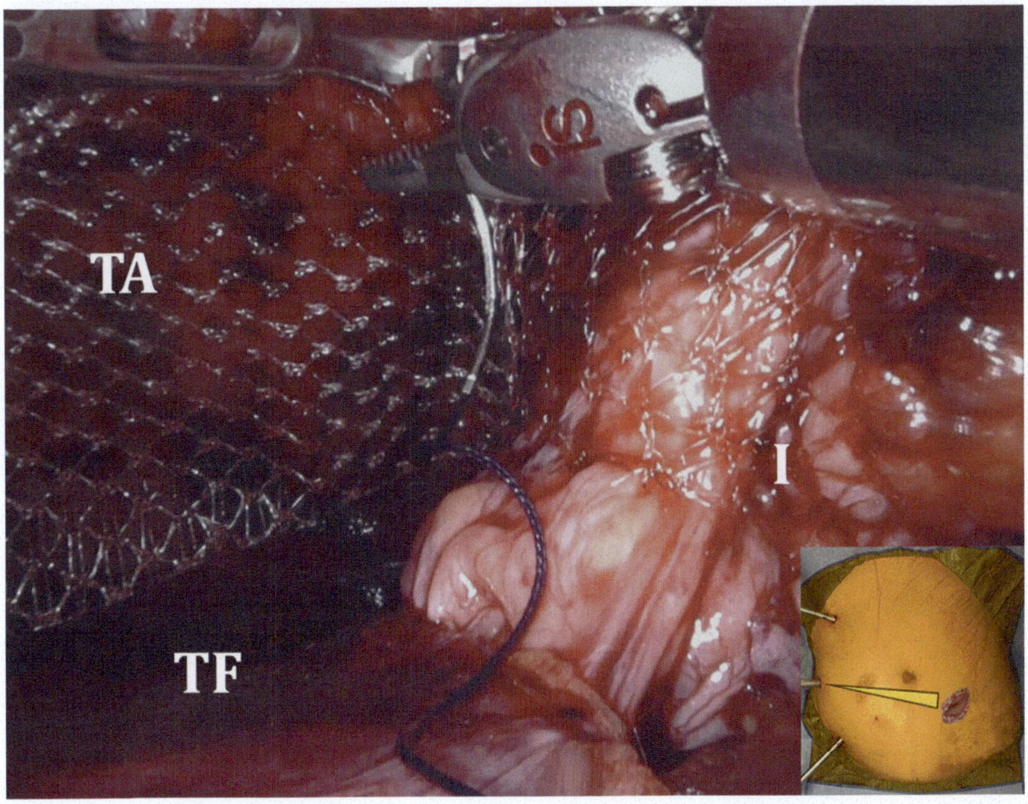


**Fig. 11.27** If desired, the mesh can be affixed to the transversus abdominis muscle superior and inferior to the ostomy, with particular care to ensure that the mesh does not exert any tension on the ostomy. These lateralizing sutures are surgeon-dependent and can be omitted

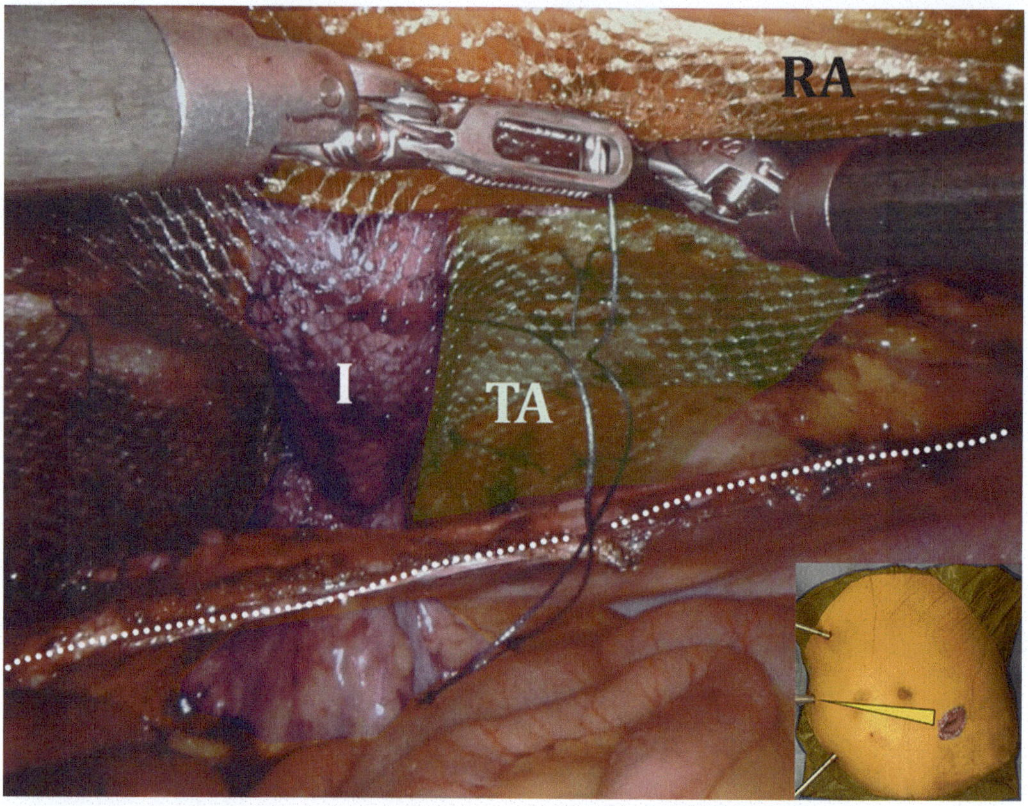


**Fig. 11.28** The mesh is further affixed to the rectus abdominis muscle within the retromuscular pocket. The sling of mesh created around the ostomy can easily be seen here, recreating a configuration similar to an intraperitoneal Sugarbaker operation. The *dotted line* indicates the cut edge of the posterior rectus sheath

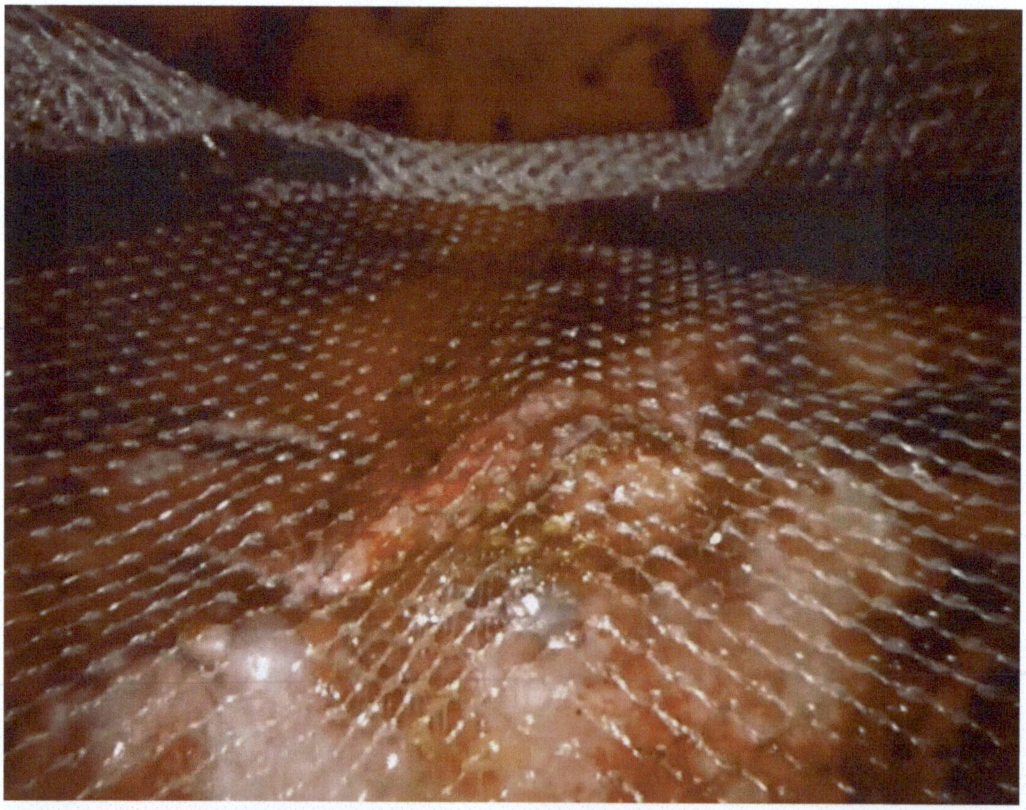

**Fig. 11.29** Alternatively, a non-fixation method of mesh positioning can be employed. Here, the mesh is laid flat on the floor of the retromuscular pocket without any suture or sealant fixation

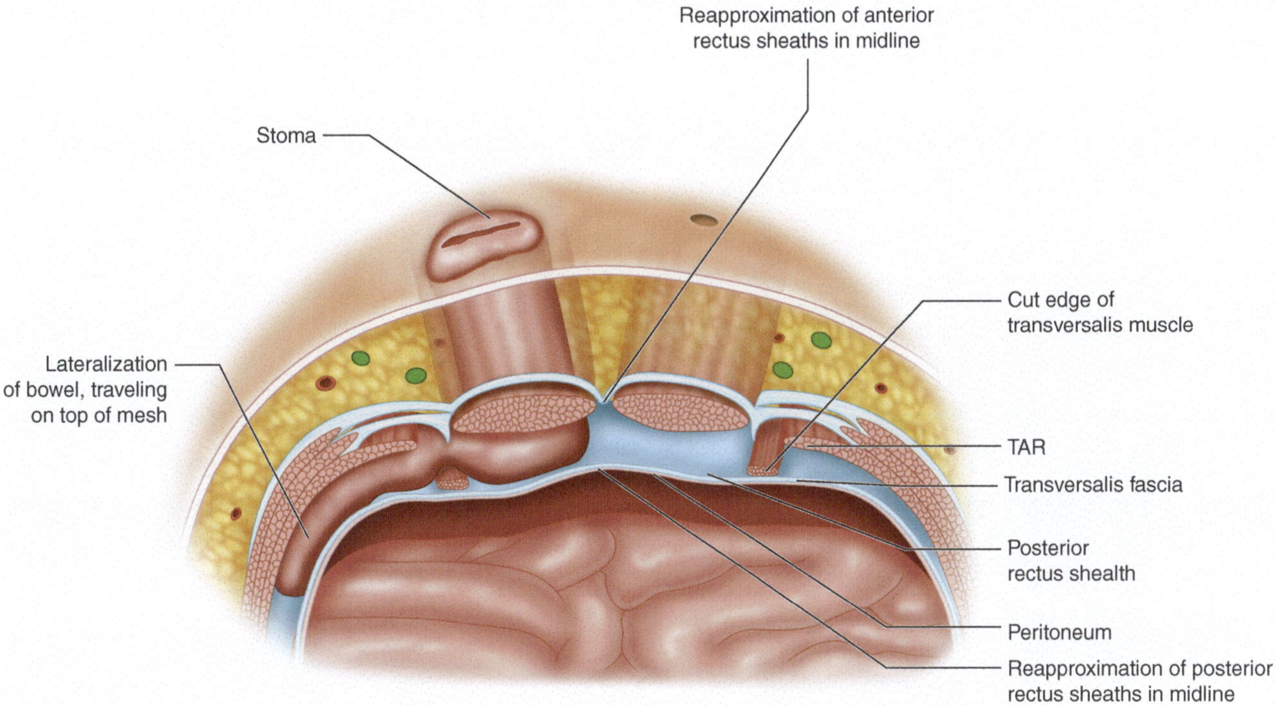


**Fig. 11.30** Diagram of mesh placement. Pictured is the position after bilateral posterior component separation and bilateral transversus abdominis release to achieve wide mesh overlap of the parastomal defect and the midline defect. The closure of the anterior rectus sheath depicted is for patients with a midline hernia defect

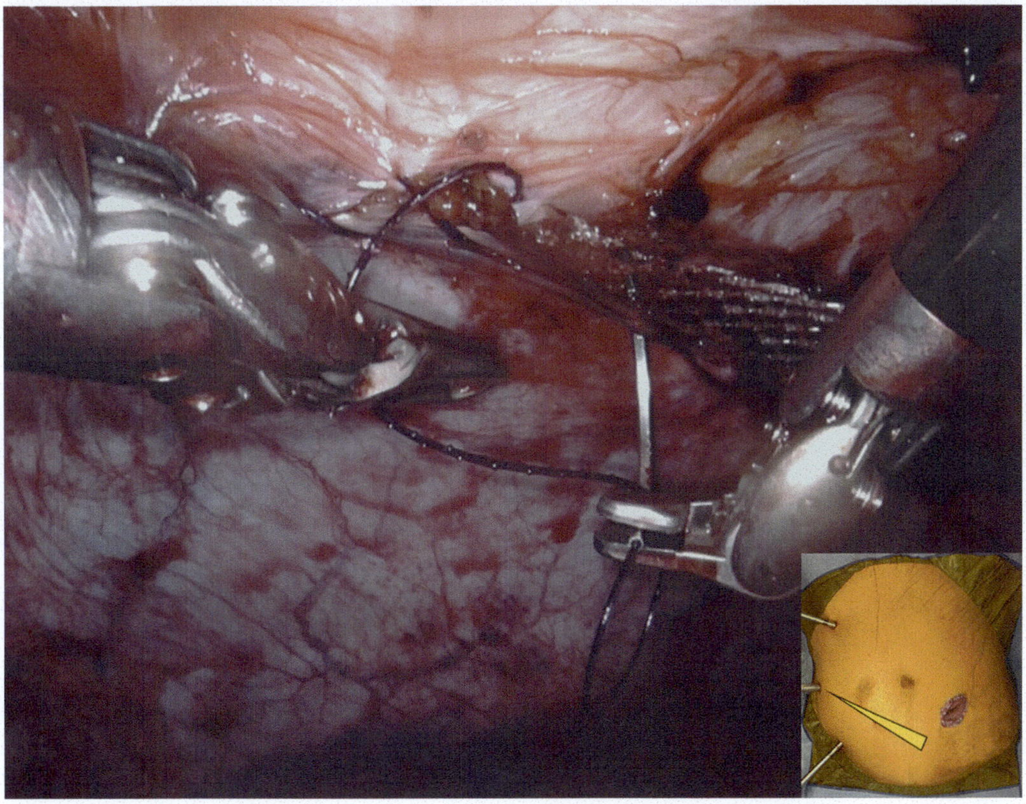

**Fig. 11.31** The retromuscular space is closed by suturing the medial edge of the posterior rectus sheath back to the abdominal wall, completely excluding the mesh from the peritoneal cavity

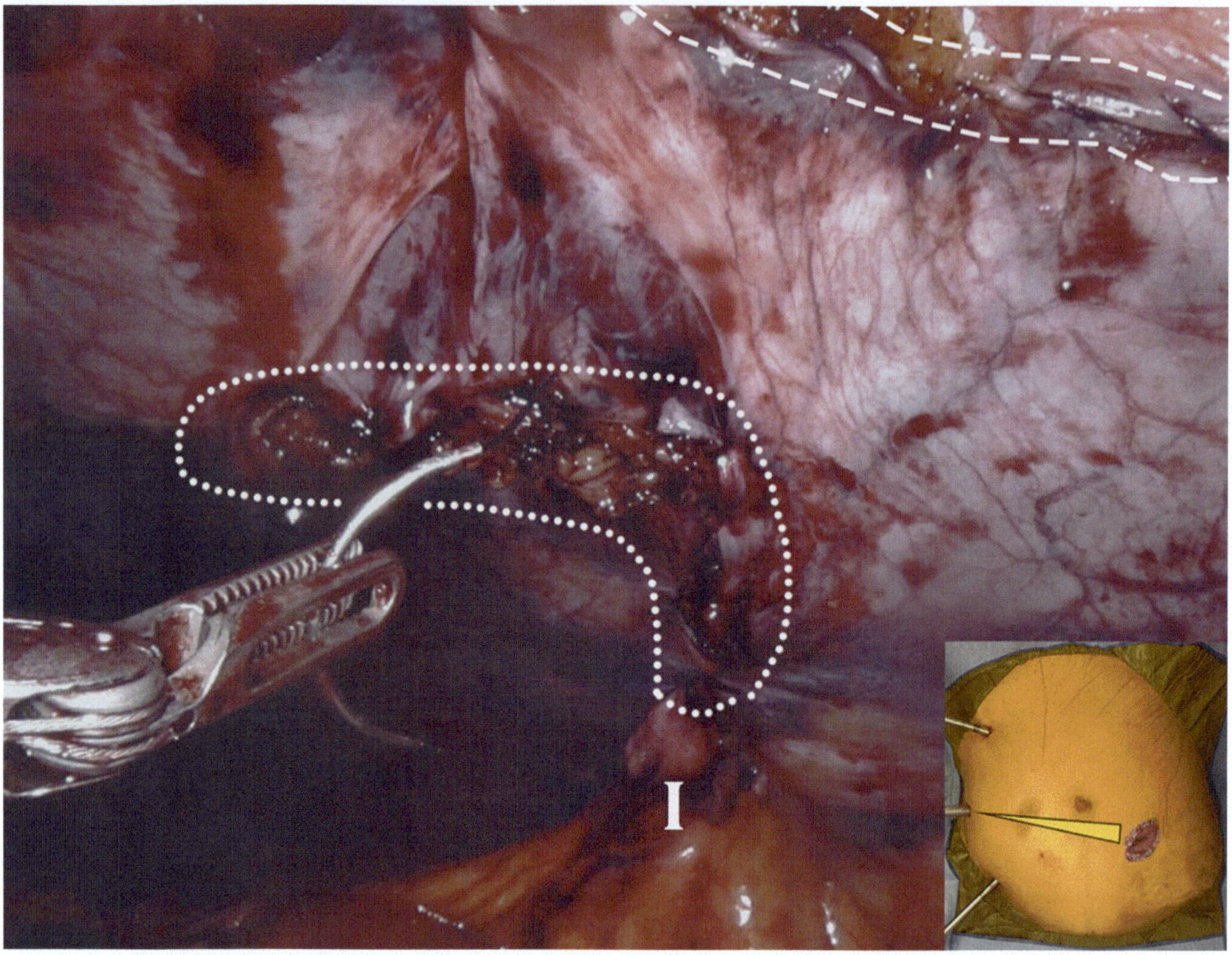


**Fig. 11.32** View of the completed closure demonstrates the ostomy entering the retromuscular plane laterally. The *dotted line* represents the joint closure of the parastomal defect in the posterior rectus sheath and the intentional cut made to lateralize the ostomy. The *dashed line* is the reapproximation of the medial cut edge of the posterior rectus sheath to the abdominal wall to exclude the mesh from the peritoneal cavity

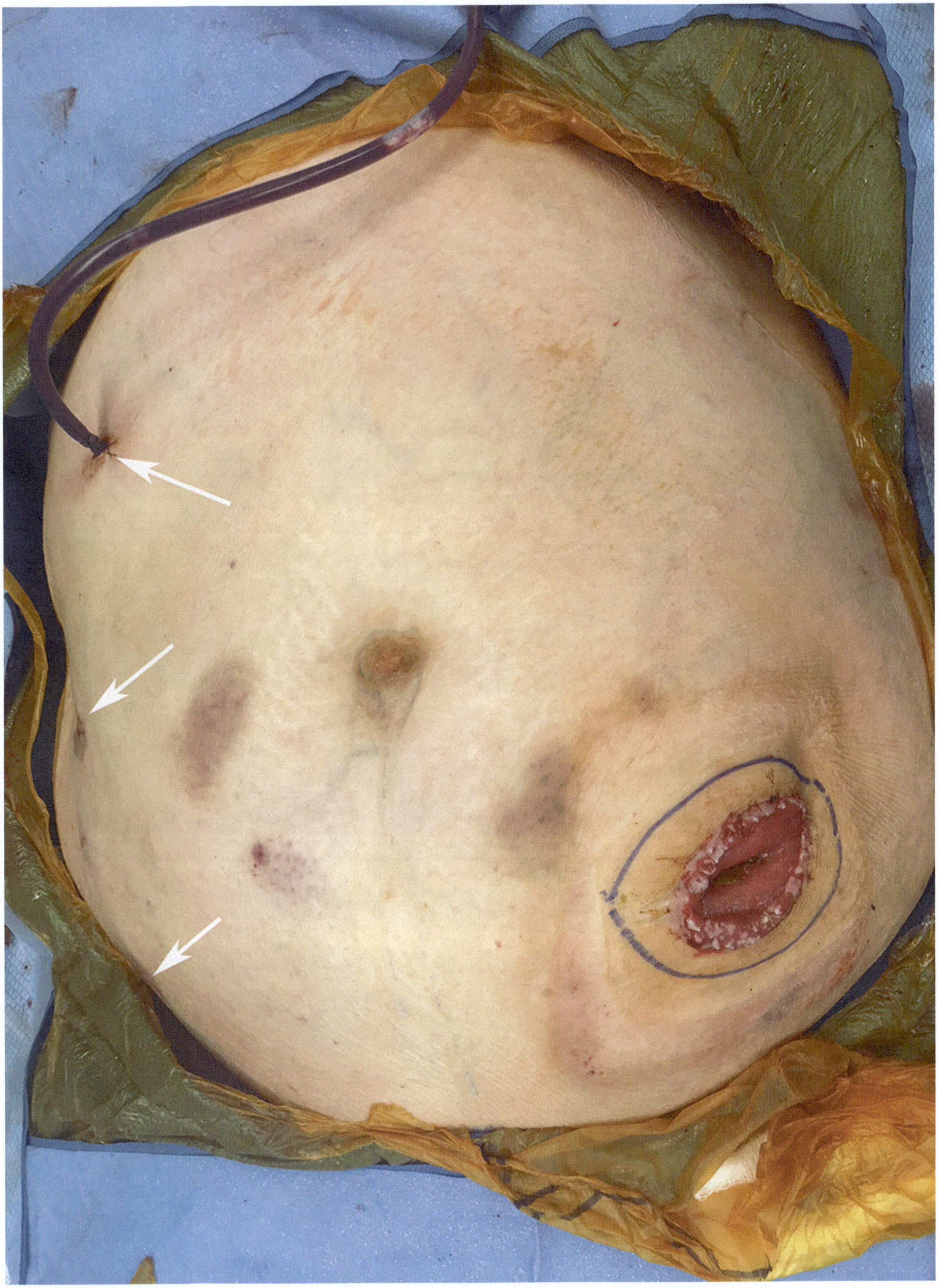

**Fig. 11.33** Immediate postoperative image (*arrows* at port incisions)

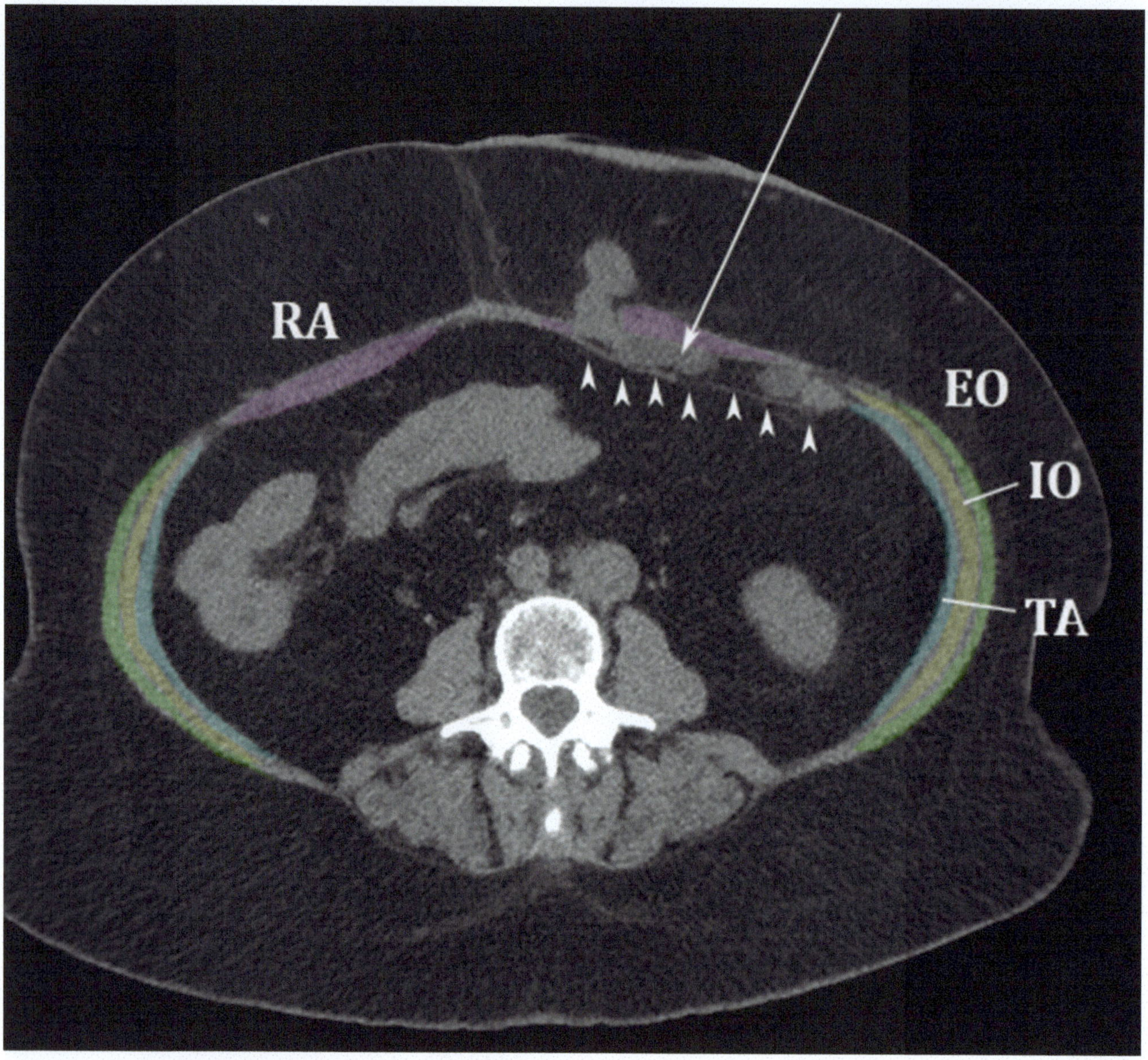


**Fig. 11.34** 1-year follow-up CT scan. The small bowel (*arrow*) is demonstrated entering the retromuscular plane running from lateral to medial. The *arrowheads* indicate the transversalis fascia, posterior rectus sheath, and sublay mesh

## Suggested Reading

Pauli EM, Juza RM, Winder JS. How I do it: novel parastomal herniorrhaphy utilizing transversus abdominis release. Hernia. 2016;20:547–52.

Raigani S, Criss CN, Petro CC, Prabhu AS, Novitsky YW, Rosen MJ. Single-center experience with parastomal hernia repair using retromuscular mesh placement. J Gastrointest Surg. 2014;18:1673–7.

Tastaldi L, Haskins IN, Perez AJ, Prabhu AS, Rosenblatt S, Rosen MJ. Single center experience with the modified retromuscular Sugarbaker technique for parastomal hernia repair. Hernia. 2017;21:941–9.

Winder JS, Pauli EM. Open parastomal hernia repair. In: Rosen MJ, editor. Atlas of abdominal wall reconstruction. 2nd ed. Philadelphia: Elsevier; 2016. p. 124–49.

# Robotic Lumbar Hernia Repair: Totally Extraperitoneal (TEP)

# 12

Engin Hatipoglu and Omar Yusef Kudsi

## Introduction

Lateral incisional hernias (LIHs) are relatively rare compared with midline hernias [1]. A number of anatomical factors may cause technical difficulties in the repair of LIH. There is less aponeurotic tissue at the lateral abdominal wall than in the midline portion of the abdomen. Additionally, hernias located close to bony prominences (such as the costal margin and the iliac crest) or close to major neurovascular structures may not allow proper mesh overlap and adequate mesh fixation, depending on the chosen surgical approach [1–3].

Several techniques using the robot have been described, including retromuscular repair with or without transversus abdominis release (TAR). The technique described most recently is a retromuscular repair using a totally extraperitoneal (TEP) access.

## Procedure: Illustrated Steps

Figures 12.1, 12.2, 12.3, 12.4, 12.5, 12.6, 12.7, 12.8, 12.9, 12.10, 12.11, 12.12, 12.13, 12.14, 12.15, 12.16, 12.17, 12.18, 12.19, 12.20, 12.21, 12.22, 12.23, 12.24, 12.25, 12.26, 12.27, 12.28, 12.29, 12.30, 12.31, 12.32, and 12.33 illustrate the technical aspects of robotic TEP-TAR repair of a lumbar incisional hernia, classified as L4 (lumbar, latero-dorsal of the anterior axillary line) [4].

E. Hatipoglu
Department of General Surgery, Cerrahpasa Faculty of Medicine, Istanbul University–Cerrahpasa/Kocamustafapasa, Istanbul, Turkey

O. Y. Kudsi (✉)
Department of Surgery, Good Samaritan Medical Center, Tufts University School of Medicine, Boston, MA, USA


O. Y. Kudsi (ed.), *Robotic Hernia Surgery*, https://doi.org/10.1007/978-3-030-46667-1_12

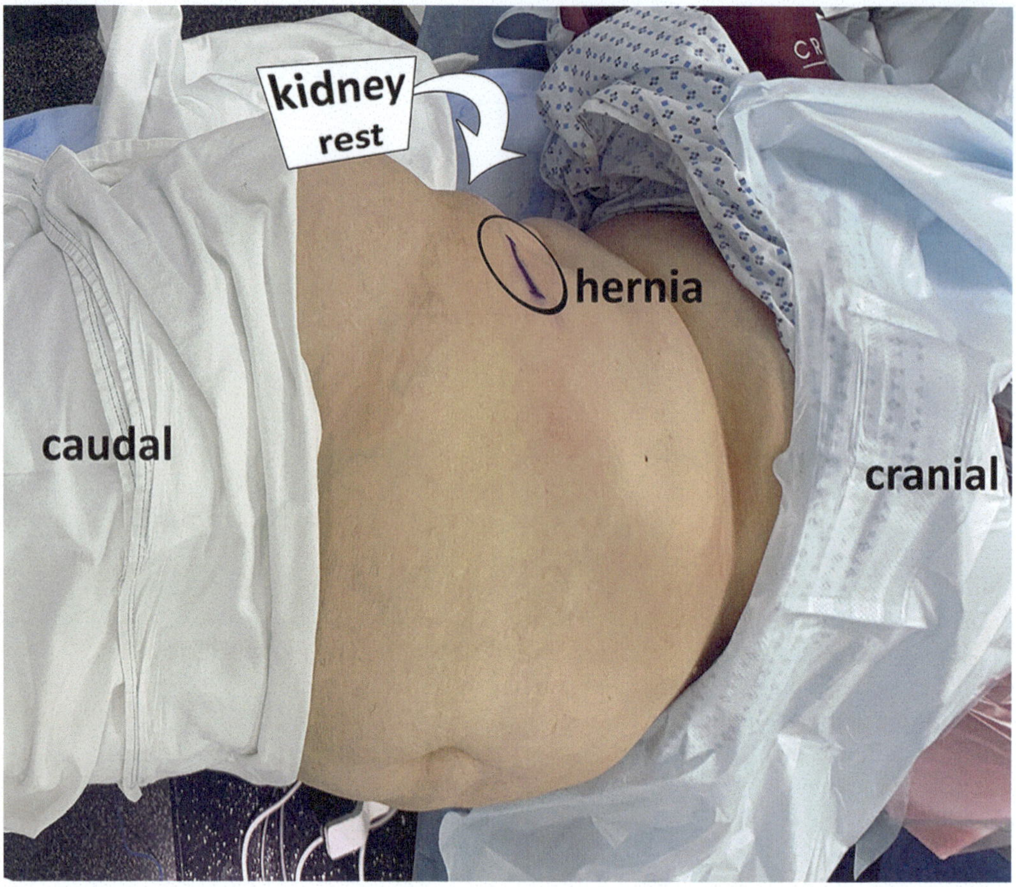


**Fig. 12.1** Patient positioning for robotic right lumbar (L4) incisional hernia repair. The patient is placed in a semilateral decubitus position with the help of kidney rest

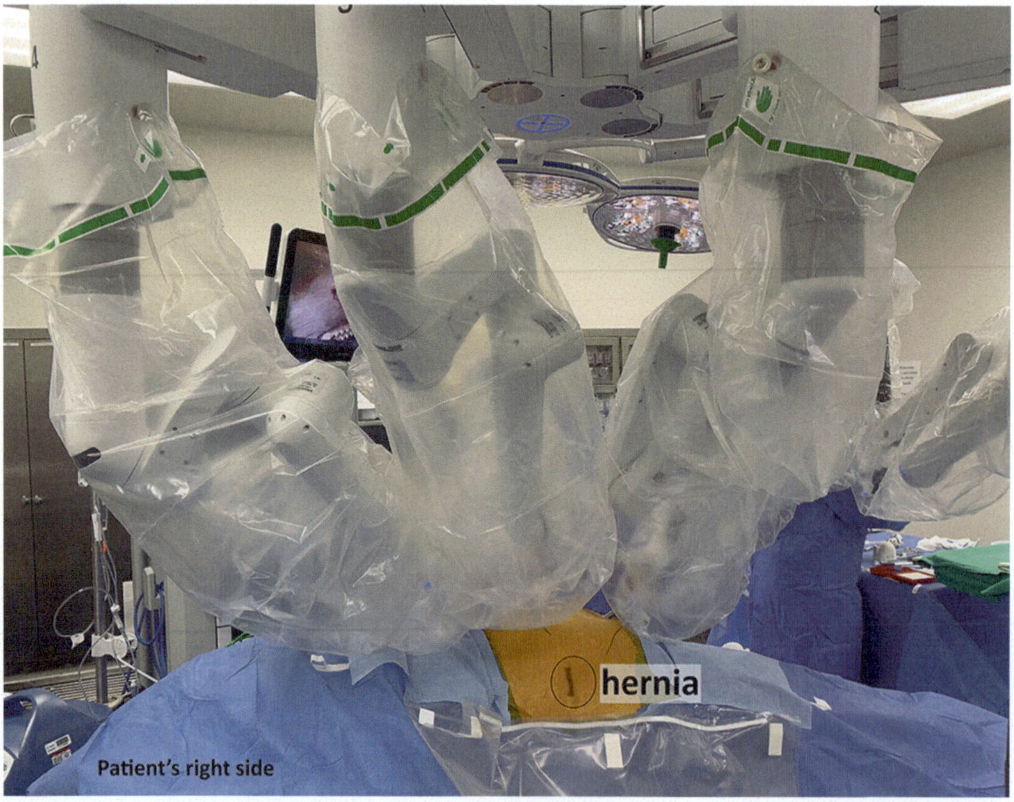


**Fig. 12.2** After proper trocar placement, the patient-side cart of the robot is docked

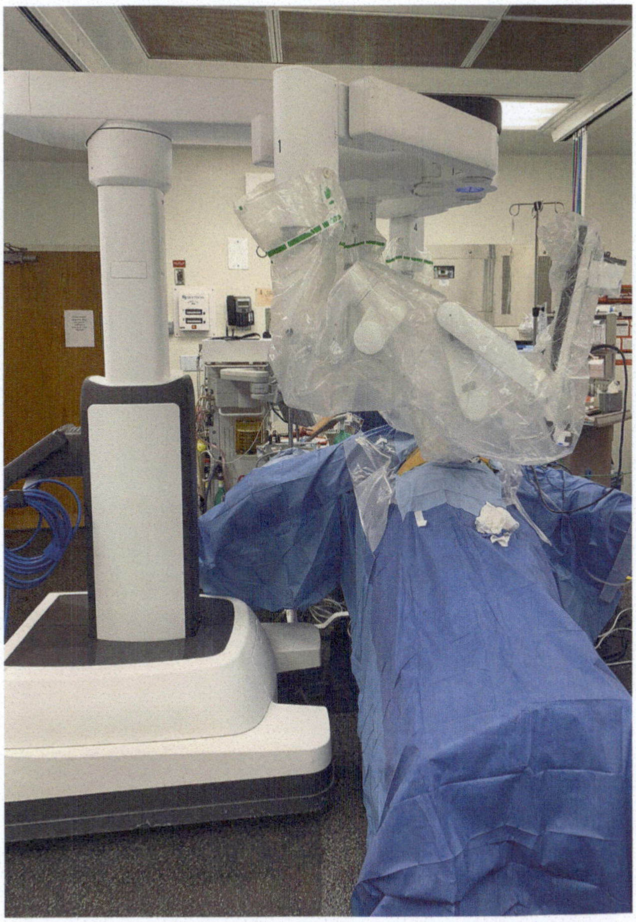

**Fig. 12.3** Side docking

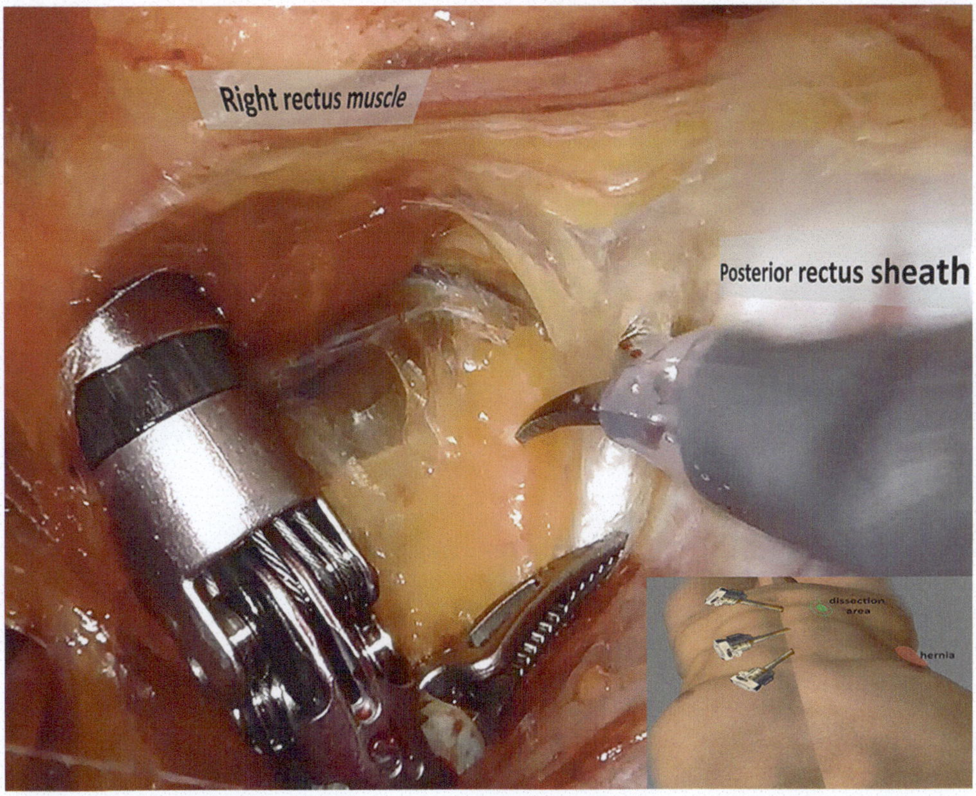


**Fig. 12.4** Initial dissection of loose connective tissues between the rectus muscle and posterior rectus sheath

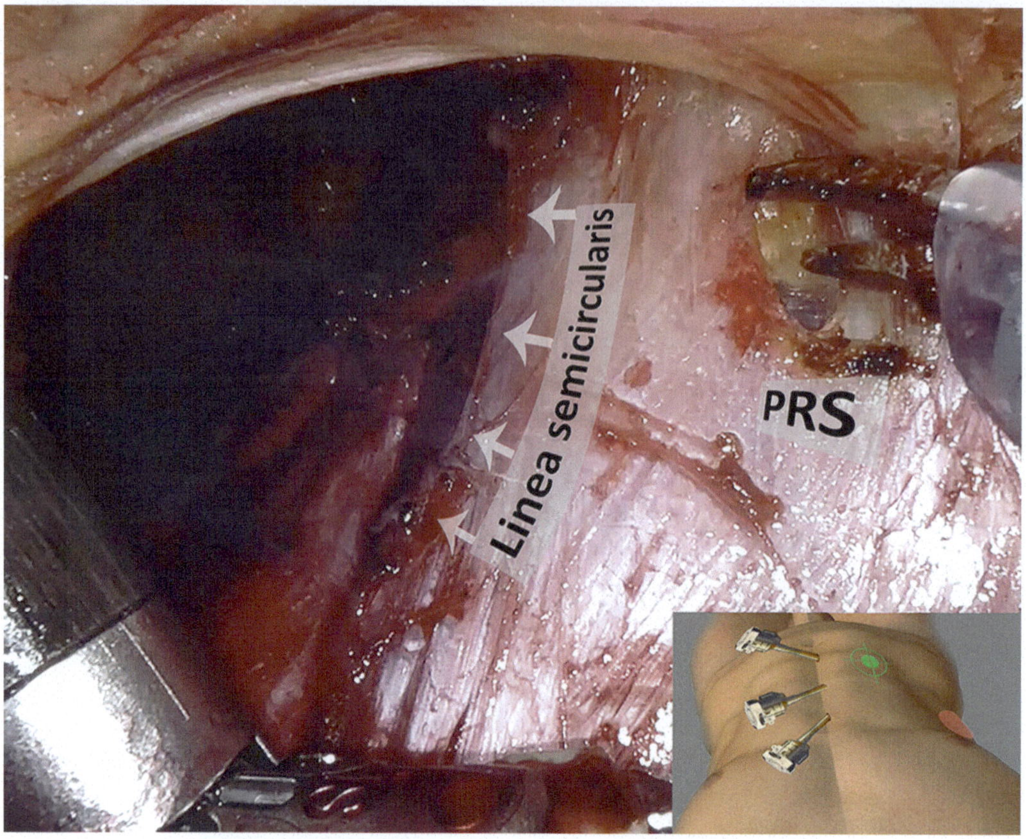


**Fig. 12.5** The dissection of the posterior lamella of the internal oblique muscle at the level of the arcuate line. The posterior lamella of the internal oblique muscle is often tightly connected to the transversus abdominis muscle's aponeurosis. PRS posterior rectus sheath

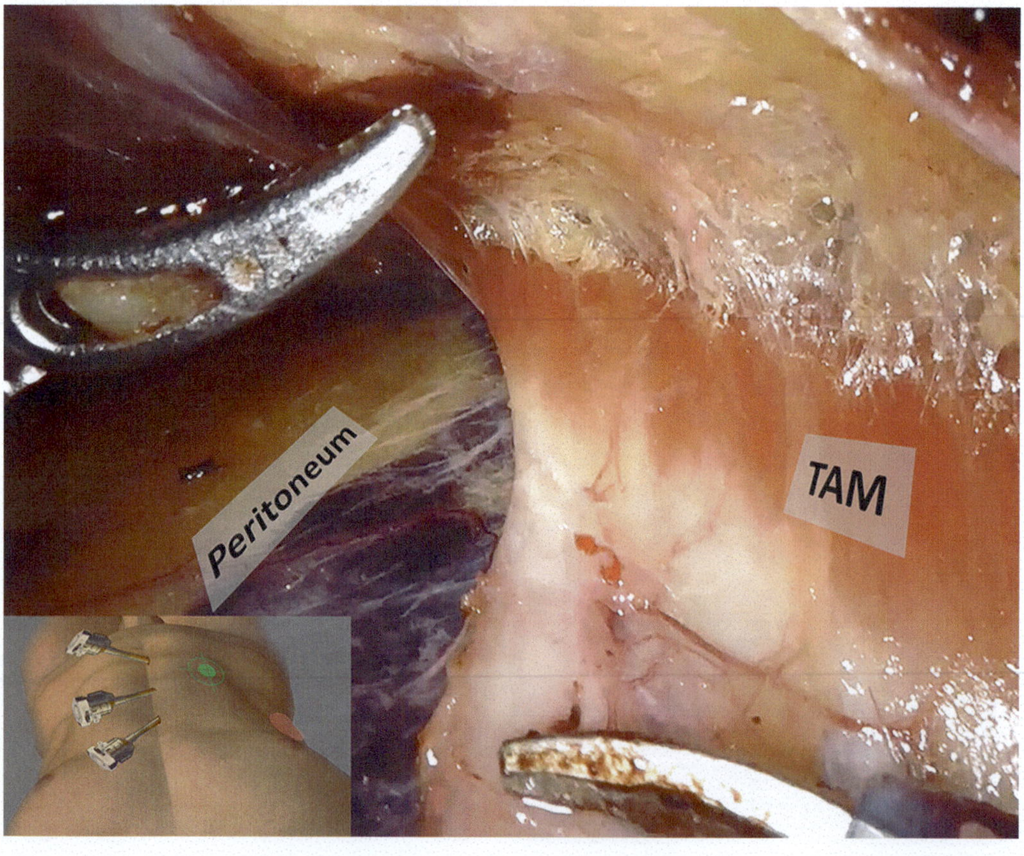


**Fig. 12.6** Exposure of fibers of the transversus abdominis muscle (TAM) at the lateral border of the rectus sheath (linea semilunaris)

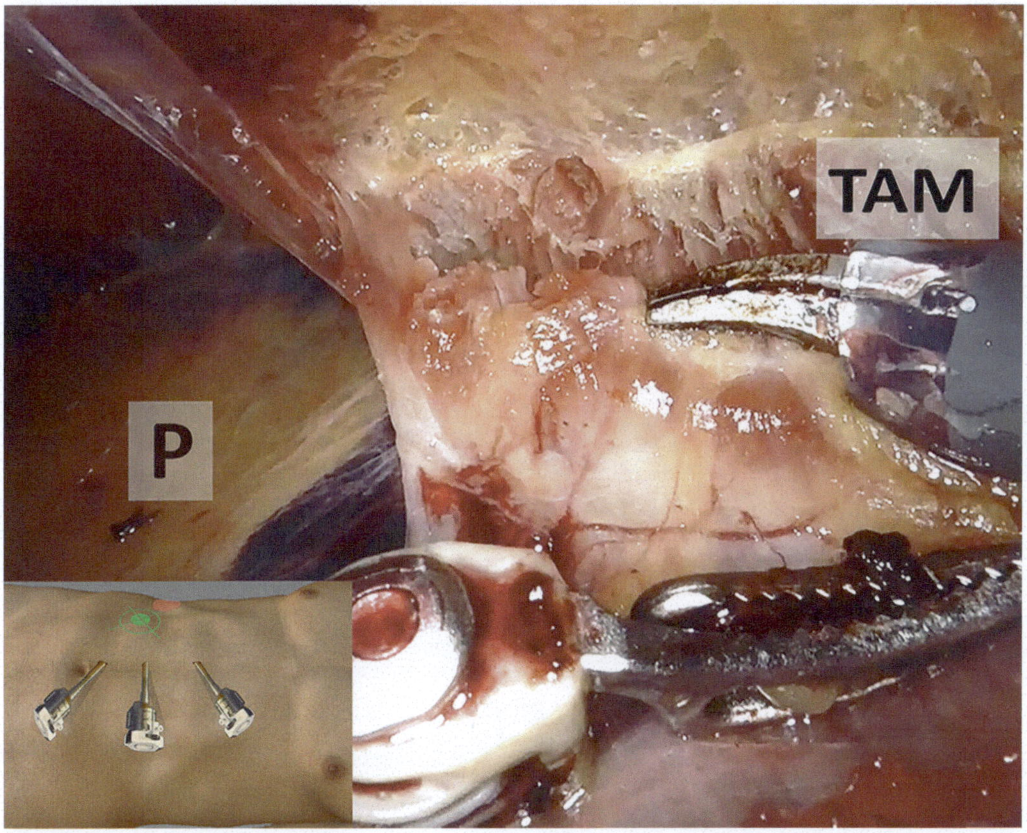


Fig. 12.7 Beginning of the transversus abdominis release (TAR). P peritoneum

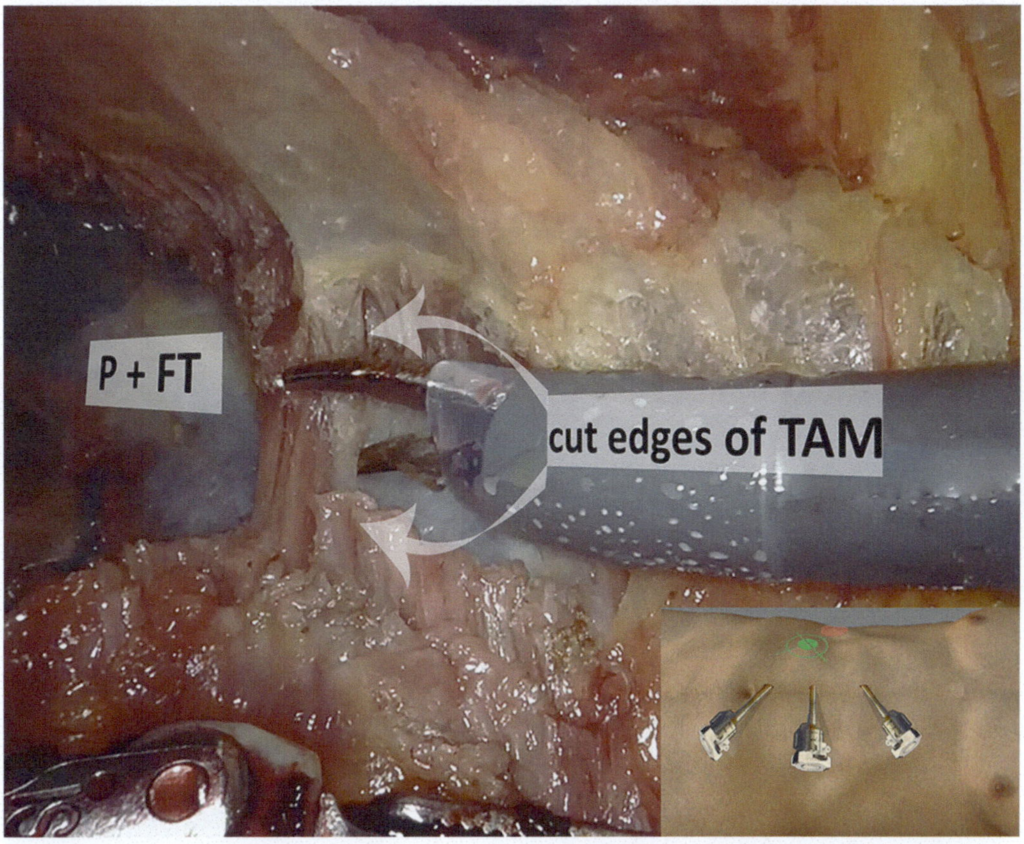


Fig. 12.8 Neurovascular bundles are preserved while performing the TAR. The peritoneum (P) and fascia transversalis (FT) are revealed during TAR

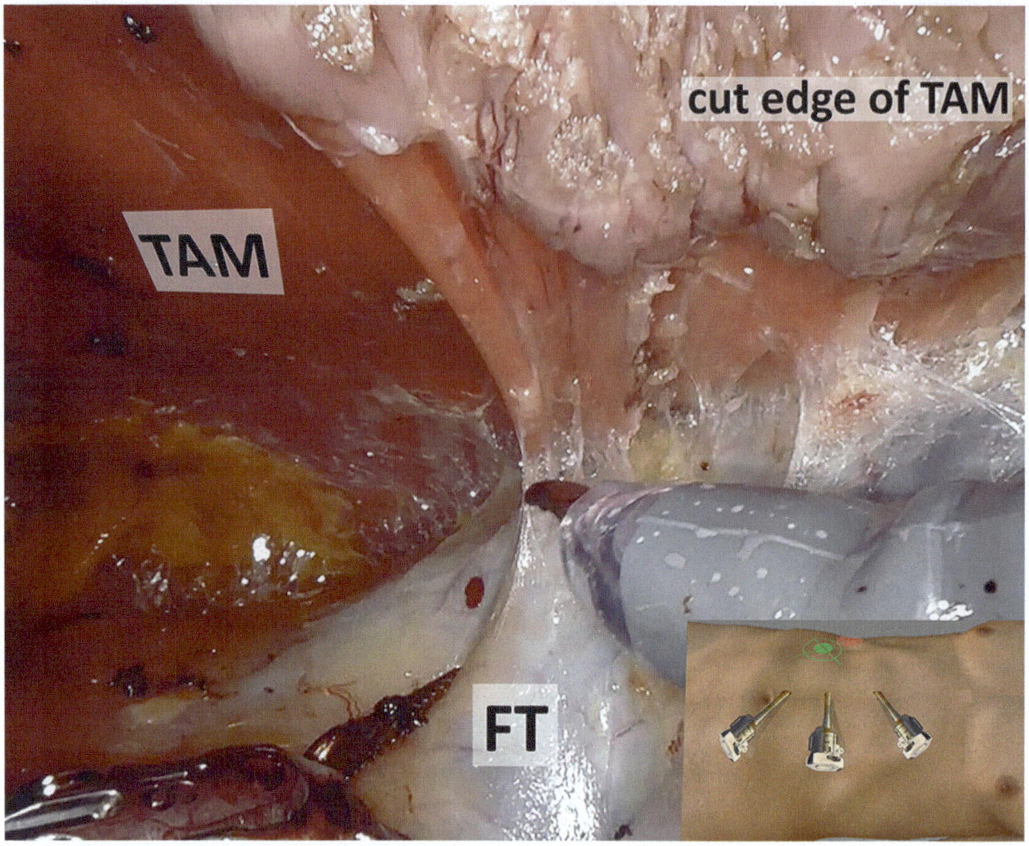


Fig. 12.9 The dissection is continued at the plane between the transversus abdominis muscle (TAM) and its fascia

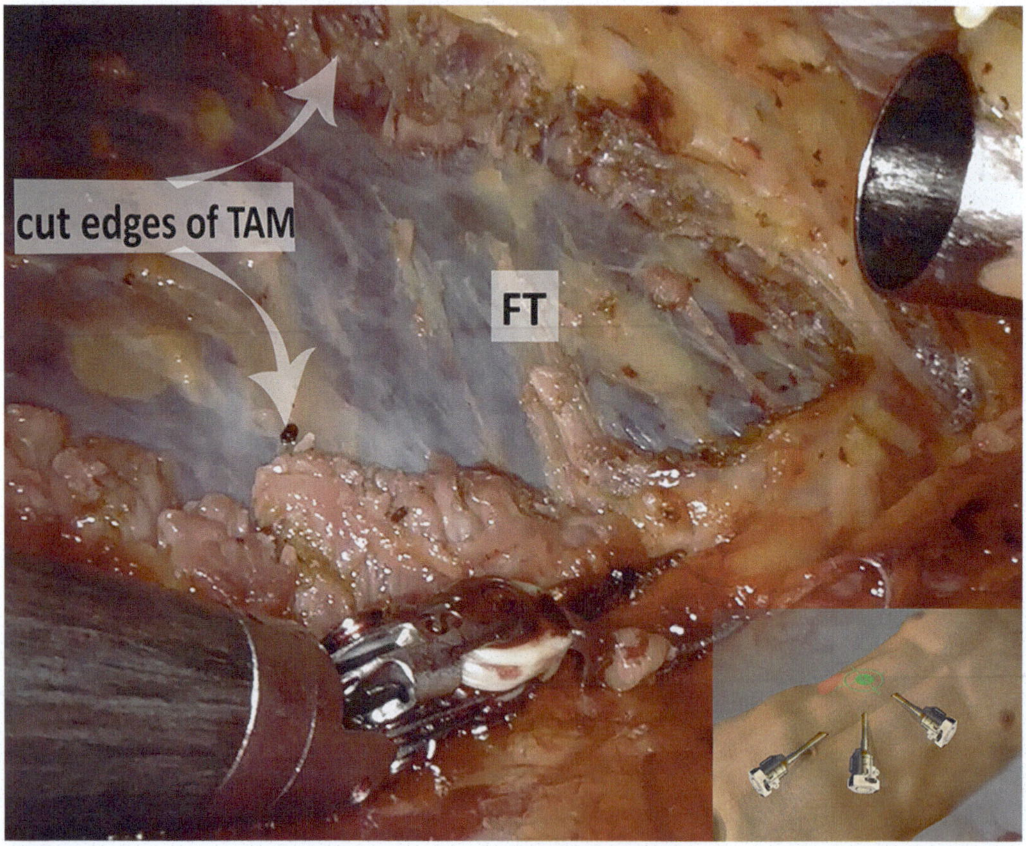


Fig. 12.10 The TAR is carried out up to the level of the rib cage. FT fascia transversalis

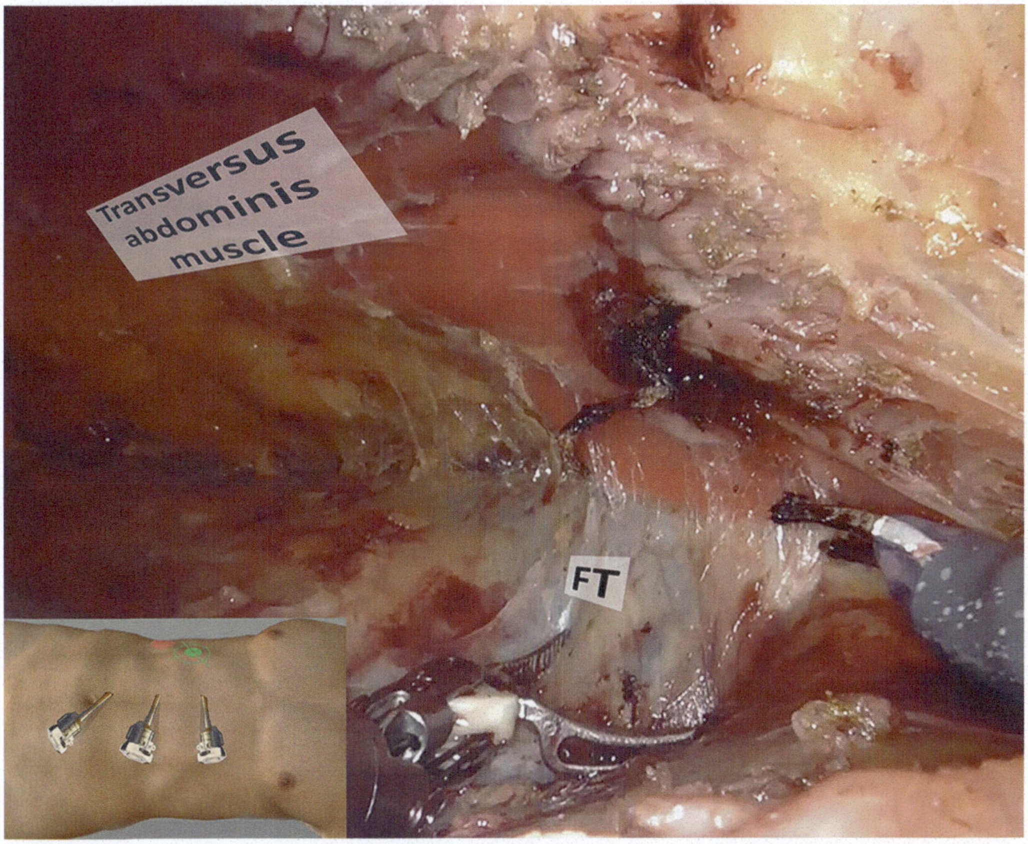


Fig. 12.11 Retromuscular dissection is continued at the level of the rib cage

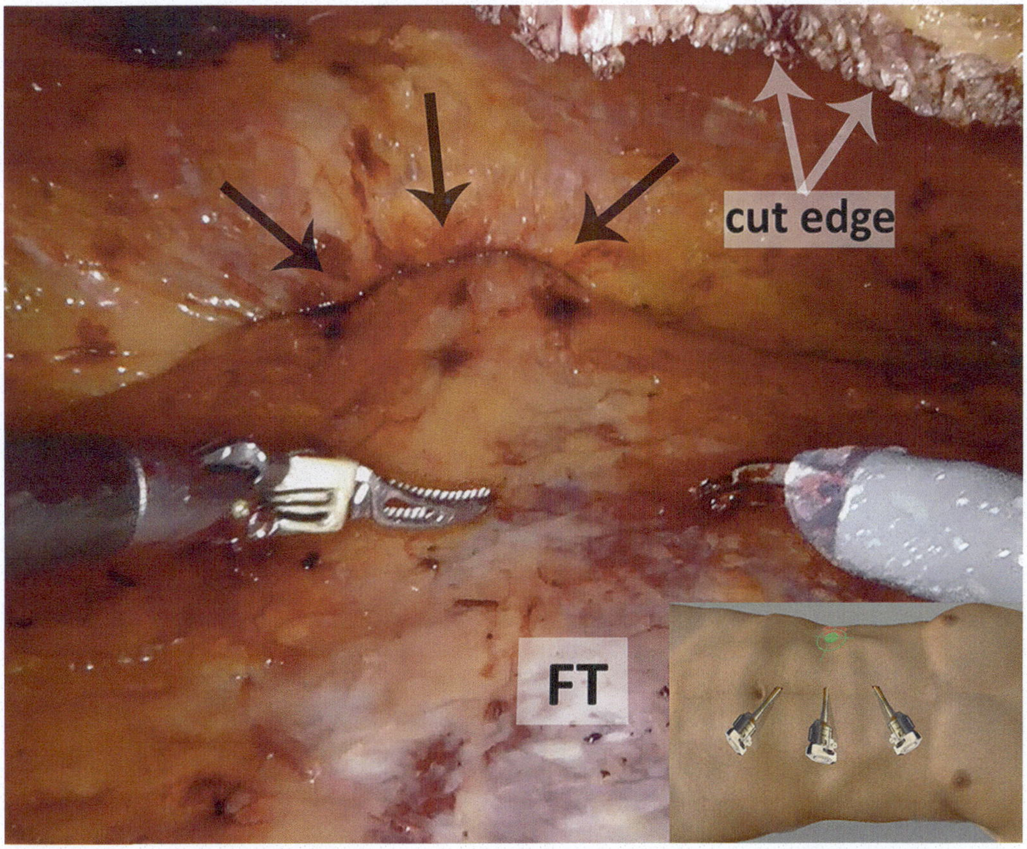


Fig. 12.12 The medial edge of the lumbar hernia (L4) (*black arrows*)

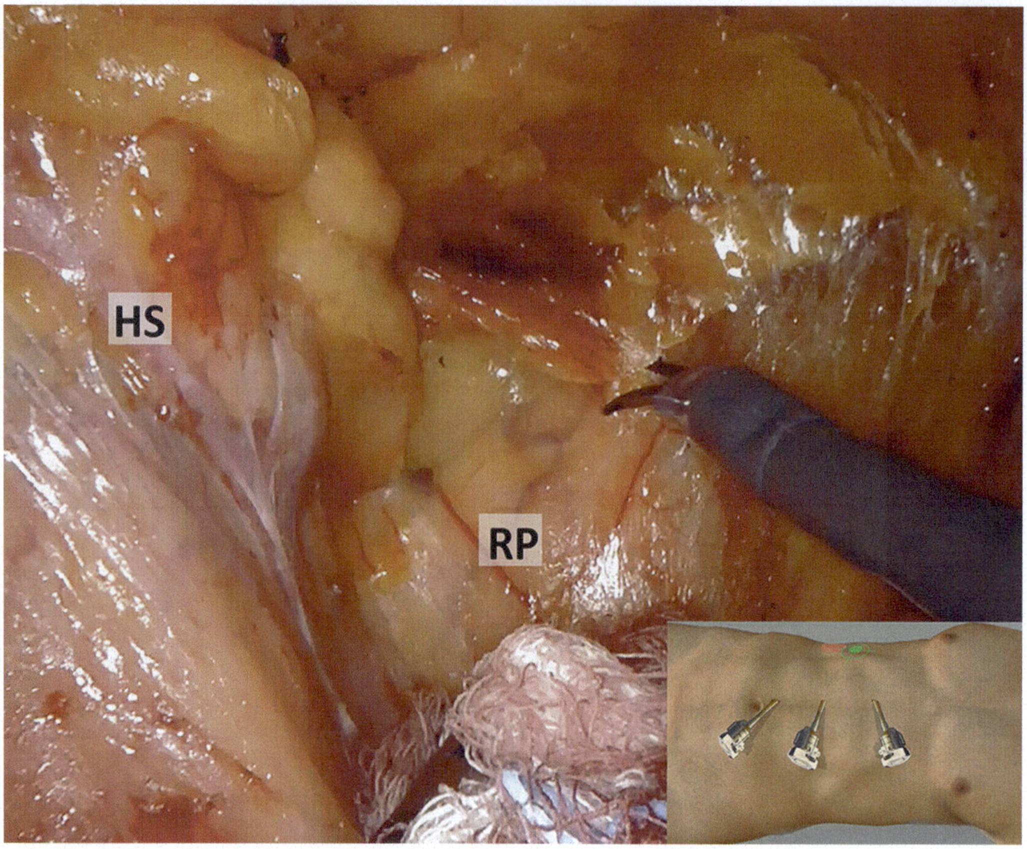


**Fig. 12.13** Extraperitoneal dissection at the level of the mid-axillary line's projection. HS hernia sac, RP retroperitoneum

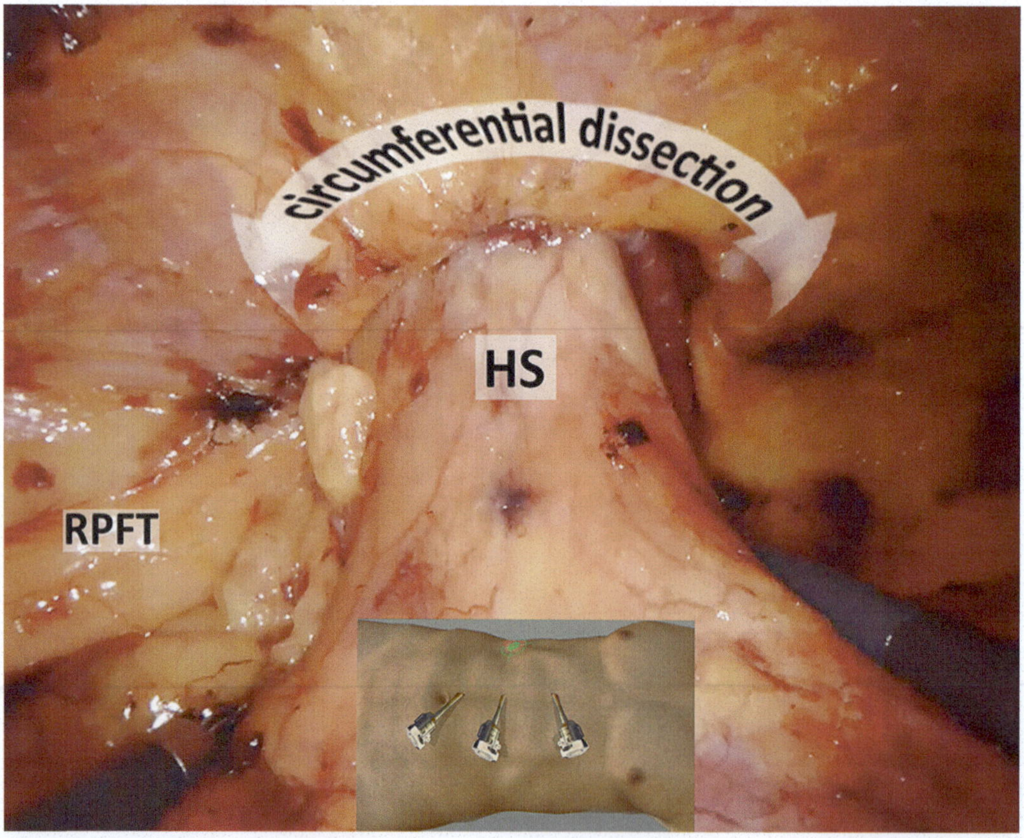


**Fig. 12.14** Circumferential dissection may prevent inadvertent tearing of the hernia sac (HS). RPFT retroperitoneal fatty tissue

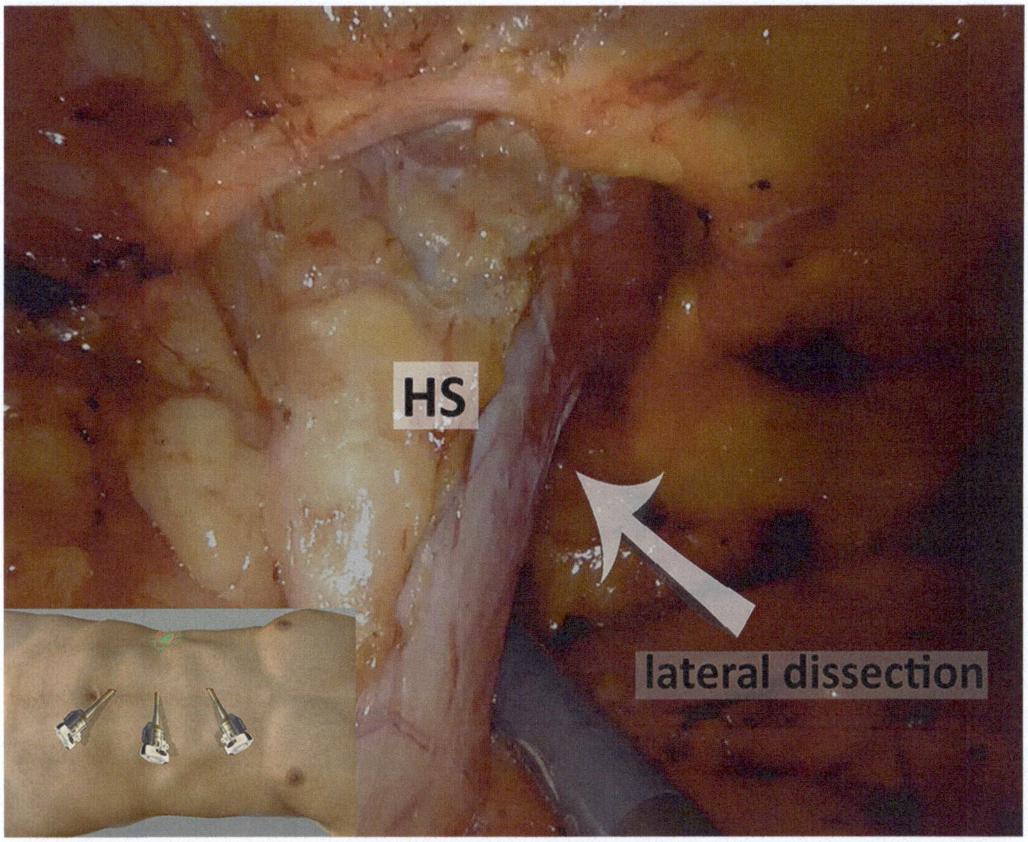


Fig. 12.15 Lateral dissection between the hernia sac (HS) and lateral abdominal wall

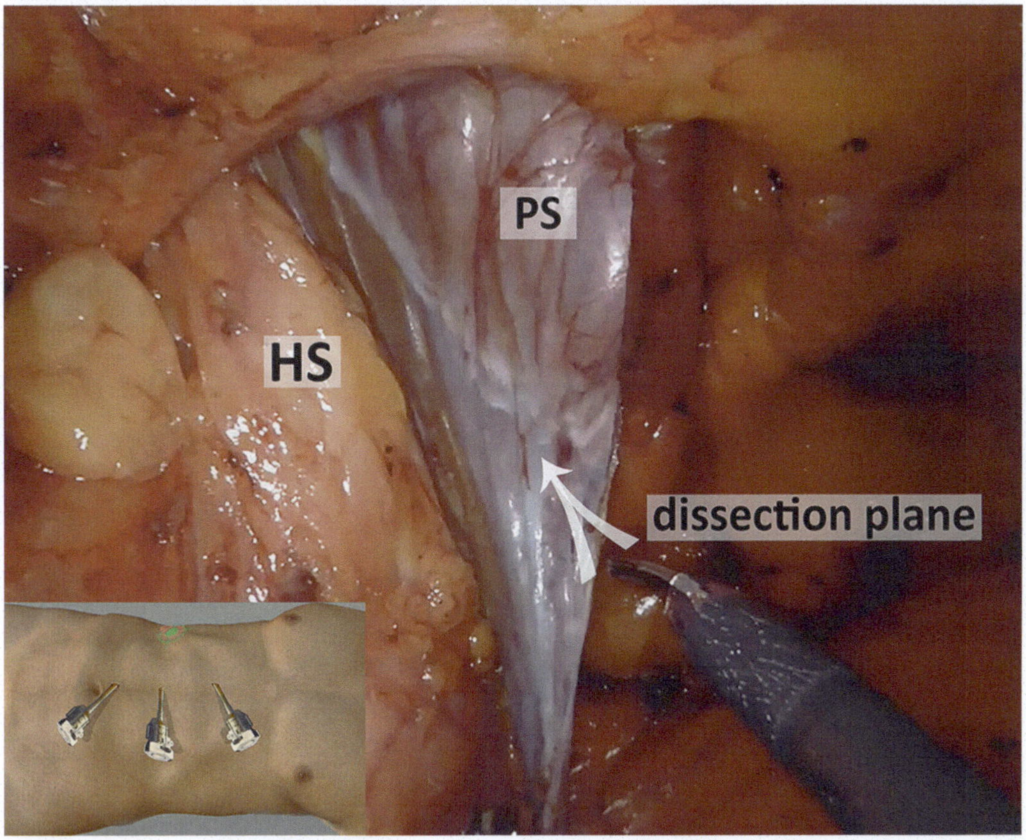


Fig. 12.16 Reducing the hernia sac from cranial to caudal direction. Gentle traction of the hernia sac may facilitate identification of the proper dissection plane between pseudo sac (PS) and hernia sac (HS)

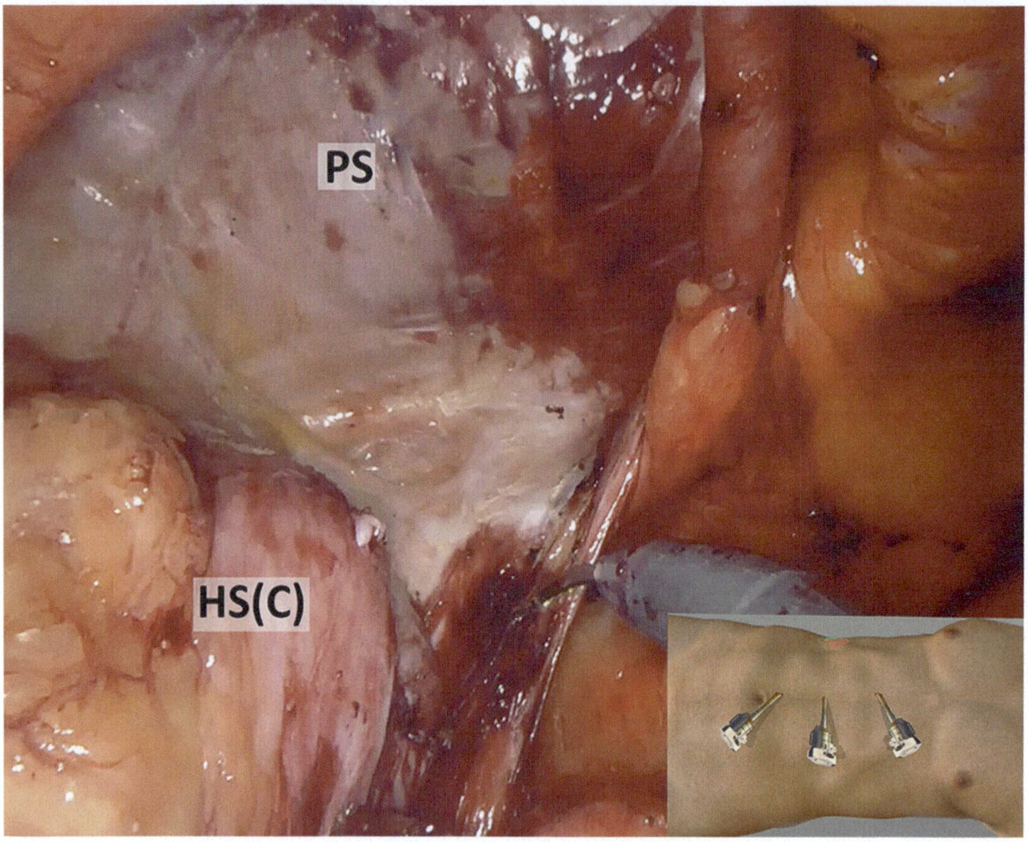


**Fig. 12.17** The dissection of lateral adhesions. HS(C) hernia sac (colon), PS pseudo sac

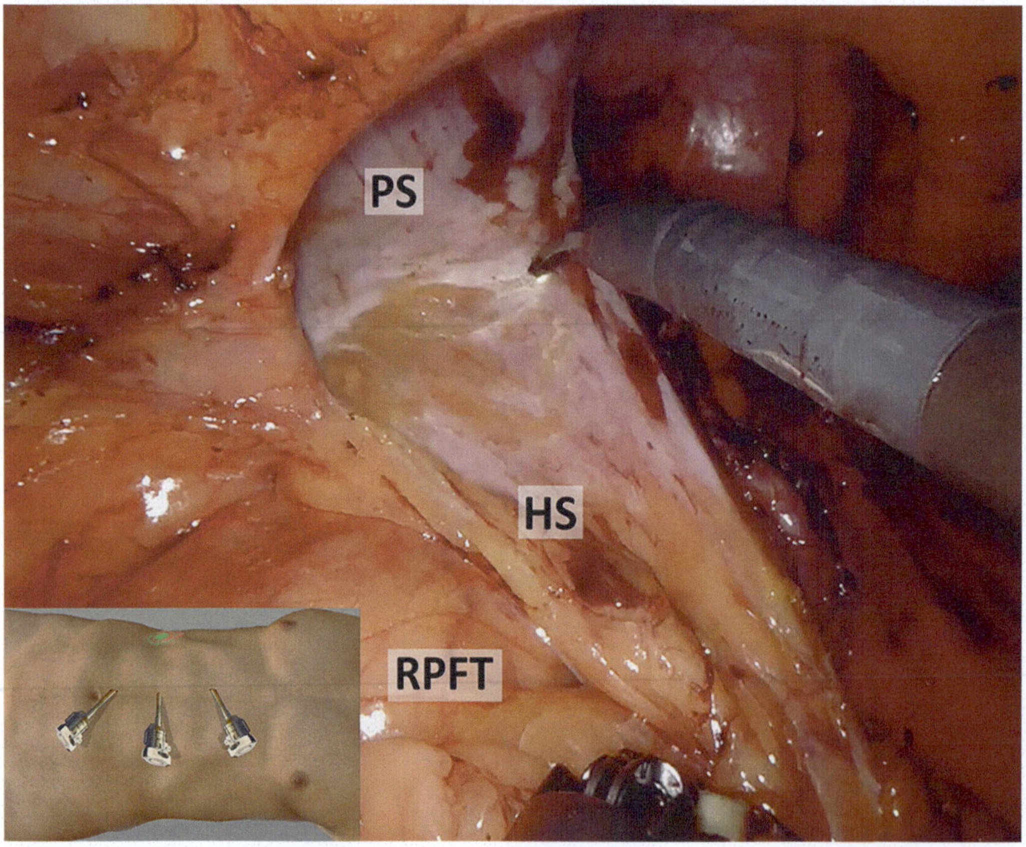


**Fig. 12.18** The dissection of inferior adhesions. RPFT retroperitoneal fatty tissue

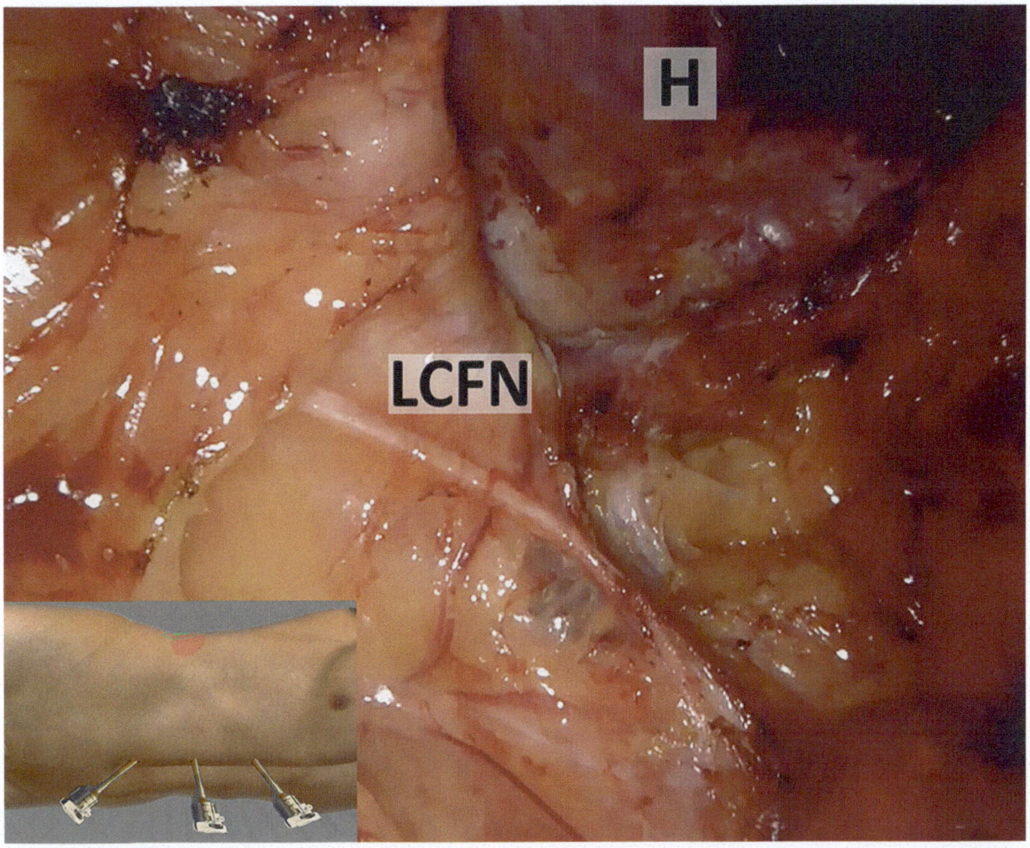


Fig. 12.19 Lateral cutaneous femoral nerve (LCFN) at the inferolateral border of the hernia (H)

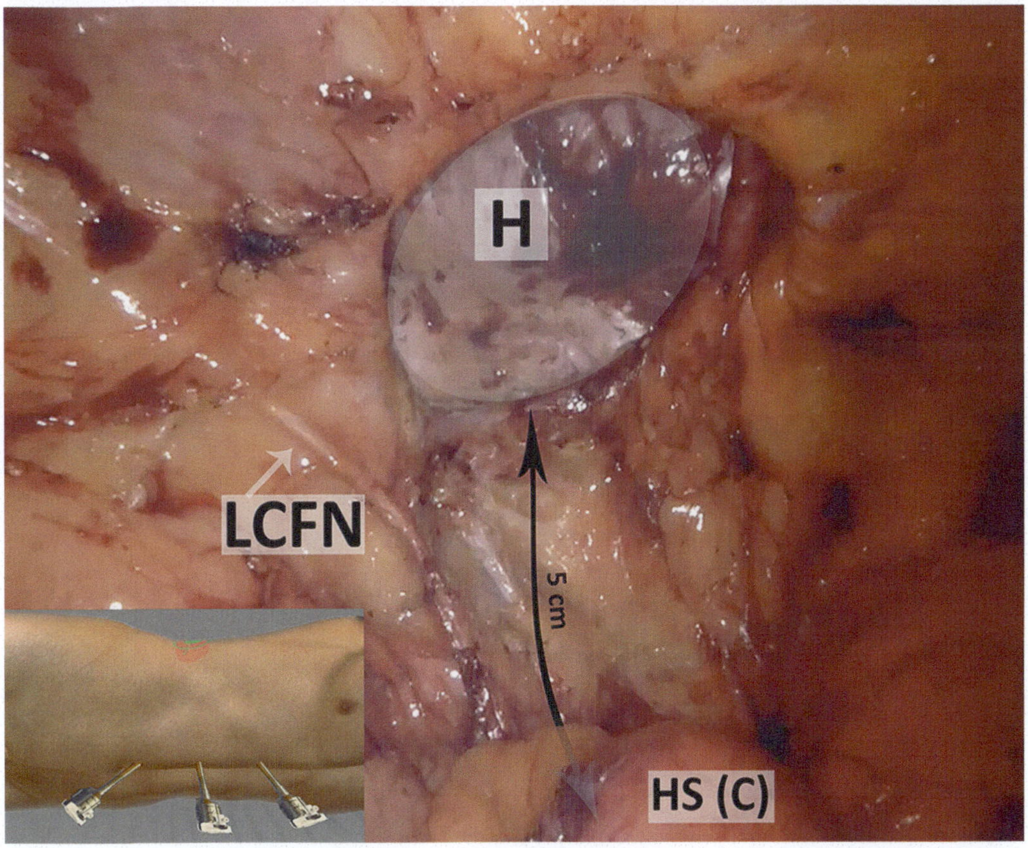


Fig. 12.20 The dissection is continued in the area surrounding the defect at least 5 cm, in order to obtain a proper mesh overlap

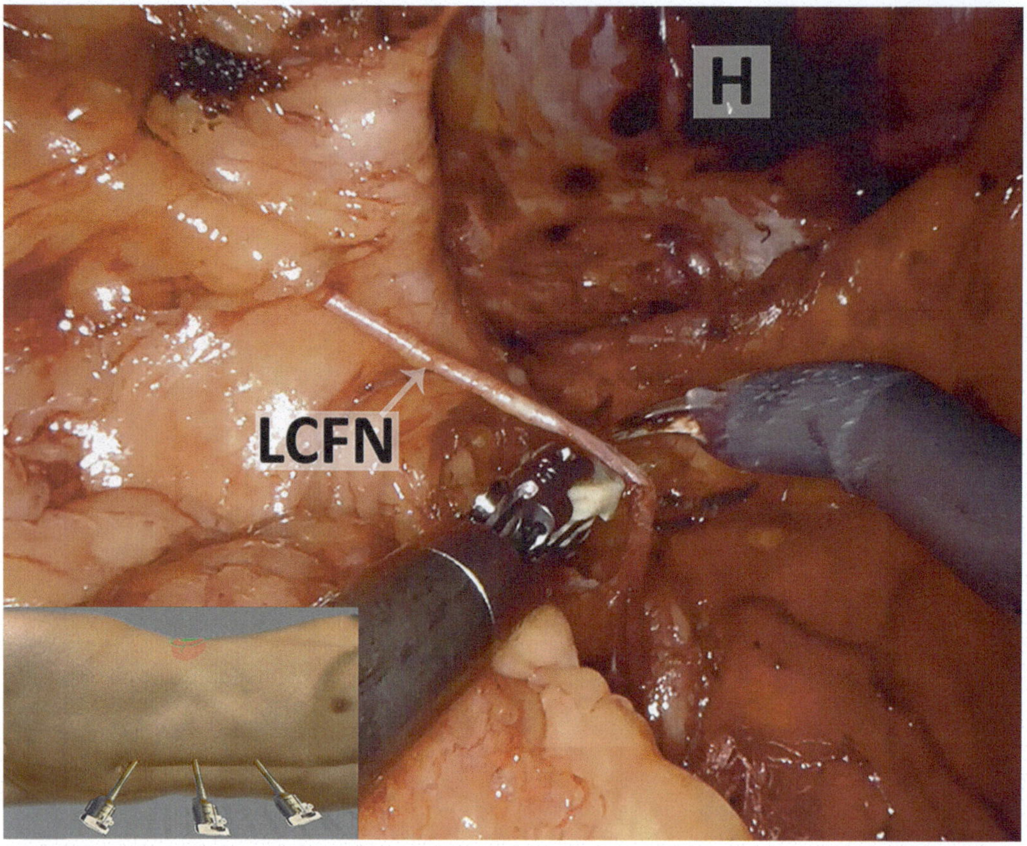


Fig. 12.21 Dividing the lateral cutaneous femoral nerve (LCFN). H hernia

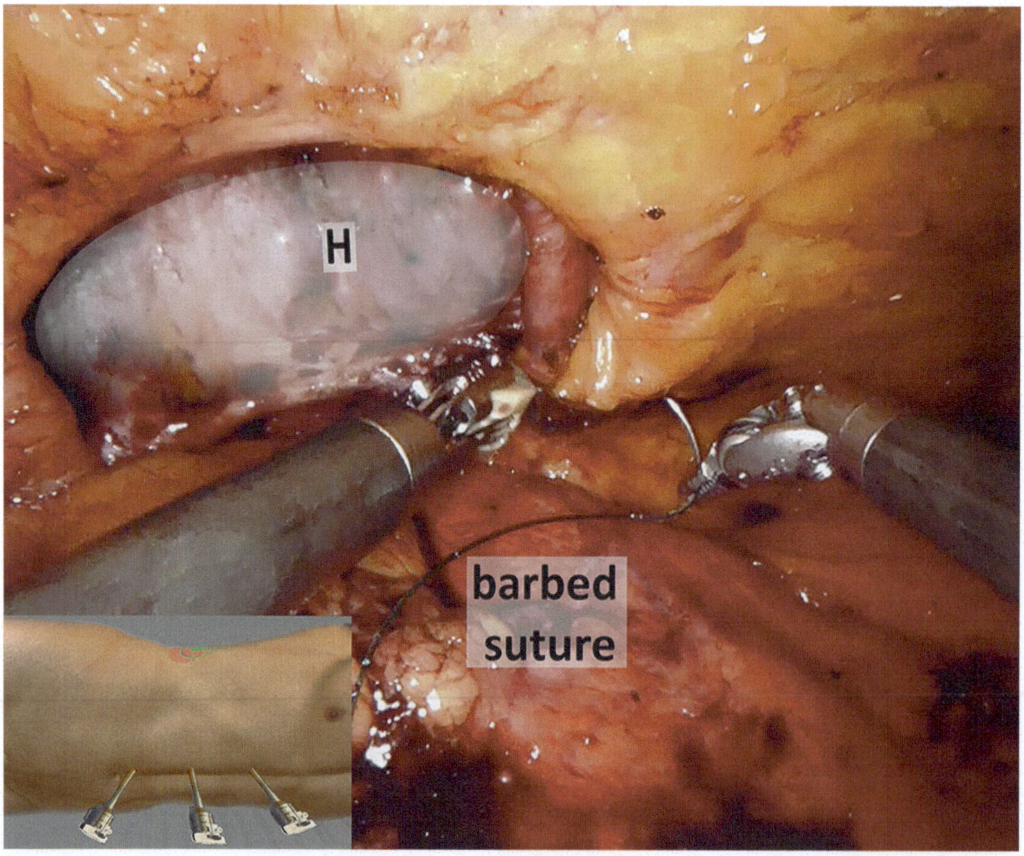


Fig. 12.22 Beginning the defect closure with a barbed suture from the cranial side

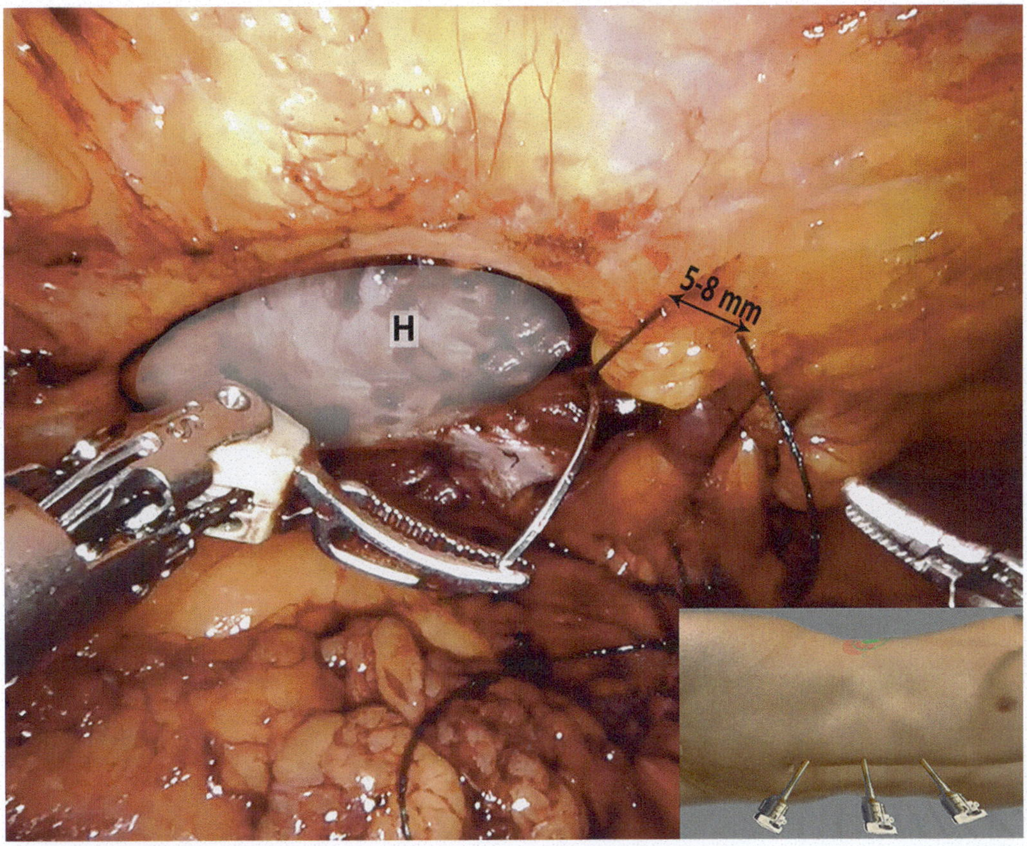


**Fig. 12.23** Small-bite closure technique is used, with a tissue bite 5–8 mm wide

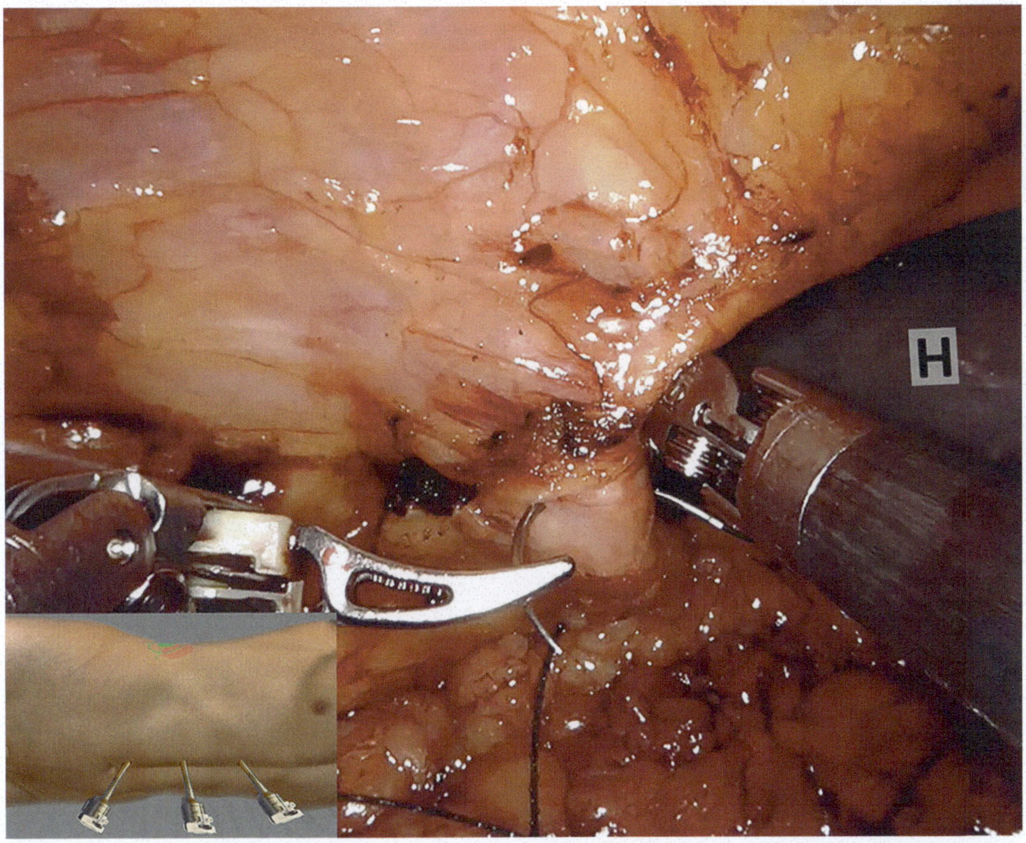


**Fig. 12.24** Closing the defect with another barbed suture, from the caudal side

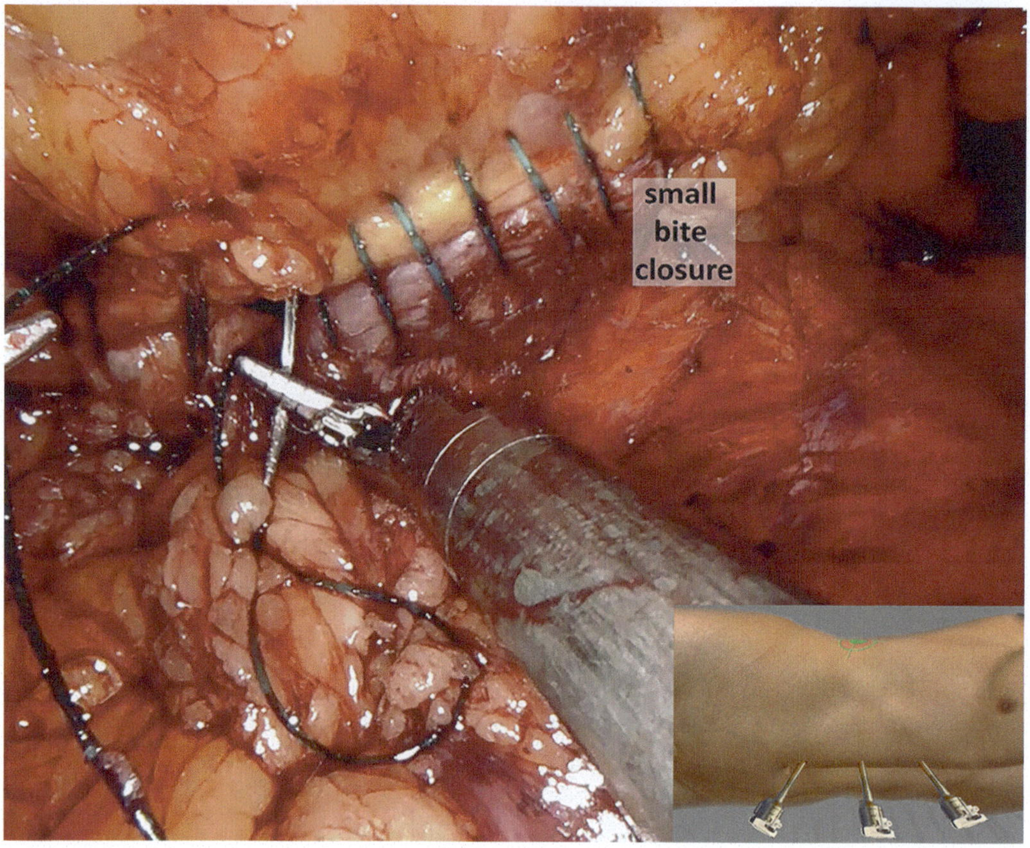


Fig. 12.25 Defect closure is complete when the two separate sutures met at the middle of the defect

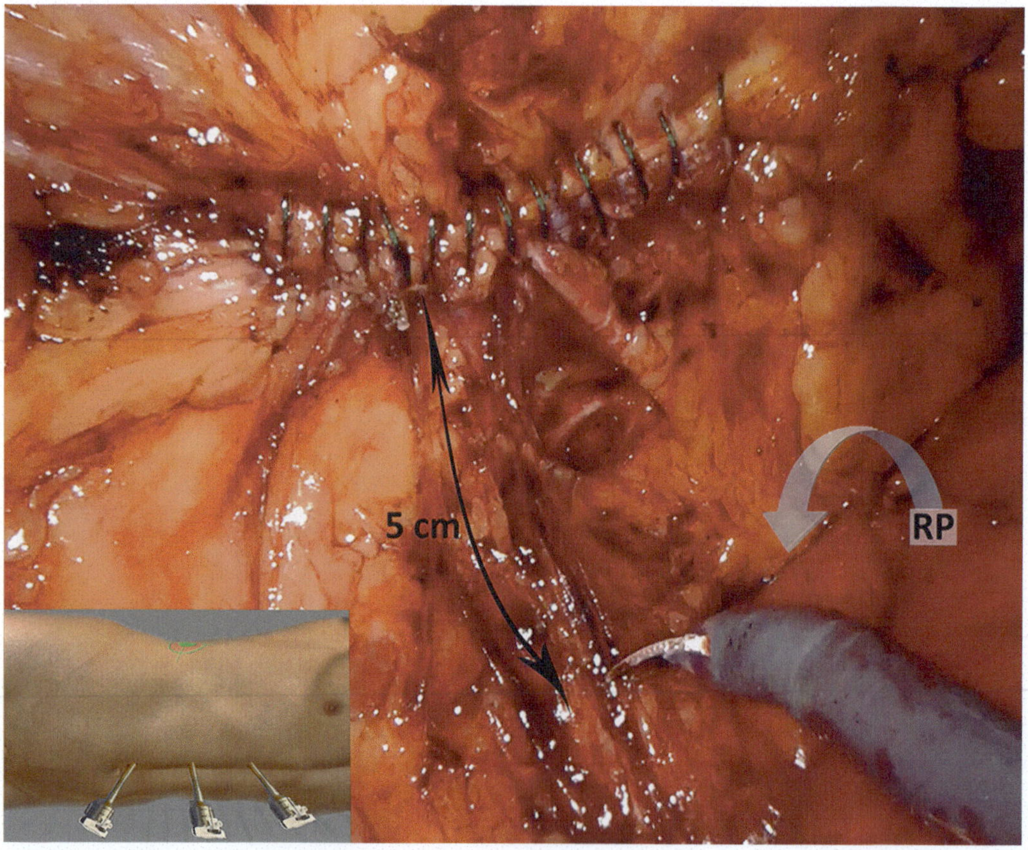


Fig. 12.26 Further dissection of the retroperitoneum (RP) may be needed in the posterolateral part of the abdominal wall

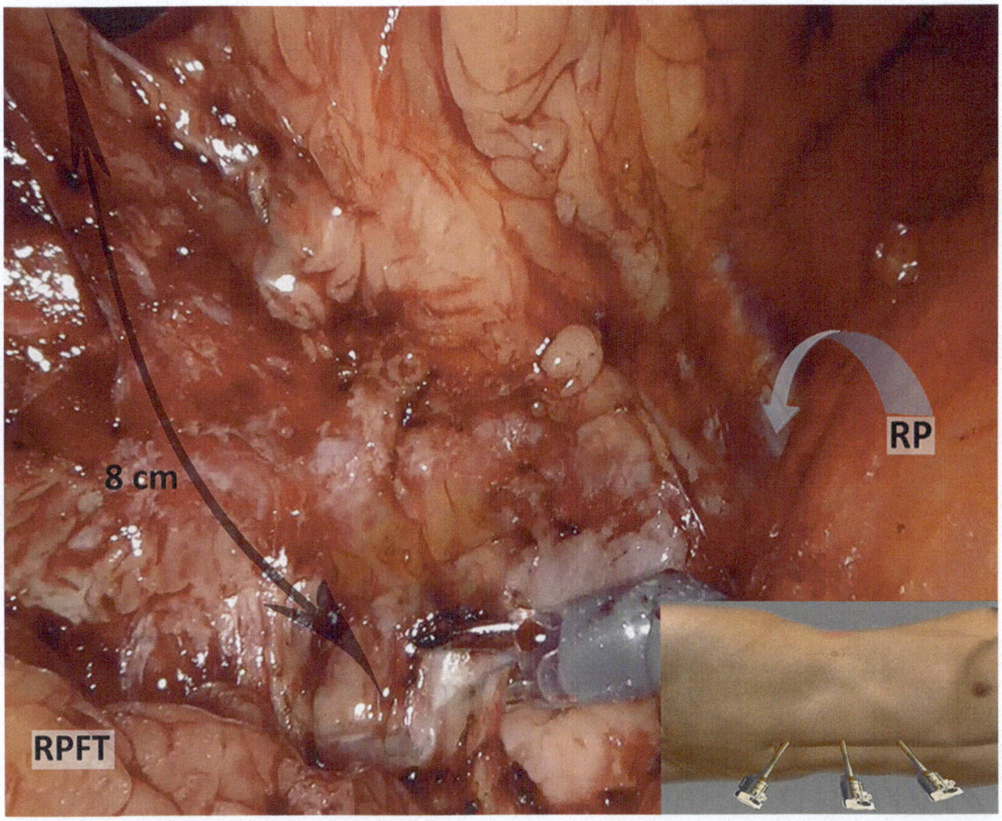


Fig. 12.27 Retroperitoneal or posterolateral dissection is carried out, approximately 8 cm away from lateral edge of the hernia defect, up to medial side of the quadratus lumborum muscle. RPFT retroperitoneal fatty tissue

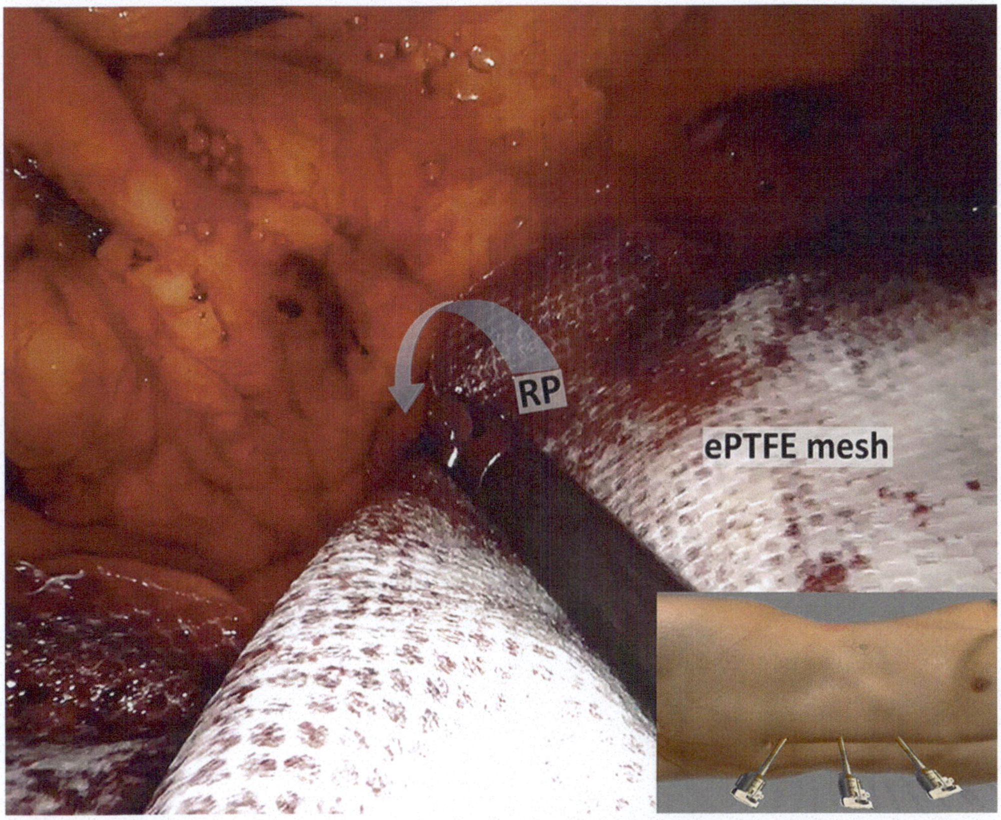


Fig. 12.28 After dissection is completed, expanded polytetrafluoroethylene (ePTFE) mesh 30 × 20 cm in size is inserted into the extraperitoneal space and deployed. RP retroperitoneum

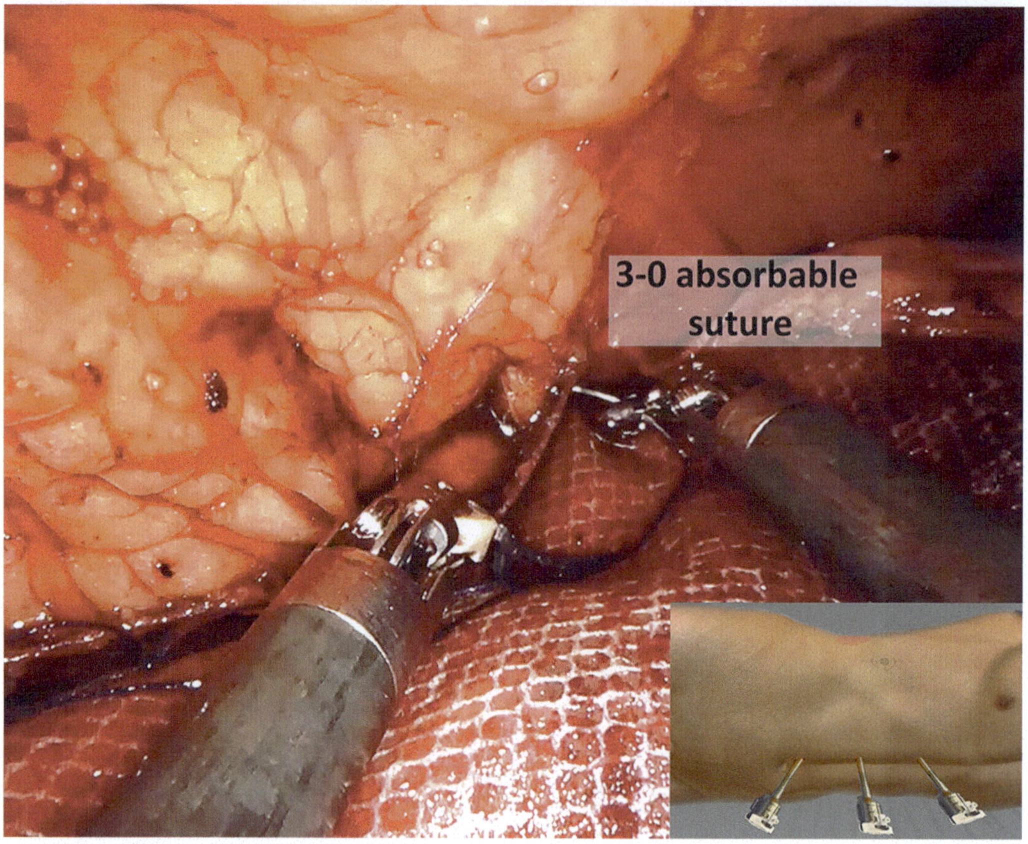


**Fig. 12.29** Mesh fixation with absorbable suture at the cranial side

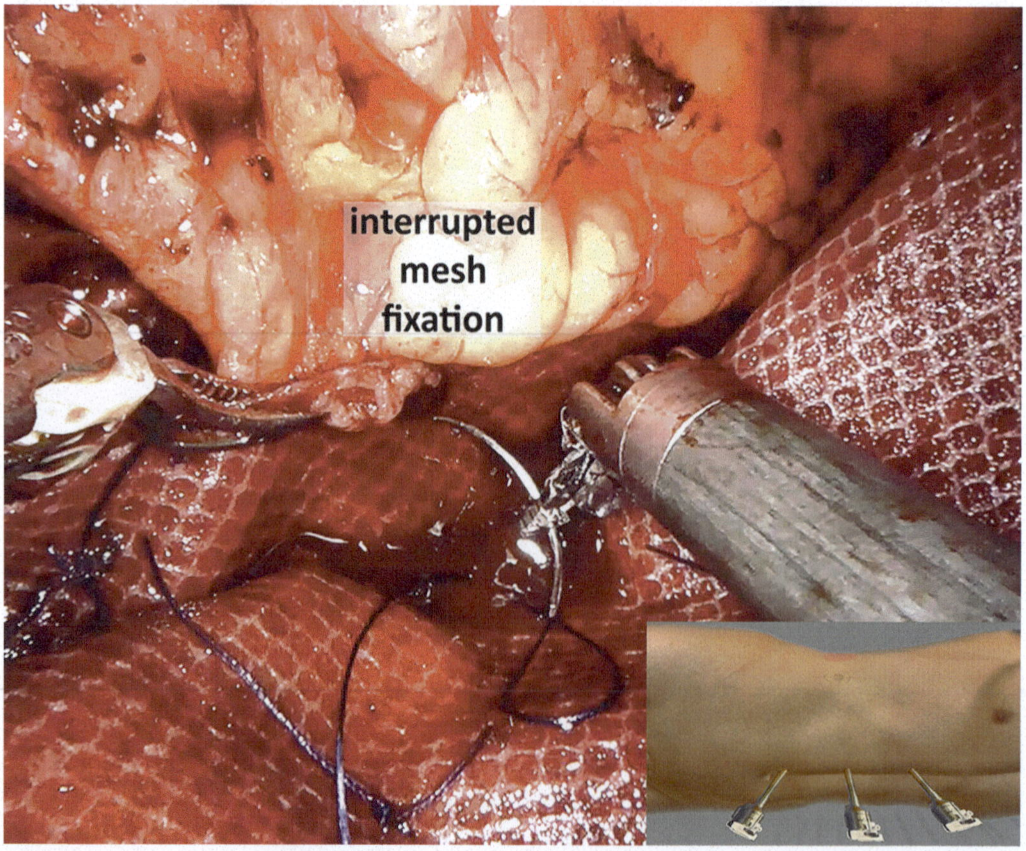


**Fig. 12.30** To prevent mesh migration, the mesh is secured with a couple of interrupted sutures

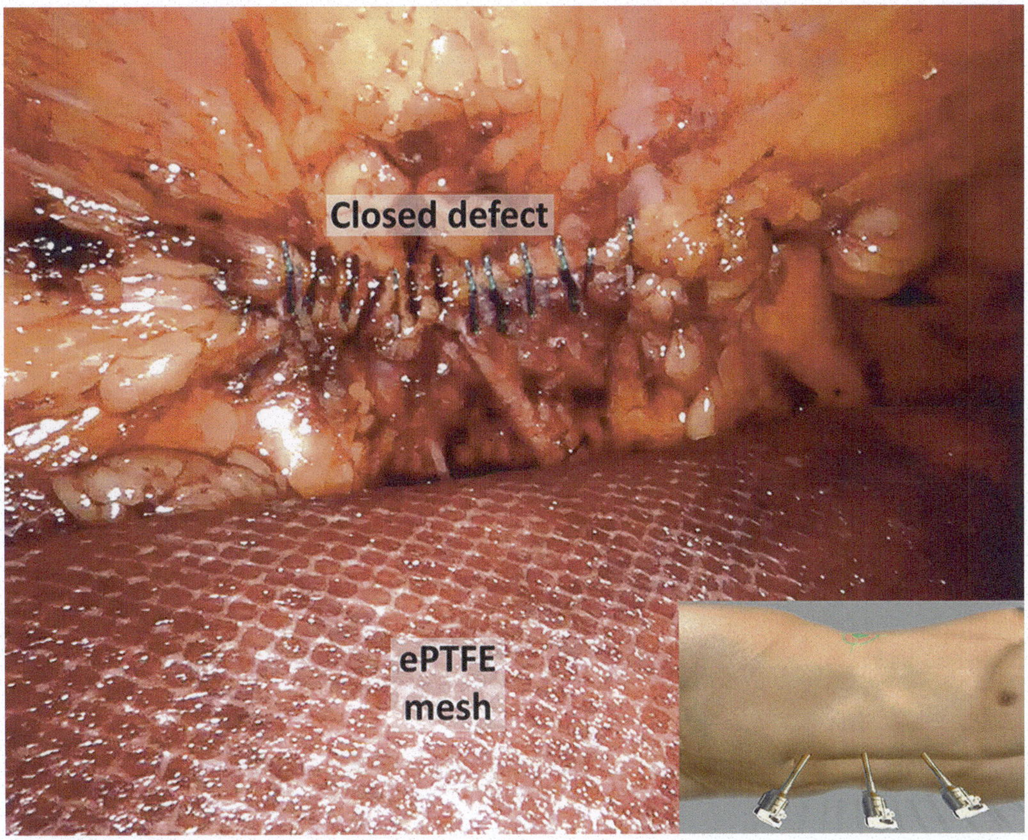


Fig. 12.31 Pneumoperitoneum is released after the mesh deployment

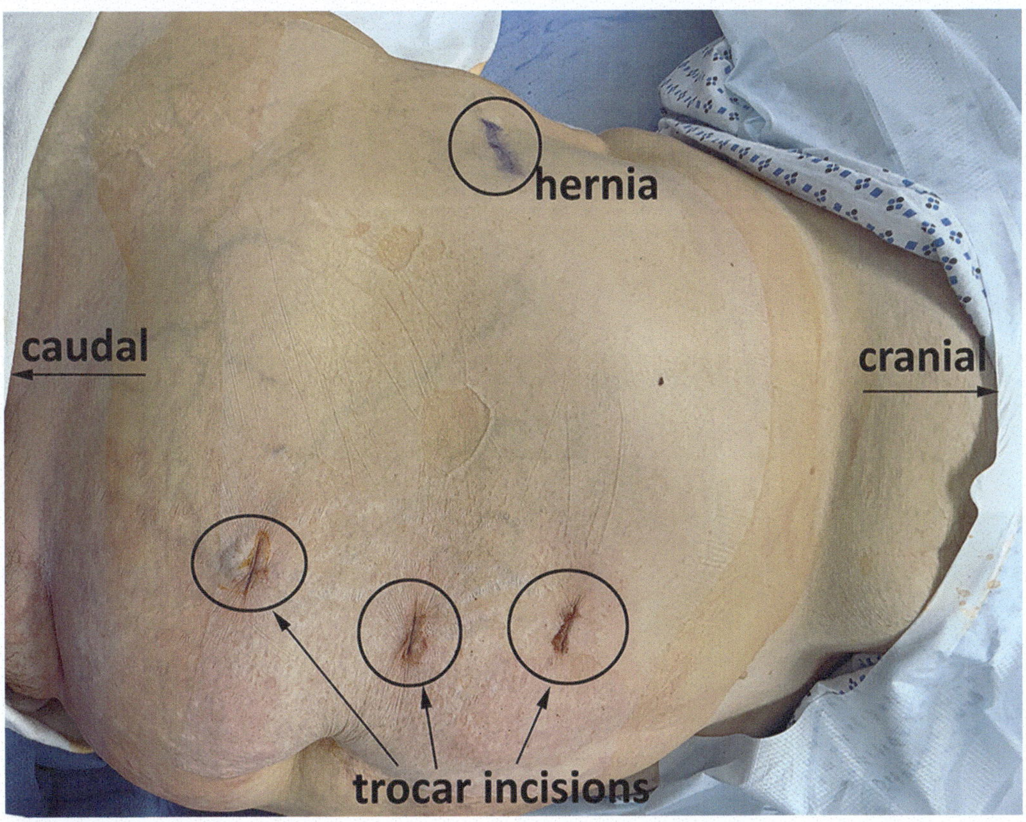


Fig. 12.32 Trocar incisions are closed

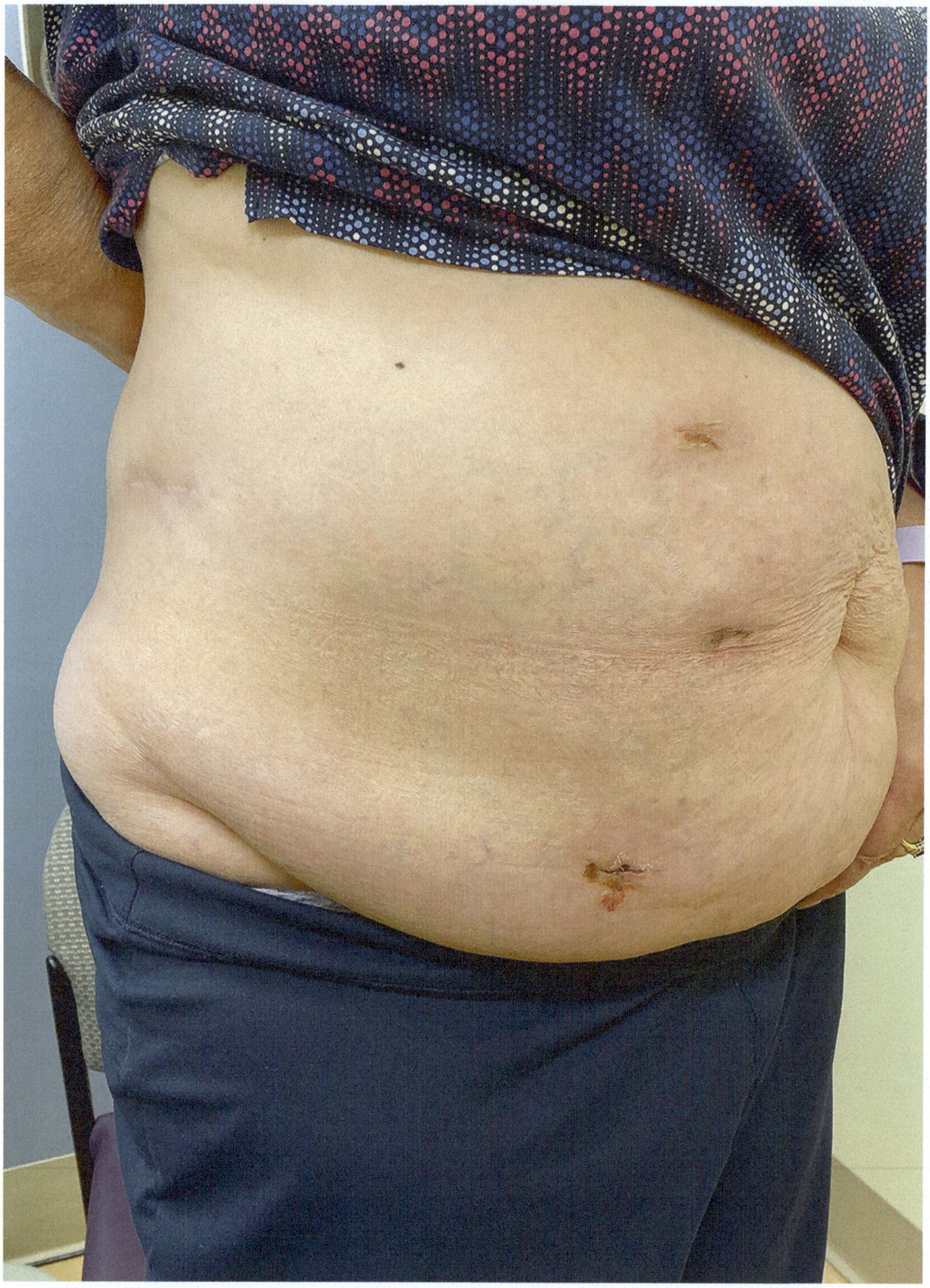

**Fig. 12.33** Follow-up visit at postoperative day 14

## References


1. Zhou DJ, Carlson MA. Incidence, etiology, management, and outcomes of flank hernia: review of published data. Hernia. 2018;22:353–61.
2. Phillips MS, Krpata DM, Blatnik JA, Rosen MJ. Retromuscular preperitoneal repair of flank hernias. J Gastrointest Surg. 2012;16:1548–53.
3. Moreno-Egea A, Torralba-Martinez JA, Morales G, Fernandez T, Girela E, Aguayo-Albasini JL. Open vs laparoscopic repair of secondary lumbar hernias: a prospective nonrandomized study. Surg Endosc. 2005;19:184–7.
4. Muysoms FE, Miserez M, Berrevoet F, Campanelli G, Champault GG, Chelala E, et al. Classification of primary and incisional abdominal wall hernias. Hernia. 2009;13:407–14.

# Robotic Iliac Hernia Repair: Totally Extraperitoneal (TEP)

13

Hakan Seyit and Omar Yusef Kudsi

## Introduction

Iliac hernias have been defined by the European Hernia Society (EHS) as those falling between a horizontal line 3 cm below the umbilicus and the inguinal region [1]. These incisional hernias are much less common than midline hernias; they often occur at colostomy sites. Challenges faced by surgeons when addressing iliac hernia repair include the scarcity of aponeurotic tissue in the lateral abdominal wall and the proximity to the iliac crest, which creates difficulty in obtaining adequate mesh overlap and increases risk of injury to nearby neurovascular structures.

Robotic repair of a lateral incisional hernia (LIH) may address these challenges effectively. Using a retromuscular approach with totally extraperitoneal access (RM-TEP), surgeons are able to create a large retrorectus space in which to work. Because these hernias lie beyond the linea semilunaris, transversus abdominis release (TAR) is then performed through careful dissection, with attention to nearby sensitive structures. After extension of the dissection laterally, surgeons can close any hernia defect and reinforce the area with mesh. Working in such a restricted area requires precise dissection and manipulation of tissues. This is where the robot may excel. It has been shown to achieve favorable postoperative morbidity and hospital length of stay (LOS) in TAR procedures for ventral hernias [2–4].

## Procedure: Illustrated Steps

Figures 13.1, 13.2, 13.3, 13.4, 13.5, 13.6, 13.7, 13.8, 13.9, 13.10, 13.11, 13.12, 13.13, 13.14, 13.15, 13.16, 13.17, 13.18, 13.19, 13.20, 13.21, 13.22, 13.23, 13.24, 13.25, and 13.26 illustrate the technical aspects of robotic totally extraperitoneal retromuscular repair with transversus abdominis release (TEP-TAR) of an iliac hernia.

H. Seyit
Department of Surgery, University of Health Sciences, Bakirkoy Dr. Sadi Konuk Training and Research Hospital, Bakirkoy, Istanbul, Turkey

O. Y. Kudsi (✉)
Department of Surgery, Good Samaritan Medical Center, Tufts University School of Medicine, Boston, MA, USA


O. Y. Kudsi (ed.), *Robotic Hernia Surgery*, https://doi.org/10.1007/978-3-030-46667-1_13

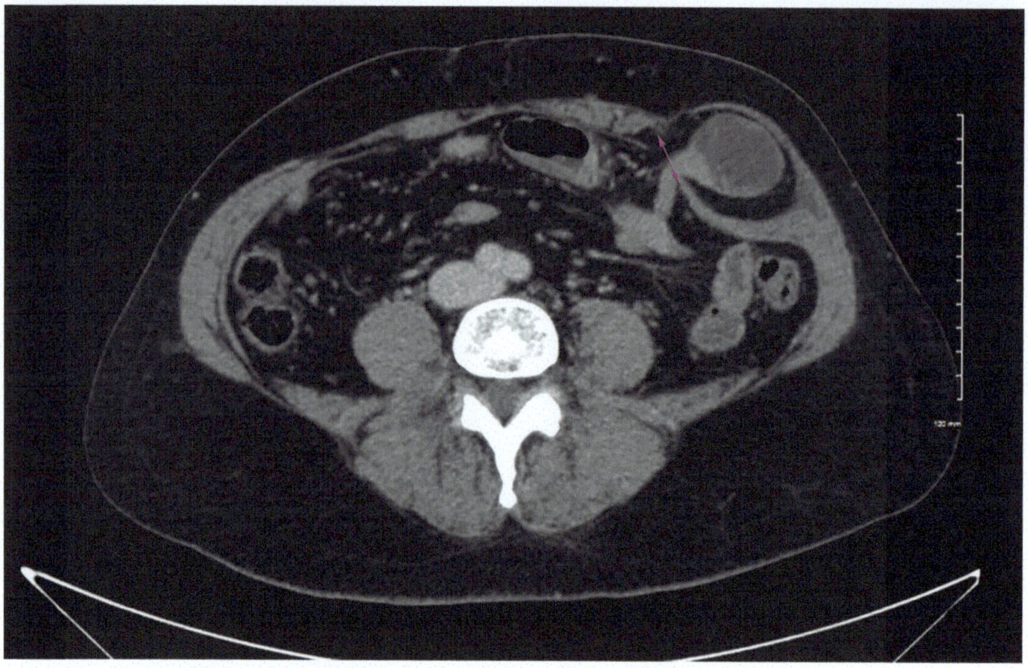

**Fig. 13.1** CT scan (transverse) showing the left-sided iliac hernia. The *arrow* points towards the hernia neck

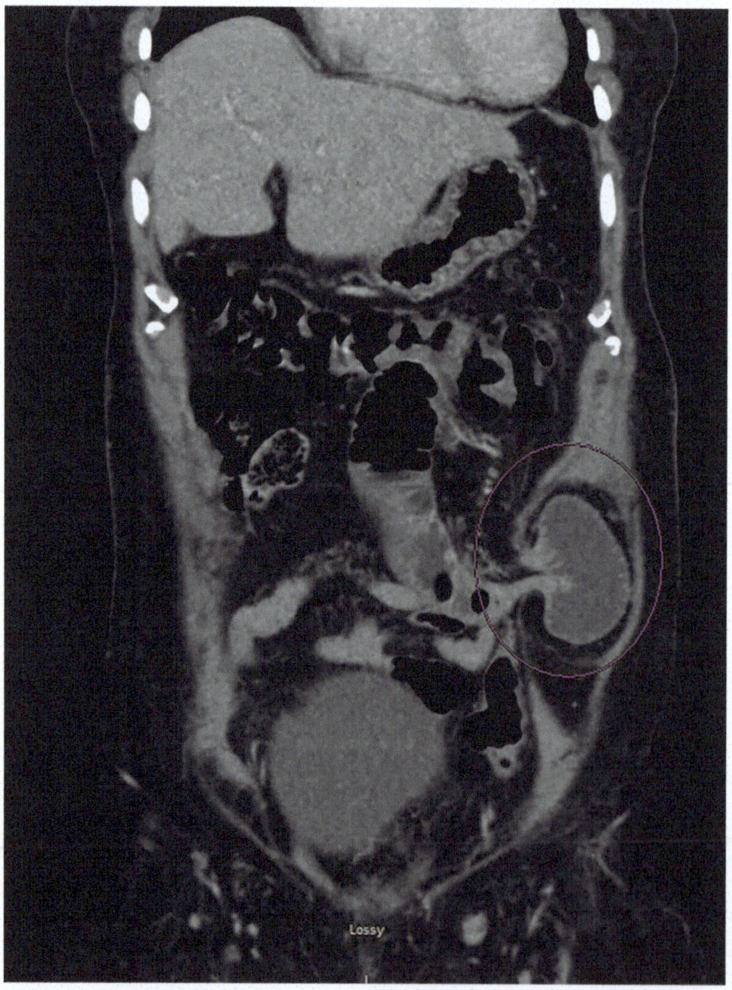


**Fig. 13.2** CT scan (coronal) showing the left-sided iliac hernia

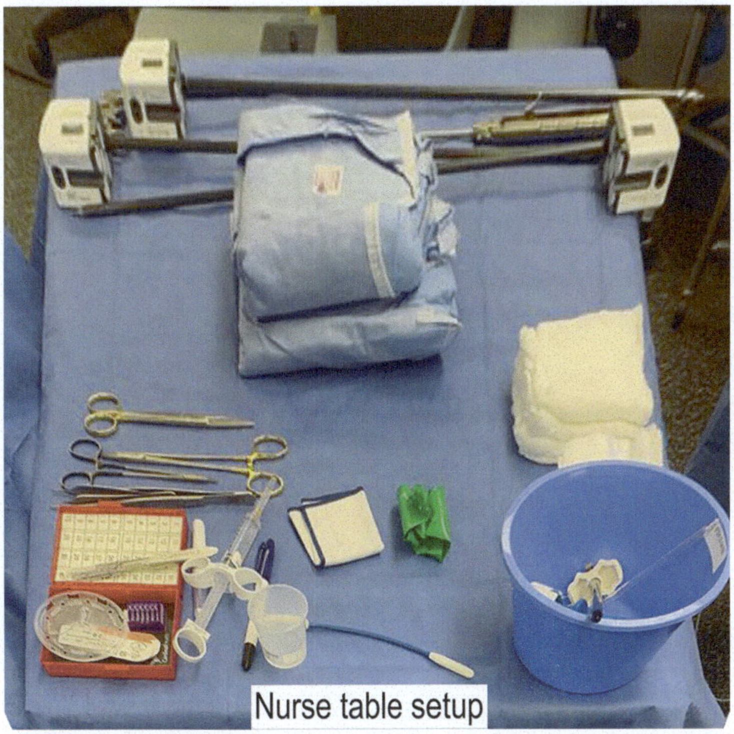


**Fig. 13.3** Scrub nurse table setup

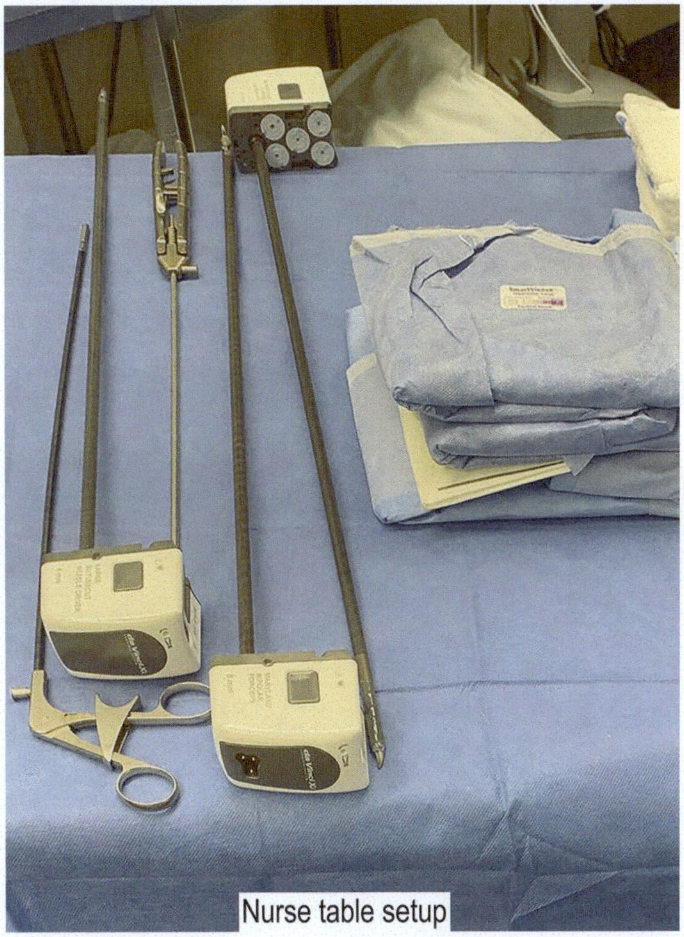


**Fig. 13.4** A total of three robotic instruments are sufficient for this operation: monopolar scissors, bipolar fenestrated forceps, and needle driver. A laparoscopic grasper and needle driver are used to transfer material into the surgical workspace

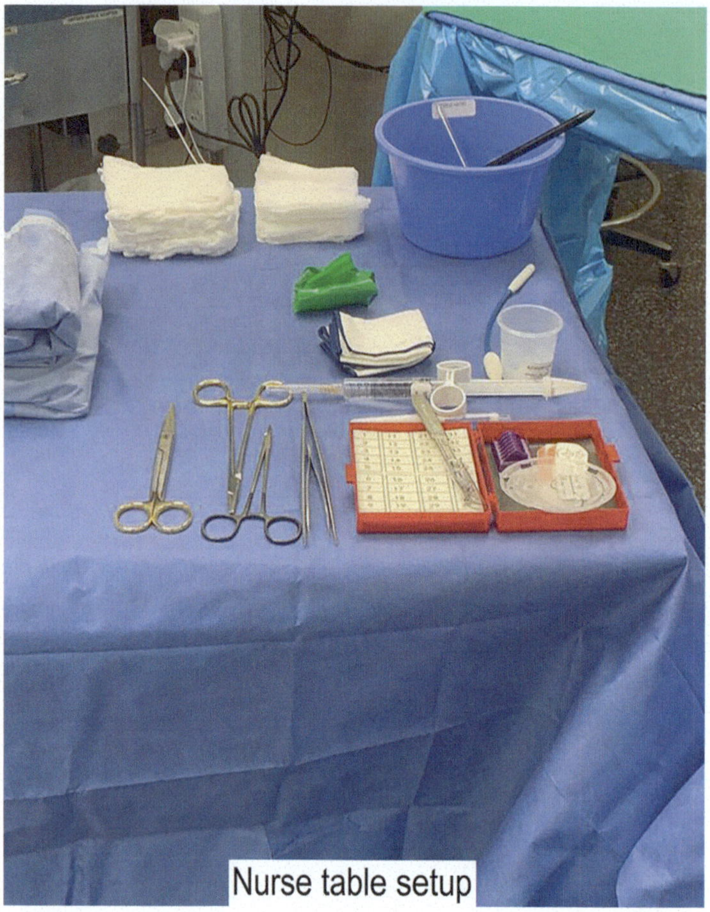


Fig. 13.5 Other surgical tools used outside of the robotic operative steps are shown

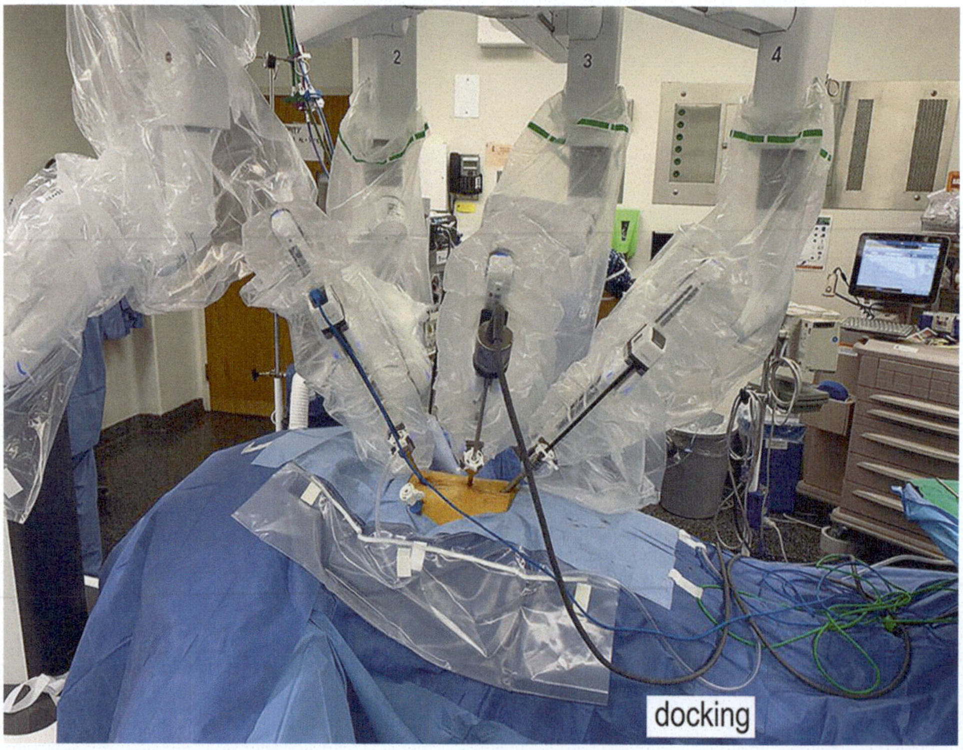


Fig. 13.6 After totally extraperitoneal (TEP) access, the patient-side cart of the robot is docked

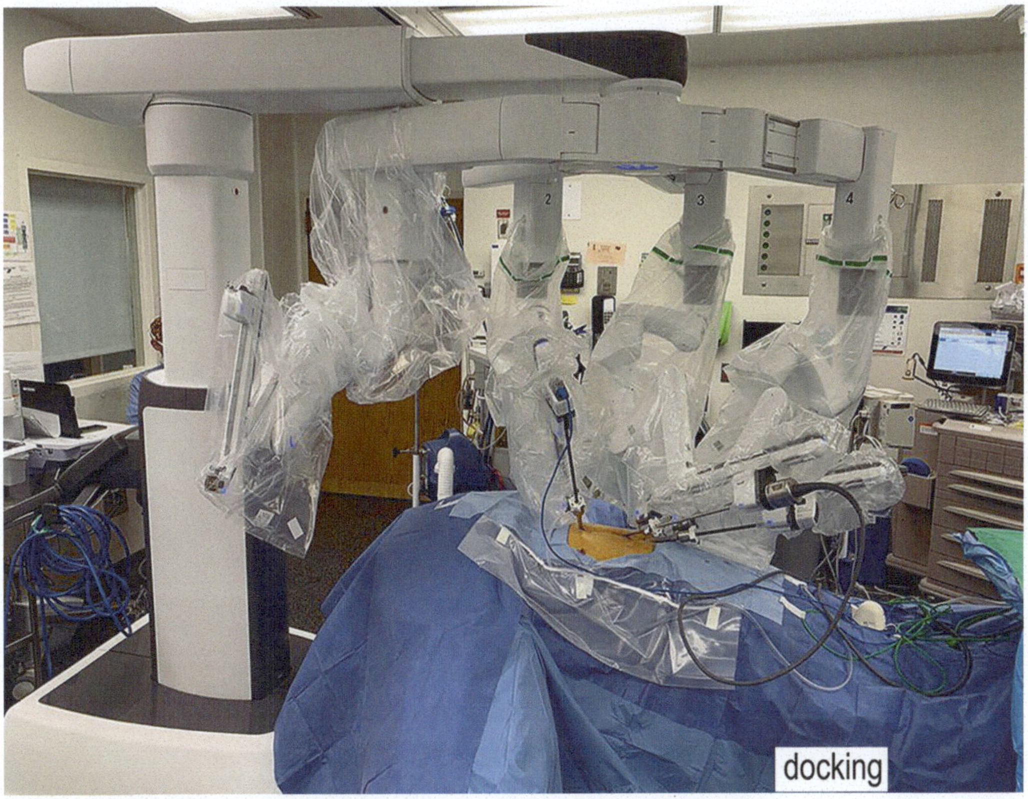


**Fig. 13.7** First, the camera arm is inserted and docked. Next, the surgical target is selected, and the system automatically positions the boom to allow for an optimal arm configuration

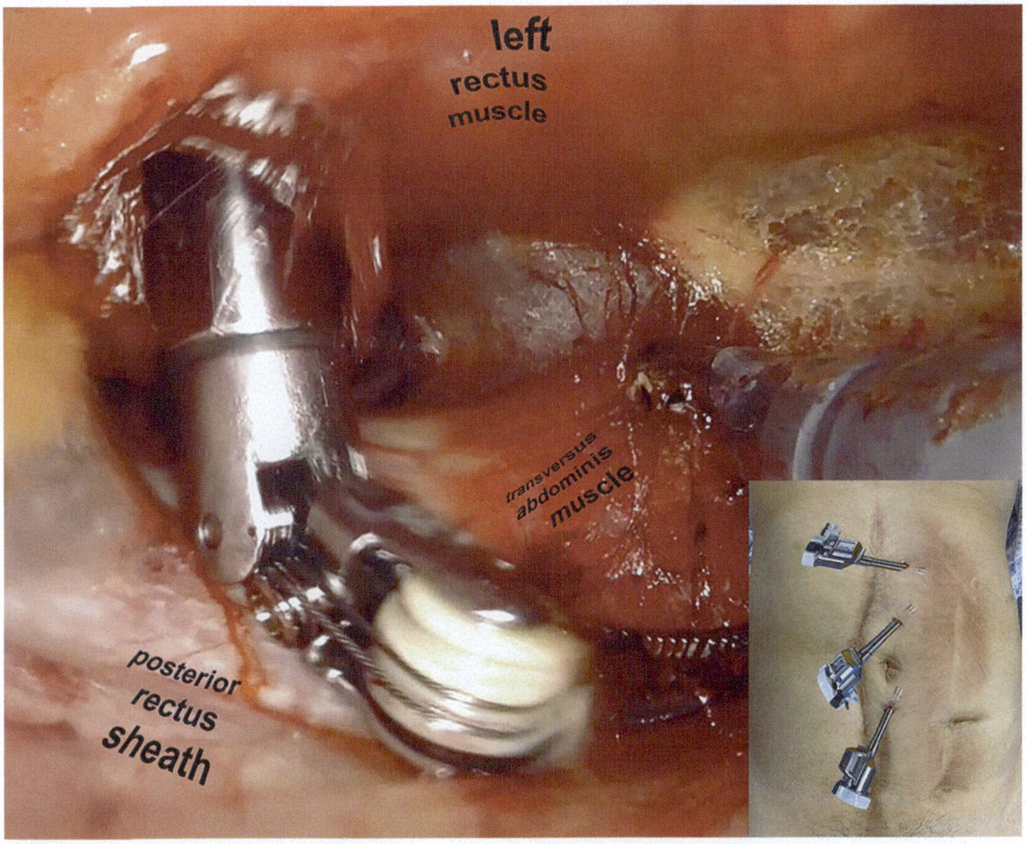


**Fig. 13.8** The ipsilateral retrorectus dissection is performed. The sub-figure shows trocar positions, captured image, and hernia location

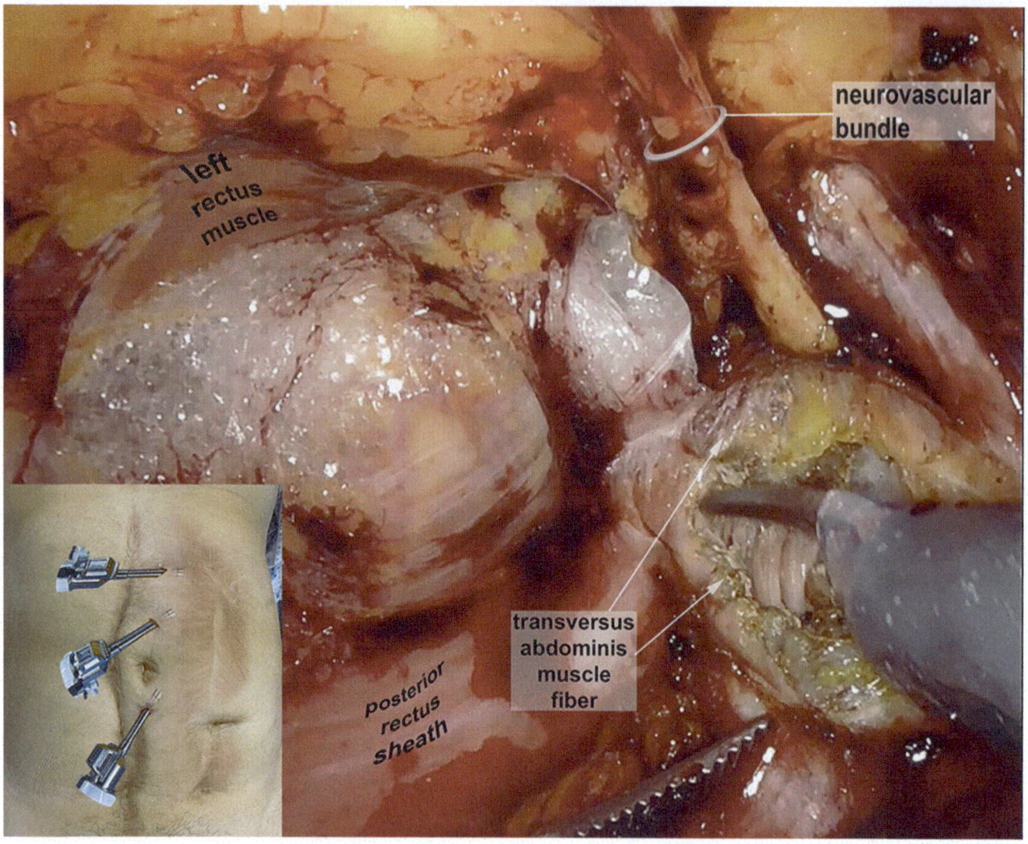


**Fig. 13.9** Ipsilateral transversus abdominis release (TAR) is initiated, proceeding in the cranial direction while preserving any encountered neurovascular bundles

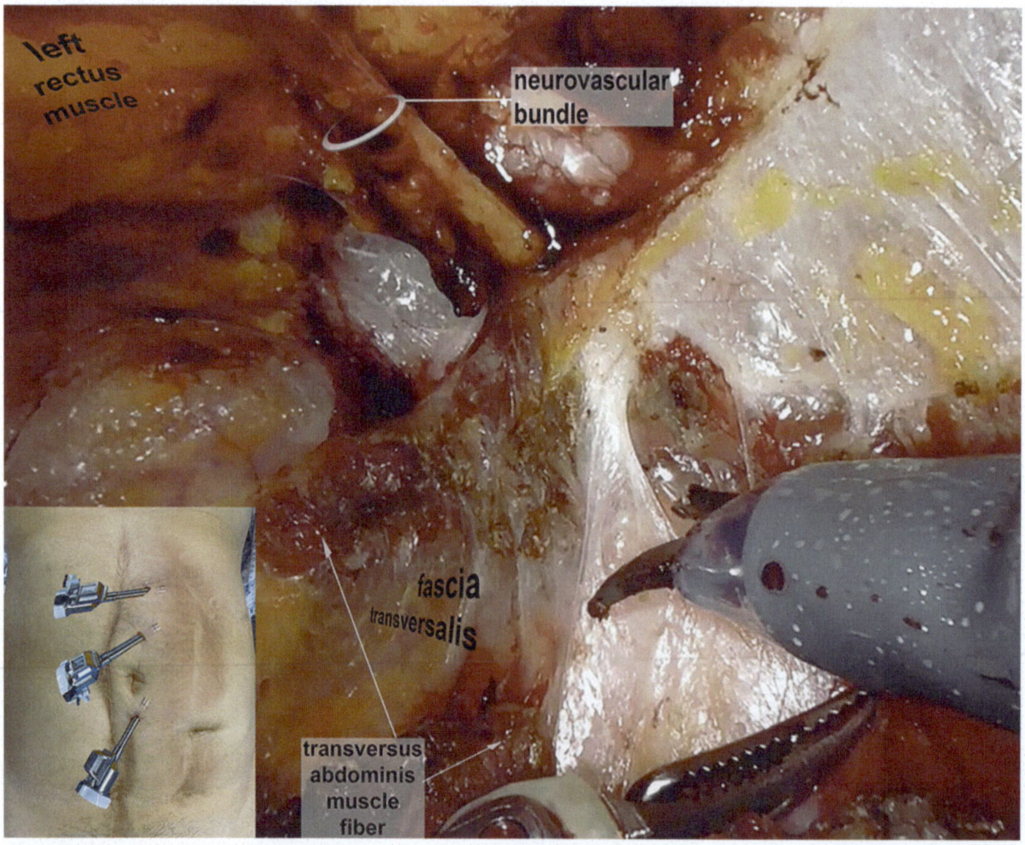


**Fig. 13.10** Continuation of TAR

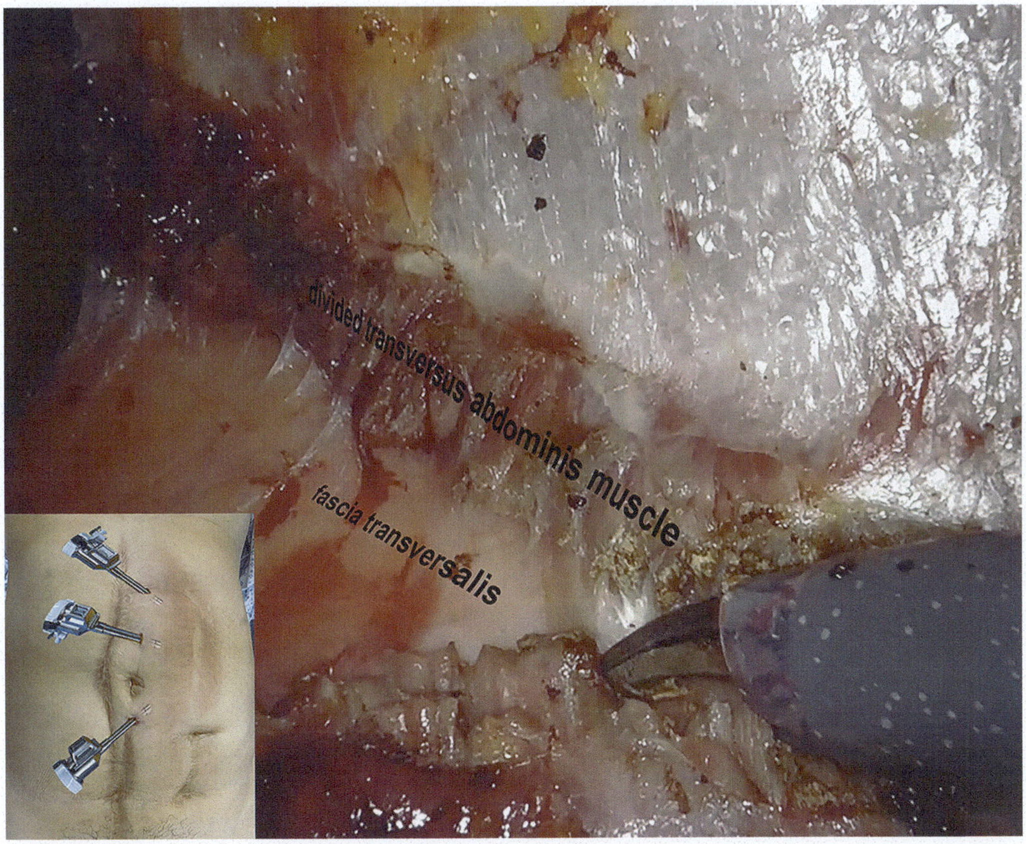


**Fig. 13.11** Once the transversus abdominis is separated, the fascia transversalis and peritoneum are visualized

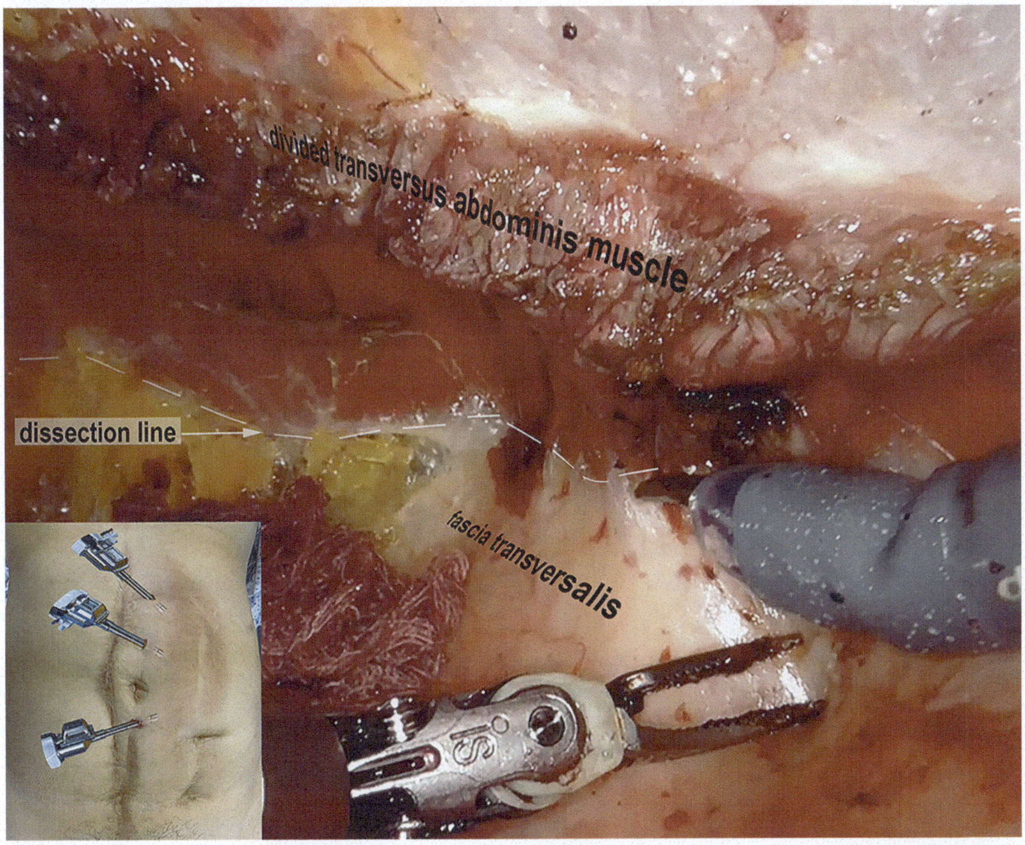


**Fig. 13.12** Gentle traction along the fascia transversalis reveals the dissection plane to be followed

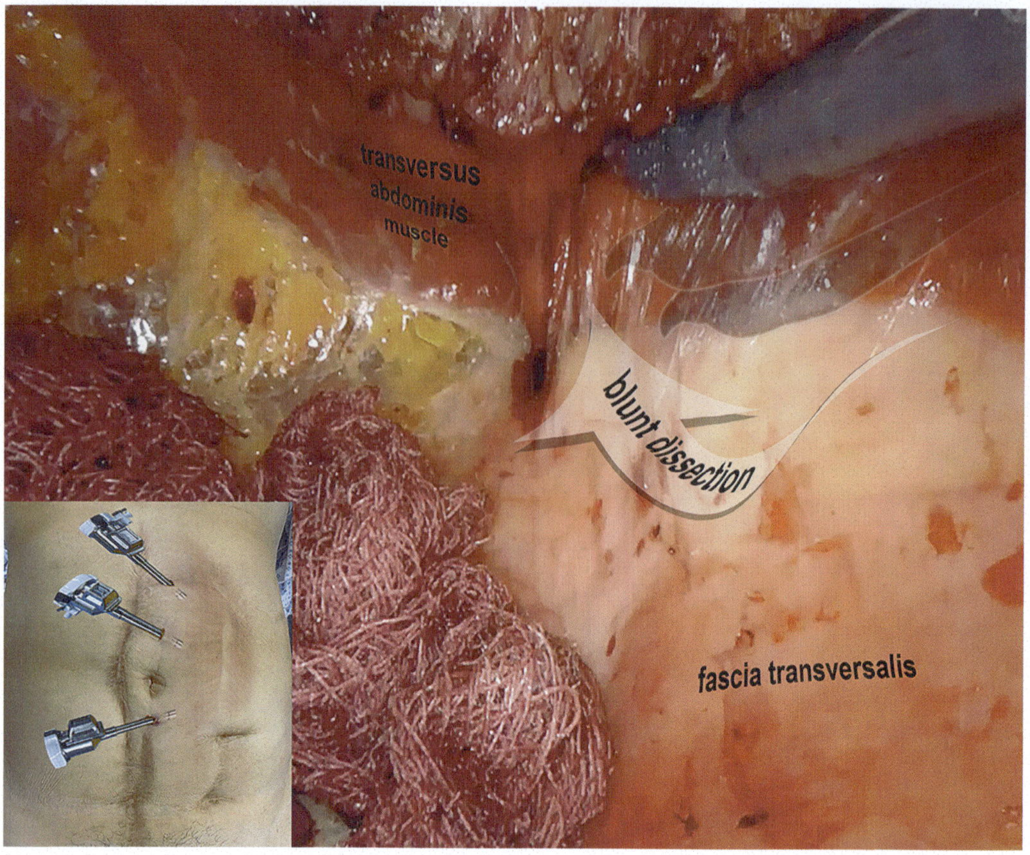


Fig. 13.13 Blunt dissection is used to help separate the transversus abdominis muscle from the fascia transversalis

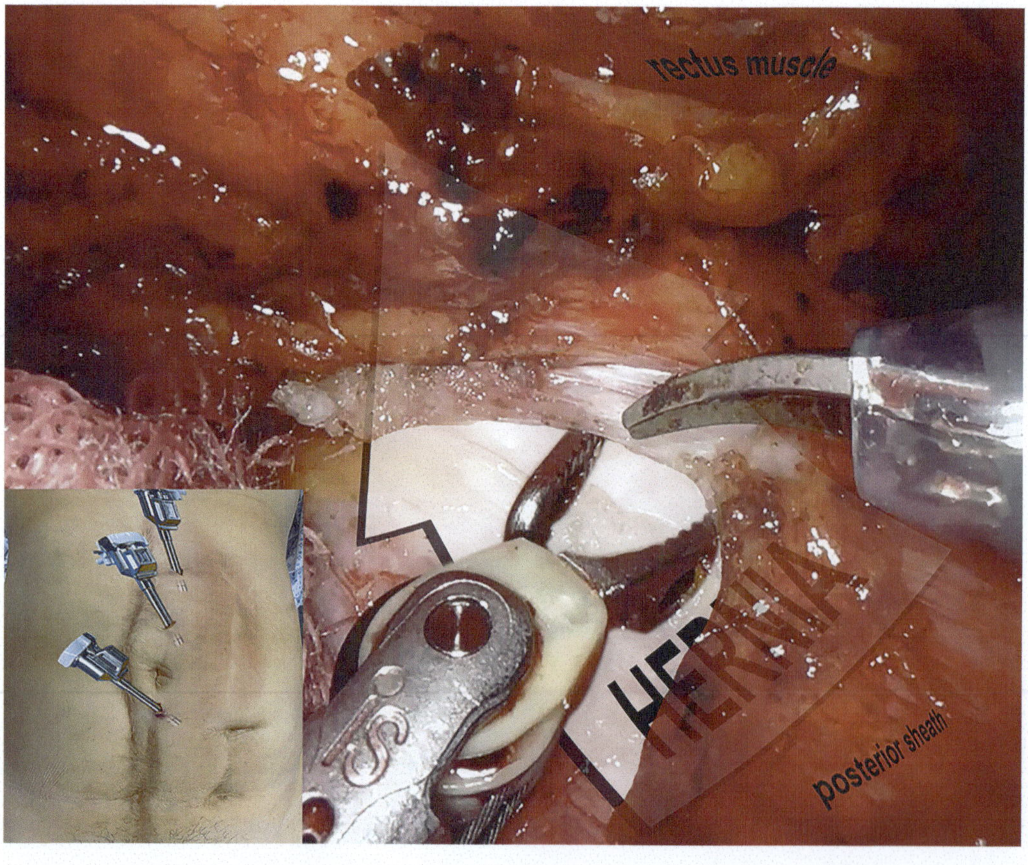


Fig. 13.14 After dissection towards the lateral abdominal wall, the hernia site is revealed below the posterior sheath

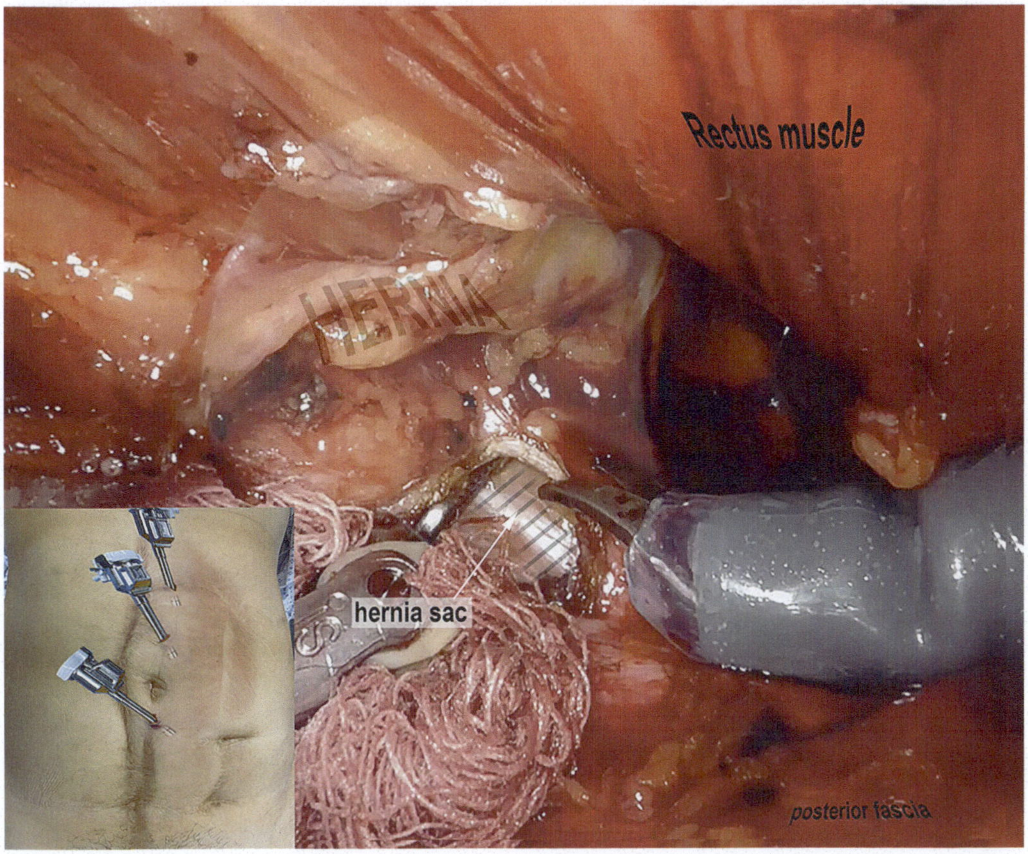


Fig. 13.15 The hernia sac is identified

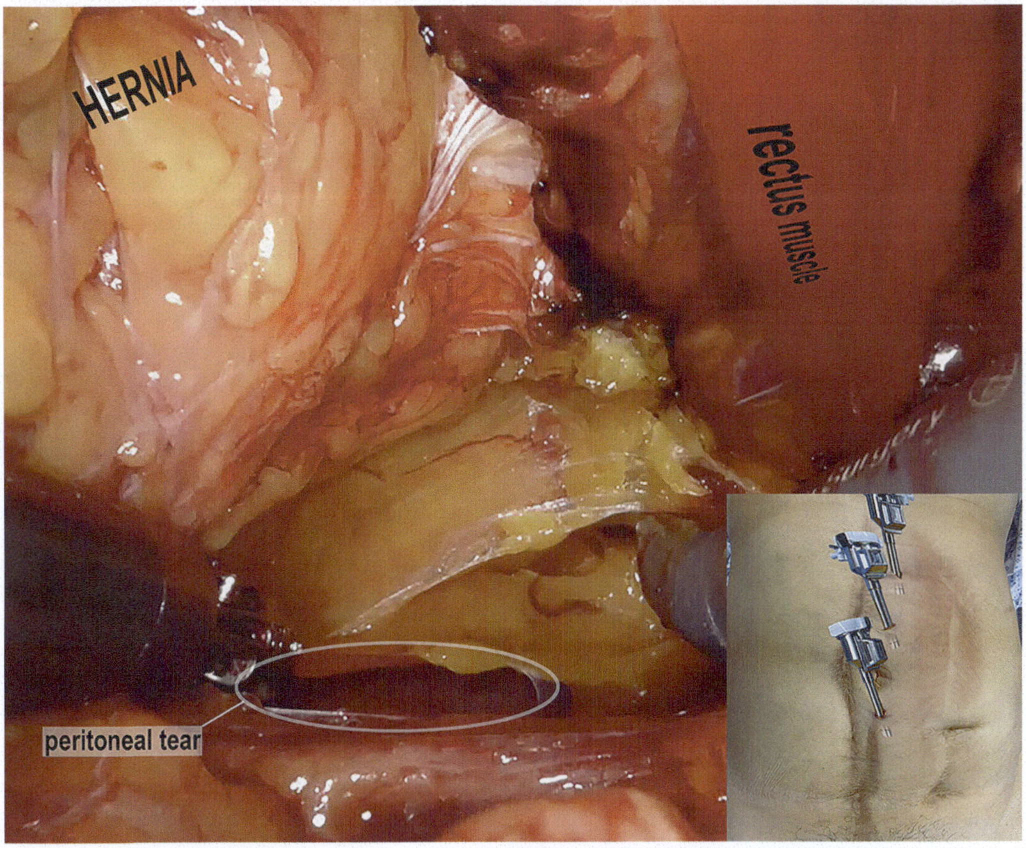


Fig. 13.16 The hernia sac is dissected circumferentially. An inadvertent peritoneal tear is to be sutured later

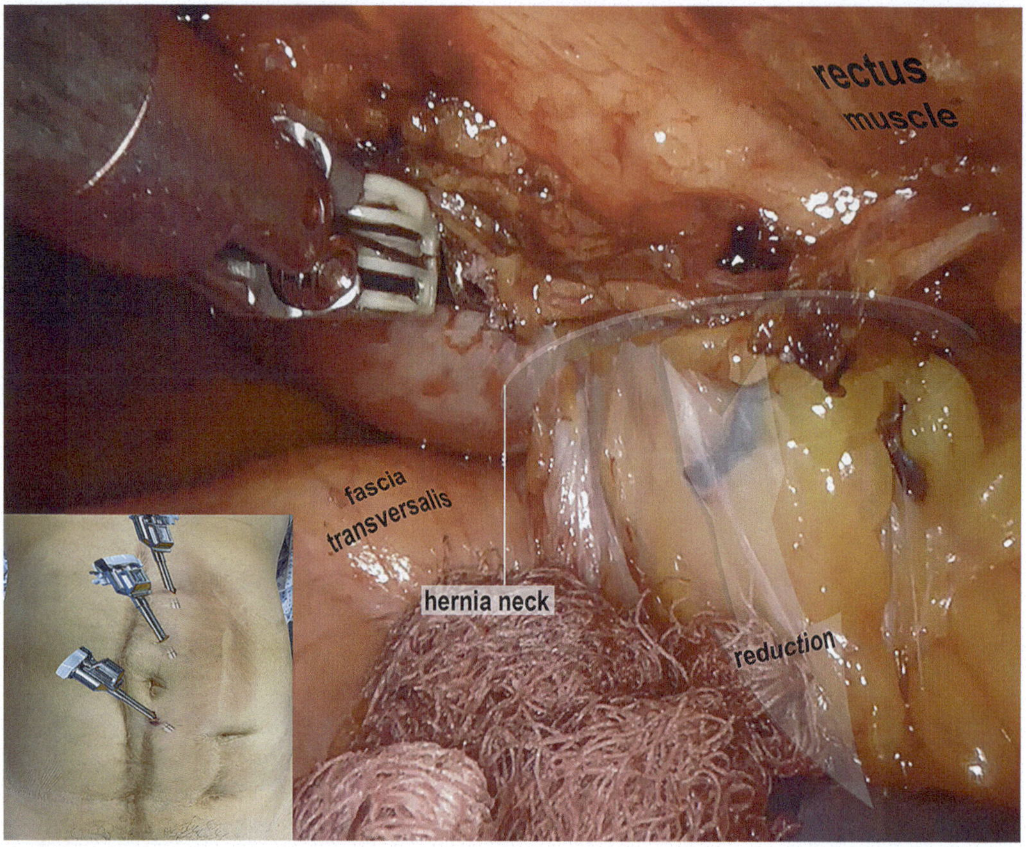


**Fig. 13.17** Next, the hernia sac is reduced through the defect

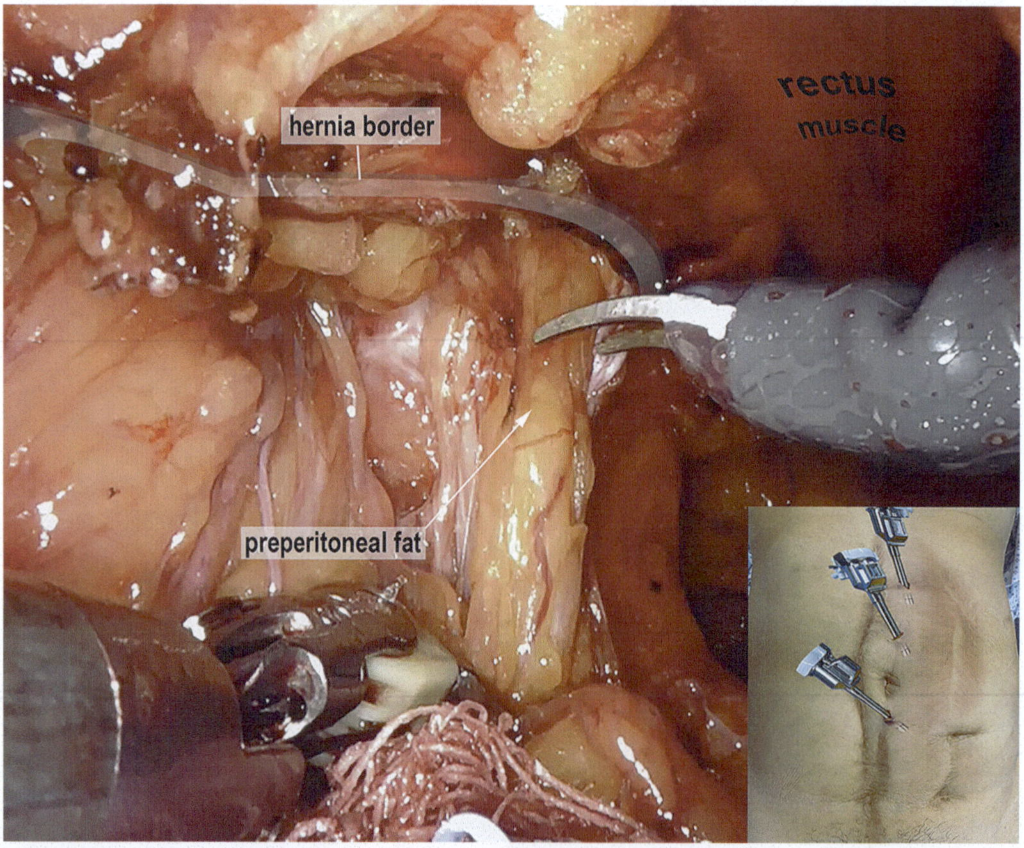


**Fig. 13.18** Hernia sac contents include preperitoneal fat; the excess of this fat is removed to facilitate reduction of the sac

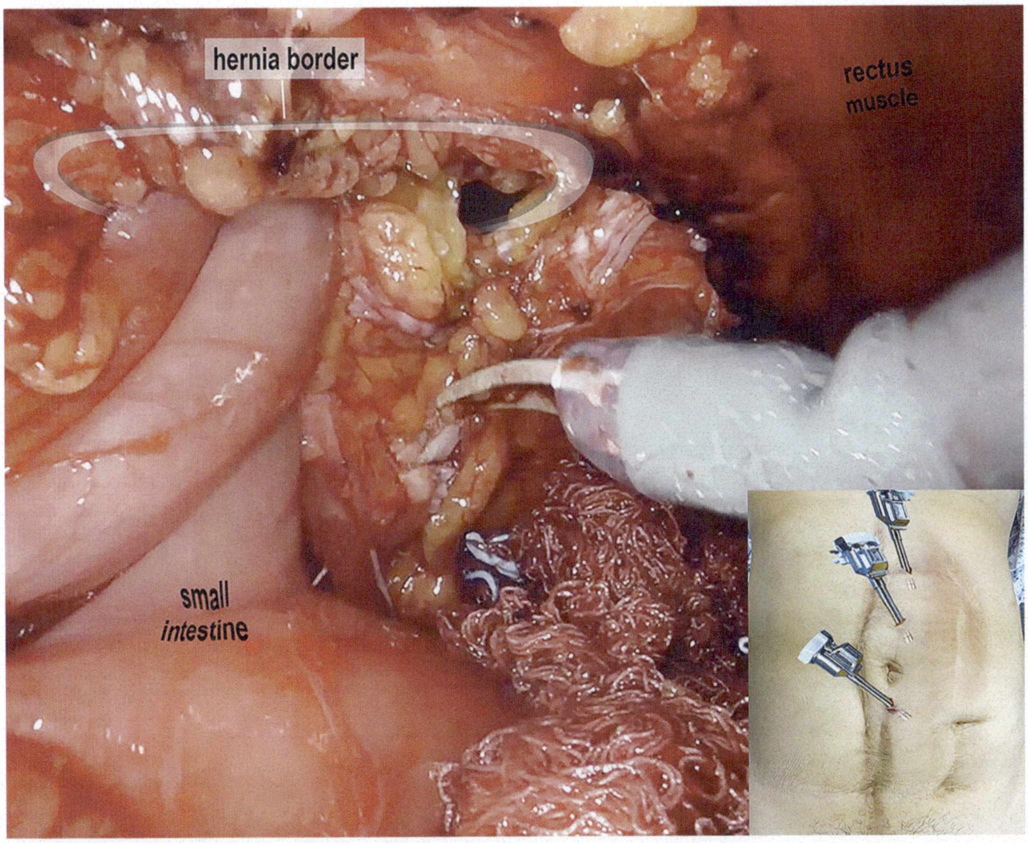


**Fig. 13.19** Small intestine is then reduced through the hernia neck

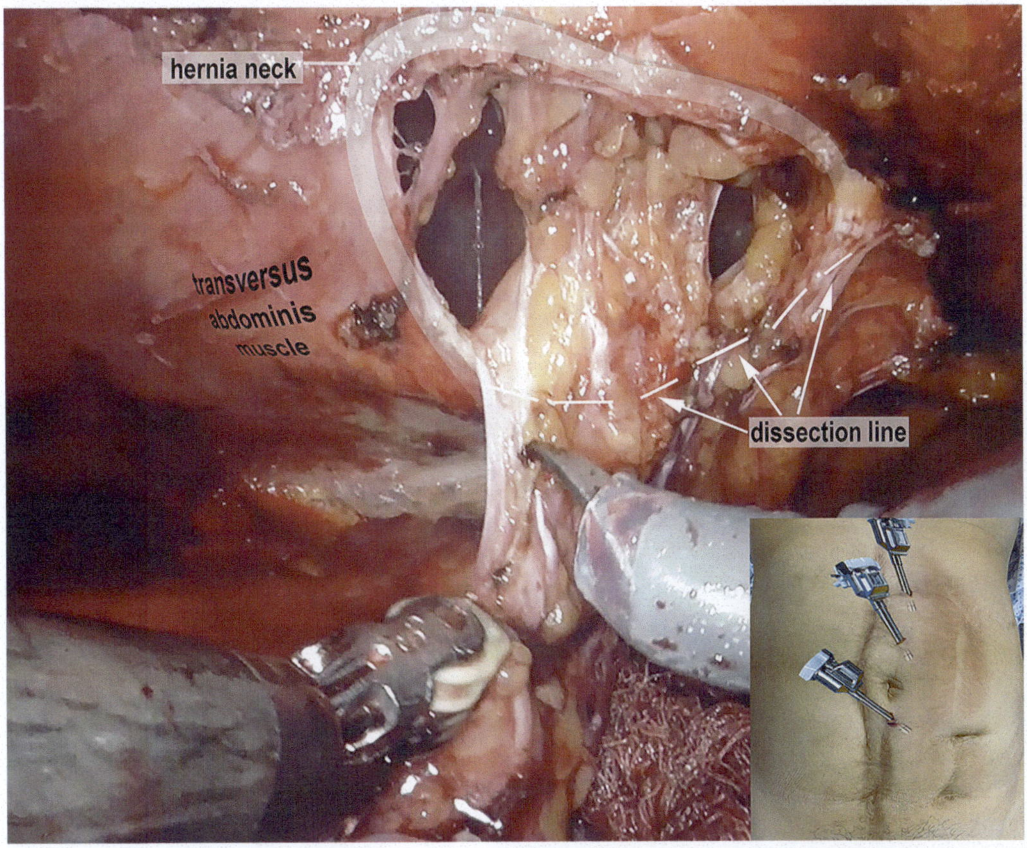


**Fig. 13.20** Pulling on the hernia sac, which is adhered to the hernia neck, reveals a dissection line to be followed in order to better visualize the hernia defect borders

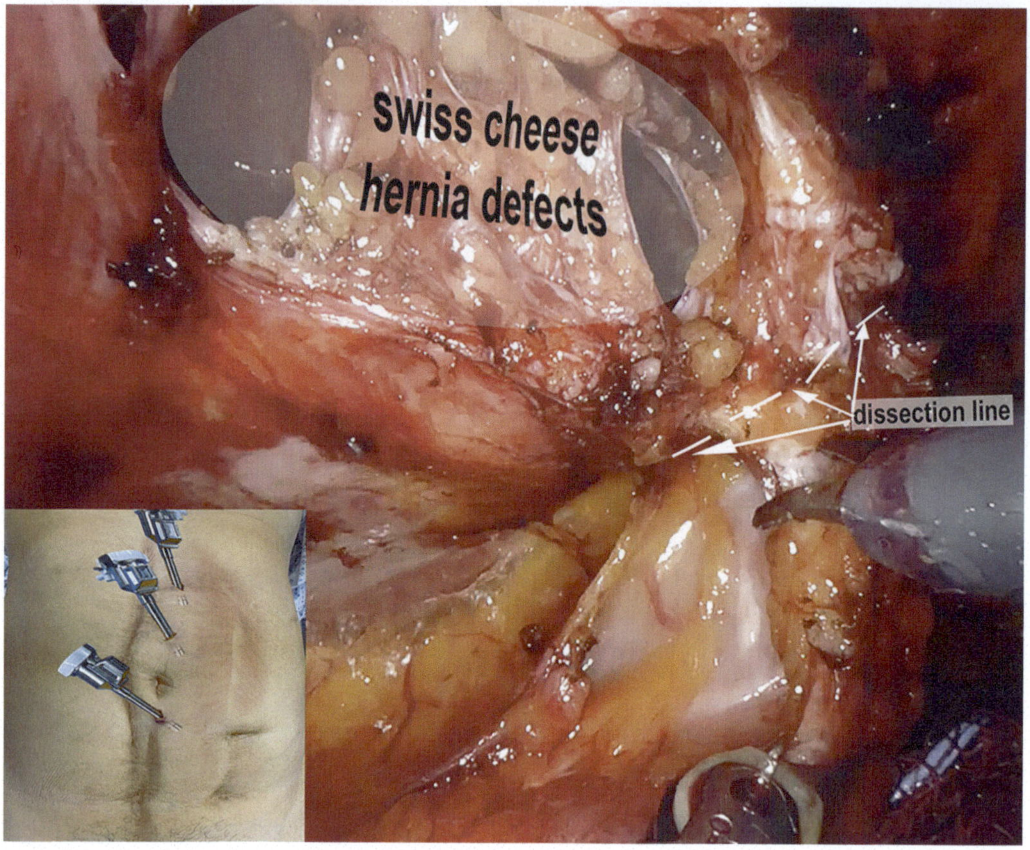


Fig. 13.21 After reducing the hernia, the hernia site is assessed and found to have multiple "Swiss-cheese" defects

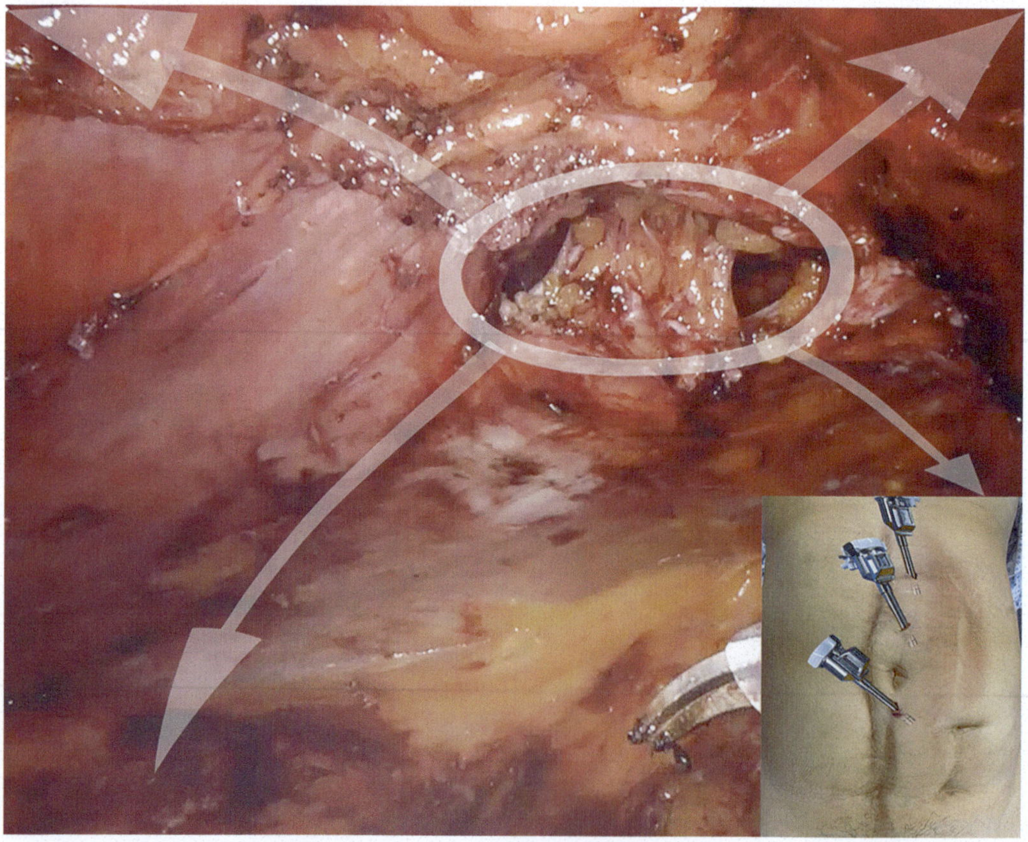

Fig. 13.22 A circumferential area of 5–8 cm from the hernia defect should be cleared of the posterior fascia, to allow for optimal mesh overlap

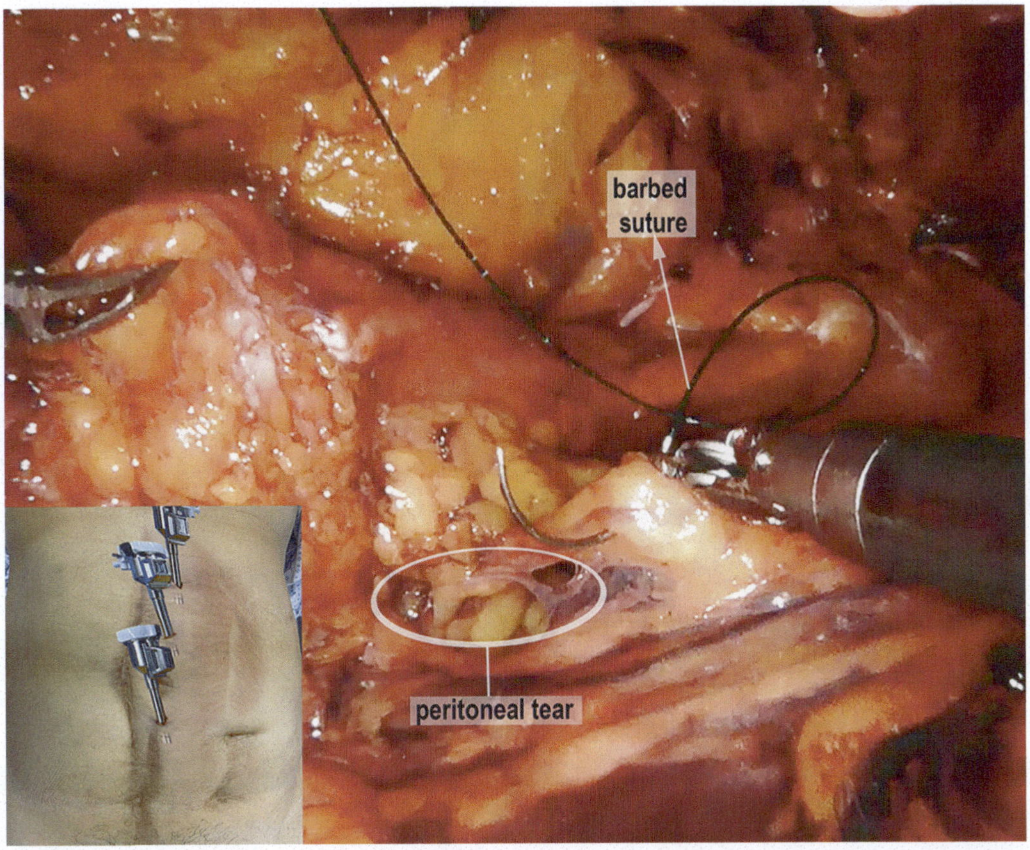


**Fig. 13.23** The peritoneal tear is closed using barbed suture

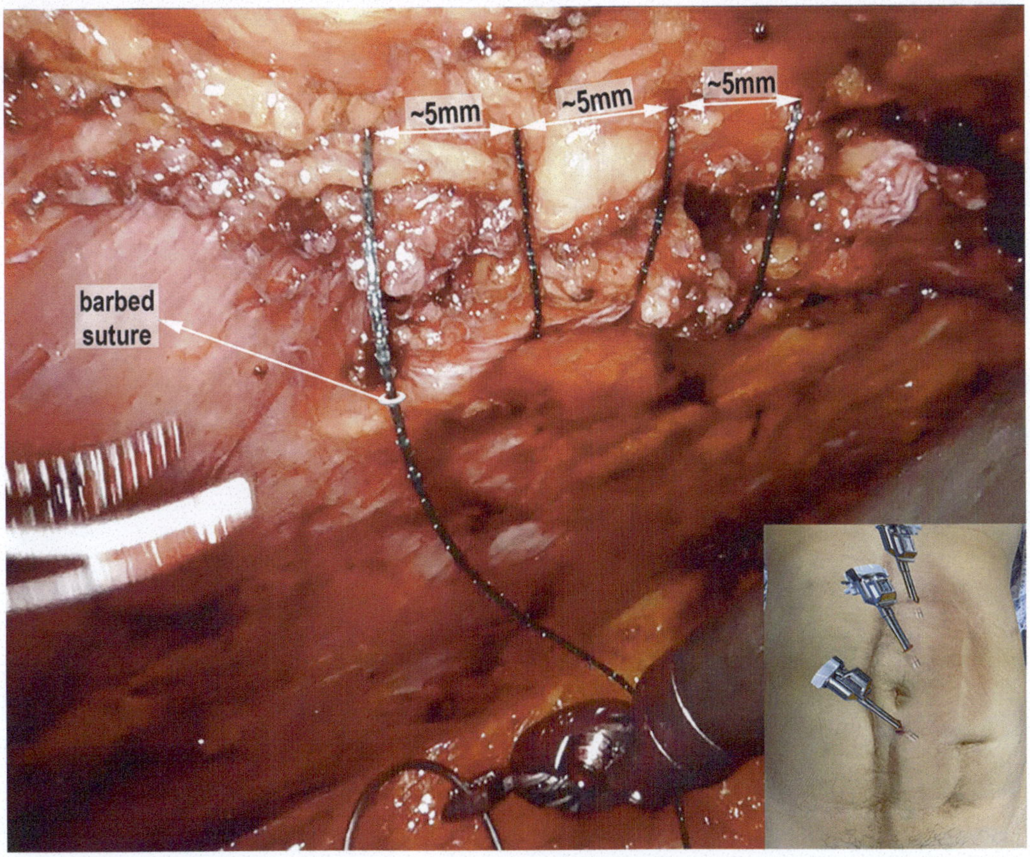


**Fig. 13.24** After addressing the peritoneal tear, the hernia defect is closed in a running fashion using barbed suture, with approximately 5-mm bites

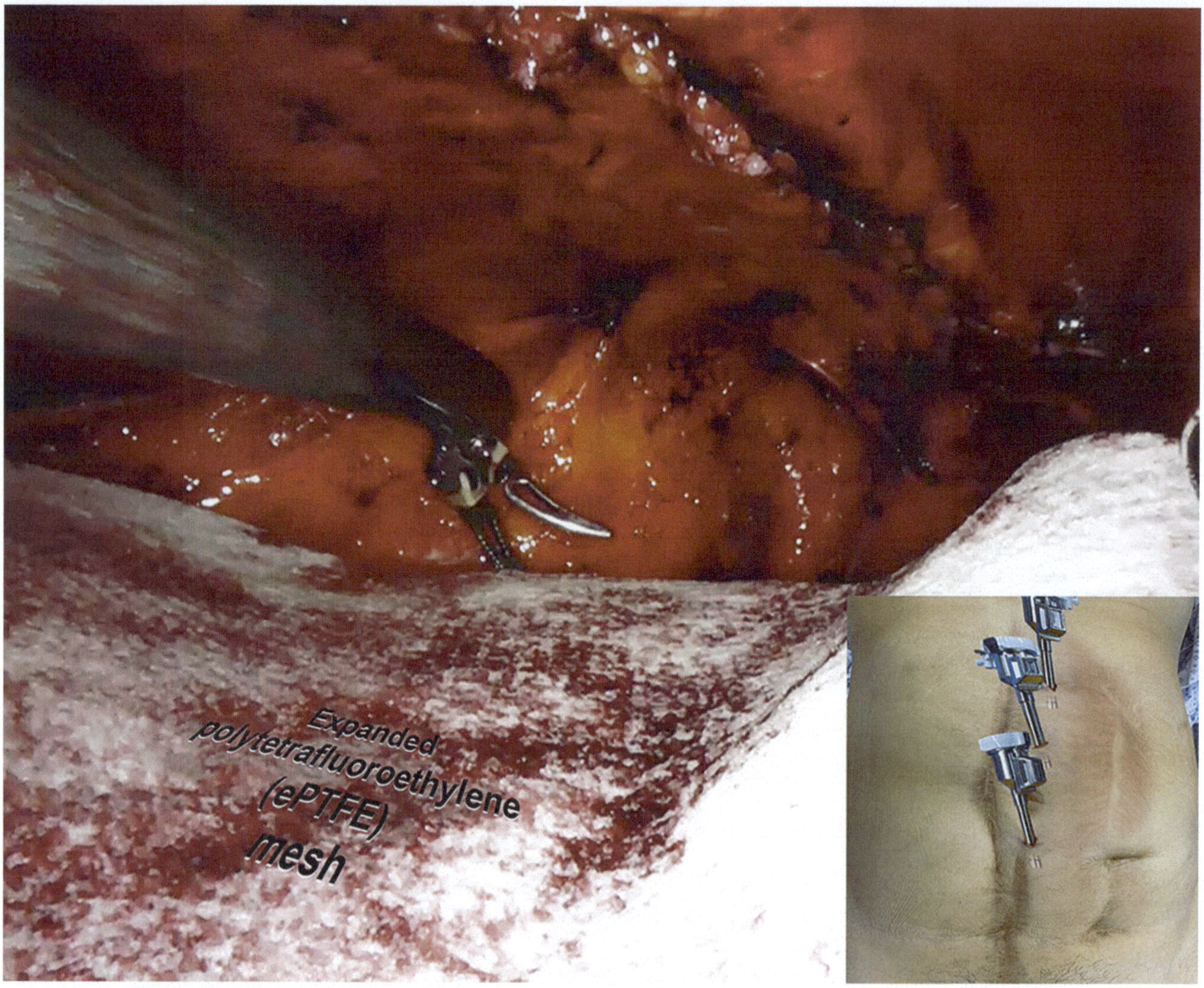


**Fig. 13.25** Expanded polytetrafluoroethylene (ePTFE) mesh is deployed and placed into position without the use of any fixation method

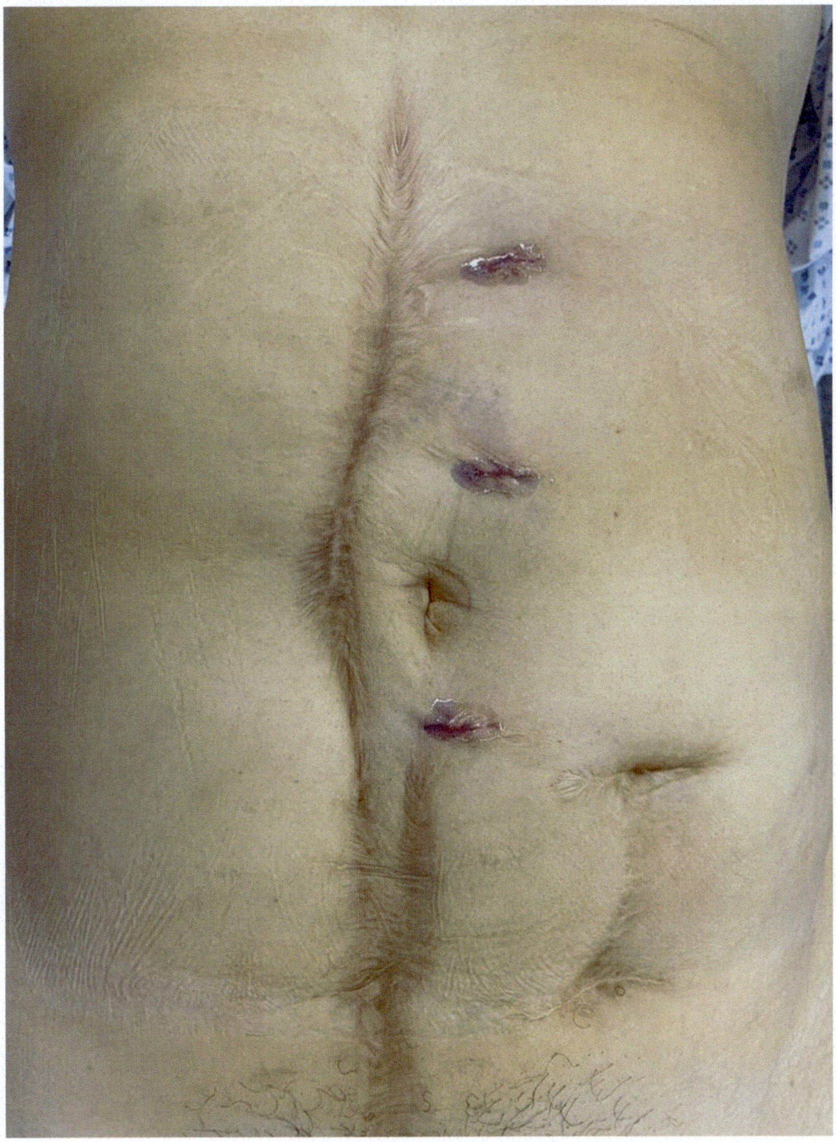

**Fig. 13.26** Trocars are removed, and skin incisions are closed after administration of a local anesthetic

## References


1. Muysoms FE, Miserez M, Berrevoet F, Campanelli G, Champault GG, Chelala E, et al. Classification of primary and incisional abdominal wall hernias. Hernia. 2009;13(4):407–14. https://doi.org/10.1007/s10029-009-0518-x.
2. Bittner JG 4th, Alrefai S, Vy M, Mabe M, Del Prado PAR, Clingempeel NL. Comparative analysis of open and robotic transversus abdominis release for ventral hernia repair. Surg Endosc. 2018;32:727–34. https://doi.org/10.1007/s00464-017-5729-0.
3. Carbonell AM, Warren JA, Prabhu AS, Ballecer CD, Janczyk RJ, Herrera J, et al. Reducing length of stay using a robotic-assisted approach for retromuscular ventral hernia repair: a comparative analysis from the Americas Hernia Society Quality Collaborative. Ann Surg. 2018;267:210–7. https://doi.org/10.1097/SLA.0000000000002244.
4. Gokcal F, Morrison S, Kudsi OY. Robotic retromuscular ventral hernia repair and transversus abdominis release: short-term outcomes and risk factors associated with perioperative complications. Hernia. 2019;23:375–85. https://doi.org/10.1007/s10029-019-01911-1.

# Robotic Inguinoscrotal Hernia Repair: Transabdominal Preperitoneal (TAPP)

14

Hakan Seyit and Omar Yusef Kudsi

## Introduction

Large indirect or scrotal hernias present several challenges for surgeons with both the open and minimally invasive approaches. Some argue that open surgery provides more benefits than laparoscopic repair in terms of ease of hernia manipulation [1], but increased wound morbidity and risk of adverse postoperative outcomes explain the choice of minimally invasive techniques for these repairs. One technique that carries over from the open and laparoscopic approaches into robotic repair is the preperitoneal method. As opposed to laparoscopic repair, the robotic platform may be favorable in terms of a superior visual field and more precise dissection in a region with surrounding delicate structures such as gonadal and iliac vessels, as well as nearby femoral nerve branches. Suturing of the peritoneal flap is also arguably facilitated with the robotic platform, and this advantage may carry over into the postoperative period, with lower rates of complications and pain [2].

When performing robotic inguinoscrotal transabdominal preperitoneal (TAPP) repair, it is important first to identify spermatic vessels, and then to dissect along these vessels towards the top of the hernia sac at the inguinal canal. After hernia and adipose tissue reduction, complete parietalization of the gonadal vessels and vas deferens, if present, should be performed, in addition to thorough dissection of the myopectineal orifice, to ensure proper placement of the mesh without folding. Any excess preperitoneal fat (cord lipoma) should be excised before closure of the peritoneal flap, as it may later mimic a recurrent hernia and become symptomatic [3].

## Procedure: Illustrated Steps

Figures 14.1, 14.2, 14.3, 14.4, 14.5, 14.6, 14.7, 14.8, 14.9, 14.10, 14.11, 14.12, 14.13, 14.14, 14.15, 14.16, 14.17, 14.18, 14.19, 14.20, 14.21, 14.22, 14.23, 14.24, 14.25, 14.26, 14.27, 14.28, 14.29, 14.30, 14.31, 14.32, 14.33, 14.34, 14.35, 14.36, 14.37, 14.38, 14.39, 14.40, 14.41, 14.42, 14.43, 14.44, 14.45, 14.46, 14.47, 14.48, 14.49, and 14.50 illustrate the technical aspects of robotic transabdominal preperitoneal (TAPP) repair of a left inguinoscrotal hernia, with right inguinal cord lipoma excision.

H. Seyit
Department of Surgery, University of Health Sciences, Bakirkoy Dr. Sadi Konuk Training and Research Hospital, Bakirkoy, Istanbul, Turkey

O. Y. Kudsi (✉)
Department of Surgery, Good Samaritan Medical Center, Tufts University School of Medicine, Boston, MA, USA


O. Y. Kudsi (ed.), *Robotic Hernia Surgery*, https://doi.org/10.1007/978-3-030-46667-1_14

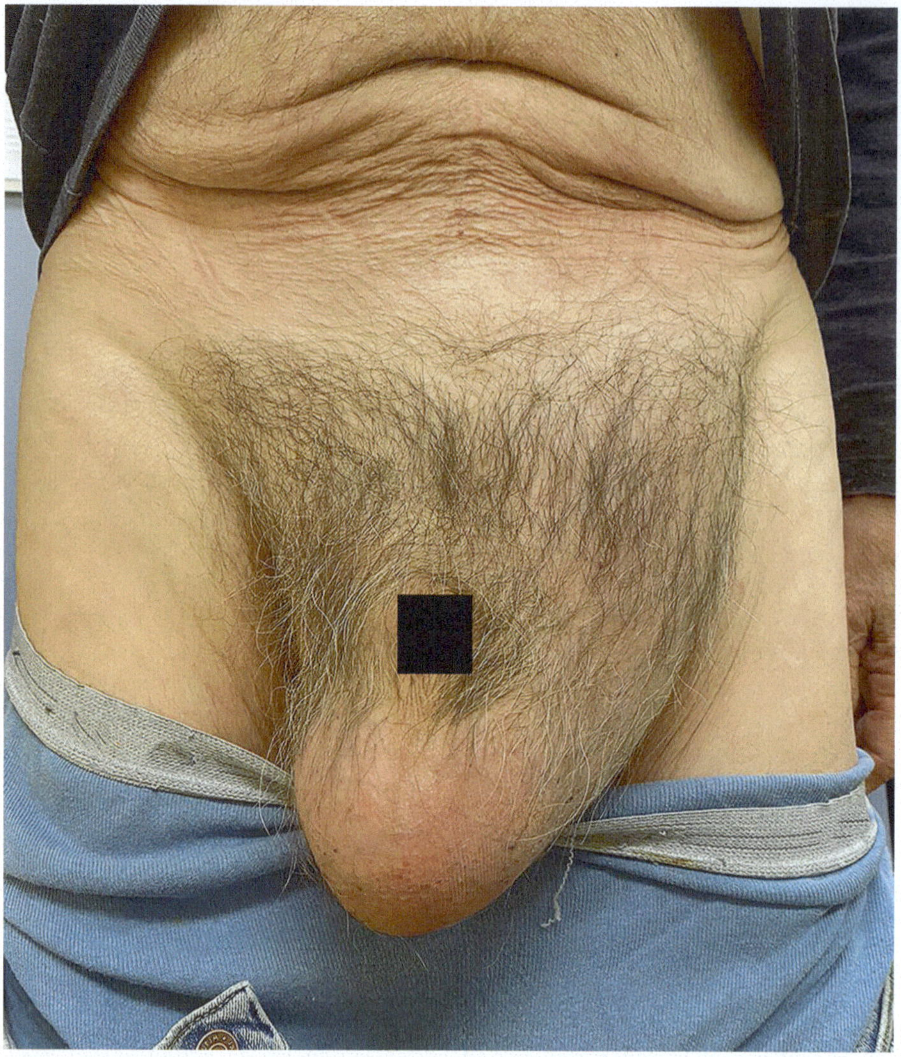

Fig. 14.1 Preoperative view of a left inguinoscrotal hernia

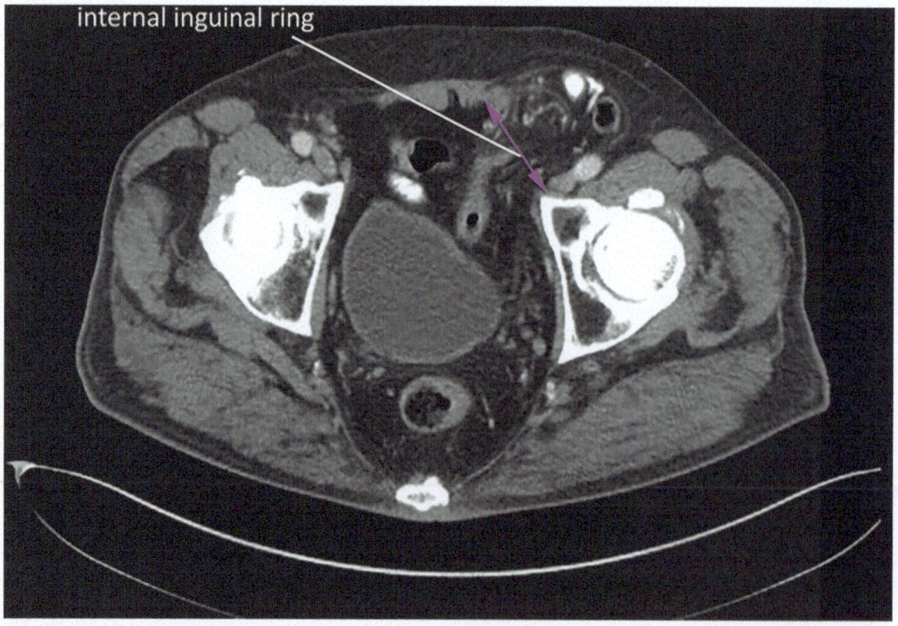


Fig. 14.2 Computerized tomography (CT) transverse image, internal inguinal ring level

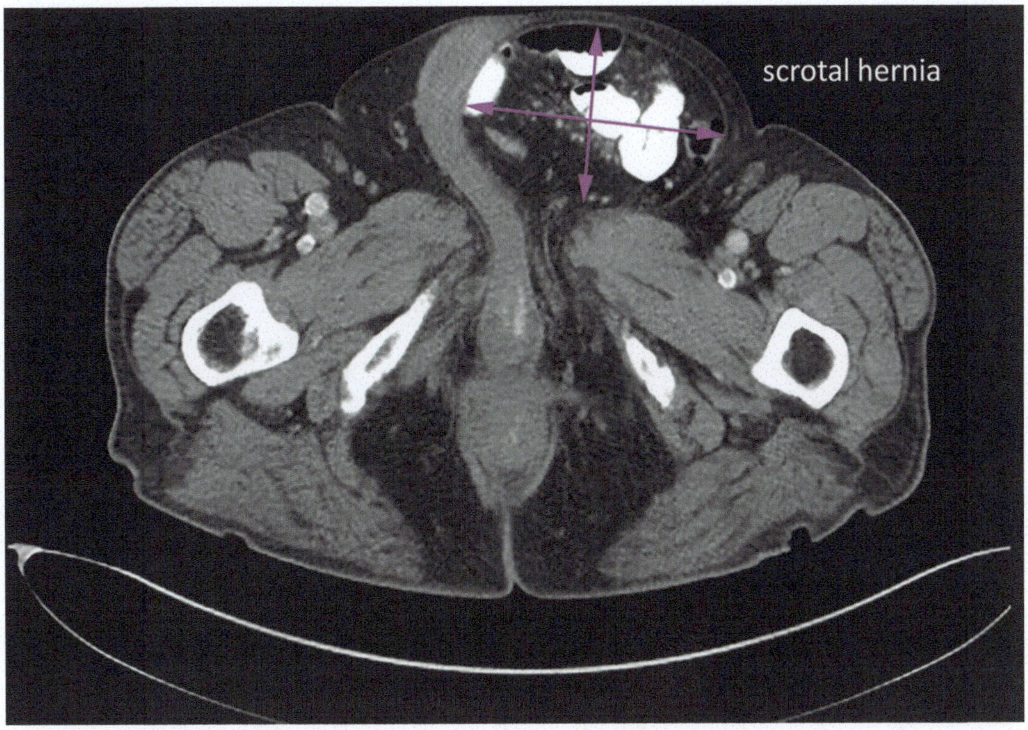


**Fig. 14.3** CT transverse image, scrotal level

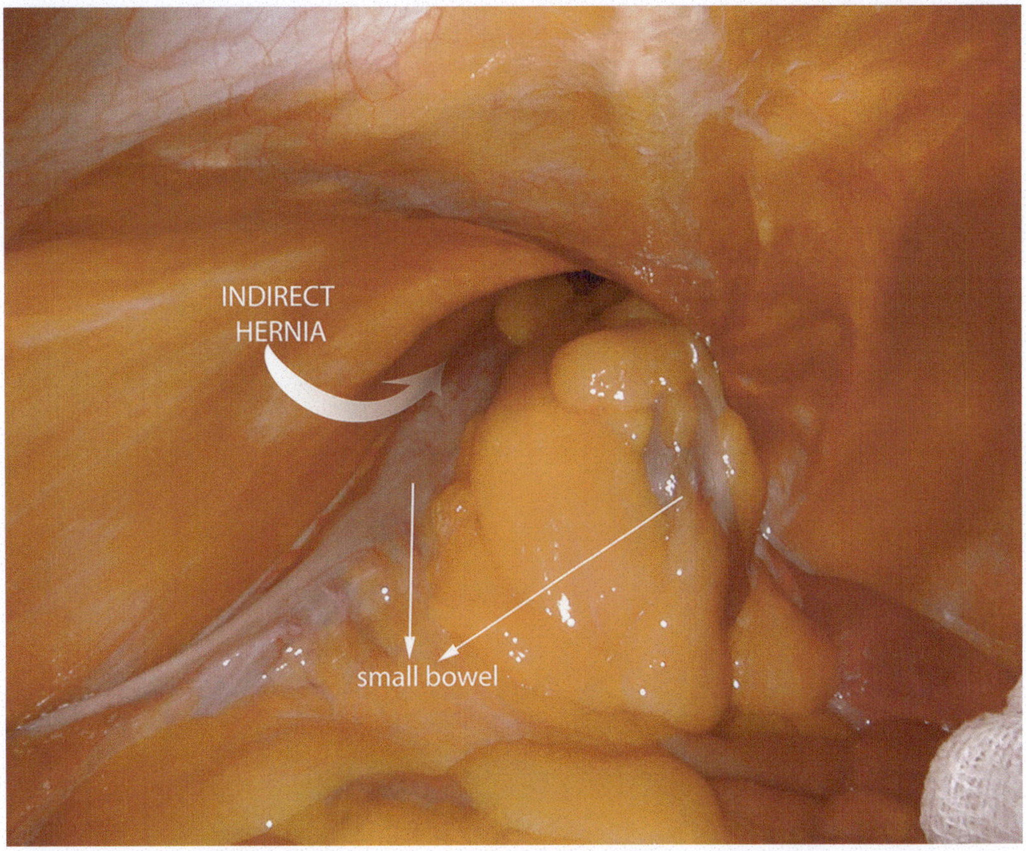


**Fig. 14.4** After the trocars are inserted, the patient-side cart of the robot is docked and the indirect inguinoscrotal hernia, which contains small bowel loops, is identified

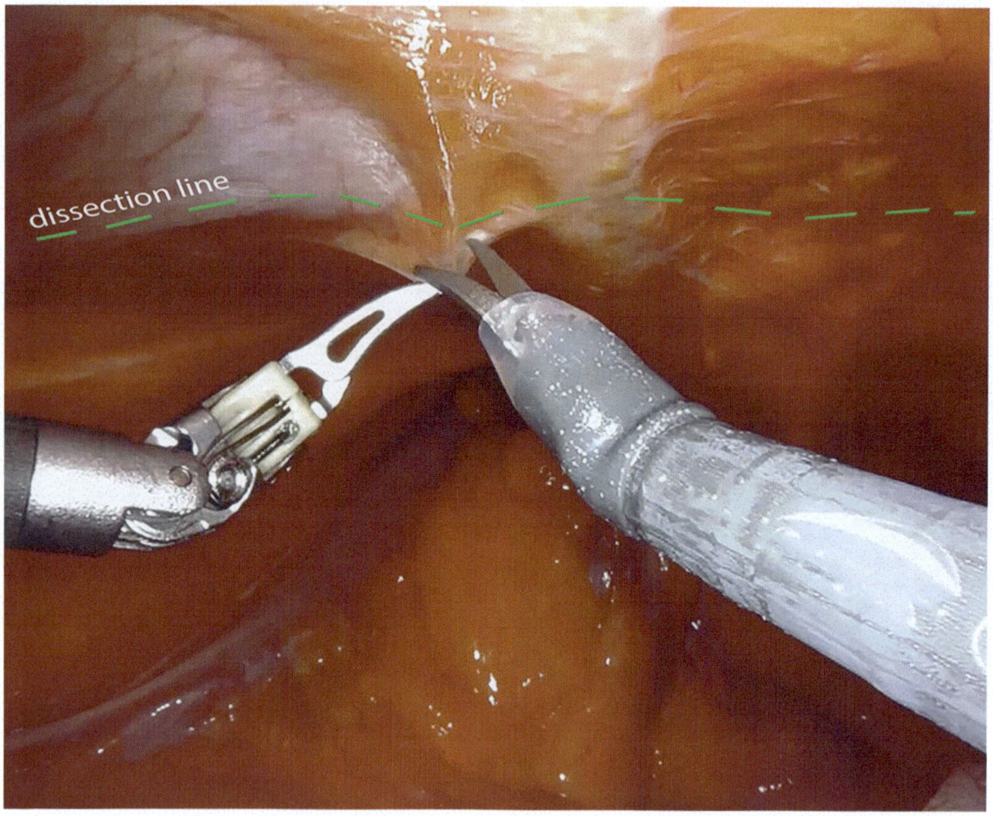


**Fig. 14.5** Any attempt to reduce the scrotal hernia content into the abdomen prior to dissection can create obstacles during the procedure. Thus, we prefer dissection first. Dissection into the peritoneum begins from the median umbilical fold and proceeds laterally, 8–10 cm above the internal inguinal ring level

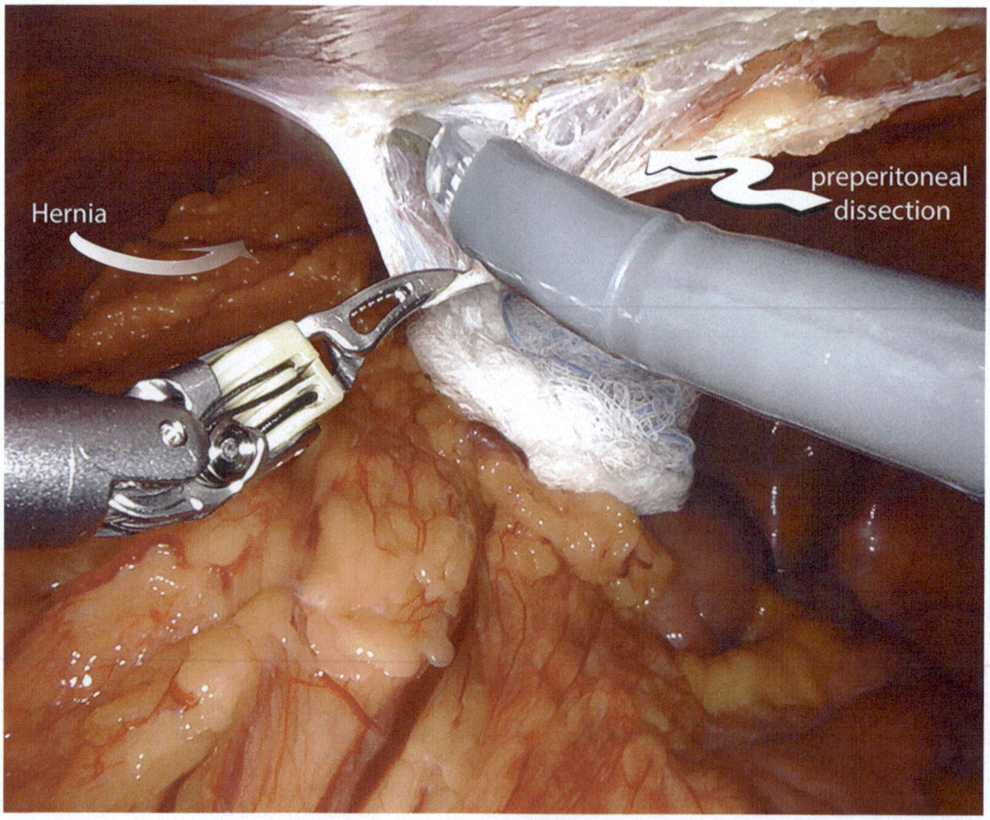


**Fig. 14.6** Once the preperitoneal plane is achieved, dissection is continued laterally

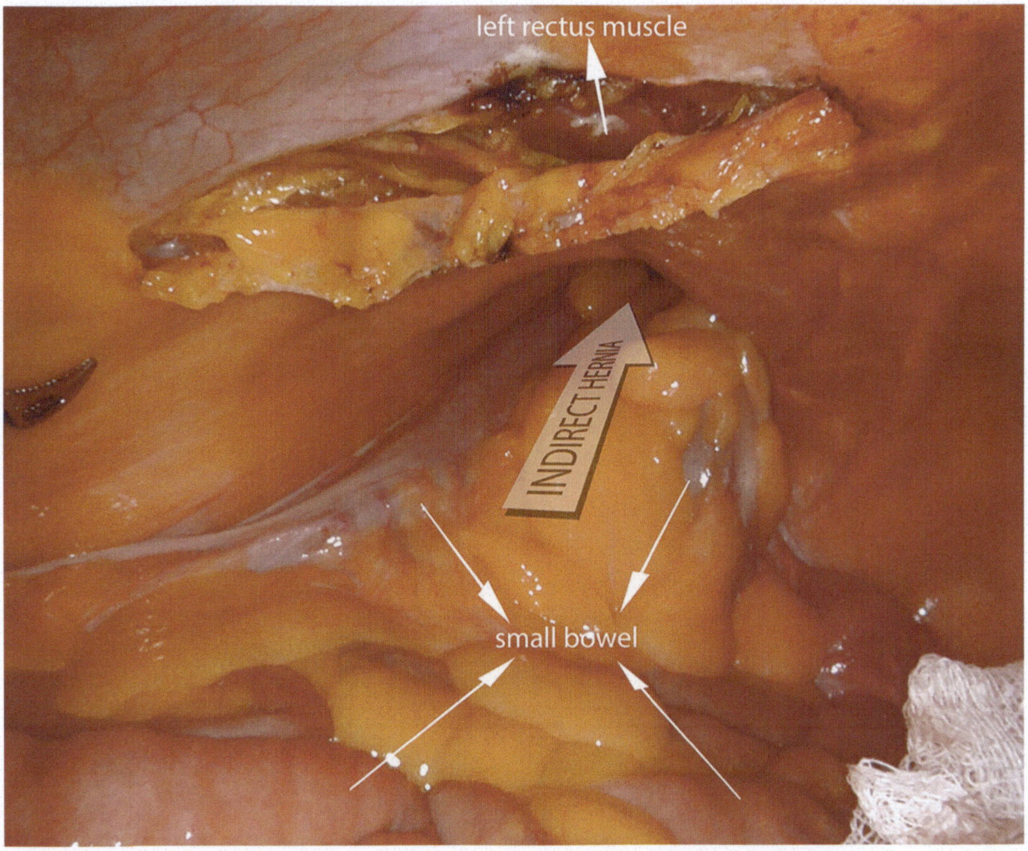


**Fig. 14.7** In case of a breach of the posterior rectus sheath, the retromuscular plane can be used instead

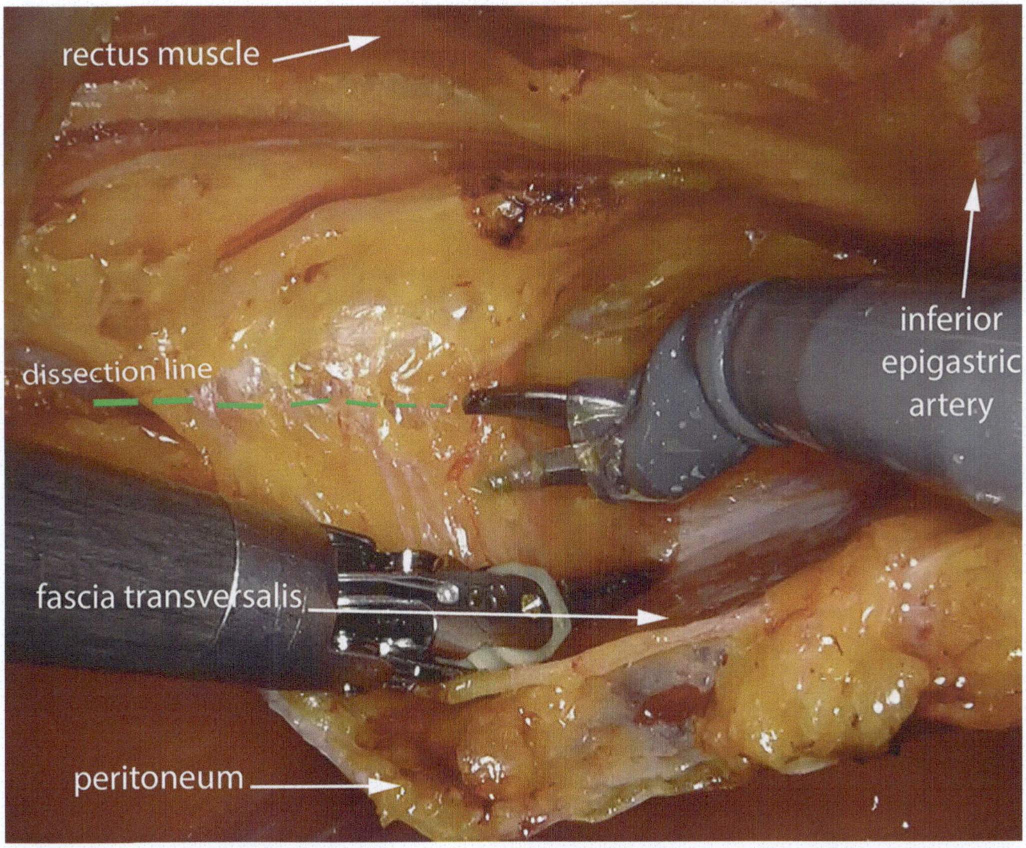


**Fig. 14.8** As lateral dissection proceeds, inferior epigastric vessels should be preserved

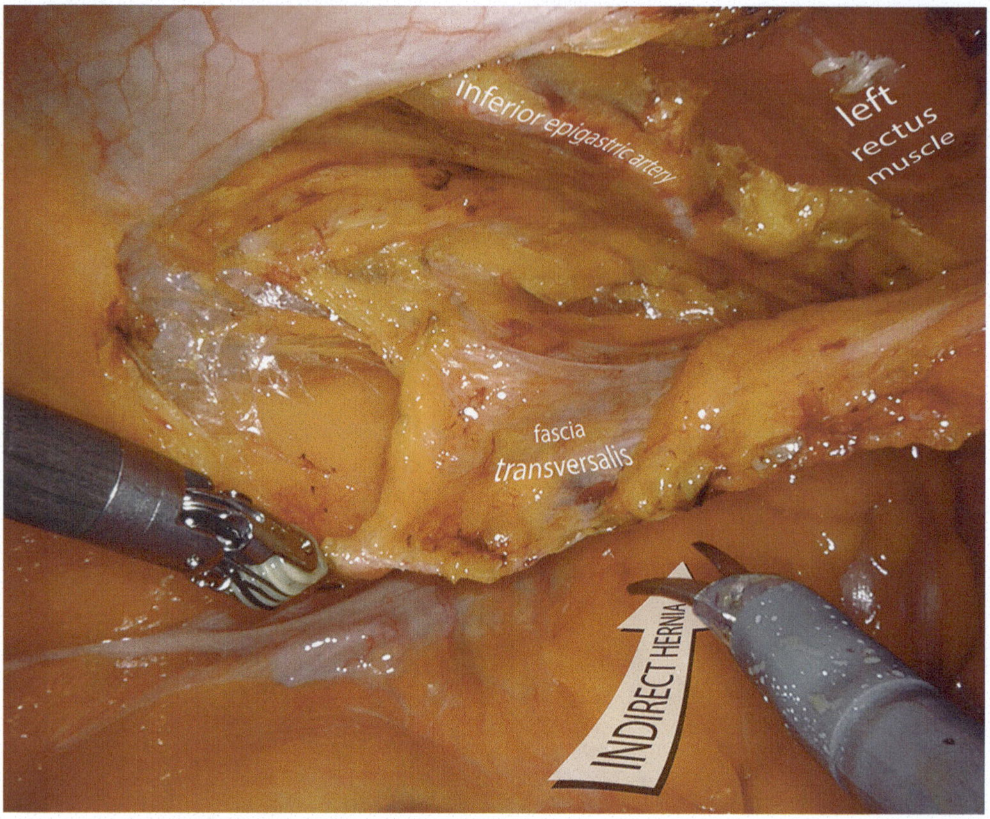


Fig. 14.9 Extension of the preperitoneal/retromuscular dissection laterally towards the transversus abdominis muscle and towards the deep inguinal ring

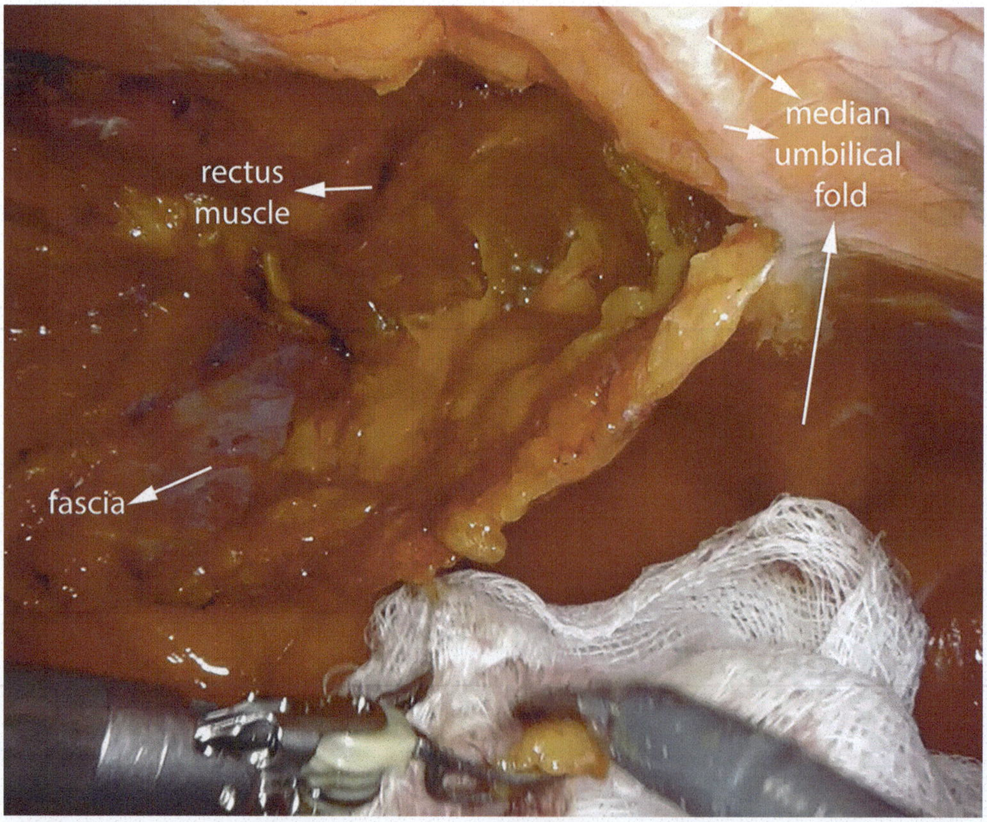


Fig. 14.10 Extension of the preperitoneal dissection medially towards the median umbilical fold

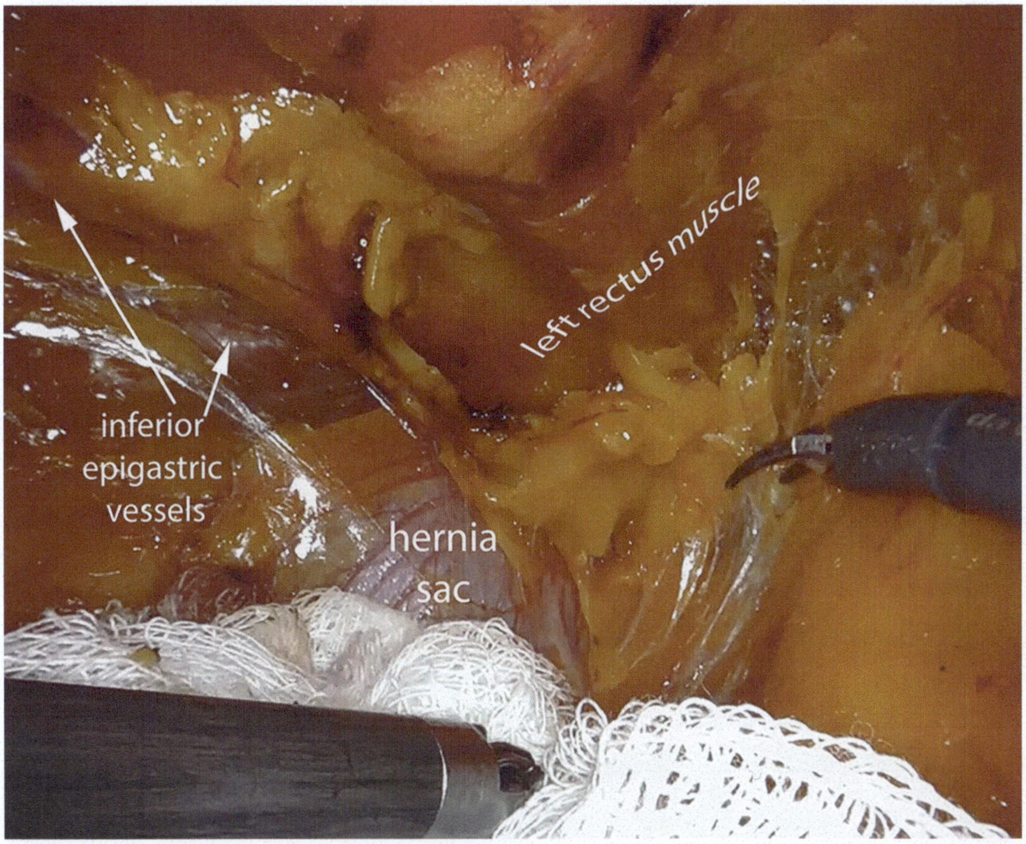


**Fig. 14.11** Dissection is continued inferiorly; gentle pressure with a sponge on the flap may help identify the dissection plane

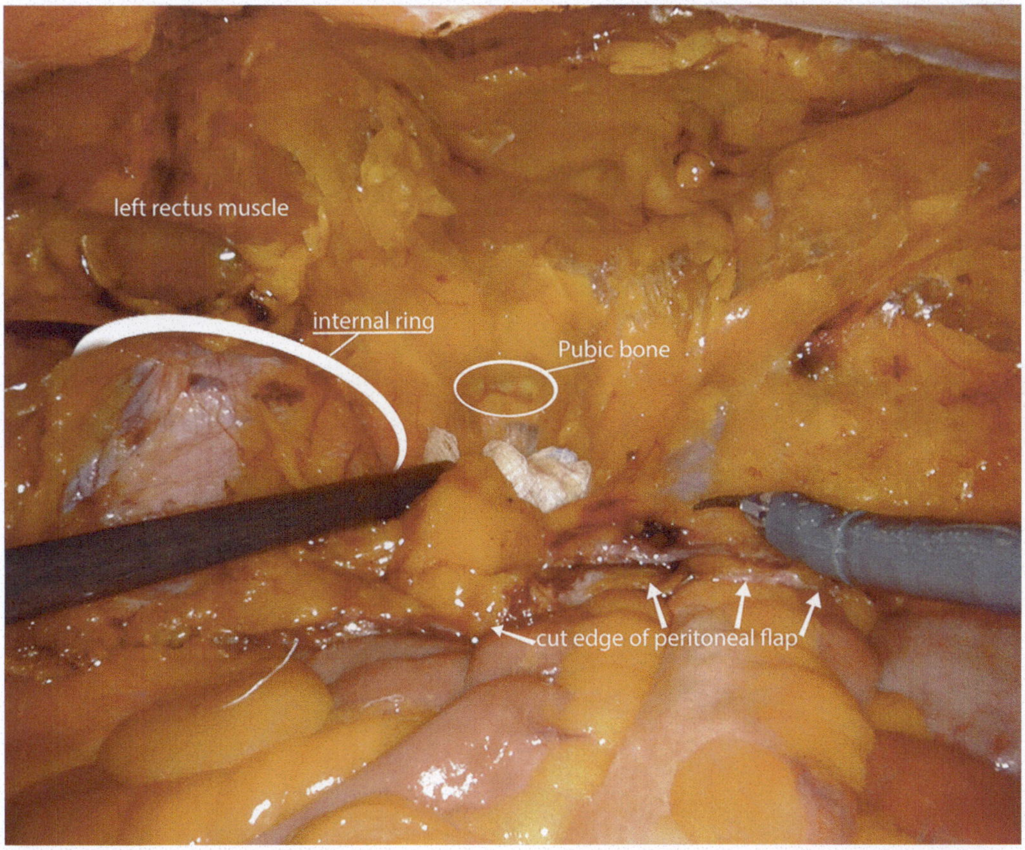


**Fig. 14.12** Pubic bone is identified medial to the inguinal ring

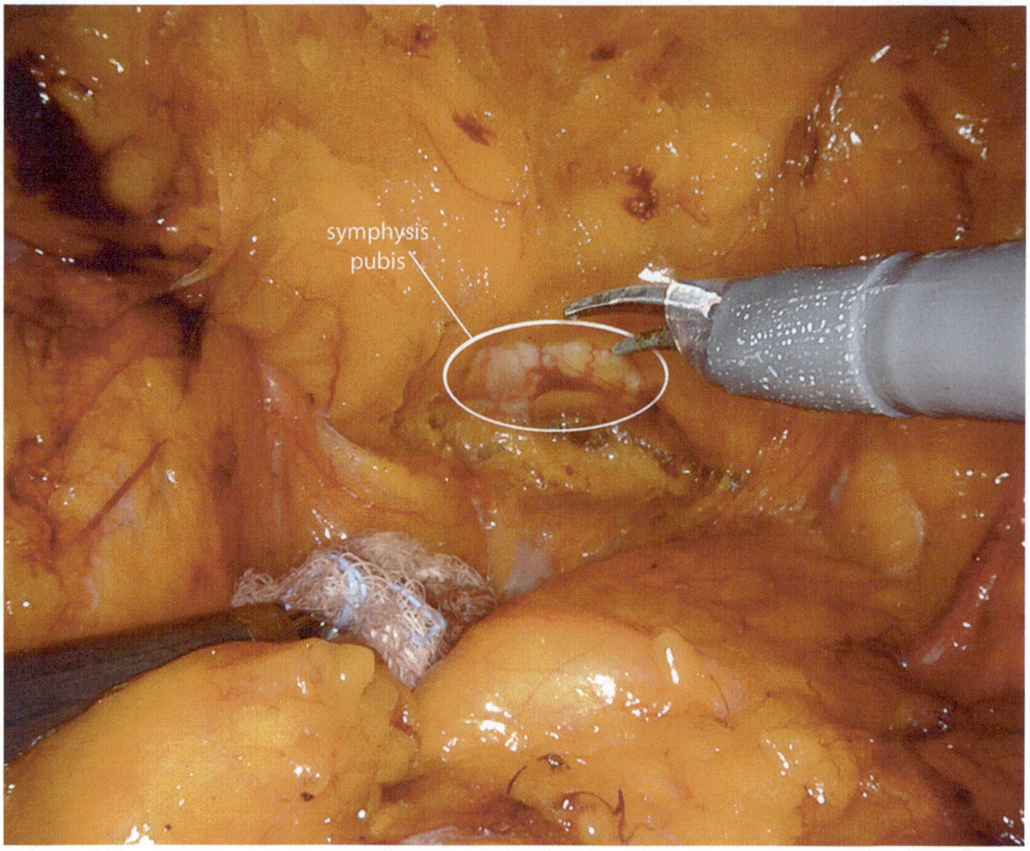


**Fig. 14.13** Preperitoneal dissection is completed at the supravesical fossa, and the symphysis pubis is identified

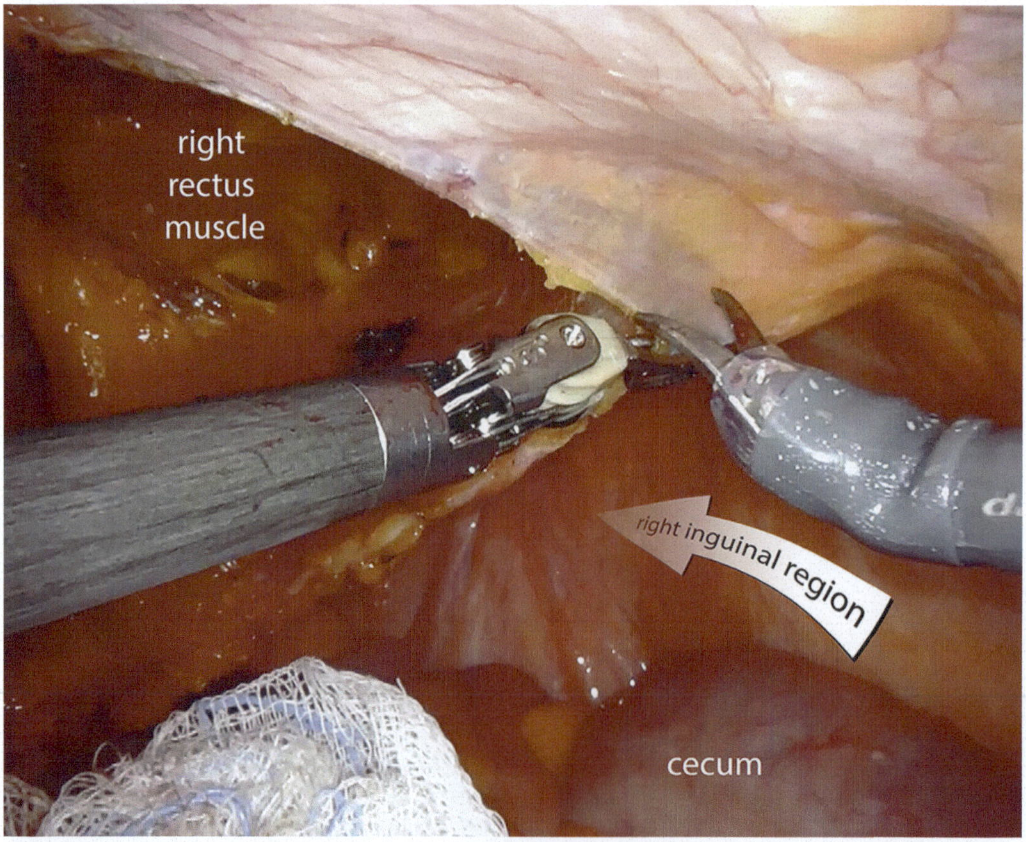


**Fig. 14.14** In some cases, enlargement of the peritoneal flap may be required; the initial peritoneal incision is extended laterally

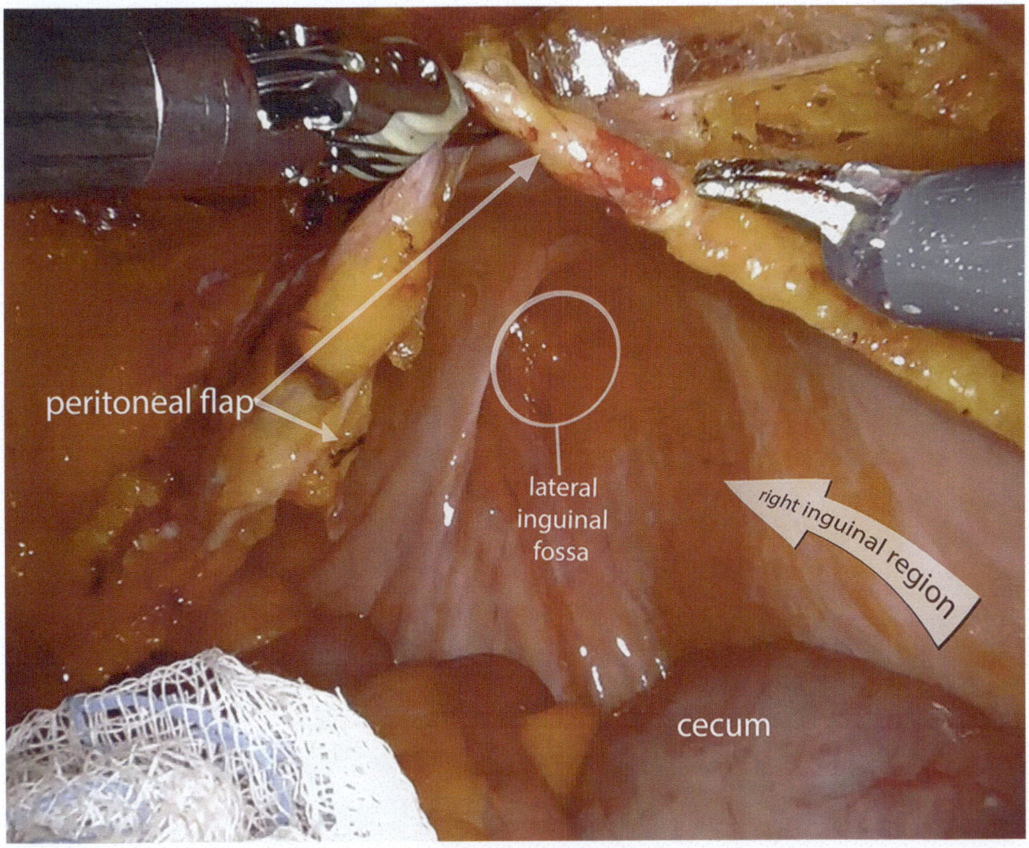


**Fig. 14.15** The right deep inguinal ring can be identified in the lateral inguinal fossa

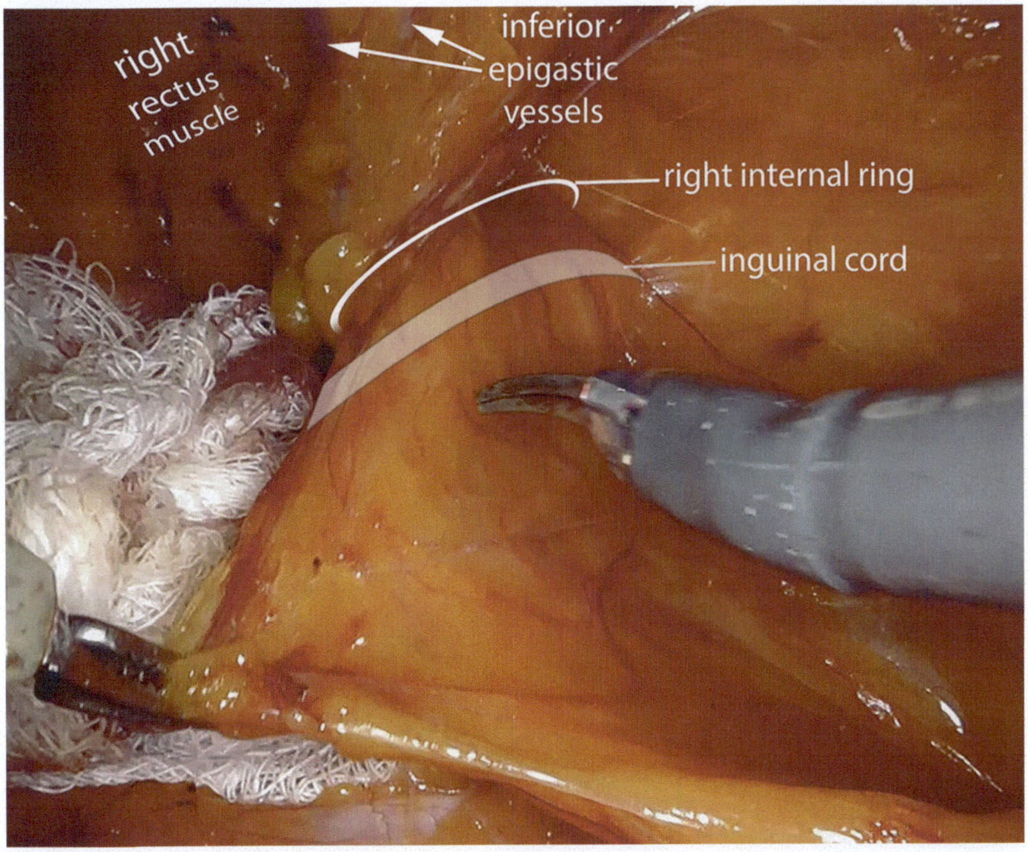


**Fig. 14.16** Once the peritoneal flap is developed at the right side, landmarks are identified: deep inguinal ring lateral to inferior epigastric vessels, and inguinal cord structures passing through the right internal ring

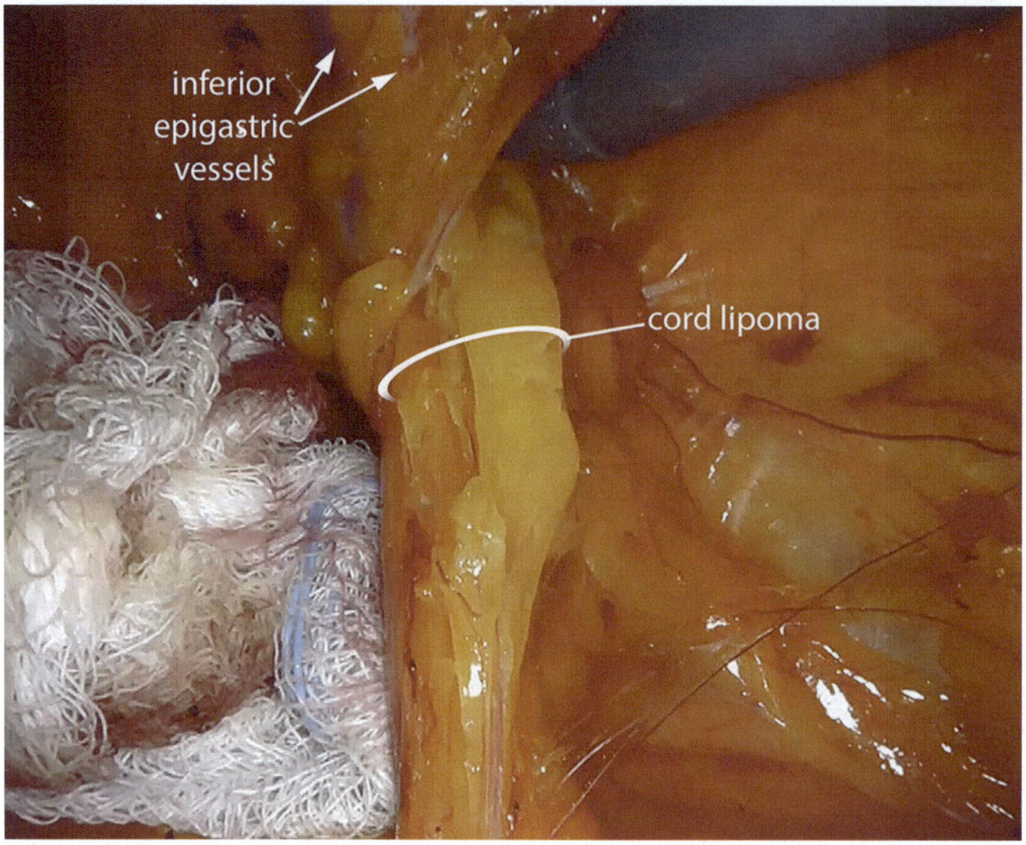


Fig. 14.17 Inguinal cord structures are separated, in order to identify the cord lipoma

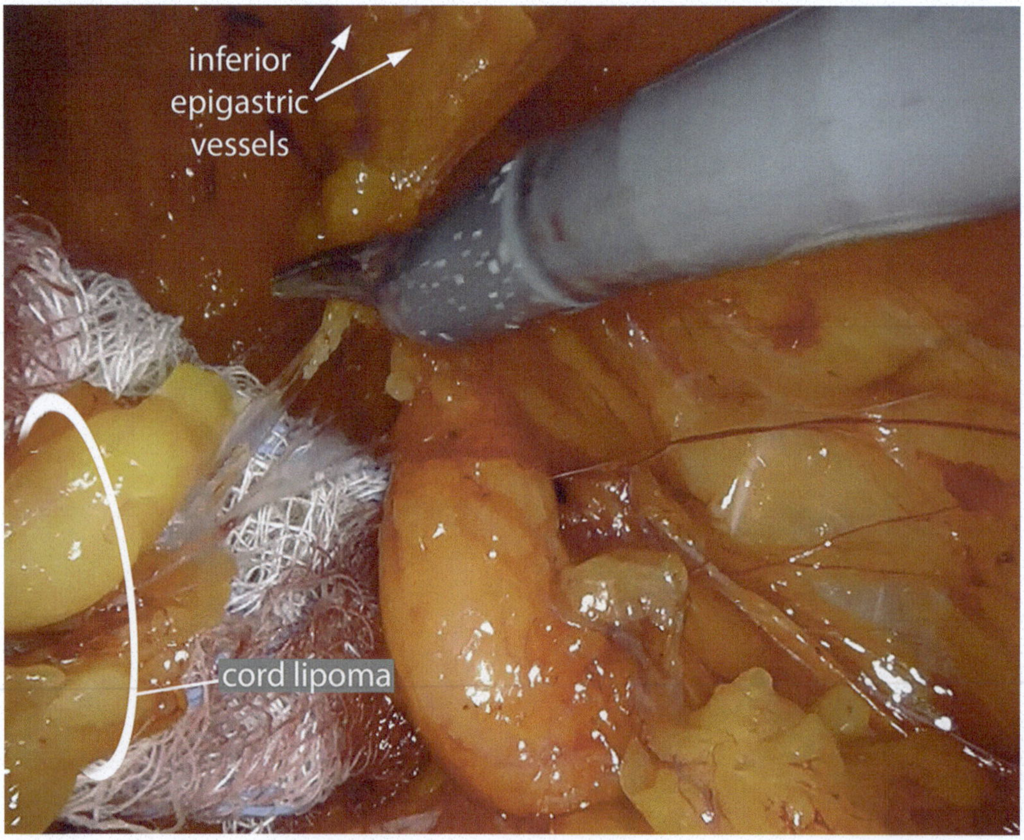


Fig. 14.18 Cord lipoma is excised from the inguinal canal

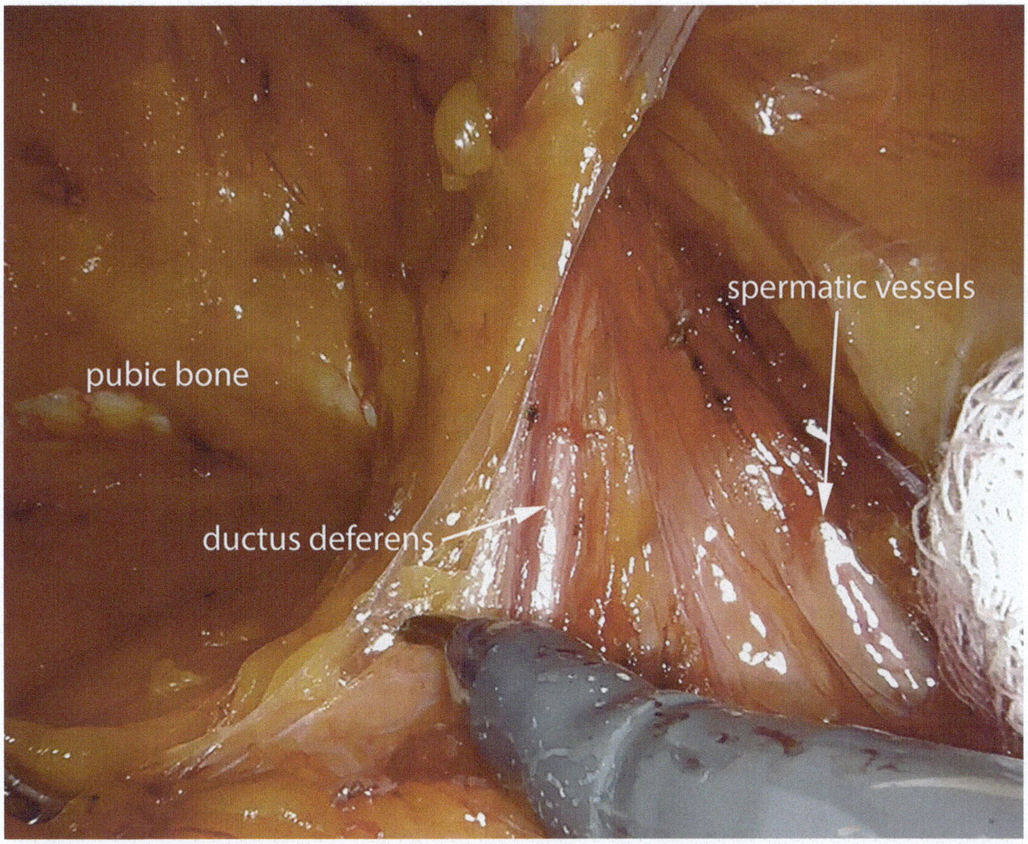


**Fig. 14.19** Surrounding structures are separated from the spermatic vessels and ductus deferens. The "triangle of doom" is identified

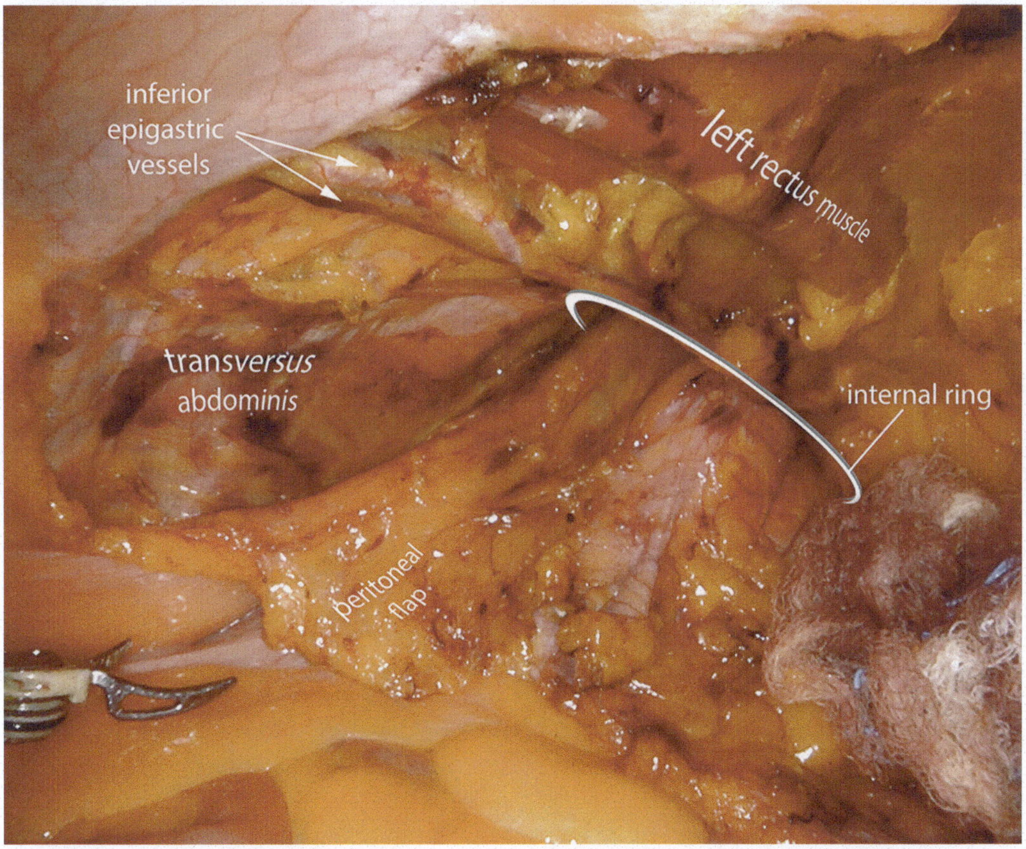


**Fig. 14.20** Preperitoneal view of the left inguinoscrotal hernia

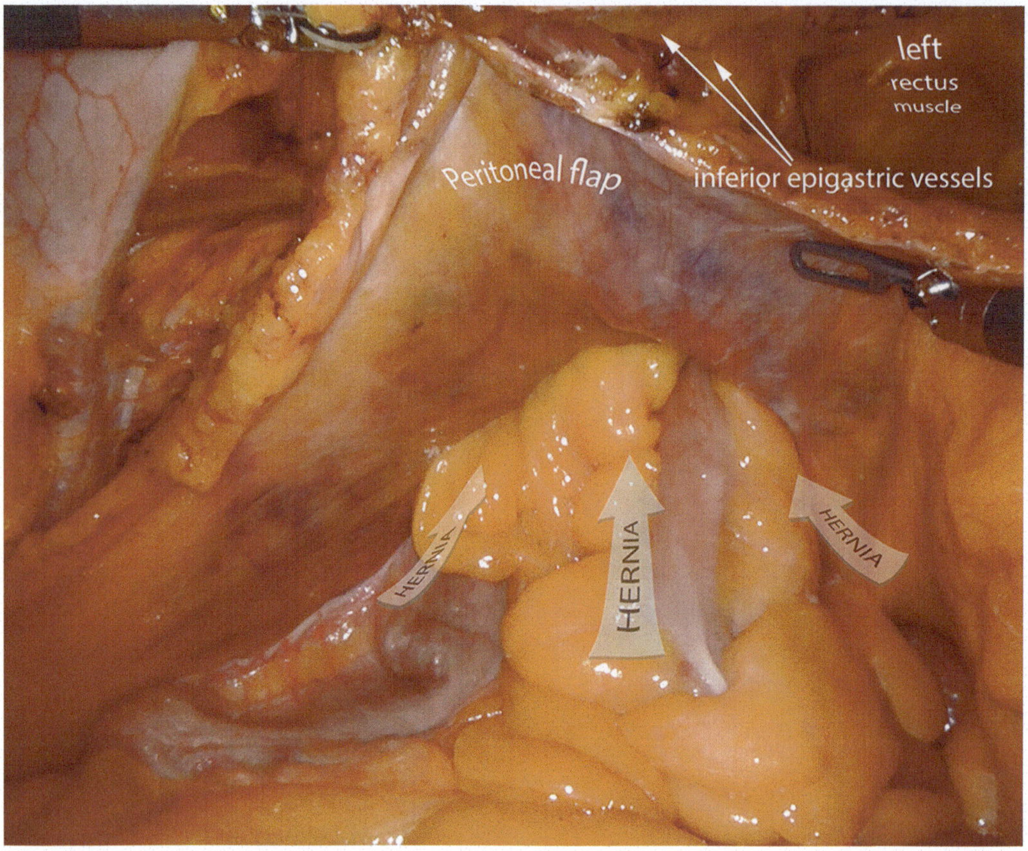


**Fig. 14.21** Intraperitoneal view, prior to reducing the hernia

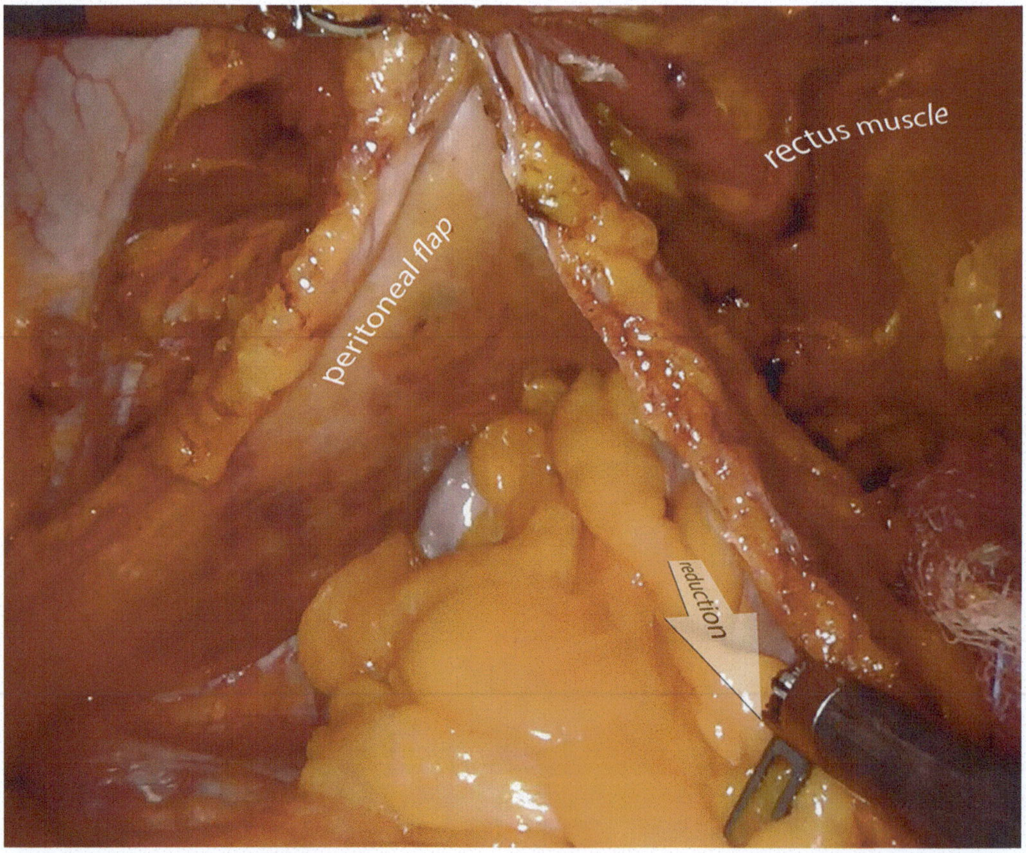


**Fig. 14.22** Beginning the hernia reduction

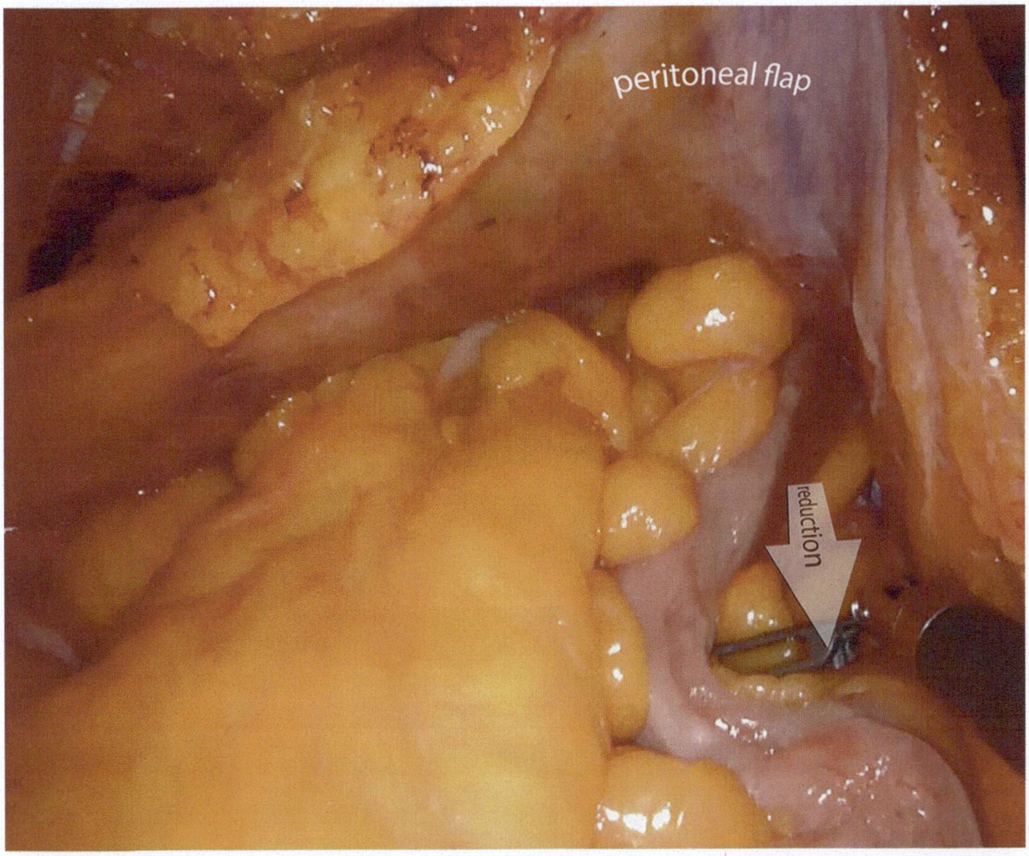


Fig. 14.23 External gentle pressure by the bedside assistant may facilitate reduction of the large amount of scrotal hernia content

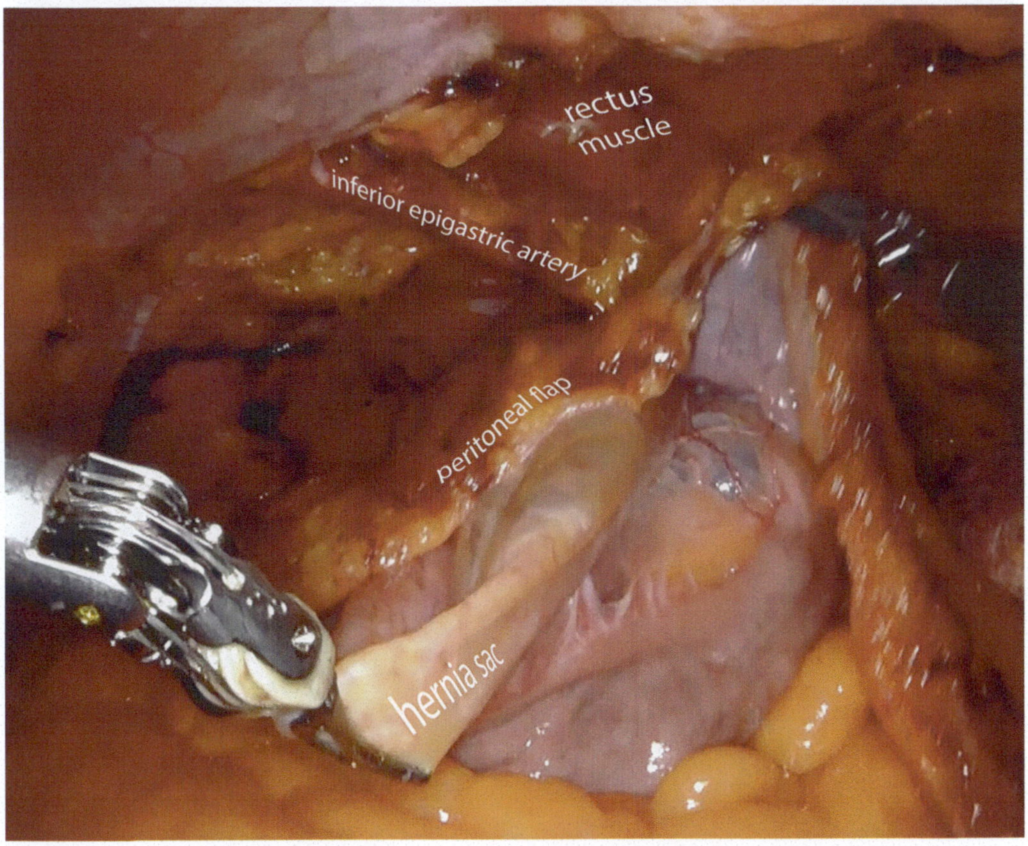


Fig. 14.24 Partially inverted hernia sac is shown after reduction of the hernia into the abdominal cavity

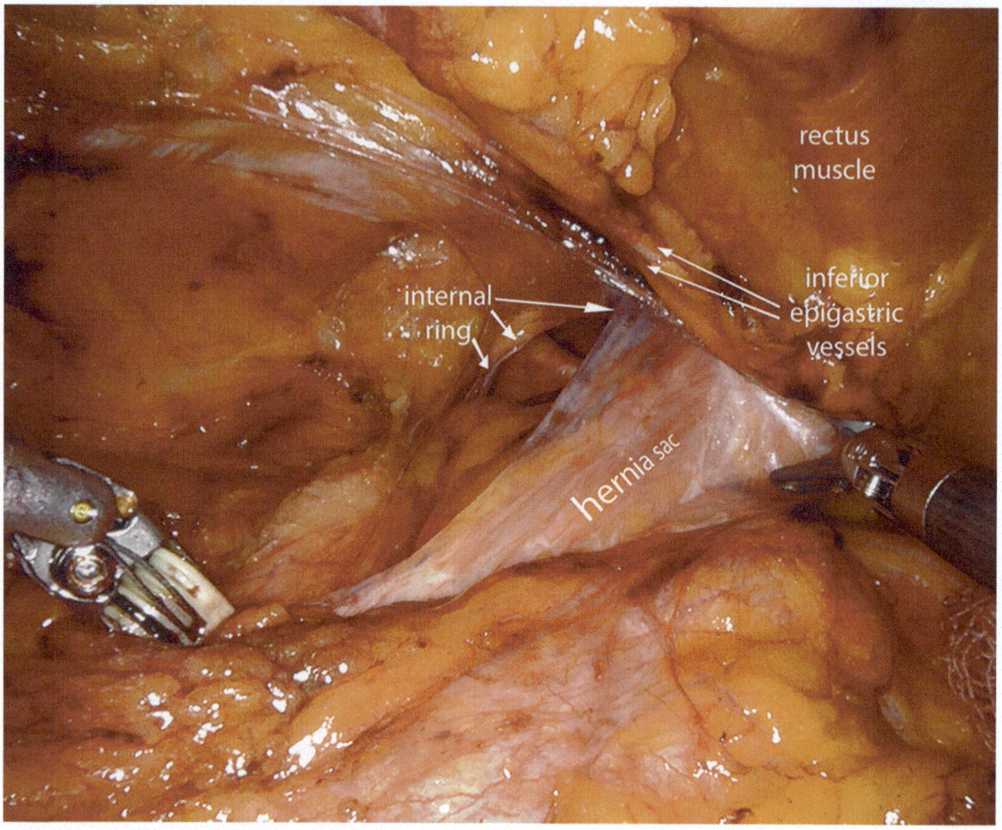


**Fig. 14.25** After the hernia is reduced, the hernia sac is identified through the internal ring

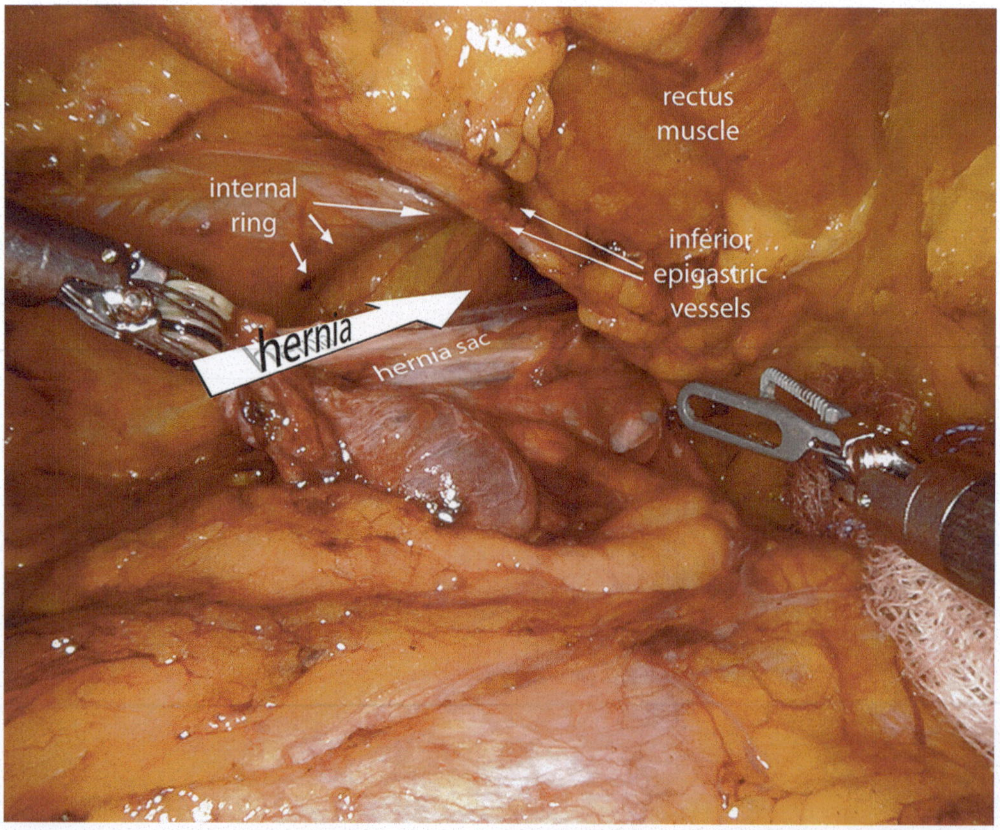


**Fig. 14.26** The hernia sac is dissected from its attachments, which are usually dense if the patient has had a long-standing history of scrotal hernia

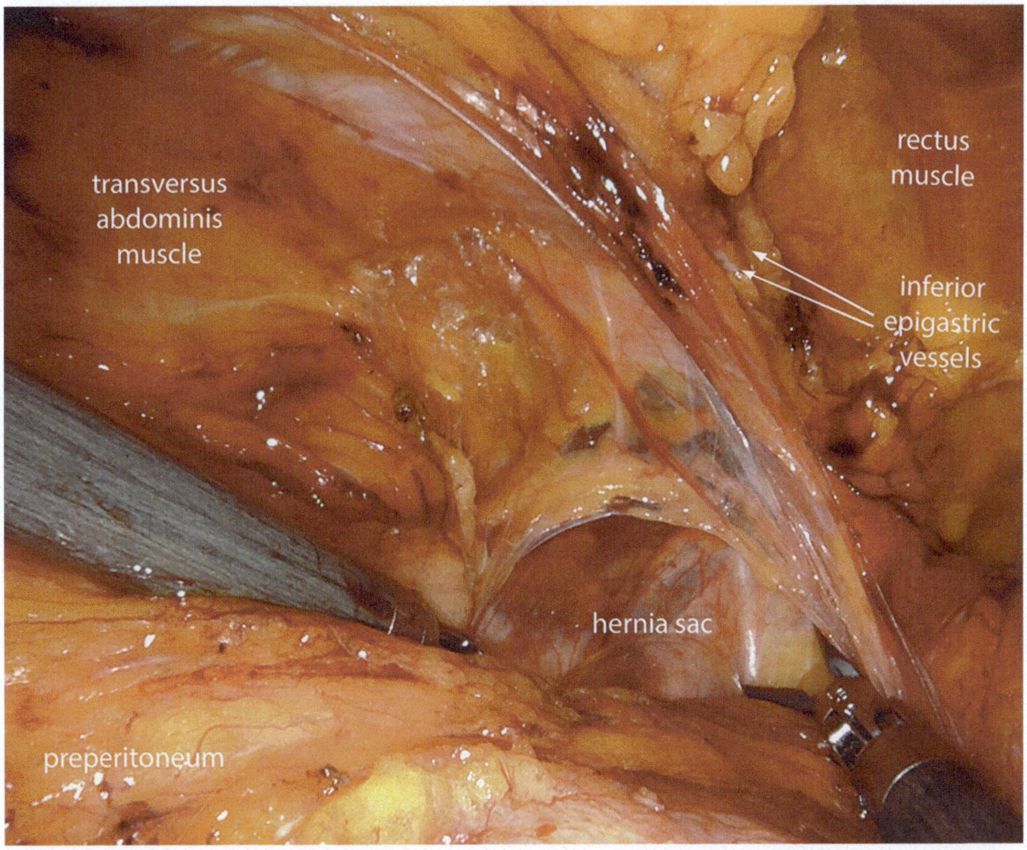


**Fig. 14.27** Careful dissection of the hernia sac is continued

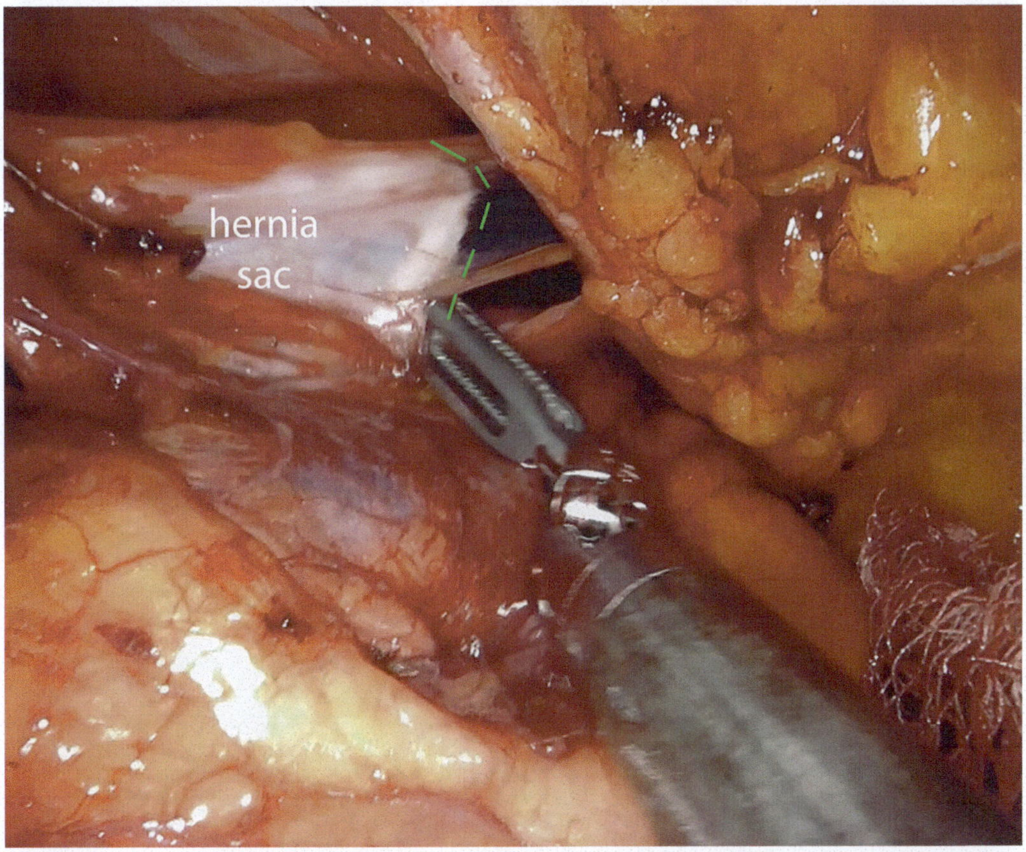


**Fig. 14.28** Gentle traction and contra-traction may facilitate identification of the border of the hernia sac and the dissection plane

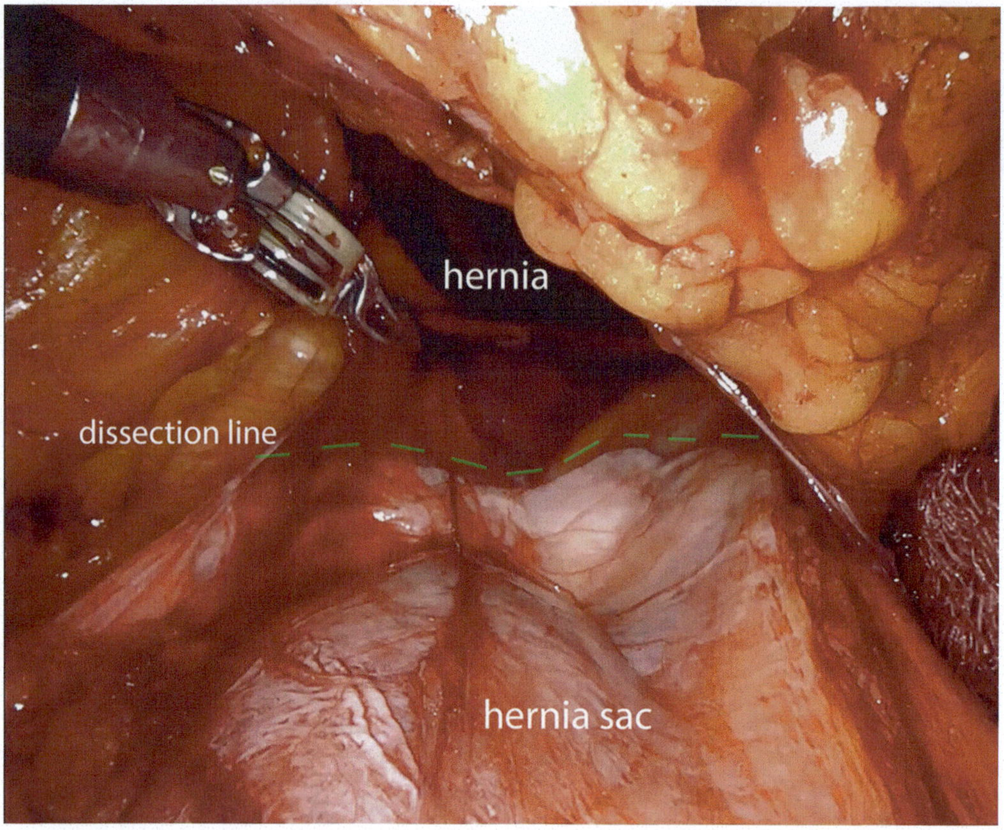


Fig. 14.29 The glistening white appearance of the peritoneum may help in recognition of the dissection line

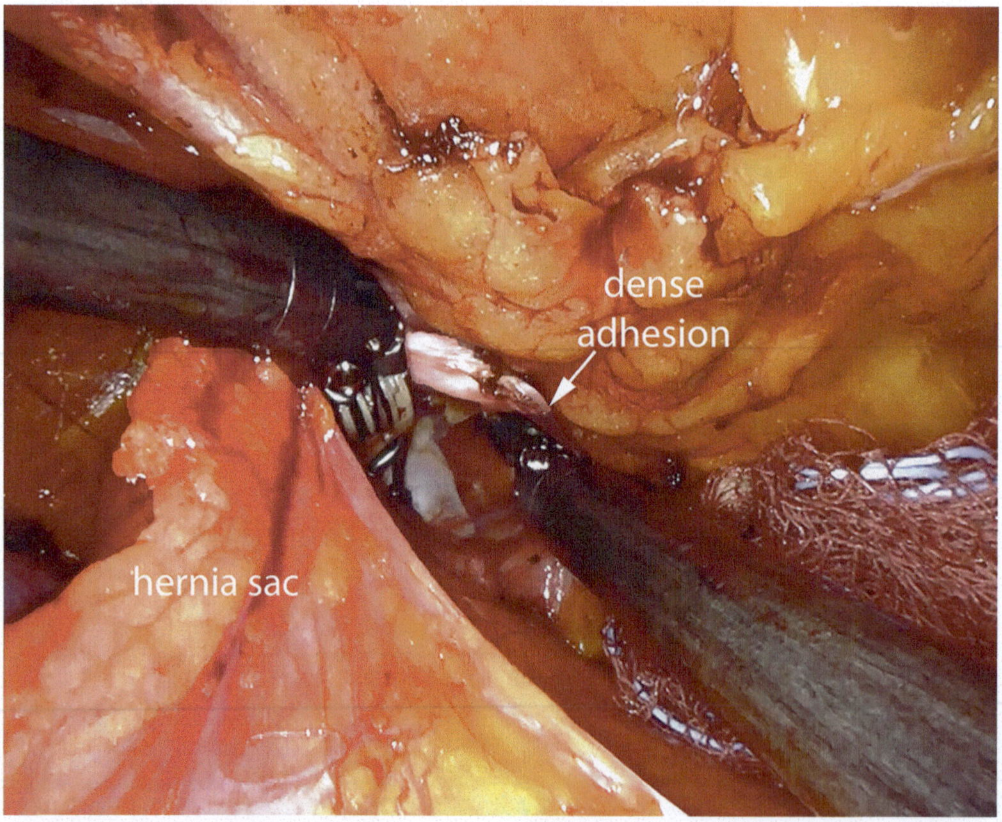


Fig. 14.30 A small window is opened at the posterior aspect of the hernia sac between the sac and the inguinal cord structures, owing to dense adhesions secondary to long-standing history of hernia

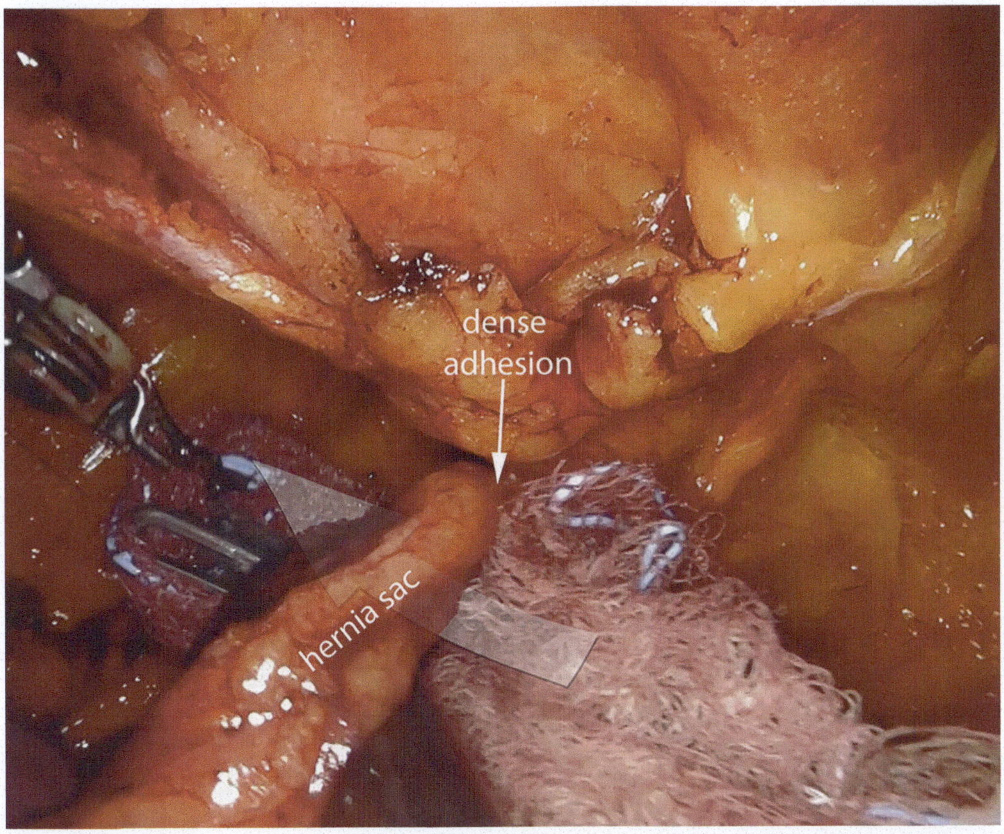


**Fig. 14.31** Throughout reduction of the hernia sac, caution is exercised so as to avoid injury to any of the structures in the triangle of doom (iliac vessels, gonadal vessels, vas deferens). Passing a sponge through the opened window can be one precautionary measure

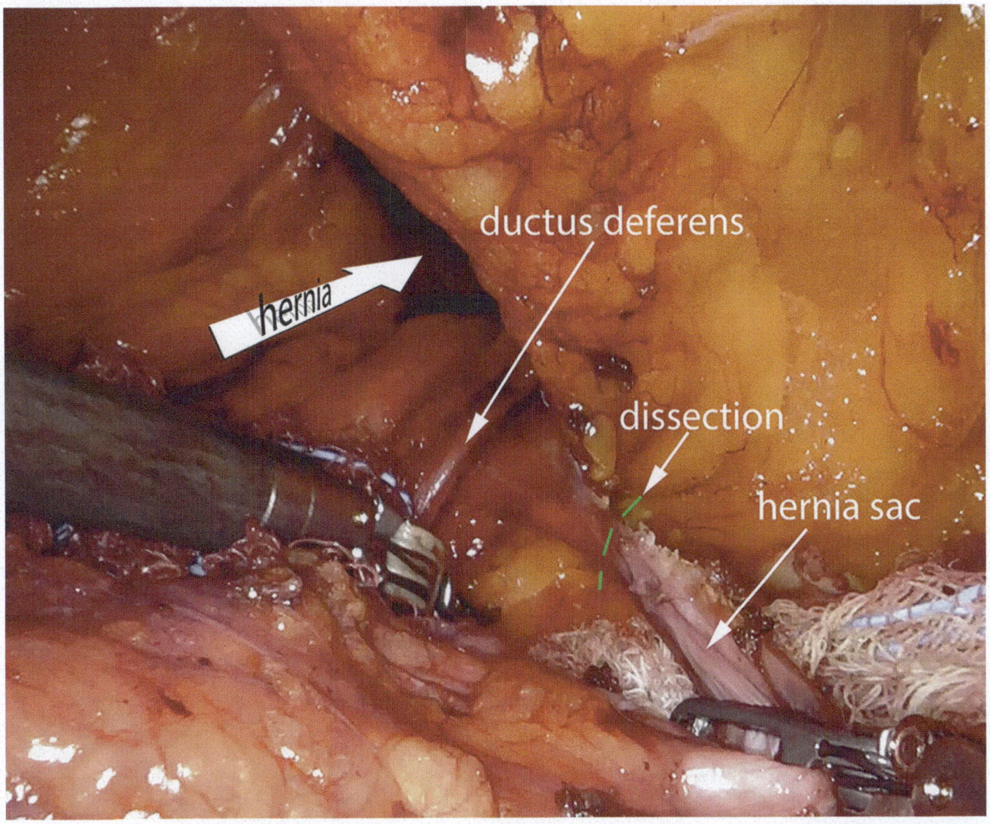


**Fig. 14.32** Dissection of dense adhesions

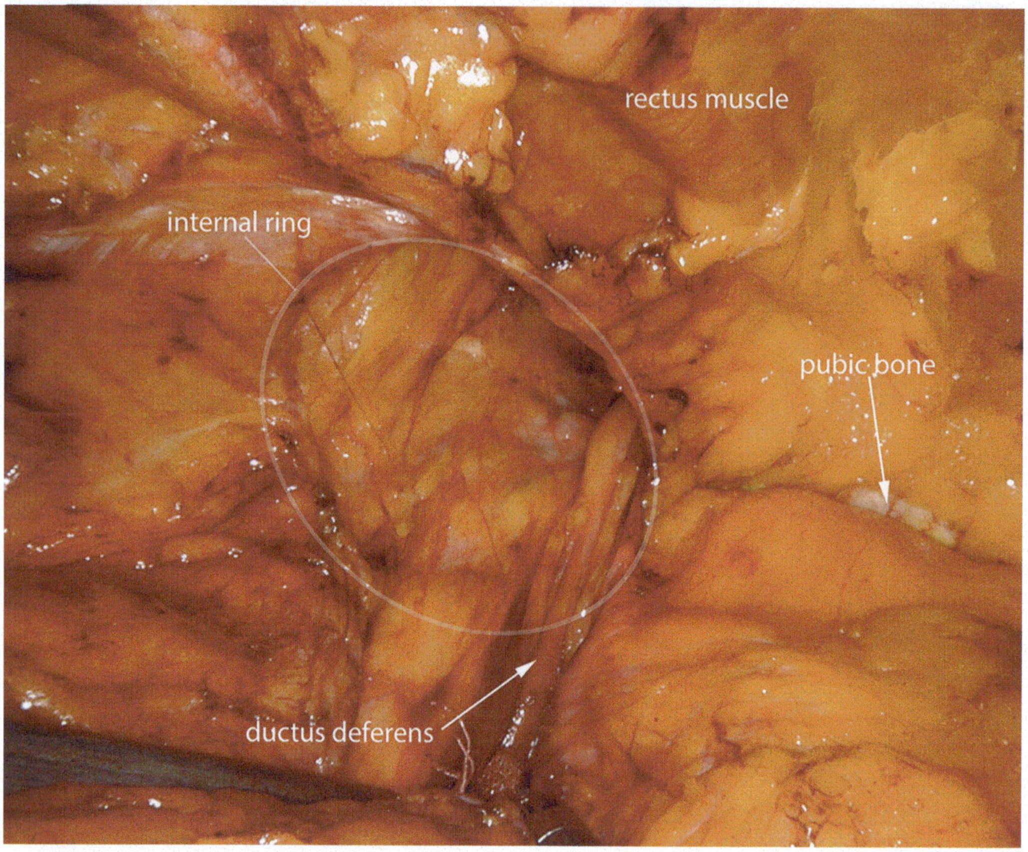


**Fig. 14.33** Posterior dissection is continued in order to obtain proper mesh overlap at the posterior side of the myopectineal orifice

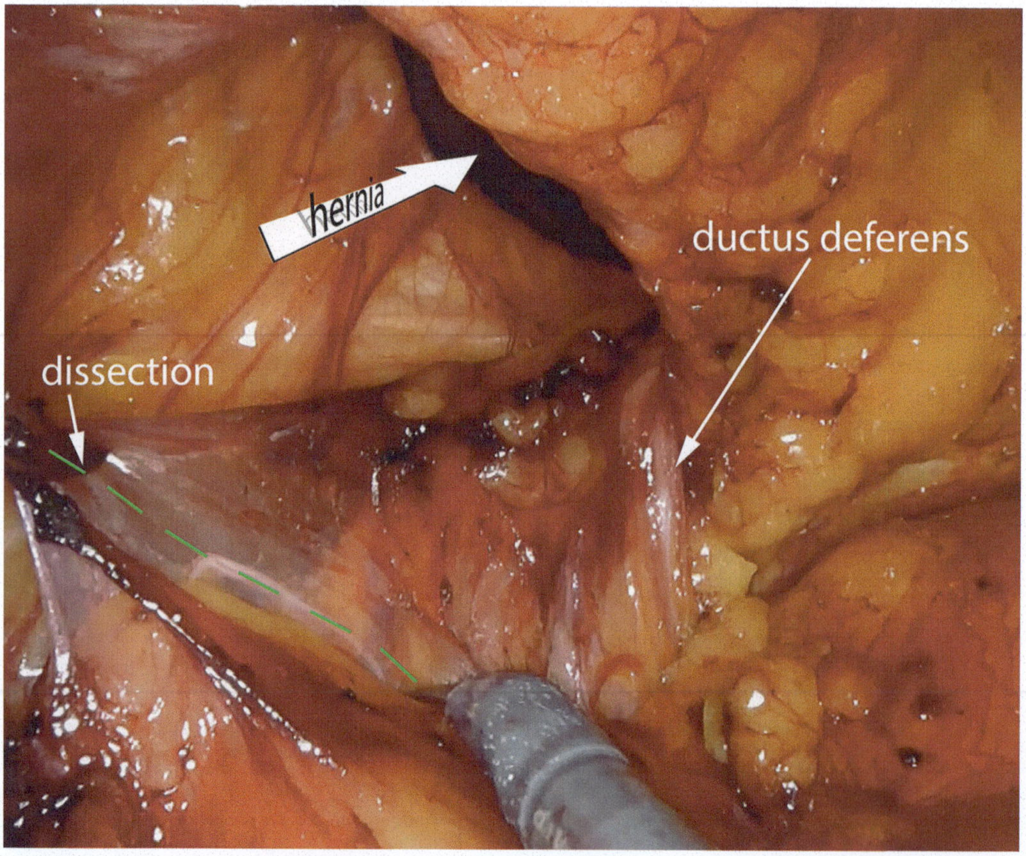


**Fig. 14.34** The inguinal cord is dissected to reveal its separate components

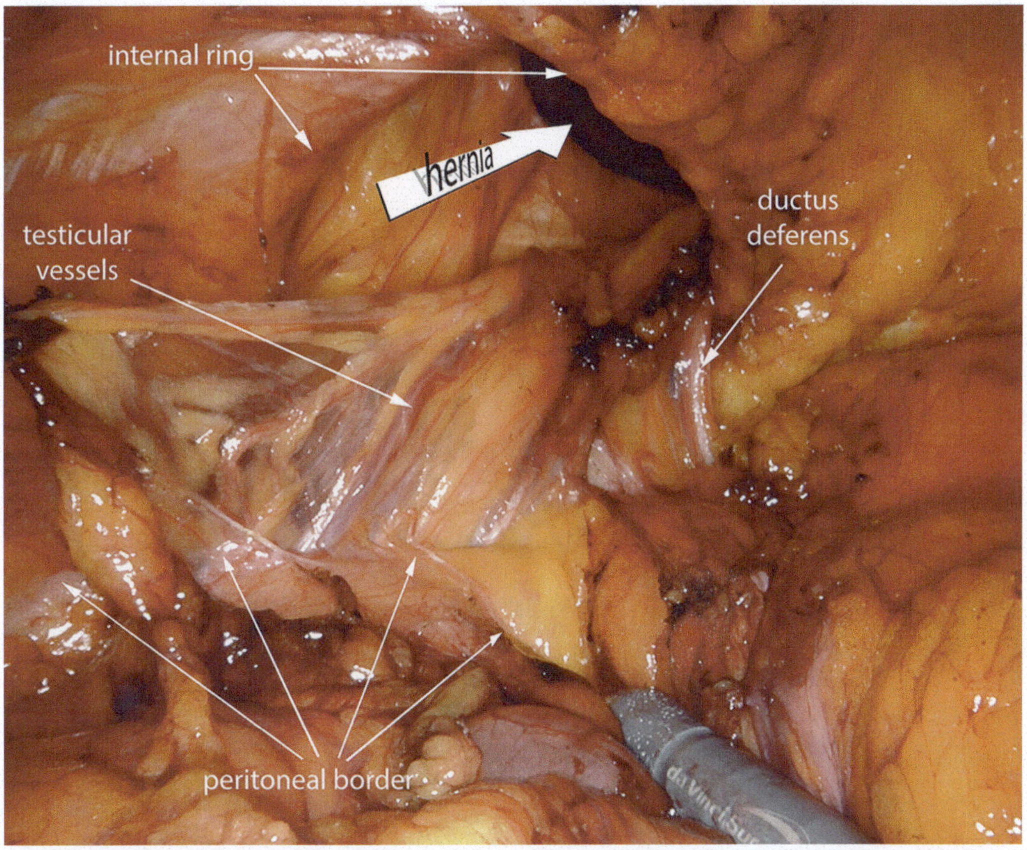


**Fig. 14.35** Continuation of the posterior dissection

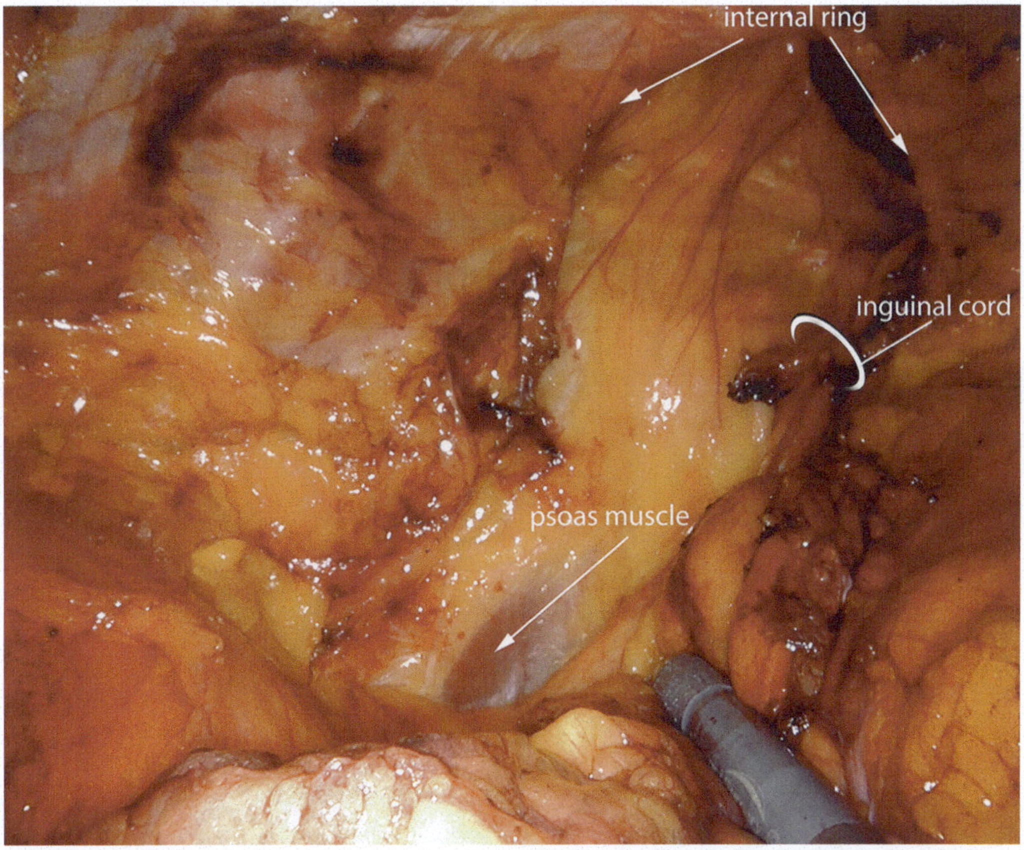


**Fig. 14.36** Psoas muscle is identified

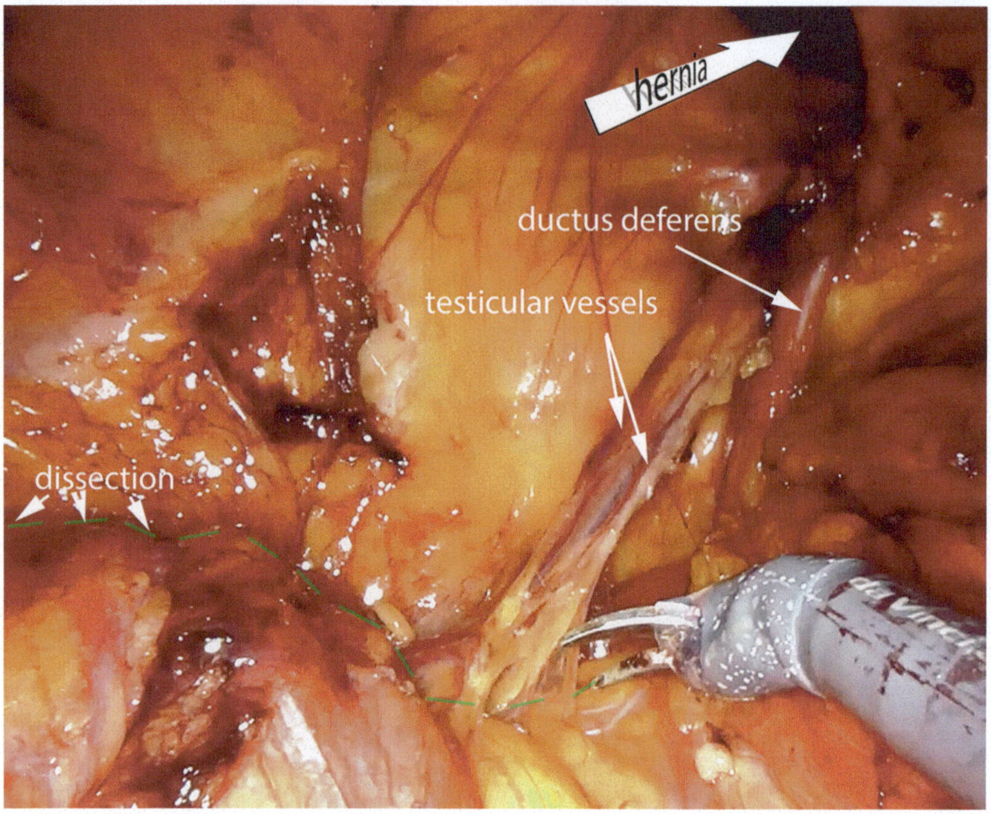


**Fig. 14.37** The hernia sac is completely dissected and separated from the spermatic vessels, ductus deferens, and other surrounding structures; the "doom triangle" is identified

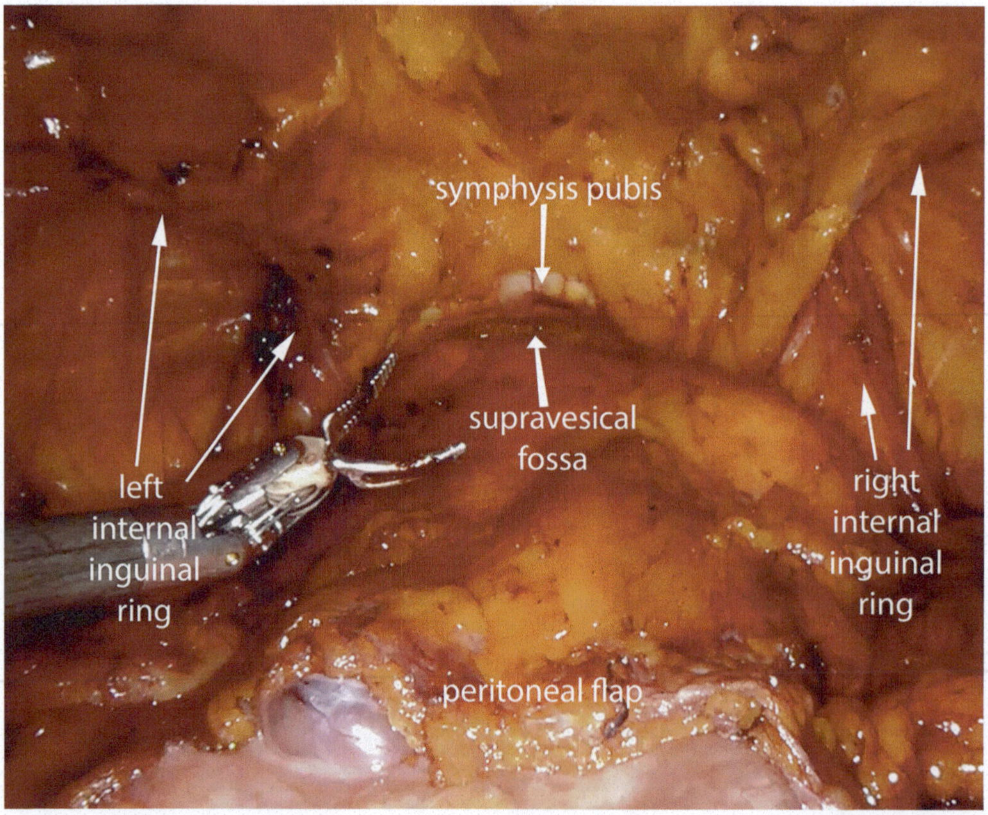


**Fig. 14.38** View of both inguinal regions

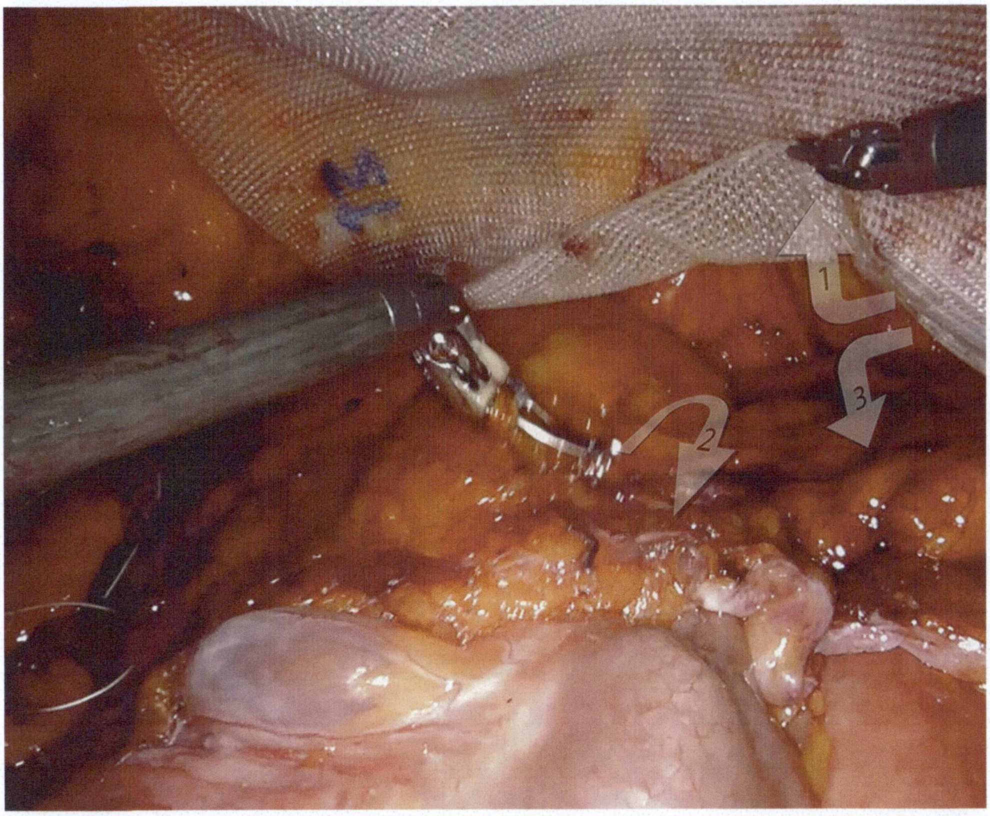


**Fig. 14.39** An anatomical mesh is inserted into the abdominal cavity and placed in its correct position (right side). 1 The inferior border of the mesh is lifted, 2 The peritoneal flap is retracted, 3 The inferior mesh border is placed between the peritoneal flap and the abdominal wall, ensuring adequate overlap across the hernia site

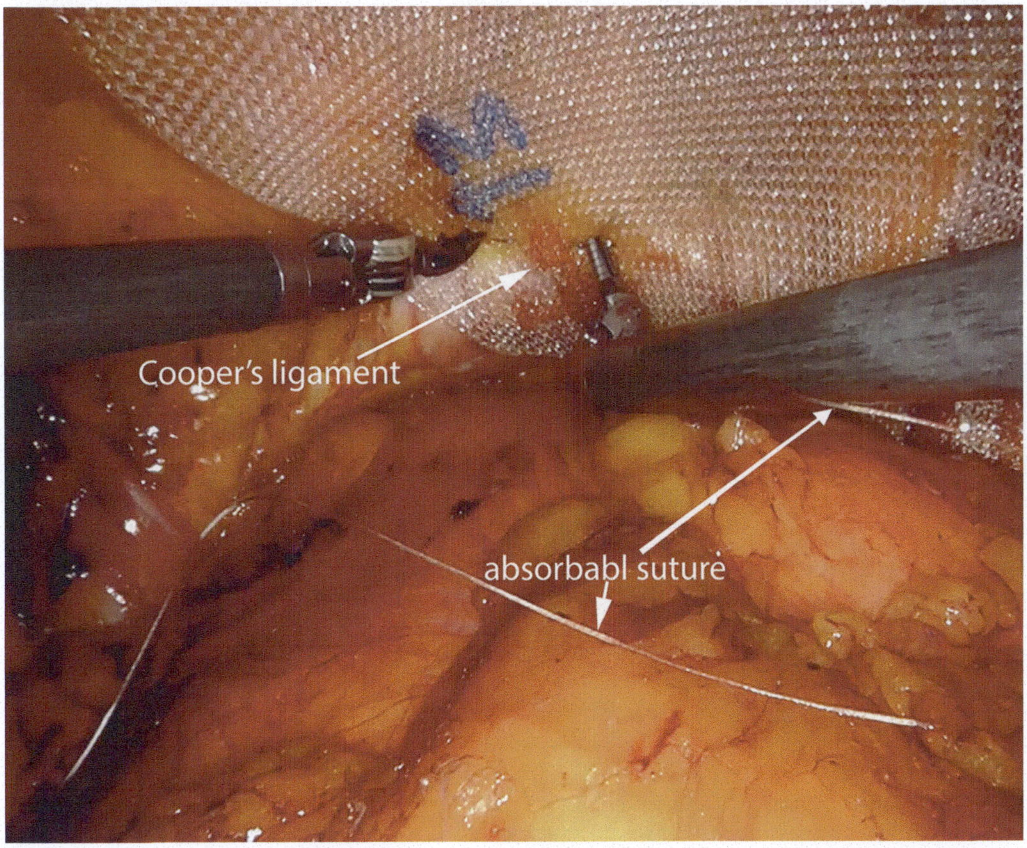


**Fig. 14.40** The mesh is fixated to Cooper's ligament using an absorbable suture

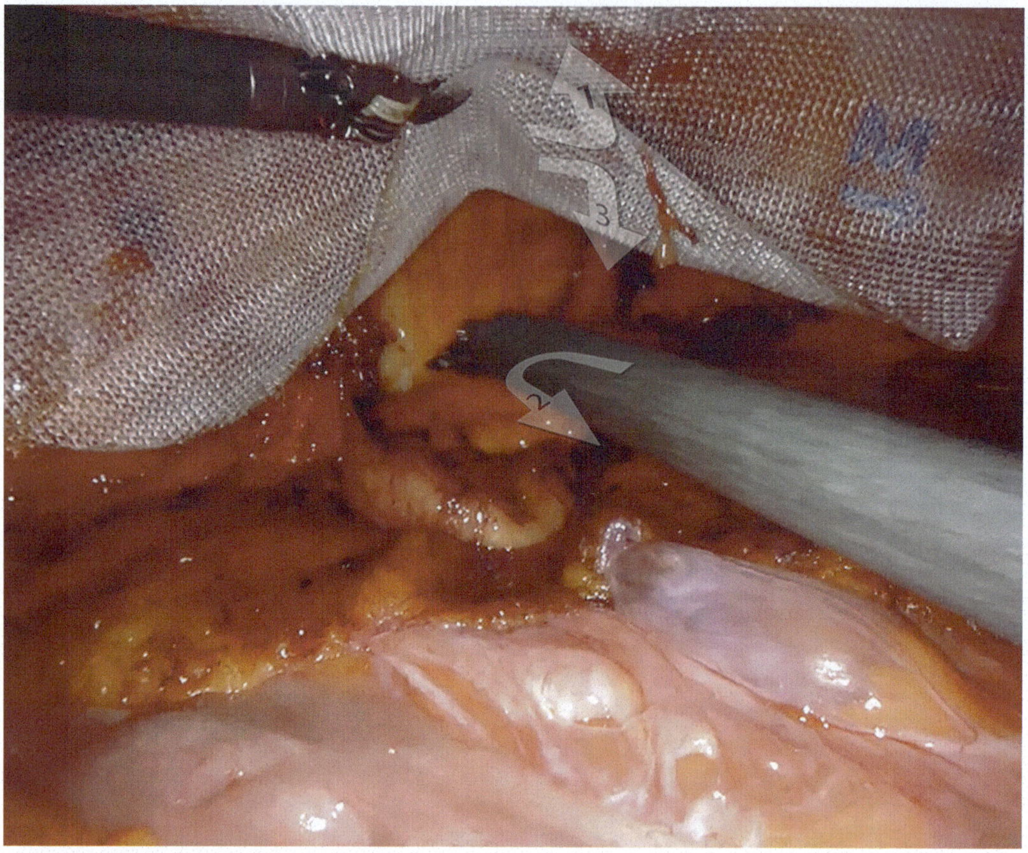


**Fig. 14.41** Another mesh is placed its correct position on the left side, following the same steps described in Fig. 14.39

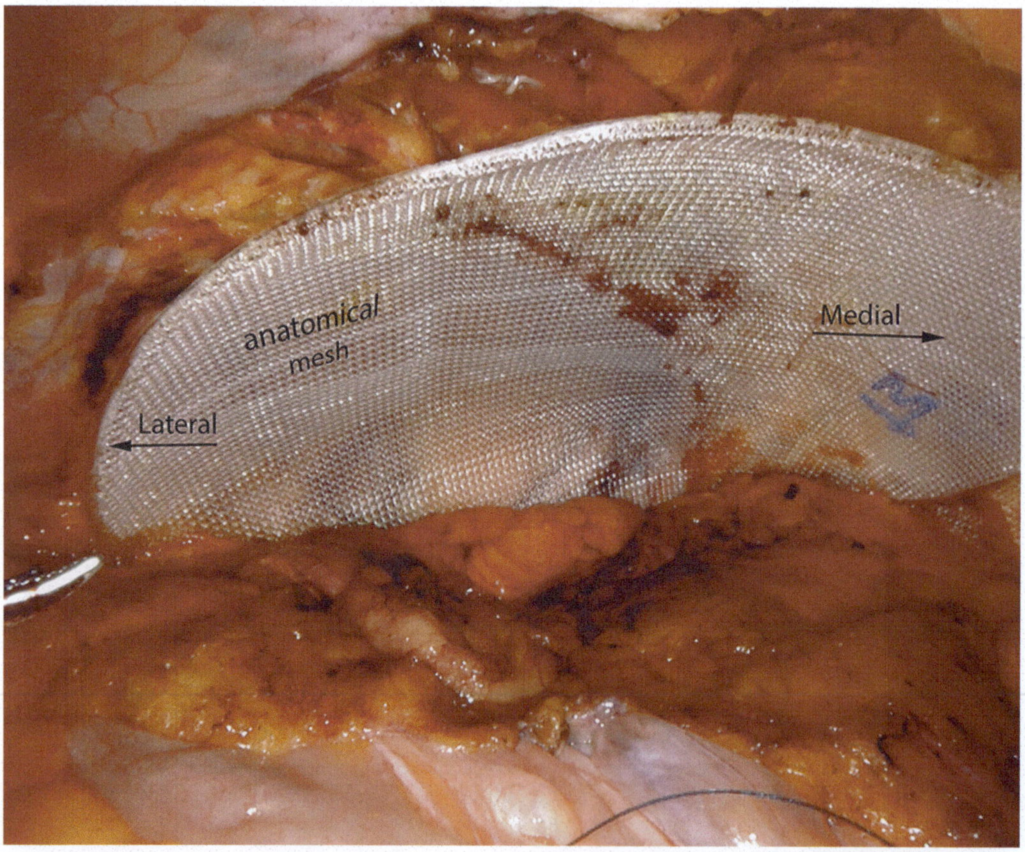


**Fig. 14.42** After the mesh is deployed, it is important to ensure that the mesh is unhindered and occupies the entire preperitoneal space

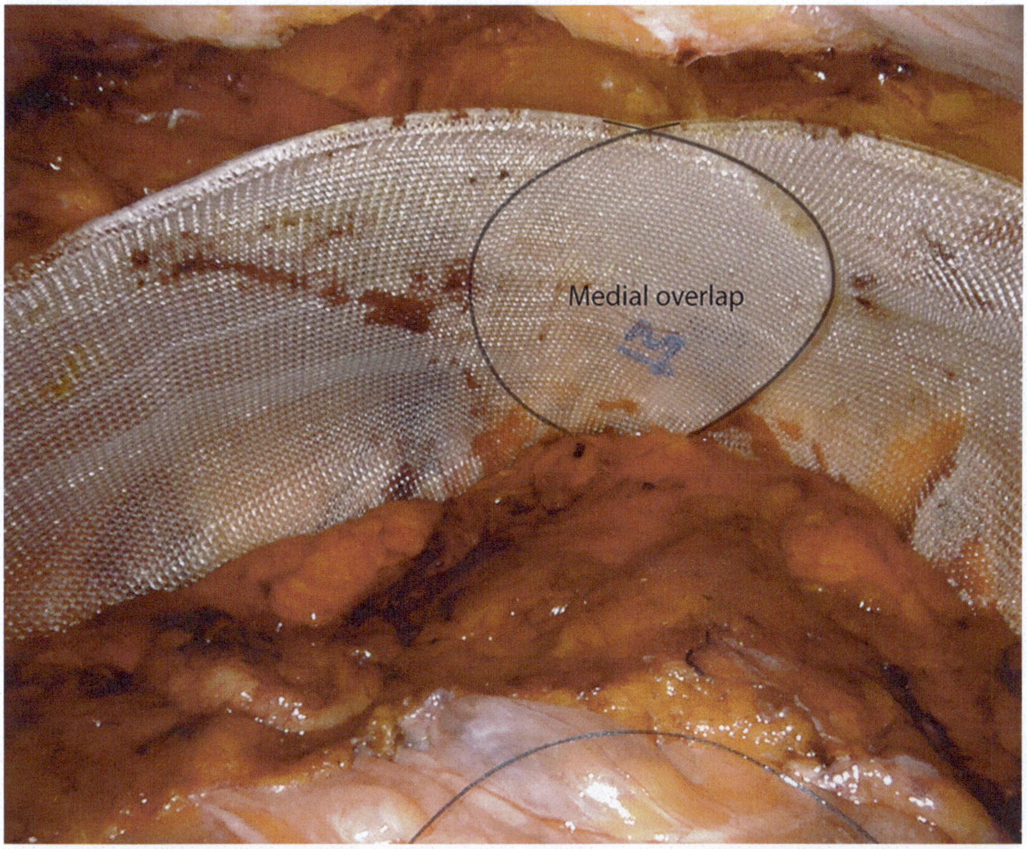


**Fig. 14.43** Medial borders of both meshes need to overlap by 2–4 cm under the symphysis pubis

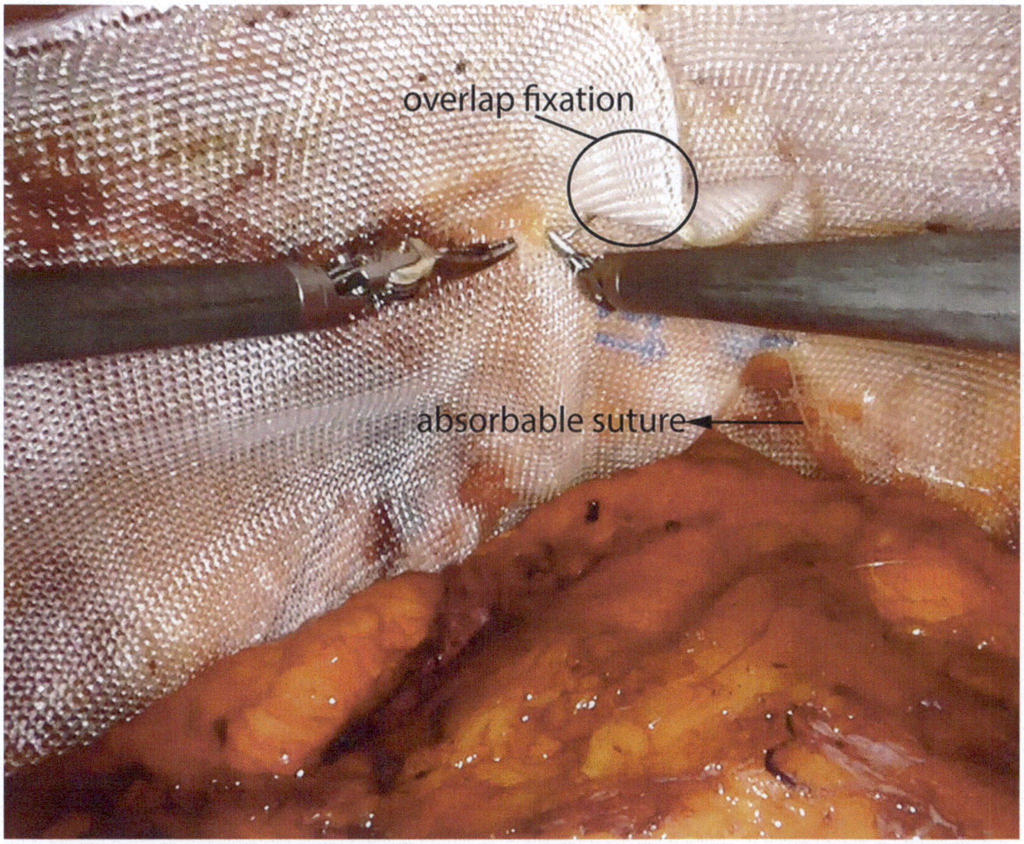


**Fig. 14.44** Medial overlap is fixated with an absorbable suture

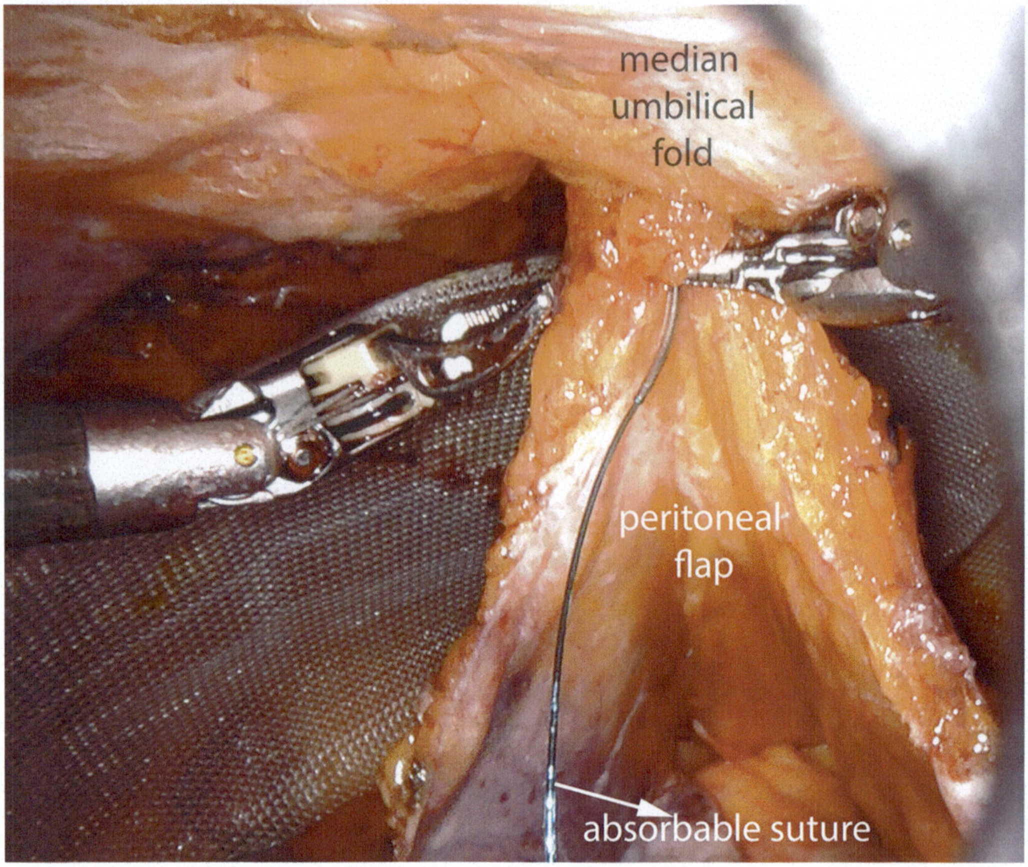


Fig. 14.45 Once the mesh is secured in place, closure of the peritoneal flap is initiated with barbed suture, starting from the median umbilical fold

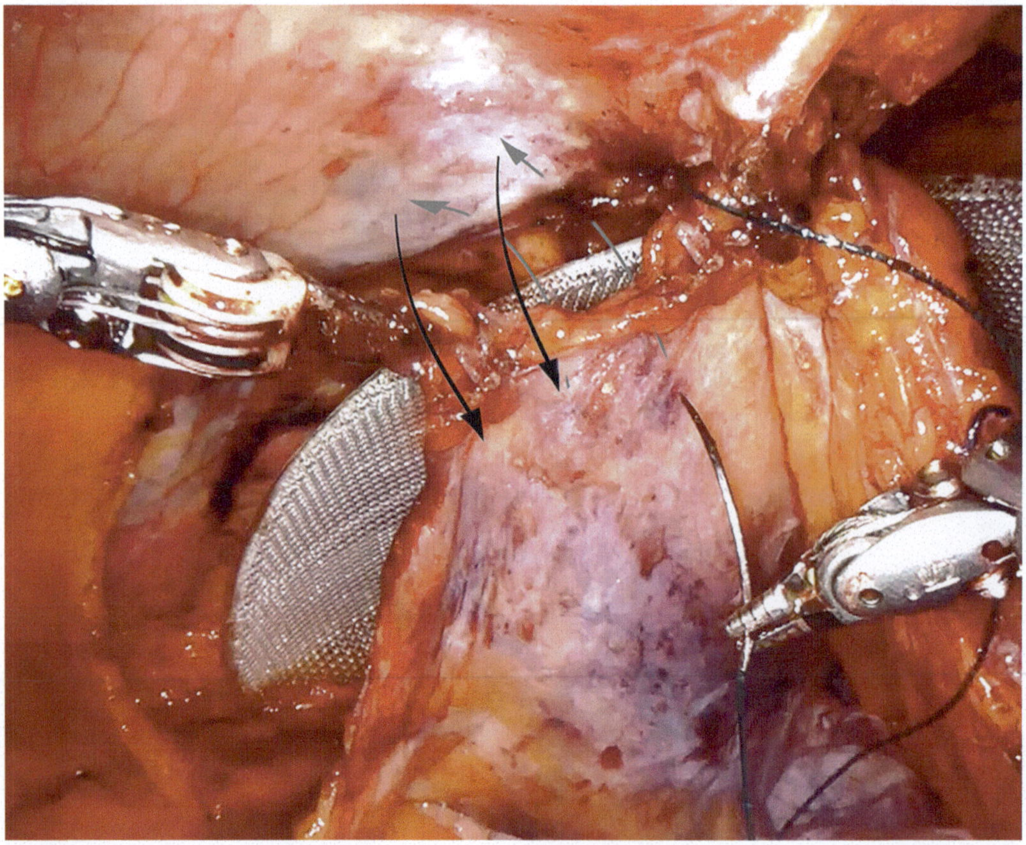

Fig. 14.46 "Backhand" suturing may facilitate closure of the peritoneal flap

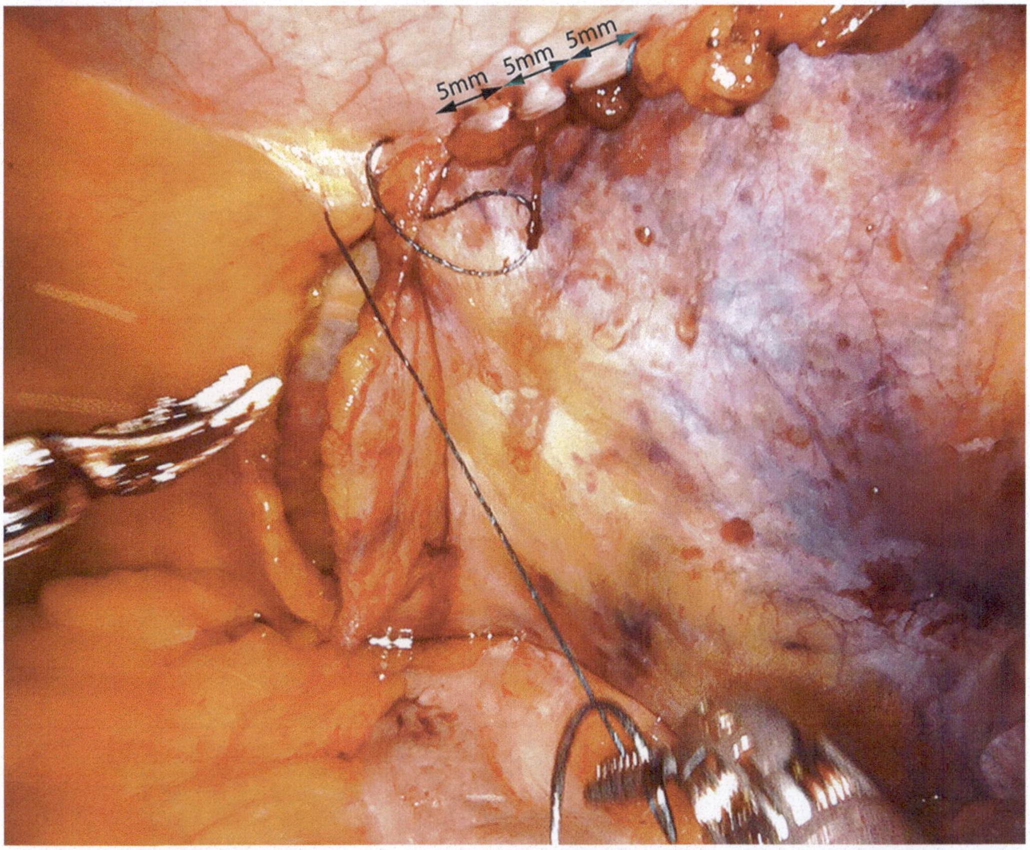


**Fig. 14.47** Suturing with small bites in a continuous fashion prevents postoperative internal herniation through the peritoneal flap

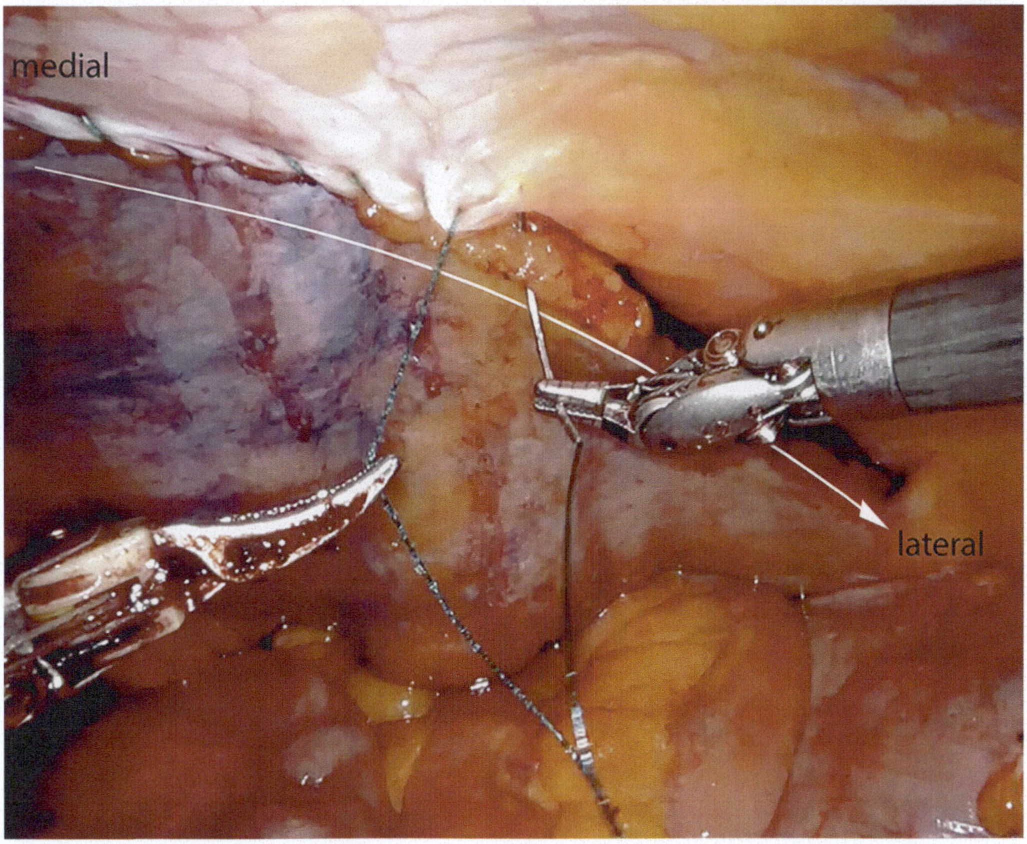


**Fig. 14.48** Similar steps are repeated for the right side

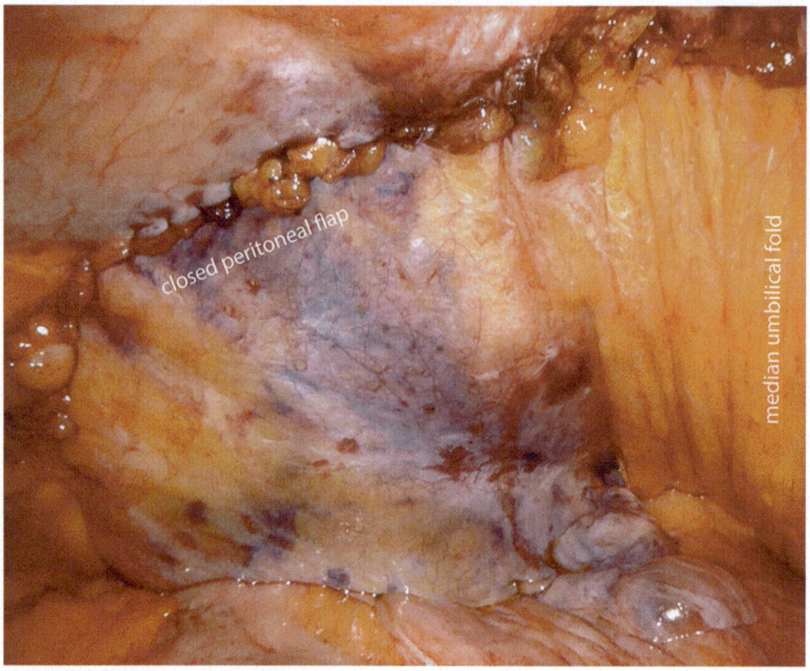


Fig. 14.49 After closure of the left side

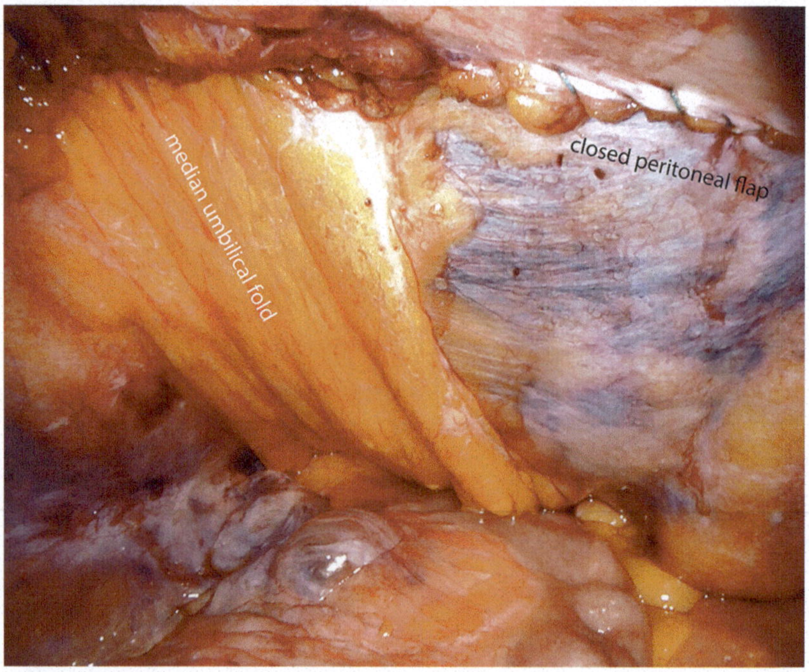


Fig. 14.50 After closure of the right side

## References

1. Roll S, Skinovsky J. Laparoscopic TAPP inguinal hernia repair. In: Novitsky YW, editor. Hernia surgery: current principles. Cham: Springer; 2016. p. 451–9.
2. Iraniha A, Peloquin J. Long-term quality of life and outcomes following robotic assisted TAPP inguinal hernia repair. J Robot Surg. 2018;12:261–9. https://doi.org/10.1007/s11701-017-0727-8.
3. Kudsi OY, McCarty JC, Paluvoi N, Mabardy AS. Transition from laparoscopic totally extraperitoneal inguinal hernia repair to robotic transabdominal preperitoneal inguinal hernia repair: a retrospective review of a single surgeon's experience. World J Surg. 2019;41:2251–7. https://doi.org/10.1007/s00268-017-3998-3.

# Robotic Direct Inguinal Hernia Repair: Transabdominal Preperitoneal (TAPP)

15

Agustin Alvarez and Omar Yusef Kudsi

## Introduction

Robotic transabdominal preperitoneal (TAPP) inguinal hernia repair (IHR) is considered analogous to the laparoscopic approach performed with different instruments. Prior experience in minimally invasive inguinal hernia repair is critical for success and the ability to reproduce a high-quality repair. If the well-established steps of TAPP IHR are not adhered to, then postoperative complications could be significant [1].

Technically, by inverting the lax fascia transversalis and closing the defect, the incidence of seroma and hematoma formation can be lessened after TAPP repair of large direct defects [2, 3]. Furthermore, proponents of closing the defects consider in theory that the greater contact surface of the prosthesis with the tissue is much better for tissue reintegration. Regarding securing of the prosthetic material, non-fixation of mesh has been recommended in minimally invasive management of all inguinal hernia types, except that mesh fixation is recommended for repair of large medial defects (direct hernias) [2].

## Procedure: Illustrated Steps

Figures 15.1, 15.2, 15.3, 15.4, 15.5, 15.6, 15.7, 15.8, 15.9, 15.10, 15.11, 15.12, 15.13, 15.14, 15.15, 15.16, 15.17, 15.18, 15.19, 15.20, 15.21, 15.22, 15.23, 15.24, 15.25, 15.26, 15.27, 15.28, 15.29, 15.30, 15.31, 15.32, 15.33, 15.34, 15.35, 15.36, 15.37, and 15.38 illustrate the technical aspects of robotic TAPP-IHR for direct hernia.

A. Alvarez
Division of Endocrine Surgery, DeWitt Daughtry Family Department of Surgery, Leonard M. Miller School of Medicine, University of Miami, Miami, FL, USA

O. Y. Kudsi (✉)
Department of Surgery, Good Samaritan Medical Center, Tufts University School of Medicine, Boston, MA, USA


O. Y. Kudsi (ed.), *Robotic Hernia Surgery*, https://doi.org/10.1007/978-3-030-46667-1_15

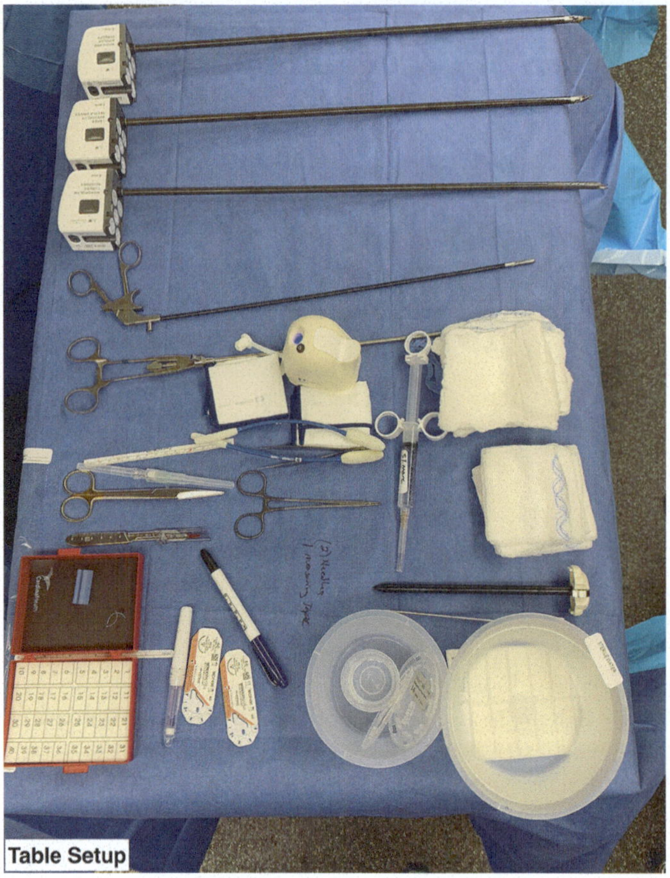


**Fig. 15.1** Robotic inguinal hernia table setup

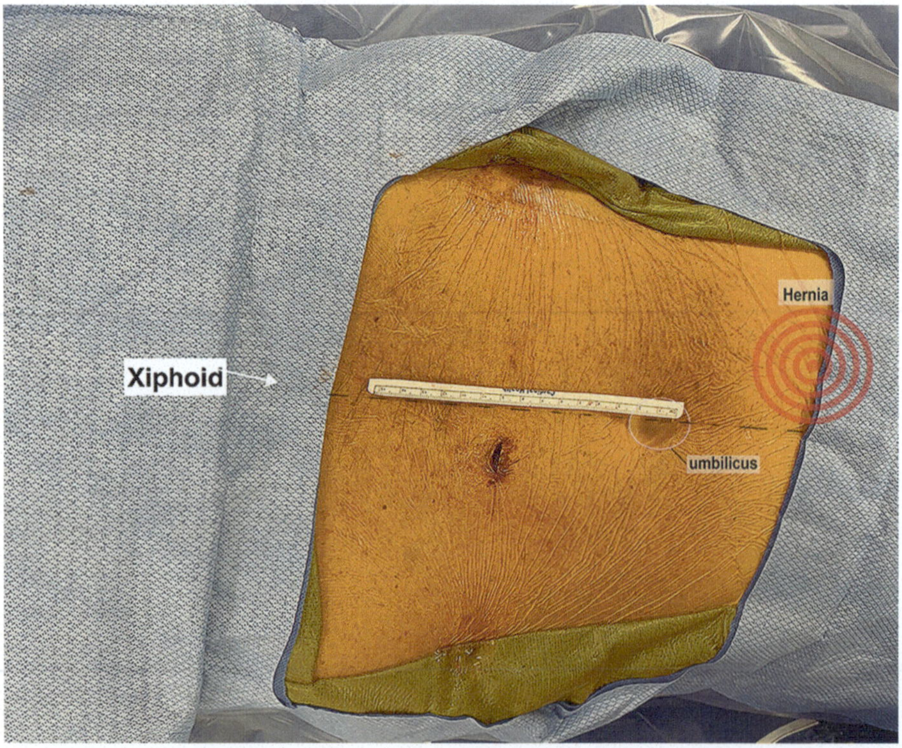


**Fig. 15.2** Incision for the first trocar (8.5 mm) is performed at approximately 8–10 cm above the umbilical level, off-midline

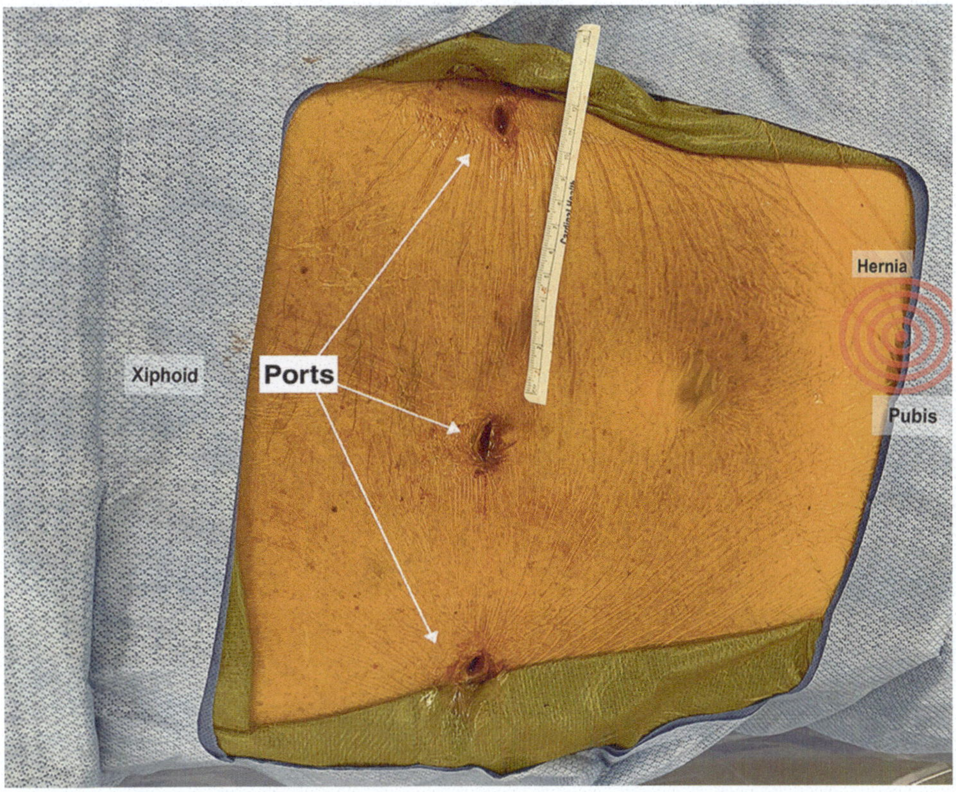


**Fig. 15.3** A minimum distance of 8 cm is recommended between trocars (8.5 mm)

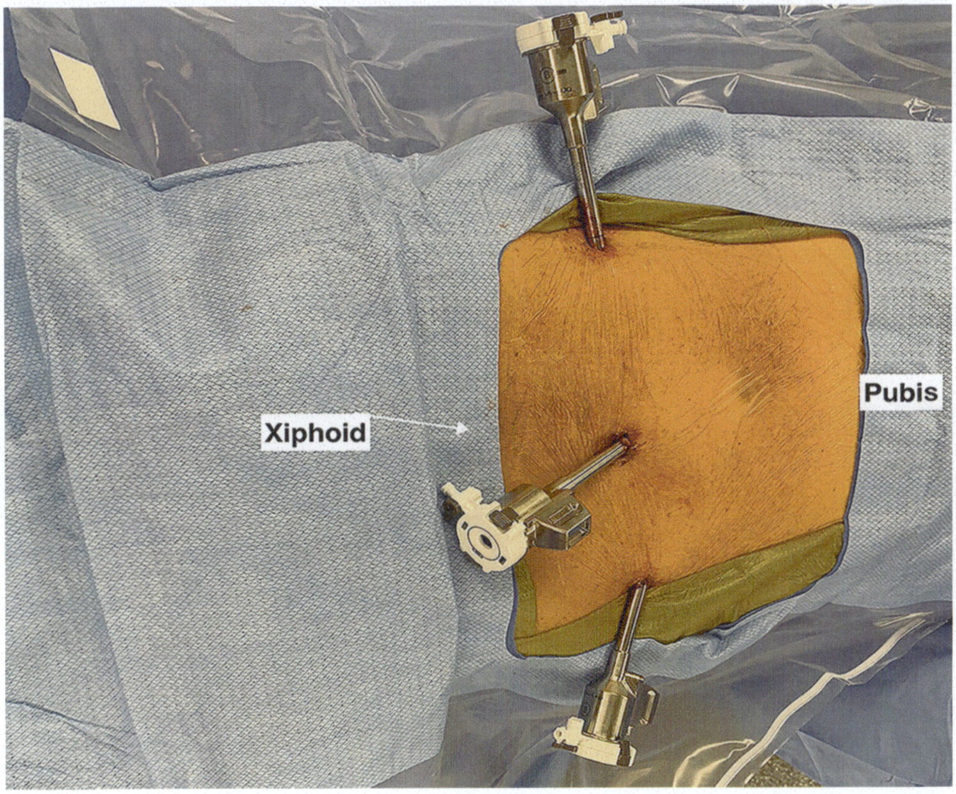


**Fig. 15.4** A total of three 8.5-mm trocars (da Vinci, Xi, Intuitive Surgical, Inc., Sunnyvale, CA) are placed

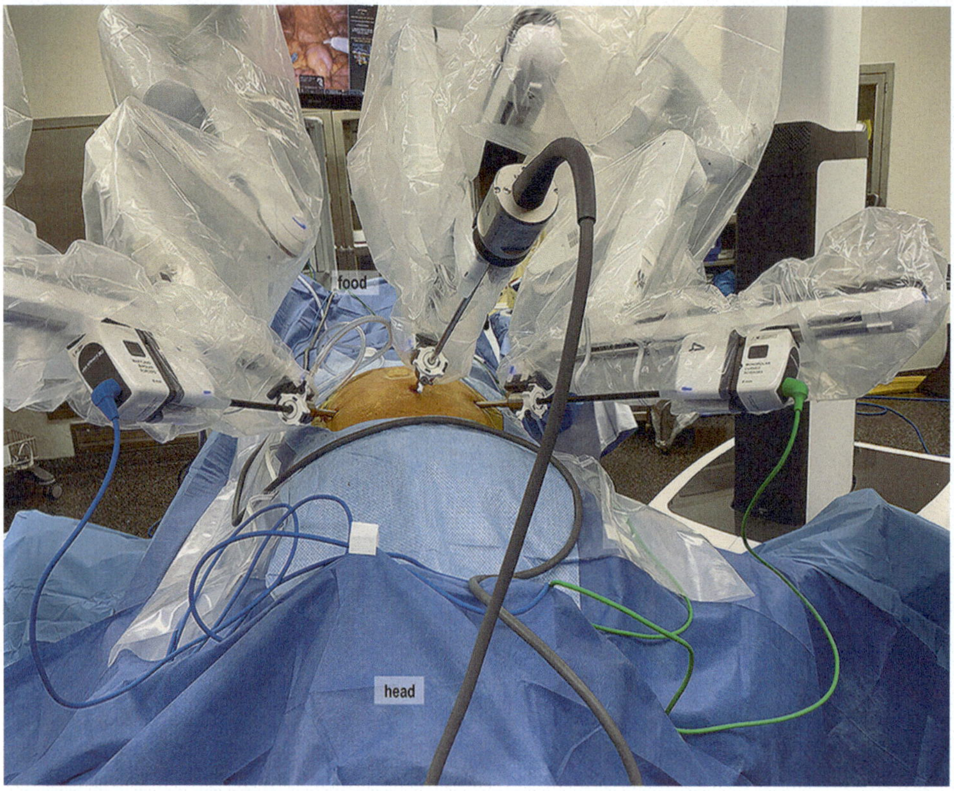


**Fig. 15.5** The patient-side cart (da Vinci, Xi, Intuitive Surgical, Inc., Sunnyvale, CA) is docked

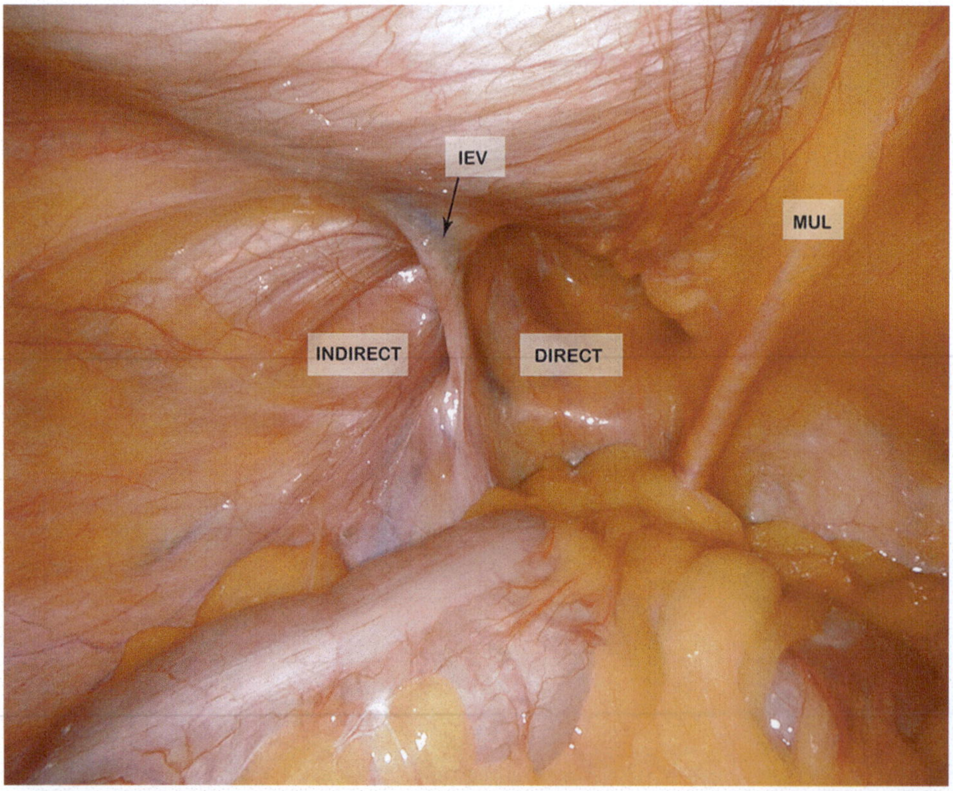


**Fig. 15.6** Posterior view of the left inguinal region. IEV inferior epigastric vessels, MUL medial umbilical ligament

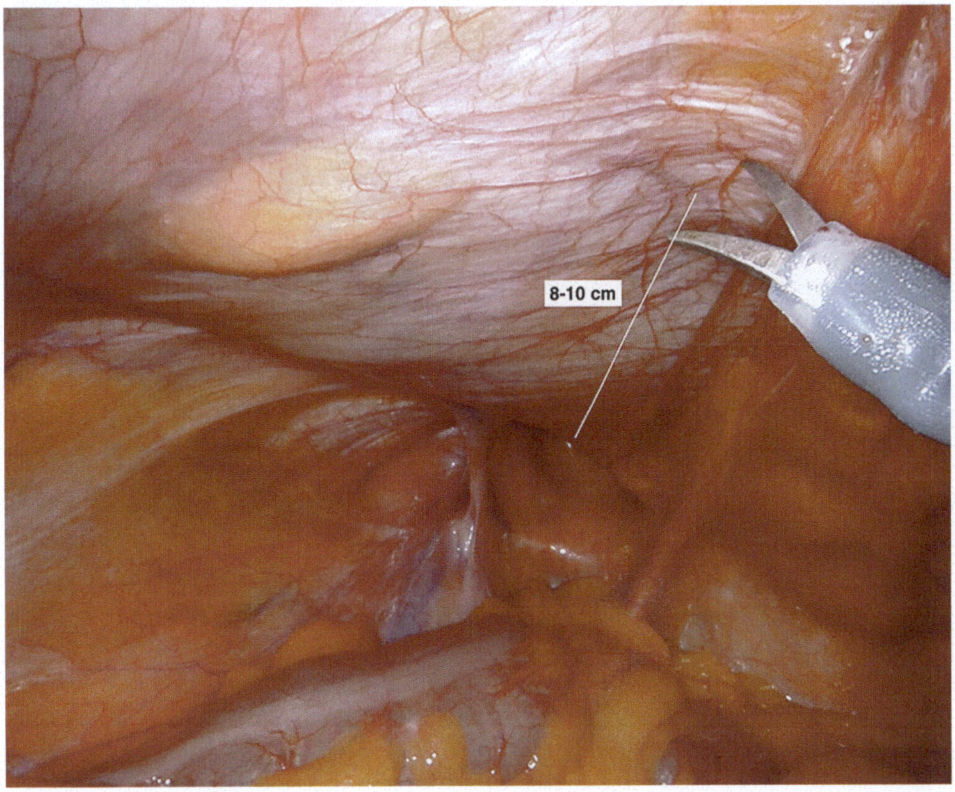


**Fig. 15.7** Preperitoneal dissection is initiated approximately 8–10 cm above the hernia defect

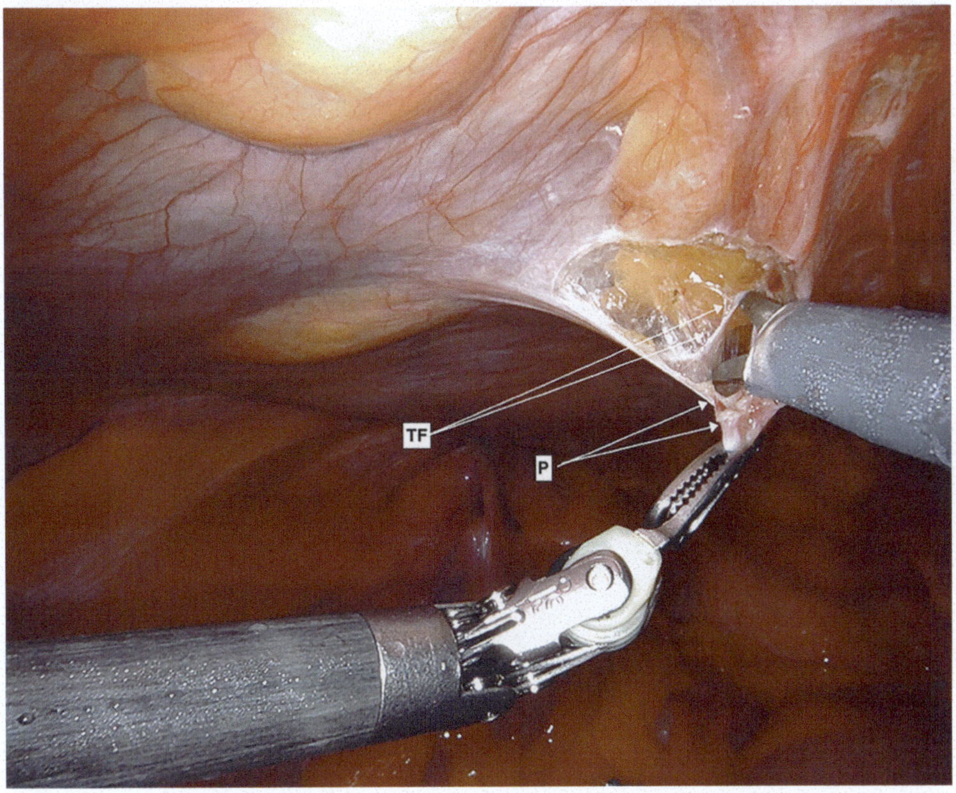


**Fig. 15.8** Initial incision is widened horizontally. In selected cases (thin peritoneum, prior mesh, prior pelvic surgery), the prefascial plane can be preferred as a dissection plane, in order to keep the posterior layer intact and able to be closed at the end of the procedure without any peritoneal tear. TF transversalis fascia, P peritoneum

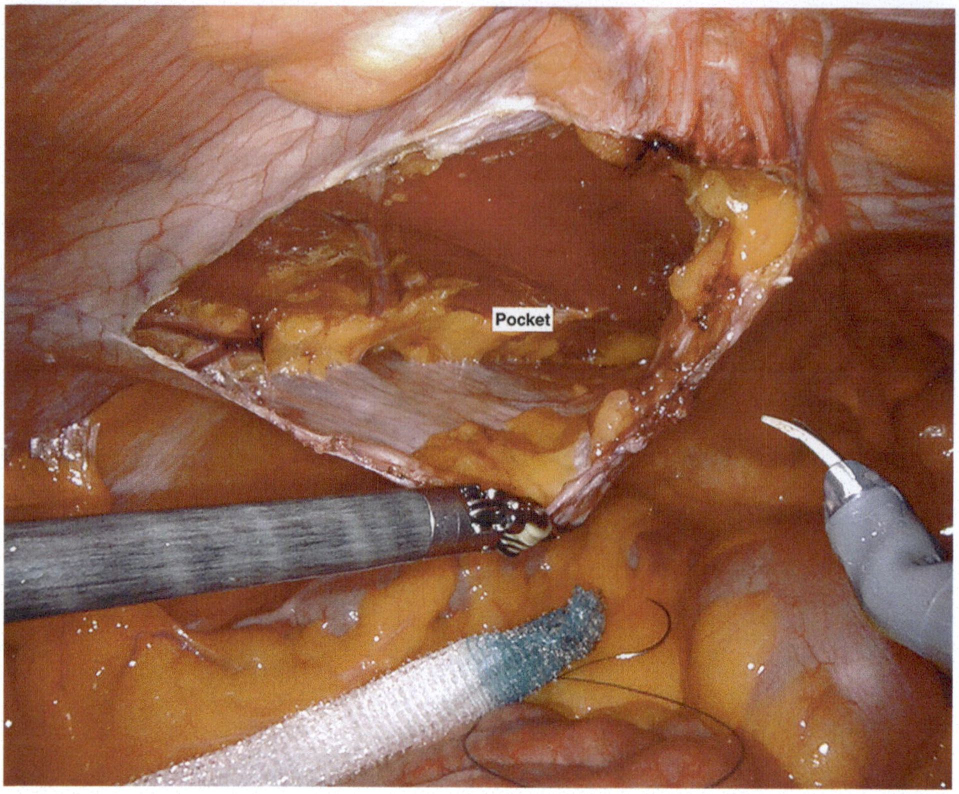


Fig. 15.9 A large peritoneal pocket is developed to place the proper-size mesh

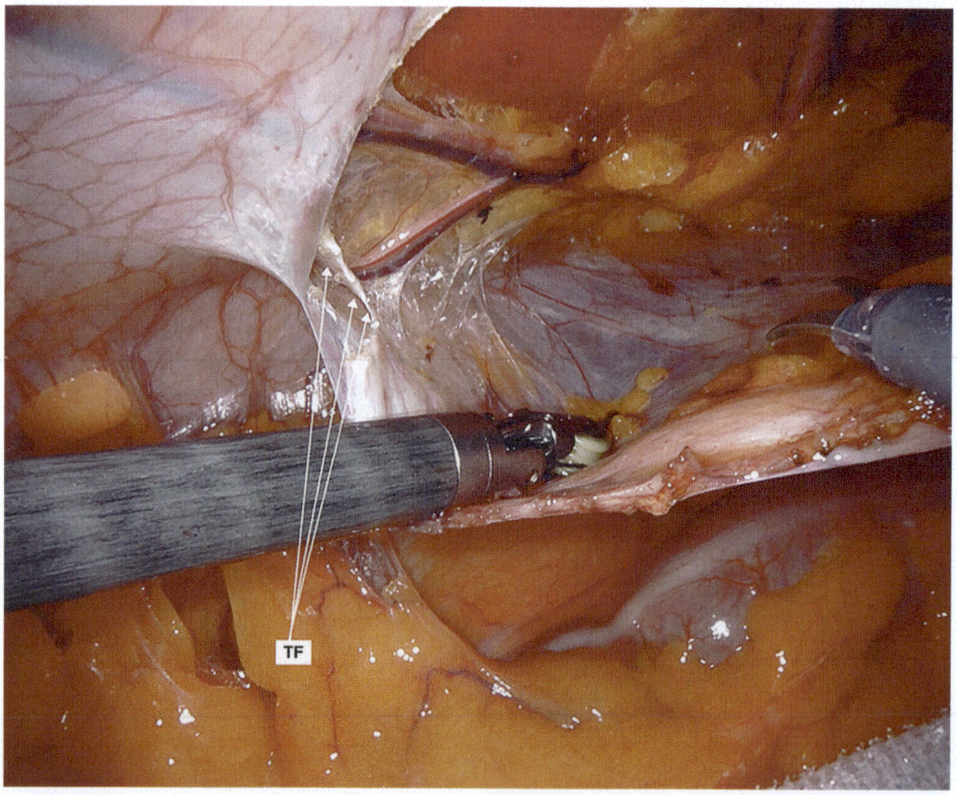


Fig. 15.10 The incision can be extended more laterally if needed. TF transversalis fascia

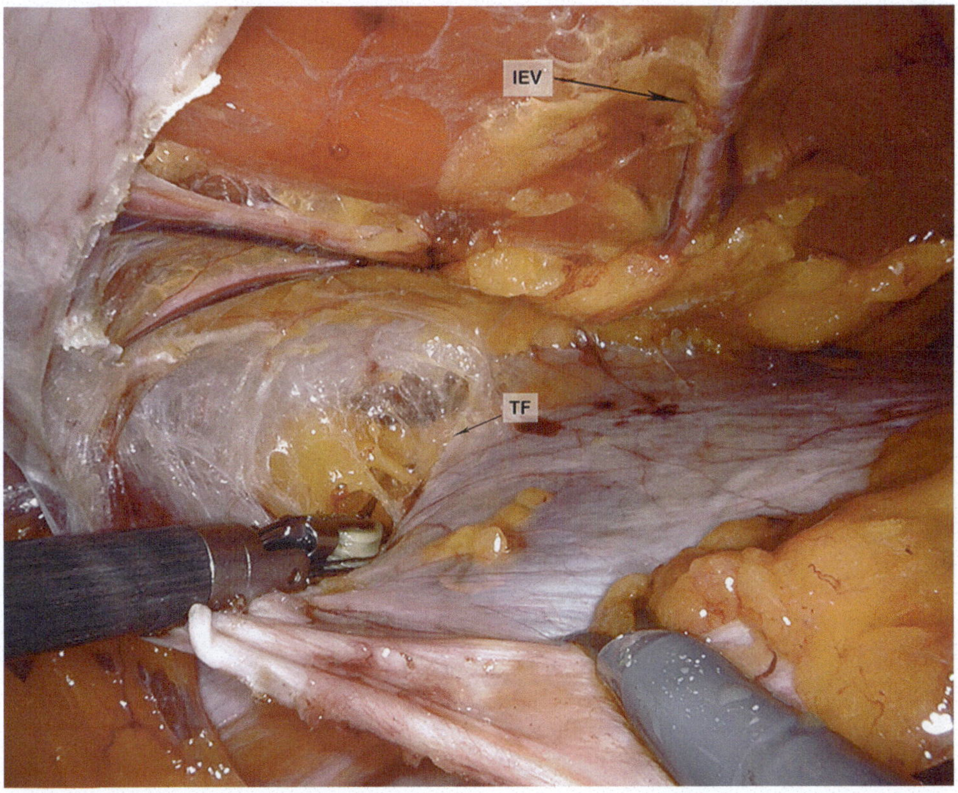


Fig. 15.11 Transversalis fascia (TF) is incised to enter the preperitoneal plane. IEV inferior epigastric vessels

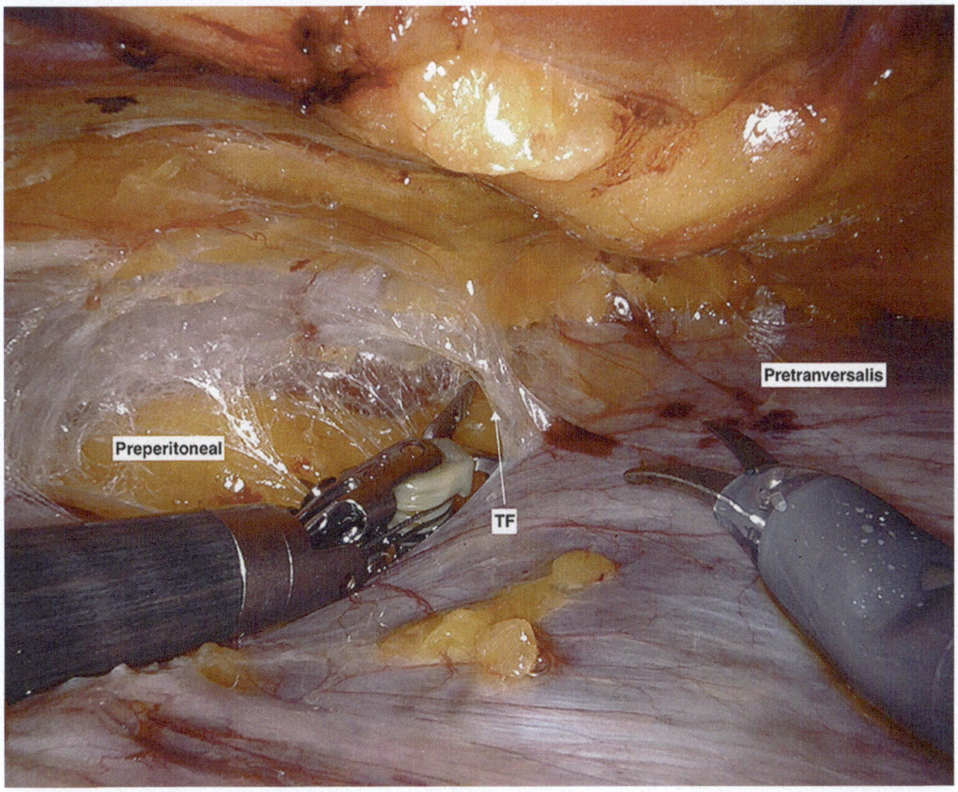


Fig. 15.12 Transition from pre-fascial to pre-peritoneal plane at the step of lateral dissection. It is crucial to dissect laterally to the level of the psoas muscle to ensure proper coverage laterally. TF transversalis fascia

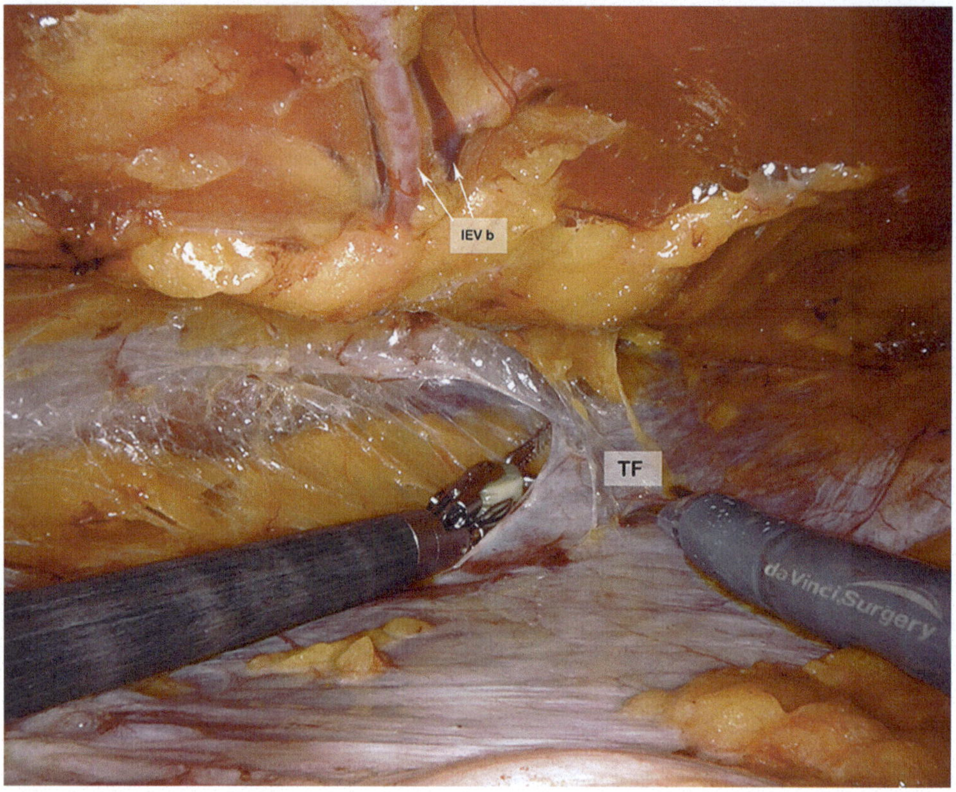


**Fig. 15.13** Transition from pre-fascial to pre-peritoneal plane at the step of caudal dissection. IEV b inferior epigastric vessel branch, TF transversalis fascia

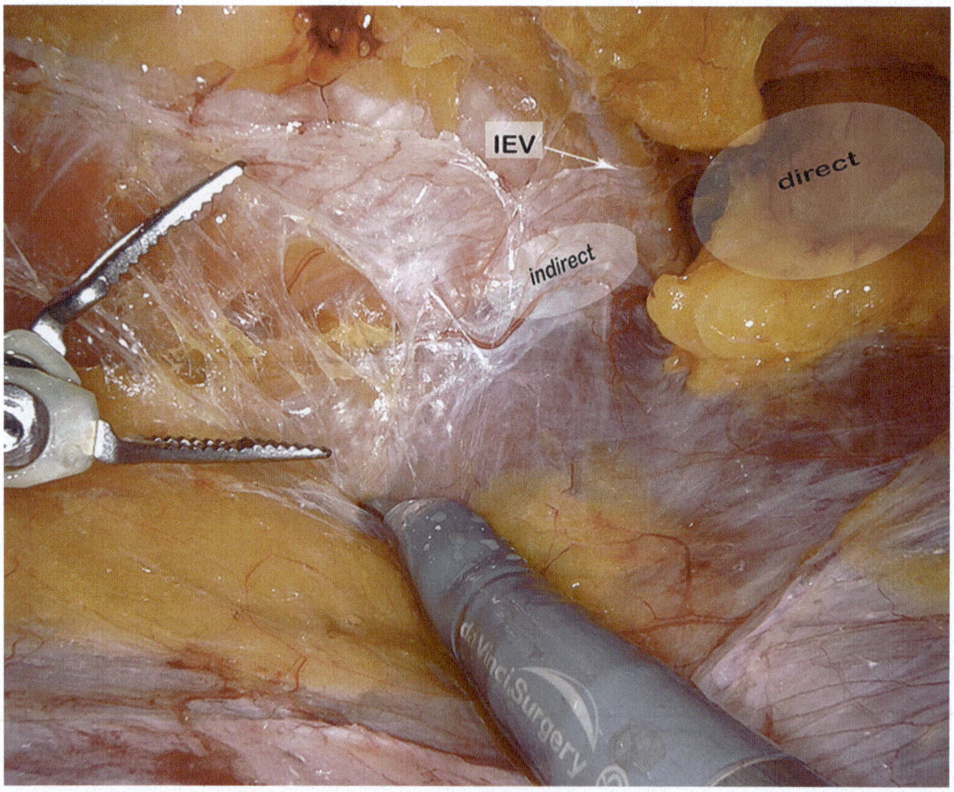


**Fig. 15.14** Recognition of hernia sites. Direct hernia is medial to the inferior epigastric vessels (IEV); the indirect hernia is lateral to the inferior epigastric vessels

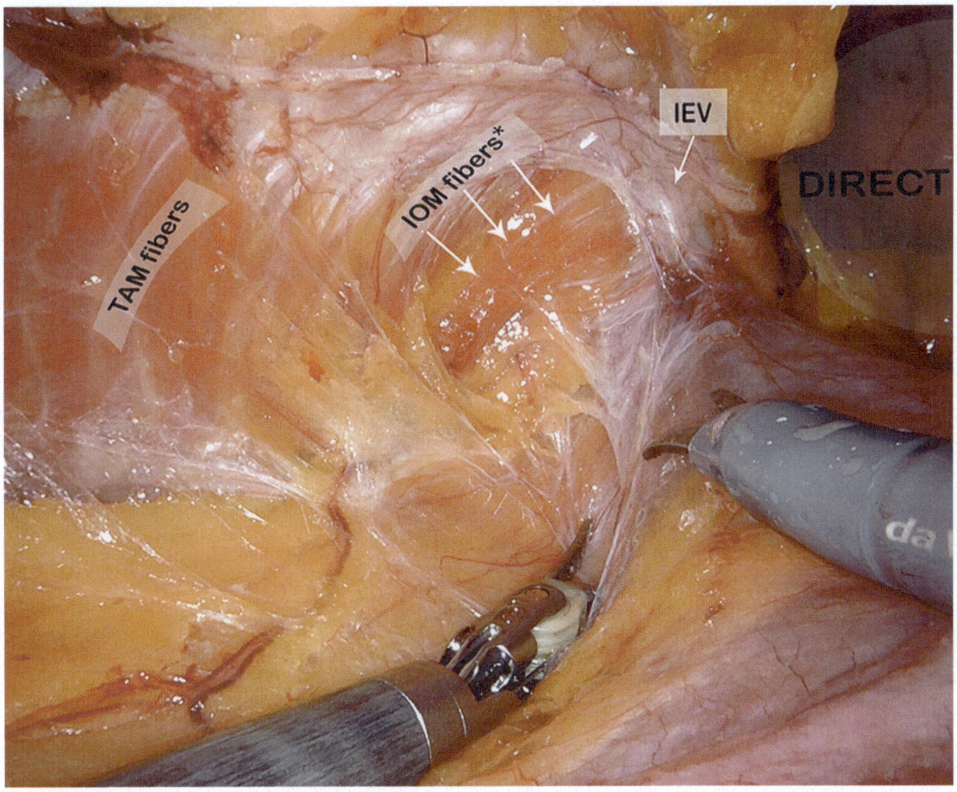


**Fig. 15.15** Dissection at the lateral aspect of inferior epigastric vessels; the fibers of internal oblique muscle join to the cremaster muscle at internal ring level (*asterisk*). IOM internal oblique muscle, TAM transversus abdominis muscle

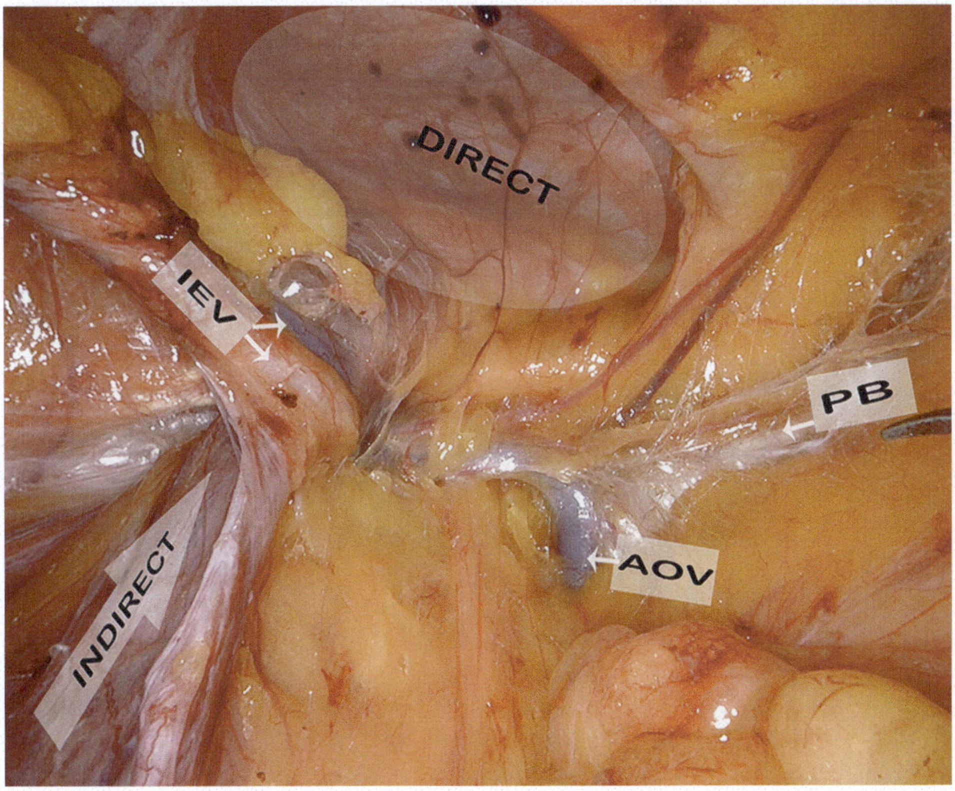


**Fig. 15.16** Direct hernia and adjacent anatomical structures. AOV aberrant obturator vein, IEV inferior epigastric vessels, PB pubic bone

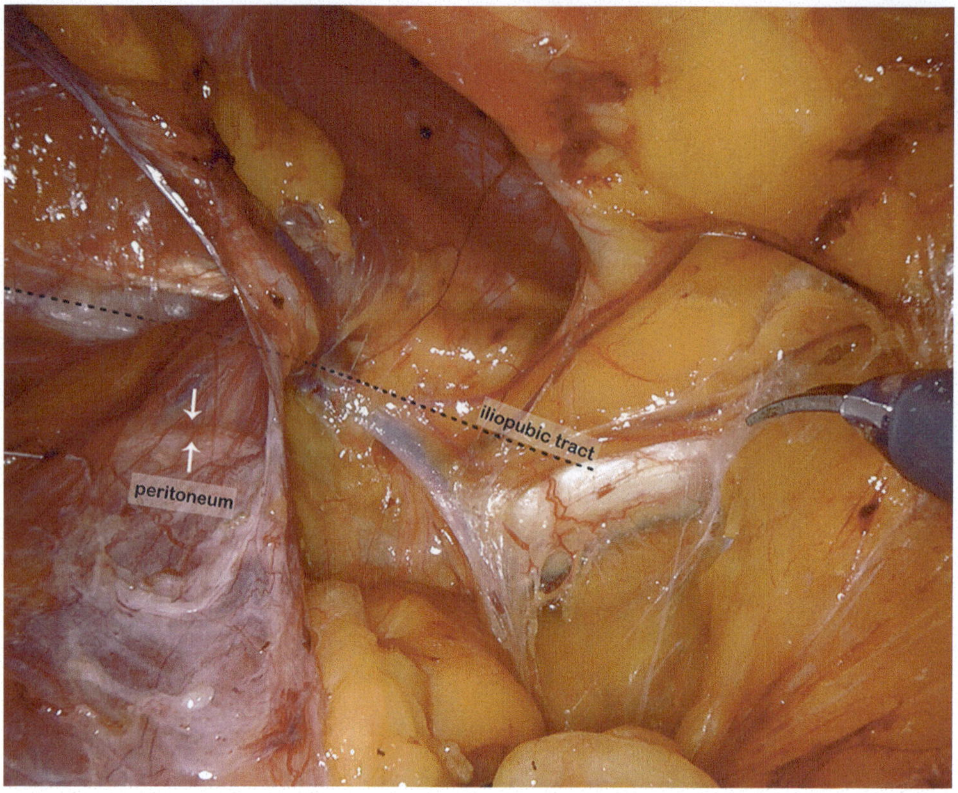


Fig. 15.17 Peritoneum is released from cord structures. (*White arrows* mark the border of the peritoneum)

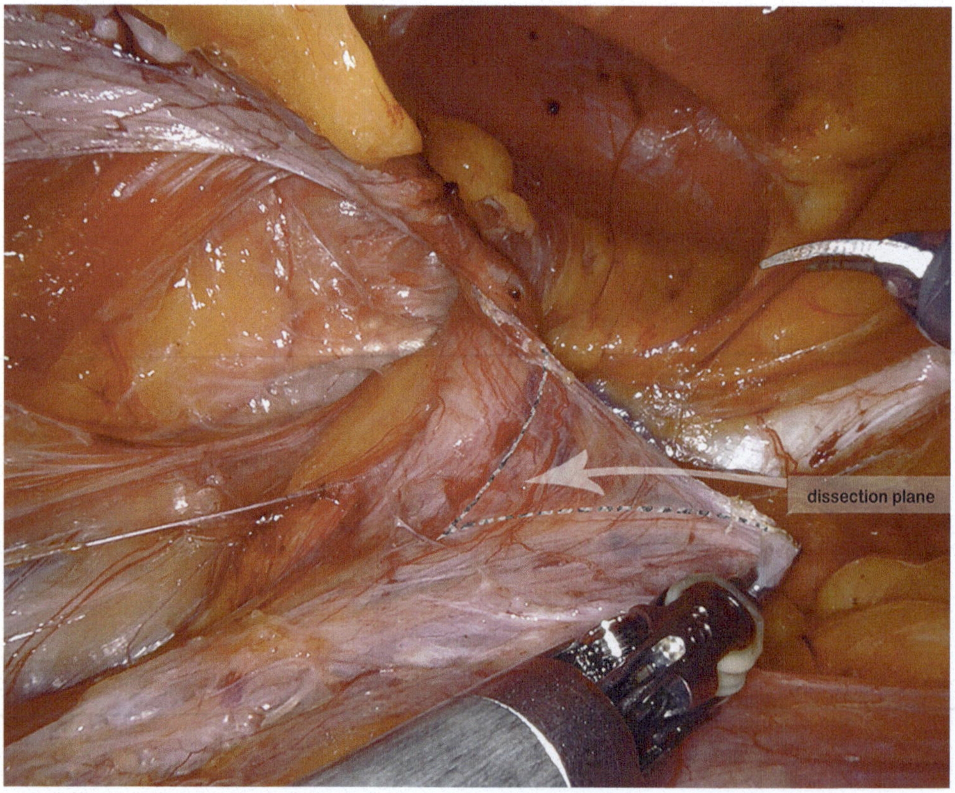


Fig. 15.18 Peritoneum is released from cord structures; the *white arrow* shows the direction of dissection

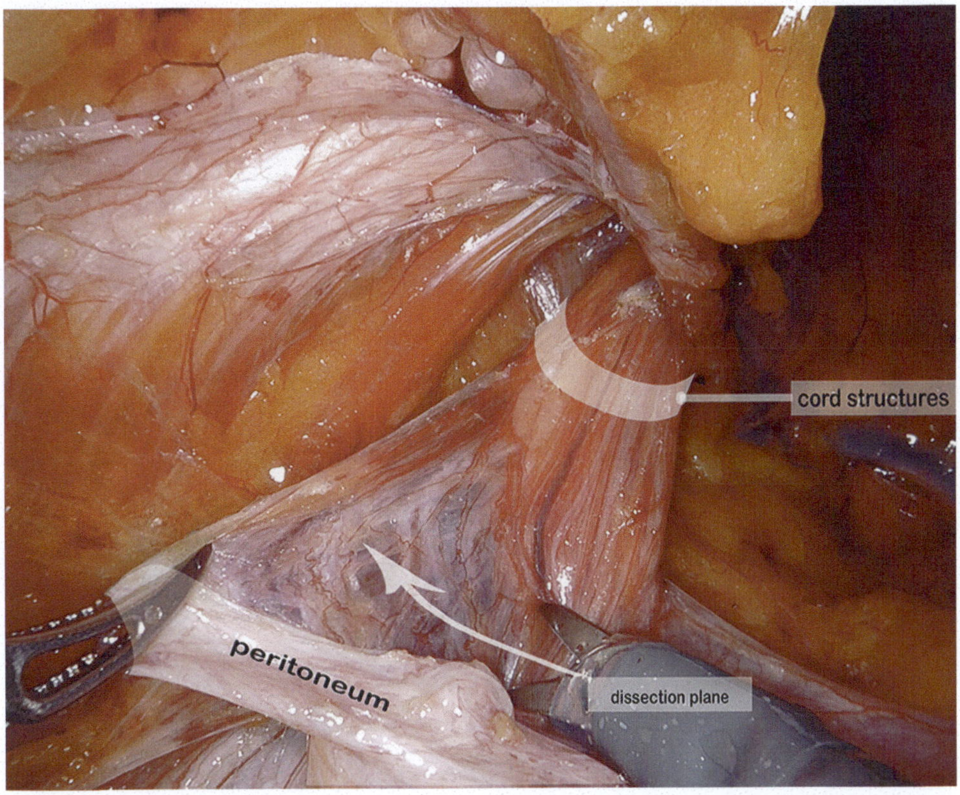


**Fig. 15.19** Continuation of releasing peritoneum from cord structures; the *white arrow* shows the direction of dissection

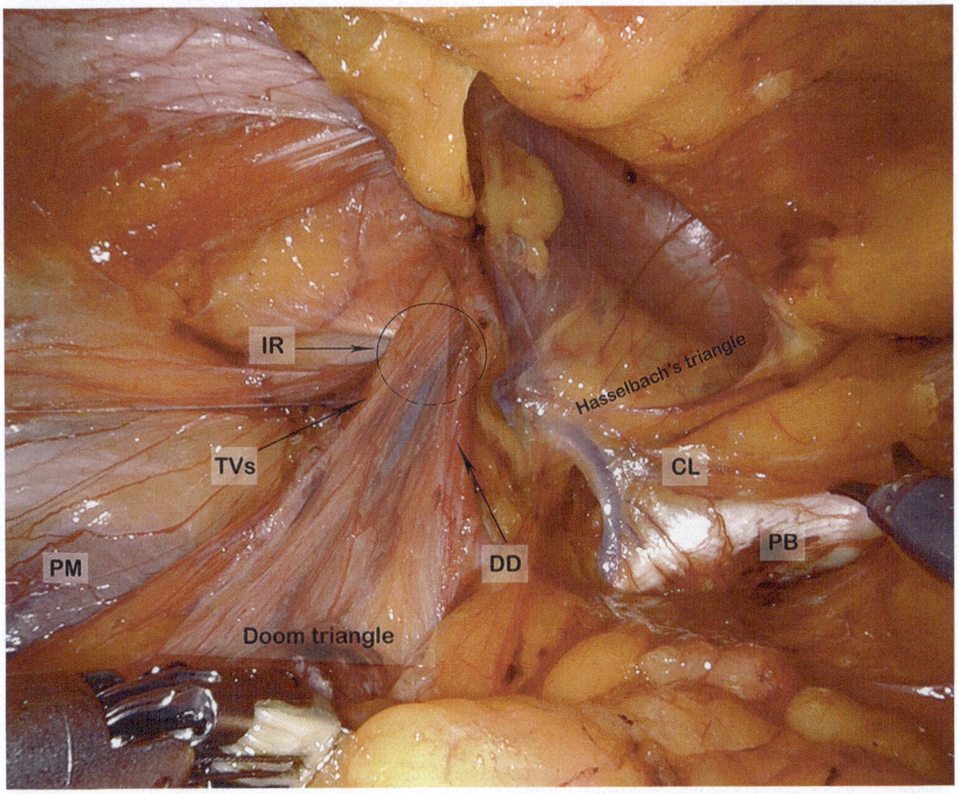


**Fig. 15.20** Eventual view to be obtained before the mesh is placed. *Doom triangle* refers to the area of the iliac vessels; *Hasselbach's triangle* refers to a direct inguinal hernia location. CL Cooper's ligament, DD ductus (vas) deferens, IR internal ring, PB pubic bone, PM psoas muscle, TVs testicular vessels

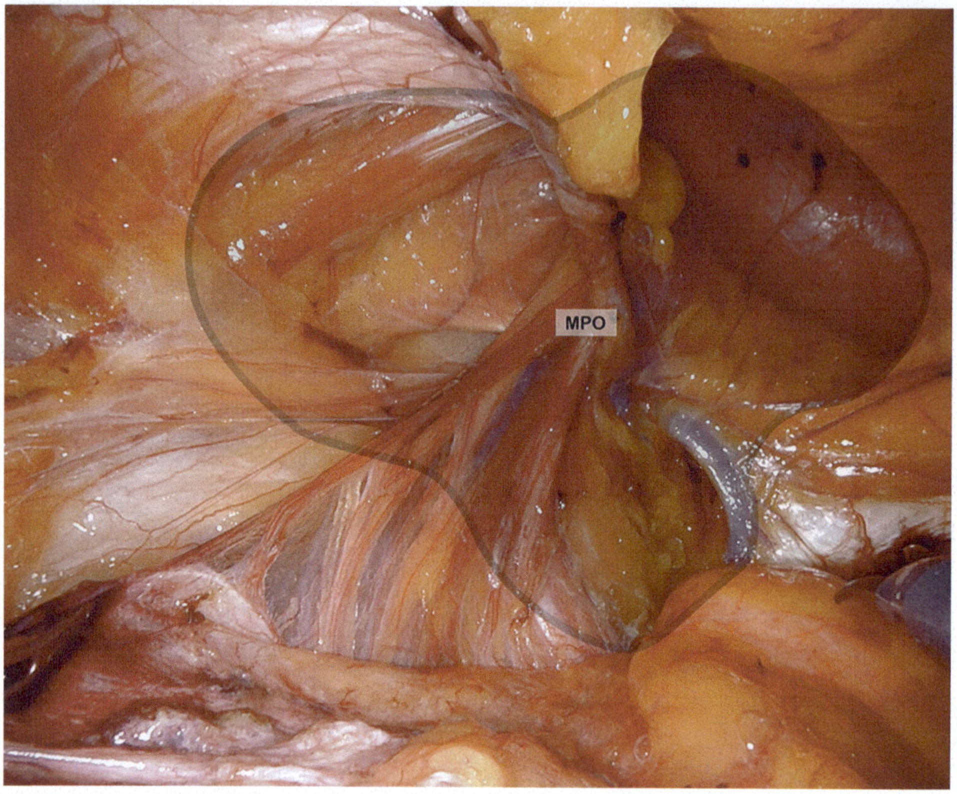


Fig. 15.21 Fruchaud's myopectineal orifice (MPO): a distinct area of weakness in the pelvic region

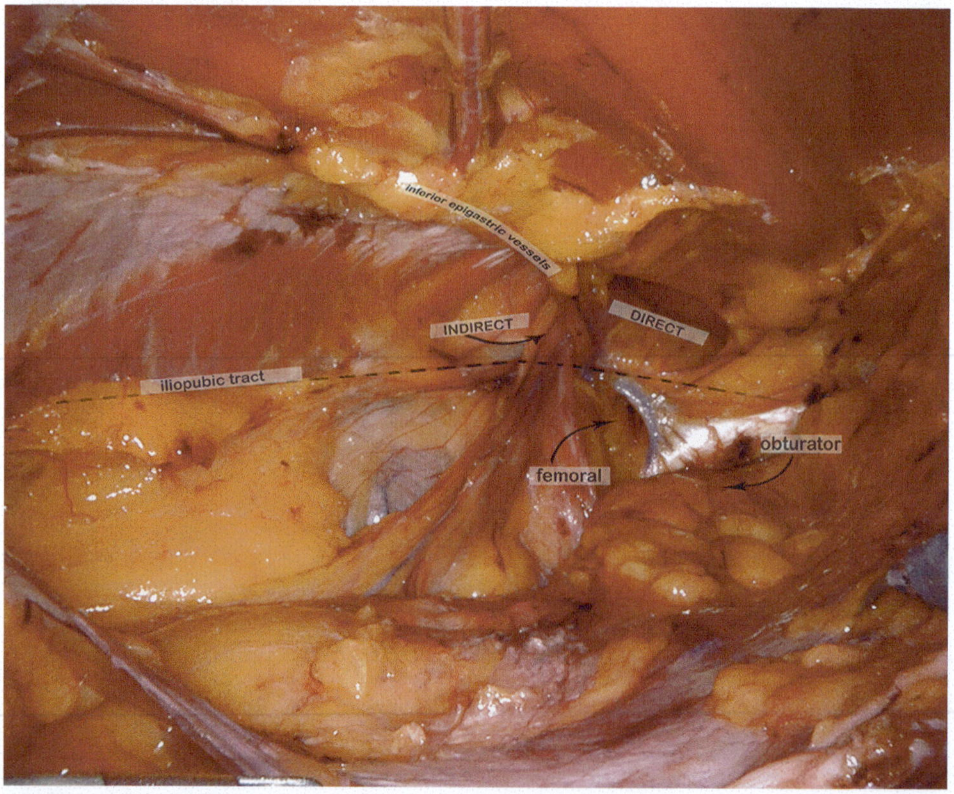


Fig. 15.22 Localizations of all potential hernias

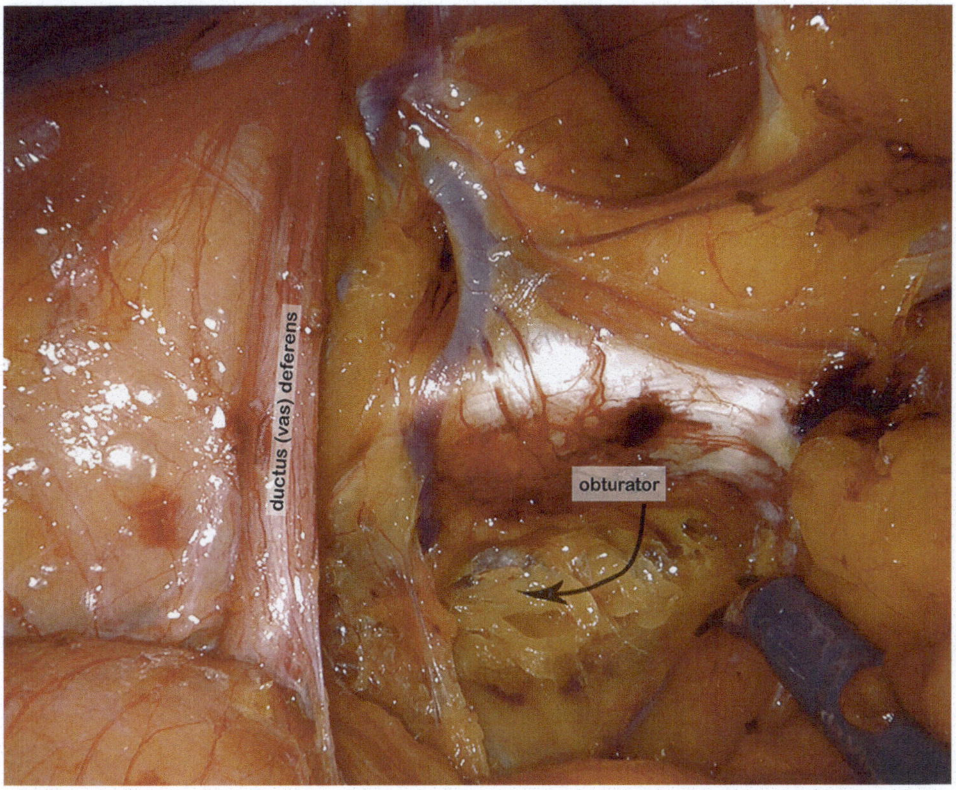


Fig. 15.23 Obturator space localization

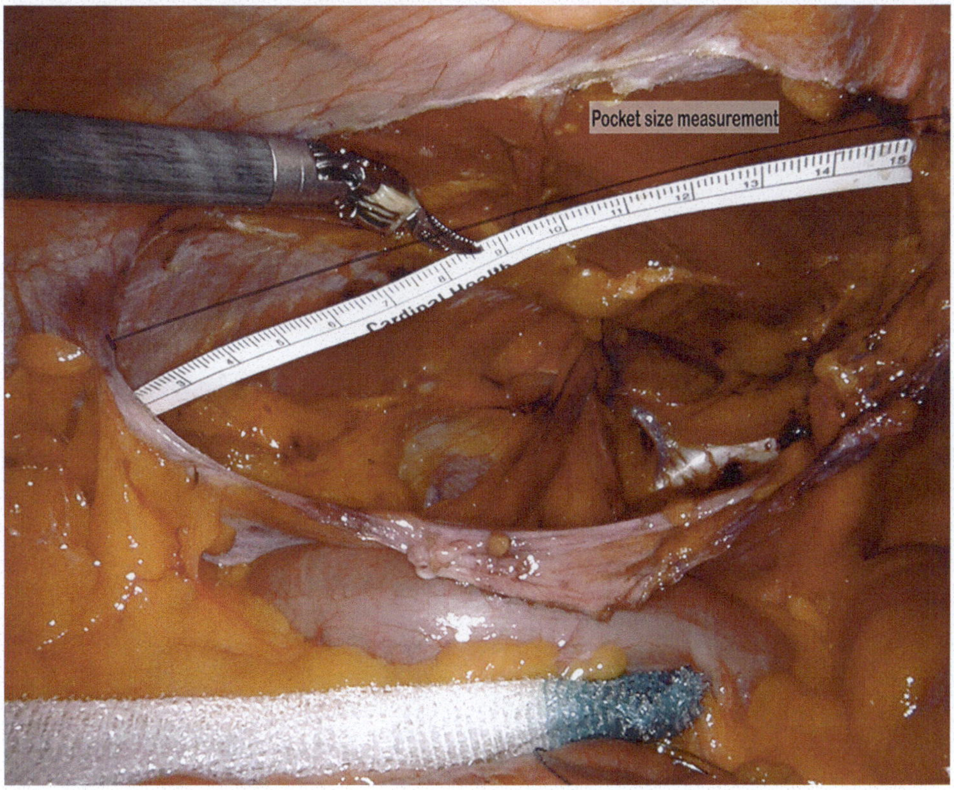


Fig. 15.24 Pocket size measurement; the mesh is measured and shaped accordingly. Size of 15 × 10 cm or larger is usually recommended

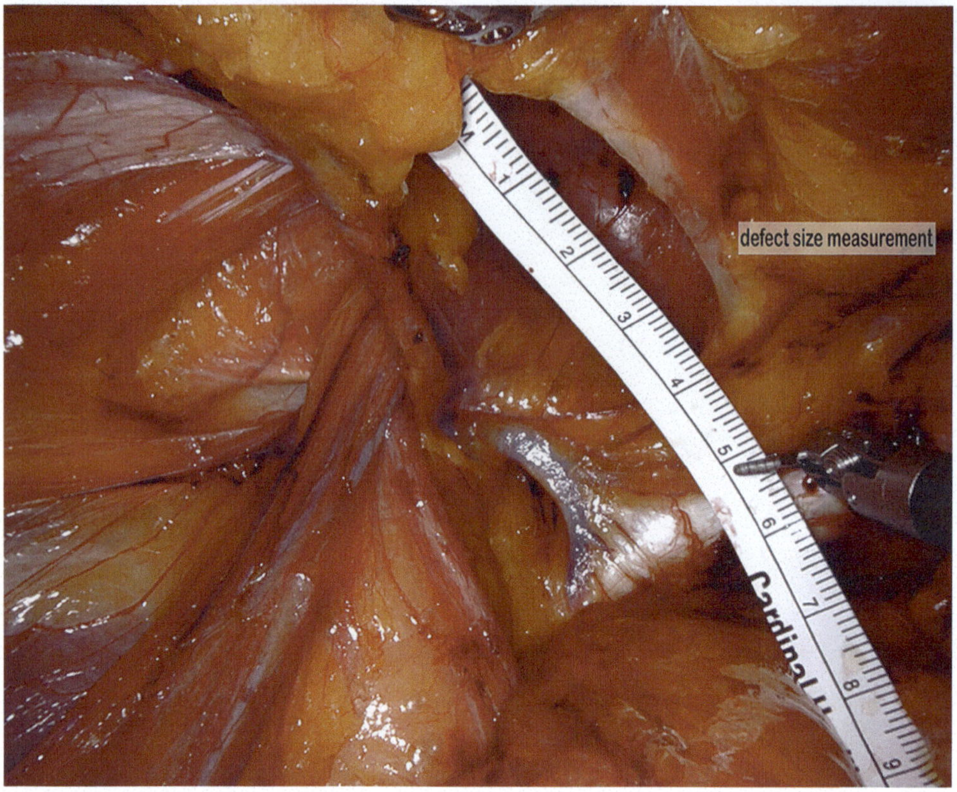


Fig. 15.25 Defect size measurement for medical records

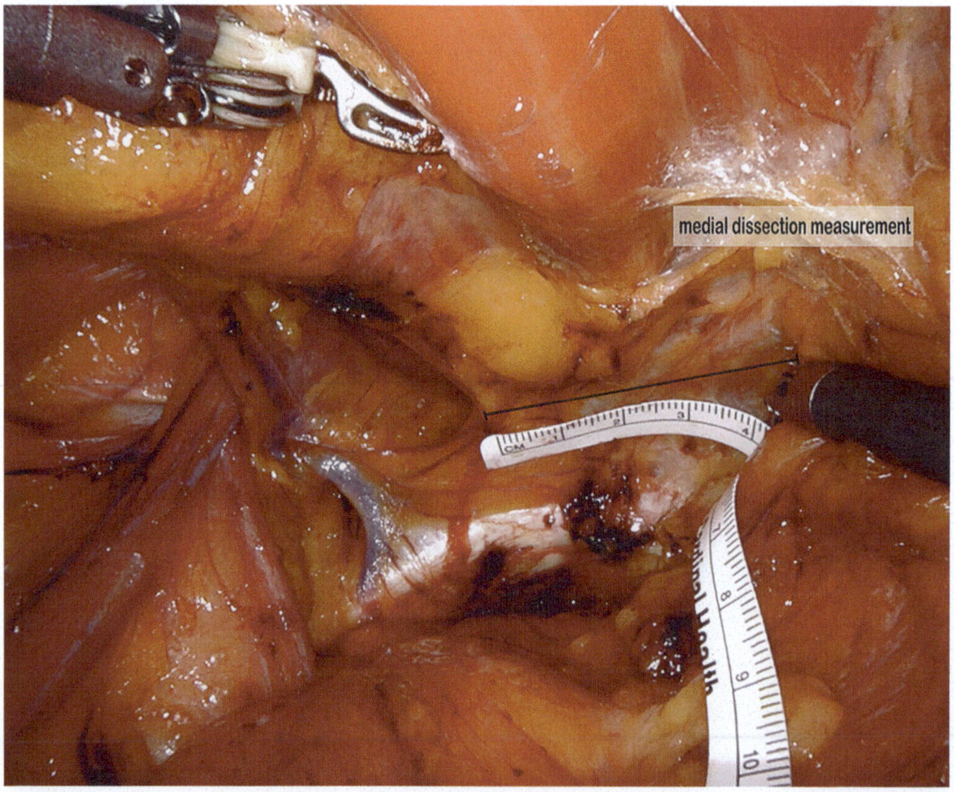


Fig. 15.26 Medial overlap of >2 cm is needed to prevent recurrence of average-sized hernia, but this overlap should be at least 4 cm for larger defects

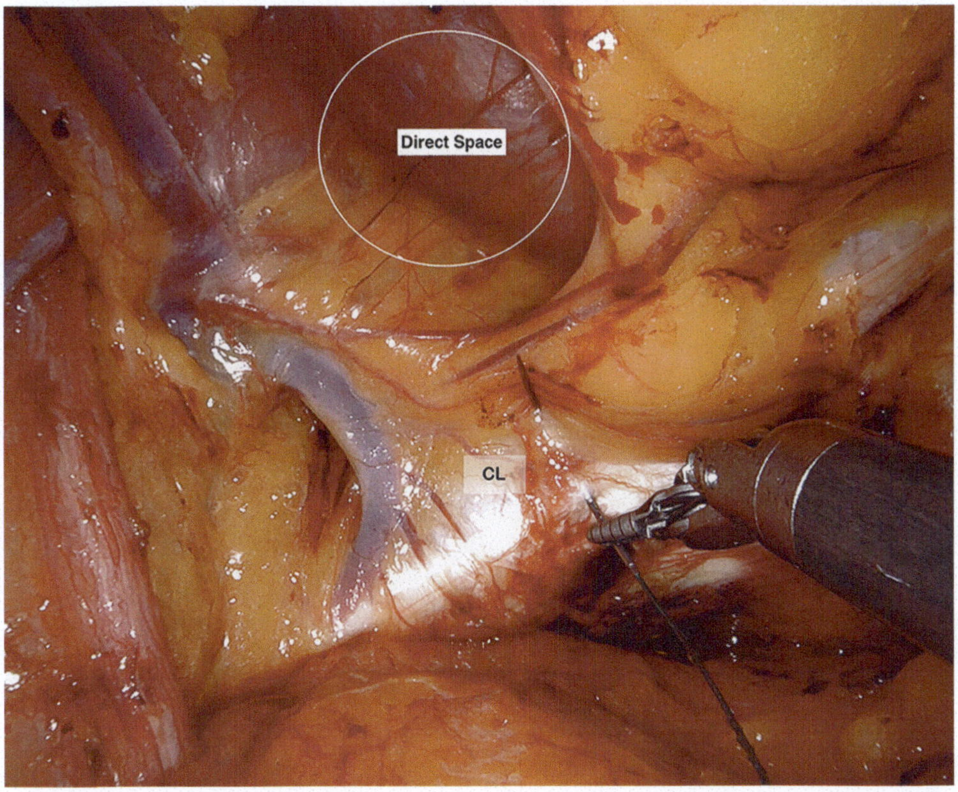


**Fig. 15.27** To invert the lax fascia transversalis and to close the defect, a barbed suture is placed initially at Cooper's ligament (CL)

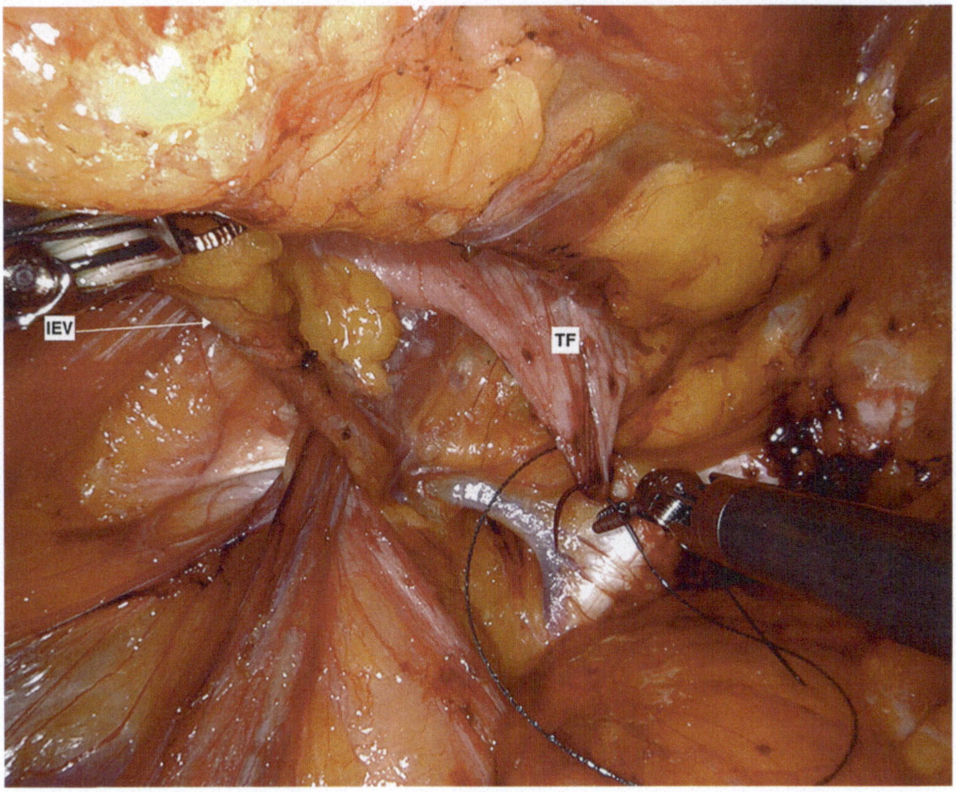


**Fig. 15.28** Continue by passing the stitch through the transversalis fascia (TF). IEV inferior epigastric vessels

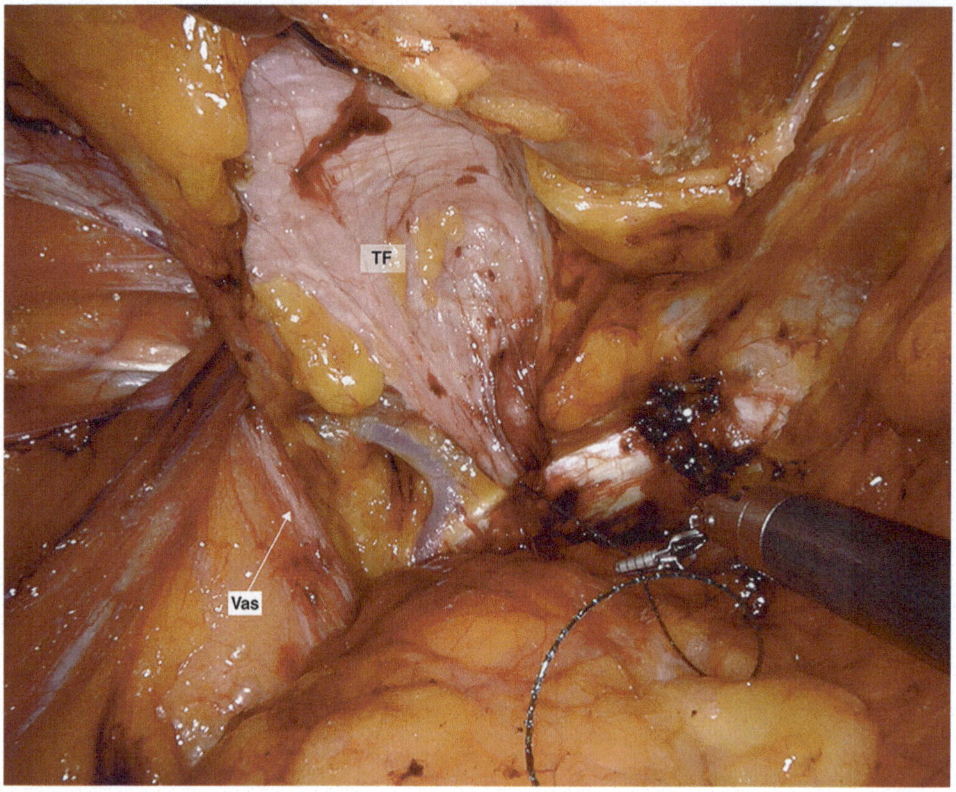


**Fig. 15.29** The lax transversalis fascia (TF) is fixed to Cooper's ligament. It is advised to pay attention to the corona mortis (anatomical variant), an anastomosis between the obturator and the external iliac or inferior epigastric arteries or veins

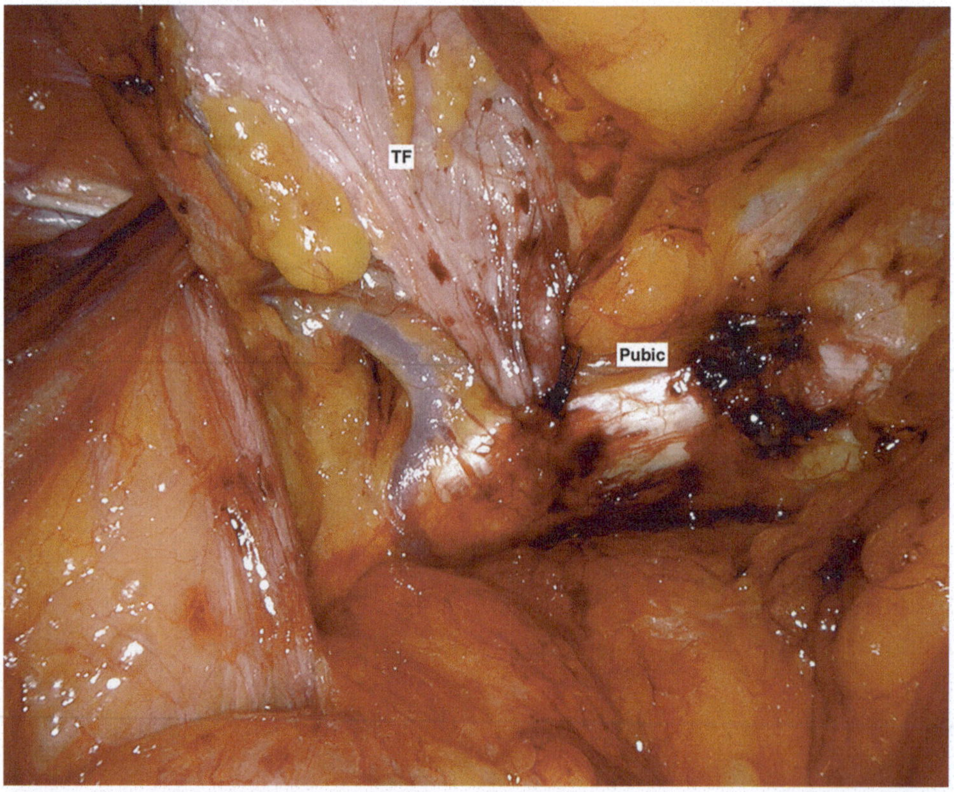


**Fig. 15.30** Eventual view of fascia transversalis inversion. TF transversalis fascia

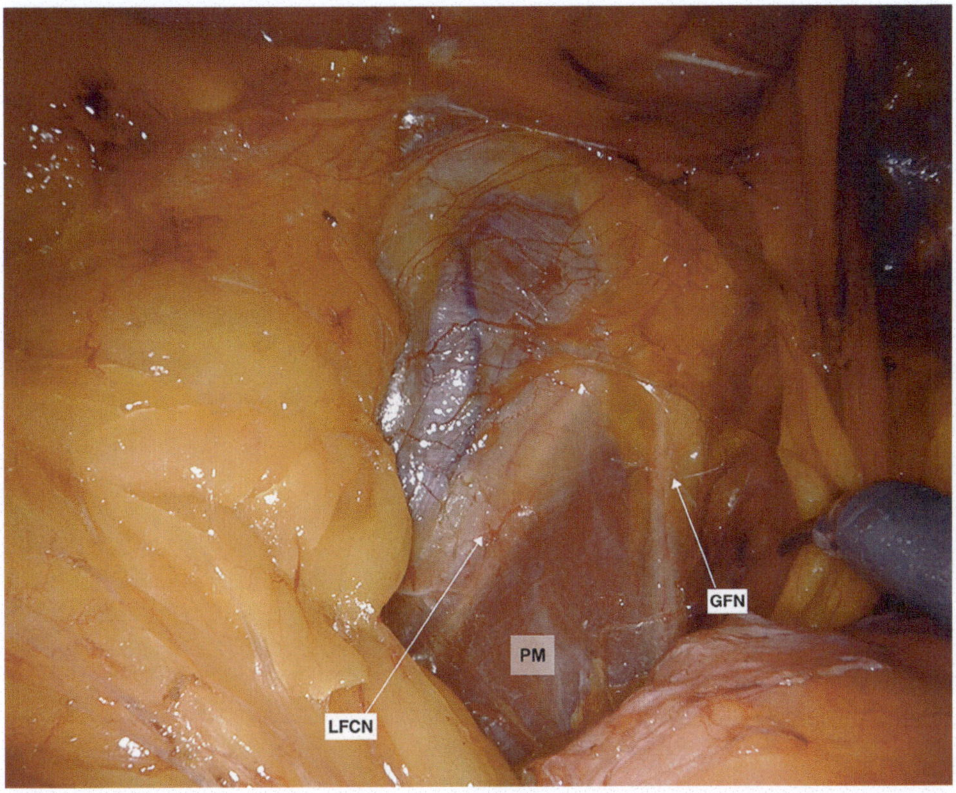


Fig. 15.31 Pain triangle. GFN genitofemoral nerve, LFCN lateral femoral cutaneous nerve, PM psoas muscle

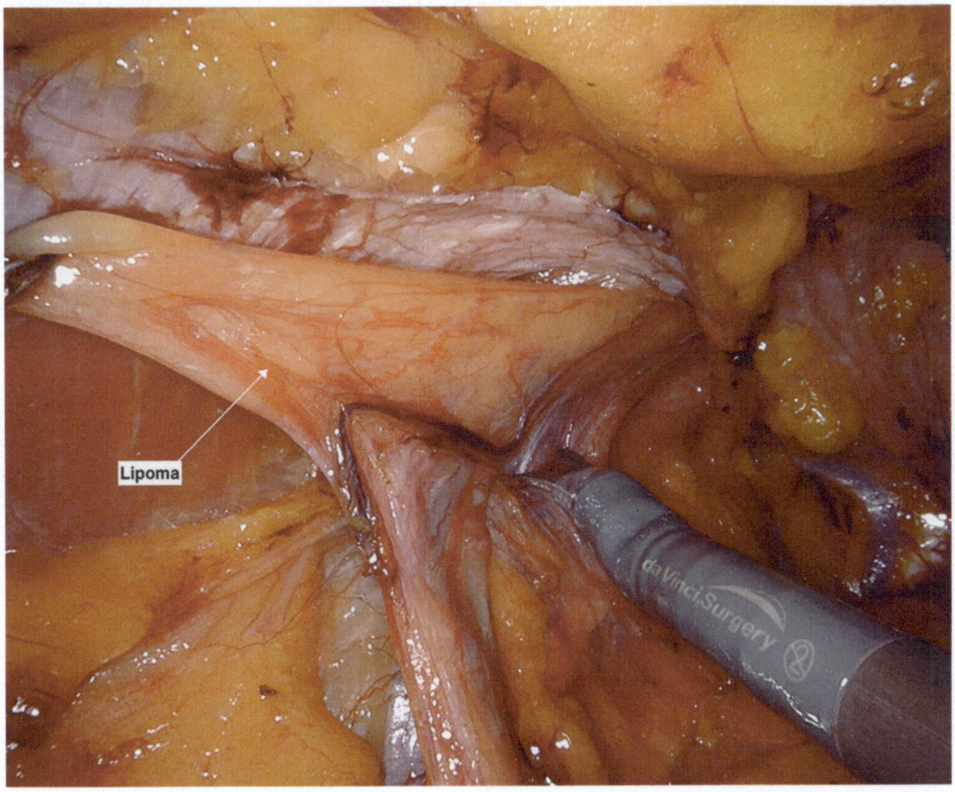


Fig. 15.32 Cord lipoma can be found within indirect hernia space

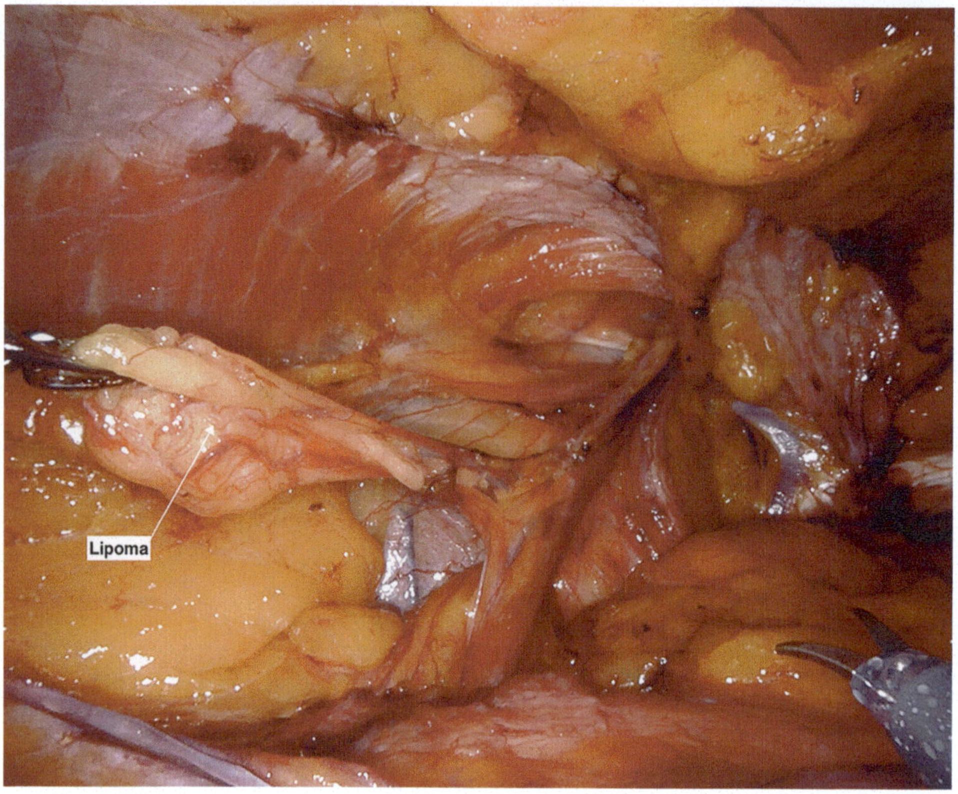


Fig. 15.33 Excision of the cord lipoma

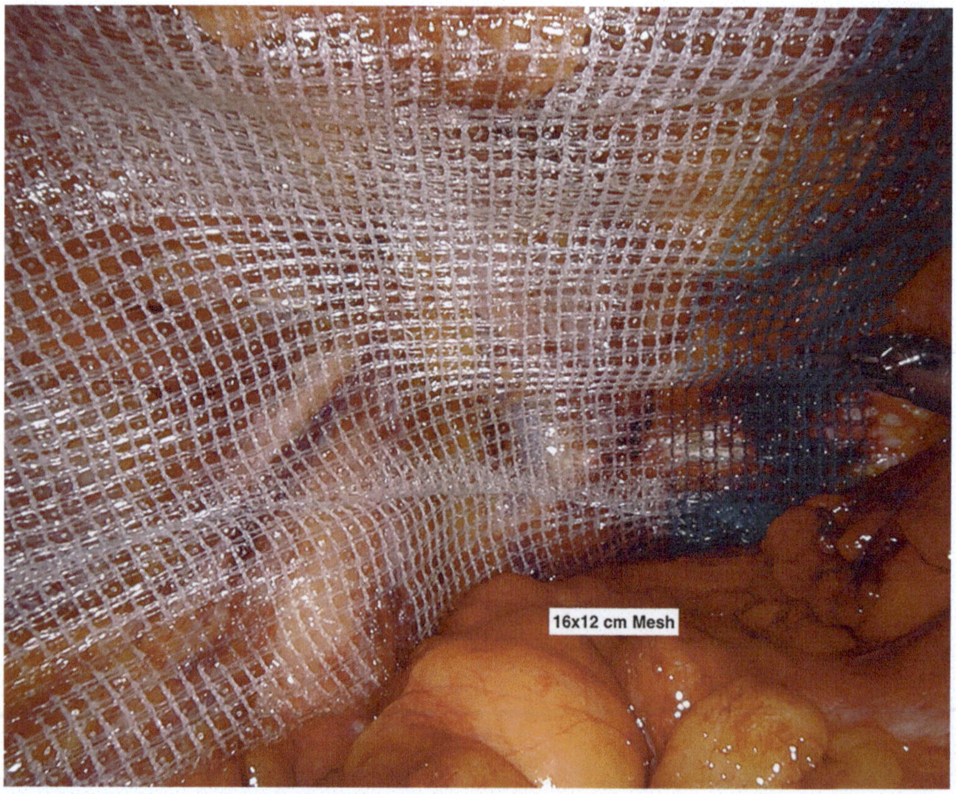


Fig. 15.34 Because of a large defect, a 16 × 12 cm mesh is used

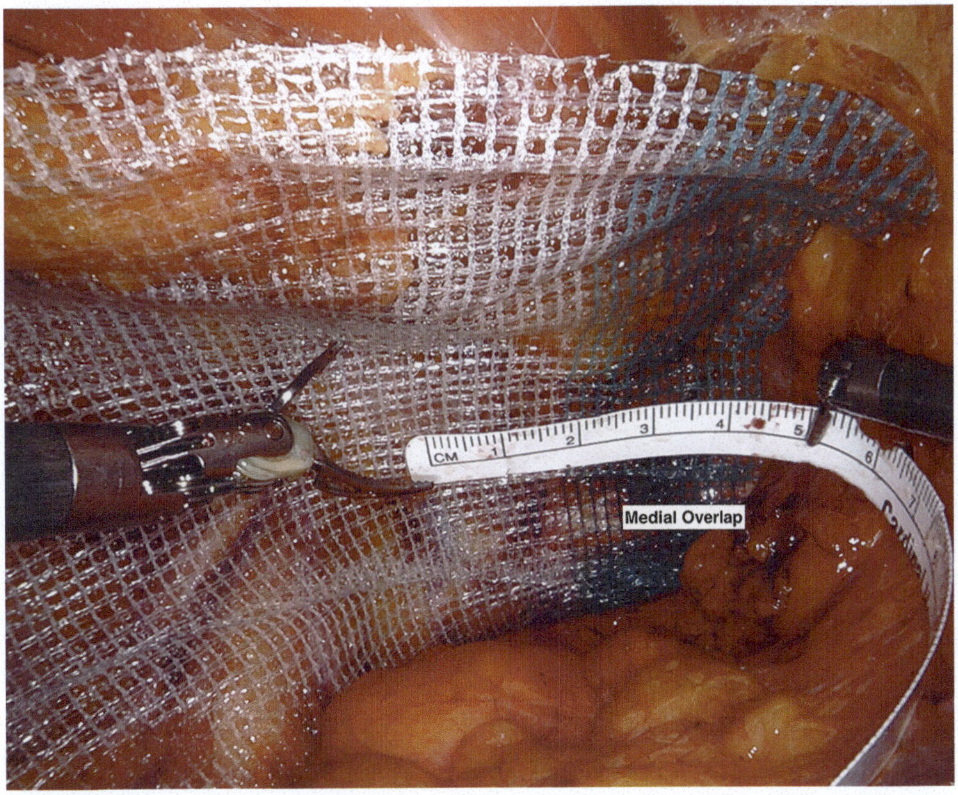


**Fig. 15.35** A minimum of 4 cm medial overlap is obtained

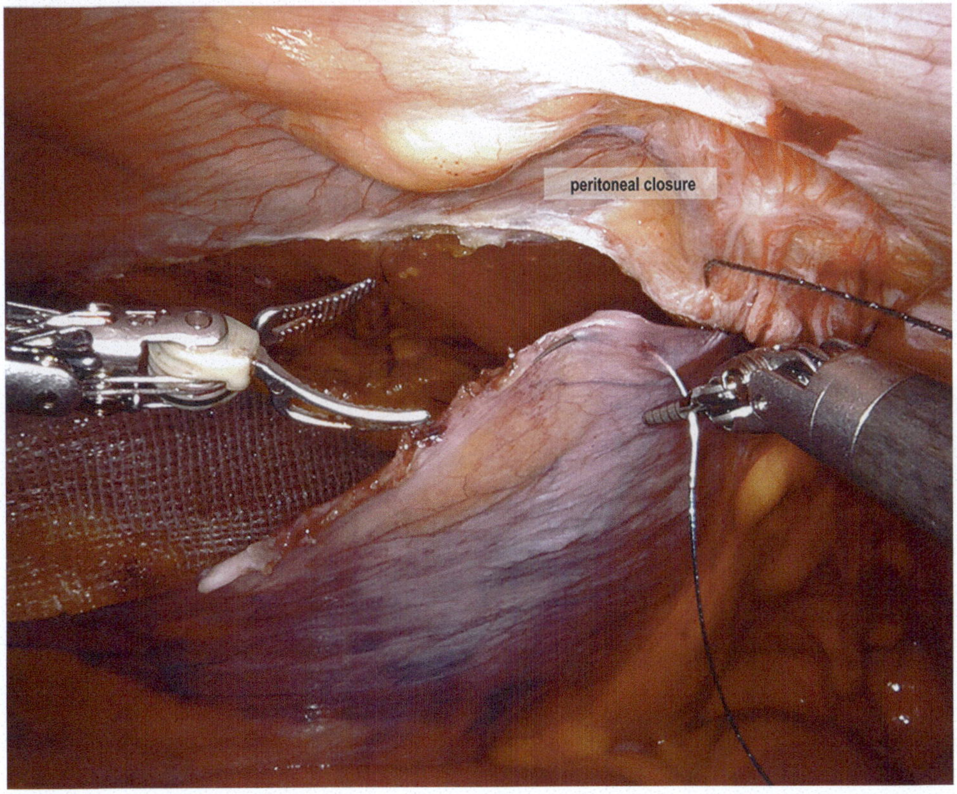


**Fig. 15.36** Peritoneal pocket is closed in a medial to lateral direction

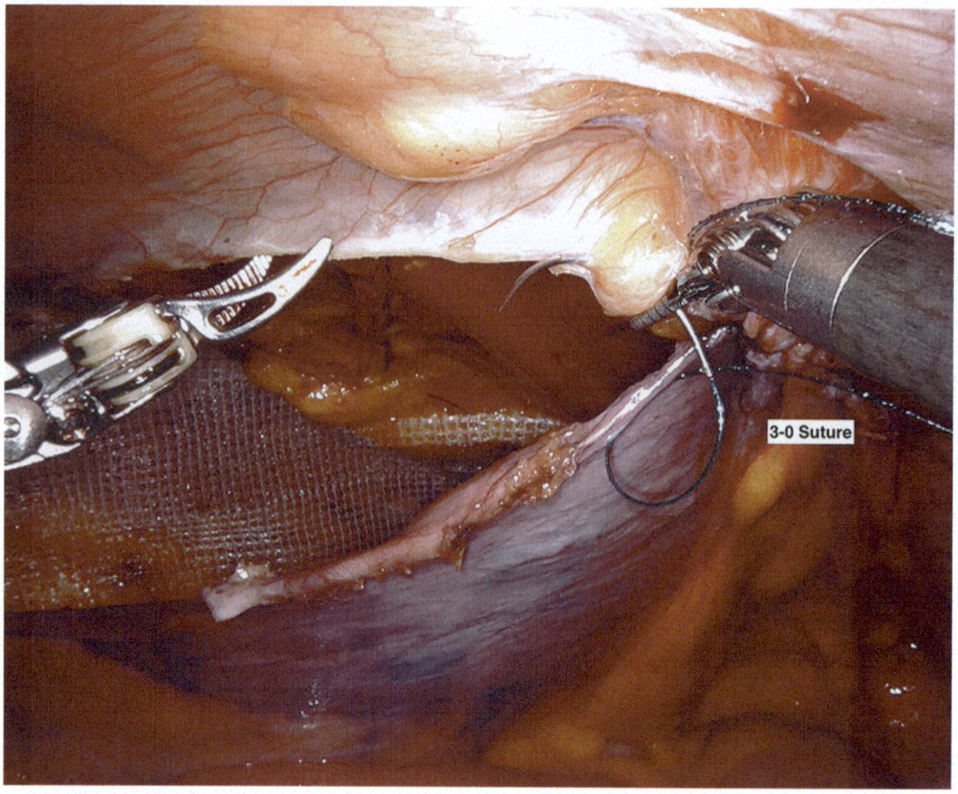


Fig. 15.37 Continue peritoneal closure with 3-0 barbed suture

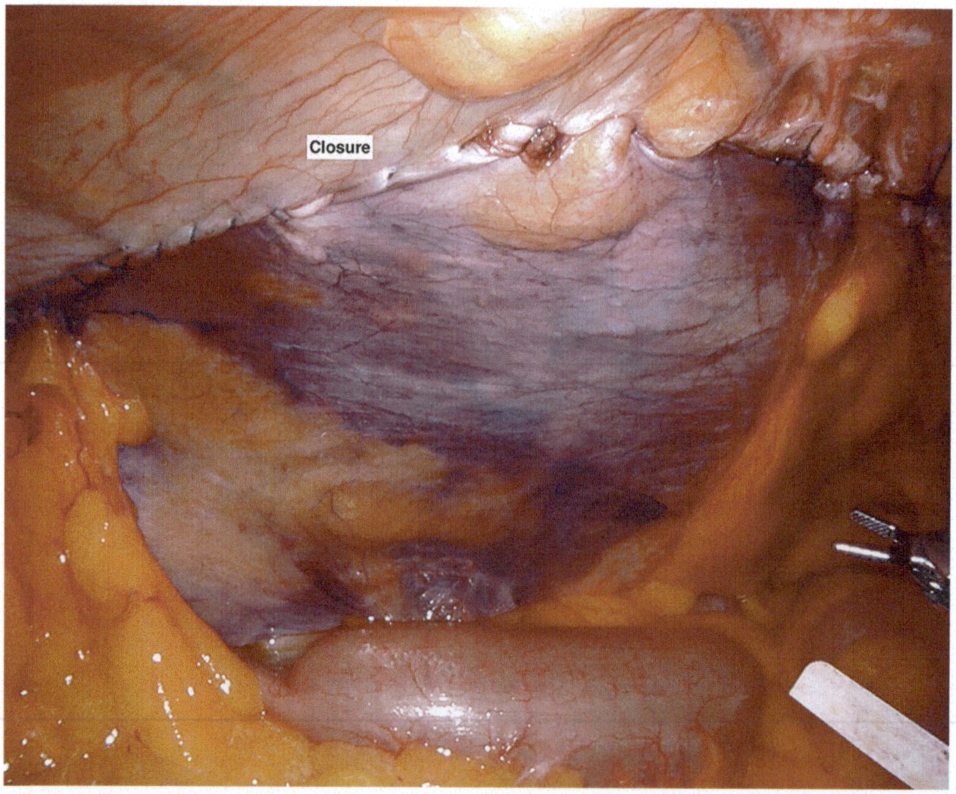


Fig. 15.38 Eventual view after peritoneal closure

## References

1. Flock BJ, Hope WW. Robotic inguinal hernia repair. In: Kudsi OY, editor. Atlas of robotic surgery. Woodbury: Ciné-Med; 2018. p. 342–60.
2. HerniaSurge Group. International guidelines for groin hernia management. Hernia. 2018;22:1–165. https://doi.org/10.1007/s10029-017-1668-x.
3. Reddy VM, Sutton CD, Bloxham L, Garcea G, Ubhi SS, Robertson GS. Laparoscopic repair of direct inguinal hernia: a new technique that reduces the development of postoperative seroma. Hernia. 2007;11:393–6. https://doi.org/10.1007/s10029-007-0233-4.

# Robotic Anterior Component Separation

# 16

Flavio Malcher, Leandro Totti Cavazzola, and Eduardo Parra-Davila

## Introduction

Ventral hernia repair with onlay mesh placement after anterior component separation is a safe alternative to sublay mesh placement after posterior component separation in low-risk patients [1]. Onlay open ventral hernia repair is still one of the most-used surgical techniques for the repair of hernias worldwide [2, 3]. It is technically easy, has relatively short surgical time, is very reproducible, and has a shorter learning curve than other repair techniques (including laparoscopic surgery) [2, 4–6].

Endoscopic surgery of the abdominal wall has its peculiarities, as intracorporeal closure of fascial defects is difficult, owing to the necessity to operate "on the roof" of the surgical field; it is not broadly accepted or widely performed because it demands advanced laparoscopic skills. Another consideration is the controversial use of synthetic mesh in contact with abdominal viscera; this is still a major point of discussion, even with technological advances on mesh-protective layers [5, 7, 8].

The Robotic Anterior Component Technique uses the surgeon's usual anatomical expertise (onlay technique) with the manipulation and advantages of minimally invasive surgery (MIS). It maintains the precepts of reestablishment of the midline integrity and insertion of mesh in the preaponeurotic space, without contact with the viscera.

In massive hernias, additional maneuvers are necessary to achieve linea alba medialization and reestablish a functional abdominal wall with autologous tissue repair. The procedure involves dividing the relatively fixed external oblique aponeurosis, elevating the rectus abdominis muscle from its posterior rectus sheath, and then mobilizing the myofascial flap consisting of the rectus, internal oblique, and transverse abdominis medially, as described originally by Ramirez in 1990. In the classic technique, prosthetic material was not necessary (a benefit in contaminated fields), but the procedure was updated to be used in more complex abdominal wall reconstruction with the use of mesh [9].

Although this technique has been shown to be a very good option for open incisional hernia repair, it has also shown some complications due to the extensive dissection required to create the subcutaneous skin flaps. Rates of complications such as flap ischemia, infection, potential formation of hematomas, seromas, and wound infections have ranged from 25% to 57% [10].

The technique described here shows a minimally invasive way to accomplish anterior component separation while trying to minimize wound complications.

## Description of Technique

The beginning of our current approach is largely based on descriptions of robotic-assisted retromuscular repairs [6, 11]. The patient is placed supine. The bed is slightly flexed, to help increase the space between the costal margin and anterior superior iliac spine. Both arms are tucked and the abdomen is prepped as usual. Pneumoperitoneum is established according to the surgeon's preference (for example, optical access from the Palmer's point). Three robotic trocars are inserted laterally under direct visualization. We typically use the 30-degree camera, a robotic fenestrated or ProGrasp™ grasper in the non-dominant hand, and robotic monopolar scissors in the dominant hand. After lysis of adhesions is completed, we identify the medial border of the rectus sheath (Figs. 16.1, 16.2, and 16.3), and start developing the subcutaneous plane anterior to the contralateral rectus muscle (Figs. 16.4, 16.5, 16.6, and 16.7).

F. Malcher (✉)
Montefiore Medical Center, Albert Einstein College of Medicine, Bronx, NY, USA

L. T. Cavazzola
Department of Surgery, Universidade Federal do Rio Grande do Sul, Porto Alegre, Rio Grande do Sul, Brazil

General Surgery Section – Hospital de Clínicas de Porto Alegre, Porto Alegre, Rio Grande do Sul, Brazil

E. Parra-Davila
Good Samaritan Medical Center, West Palm Beach, FL, USA


O. Y. Kudsi (ed.), *Robotic Hernia Surgery*, https://doi.org/10.1007/978-3-030-46667-1_16

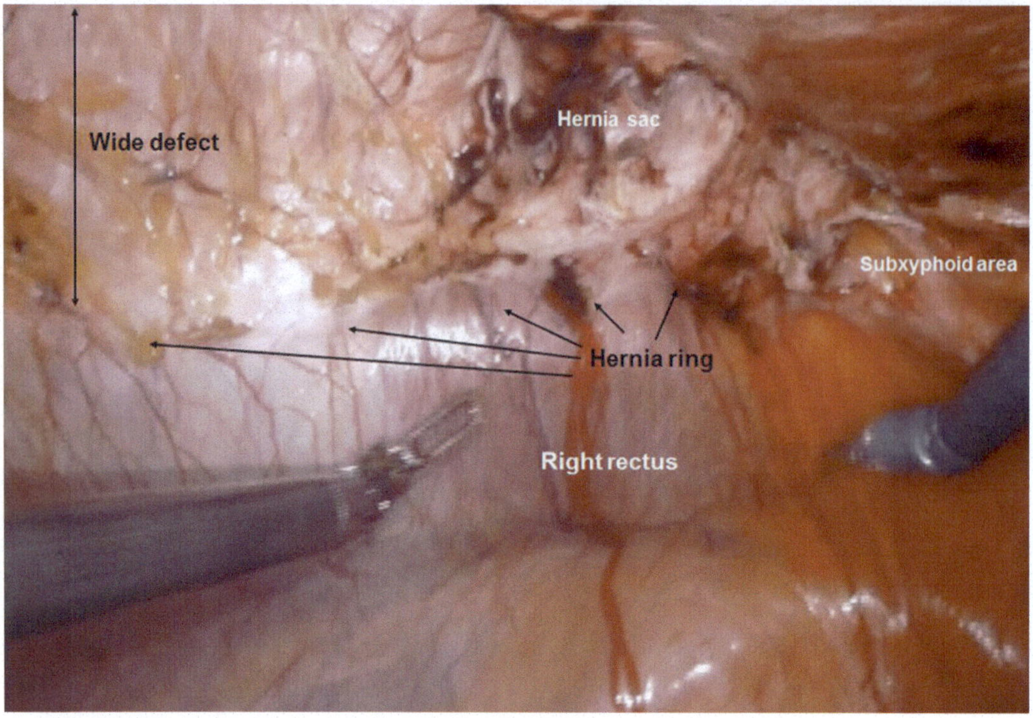


**Fig. 16.1** Initial exposure of right side hernia ring after adhesiolysis with lateral left side ports

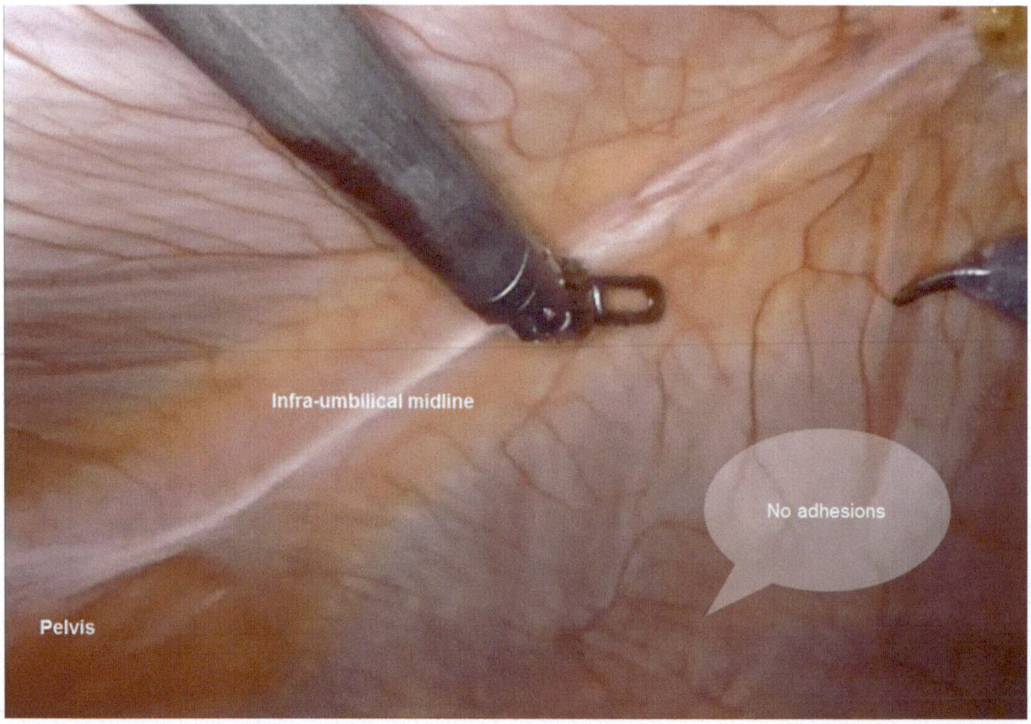


**Fig. 16.2** Adhesiolysis completed on the abdominal wall

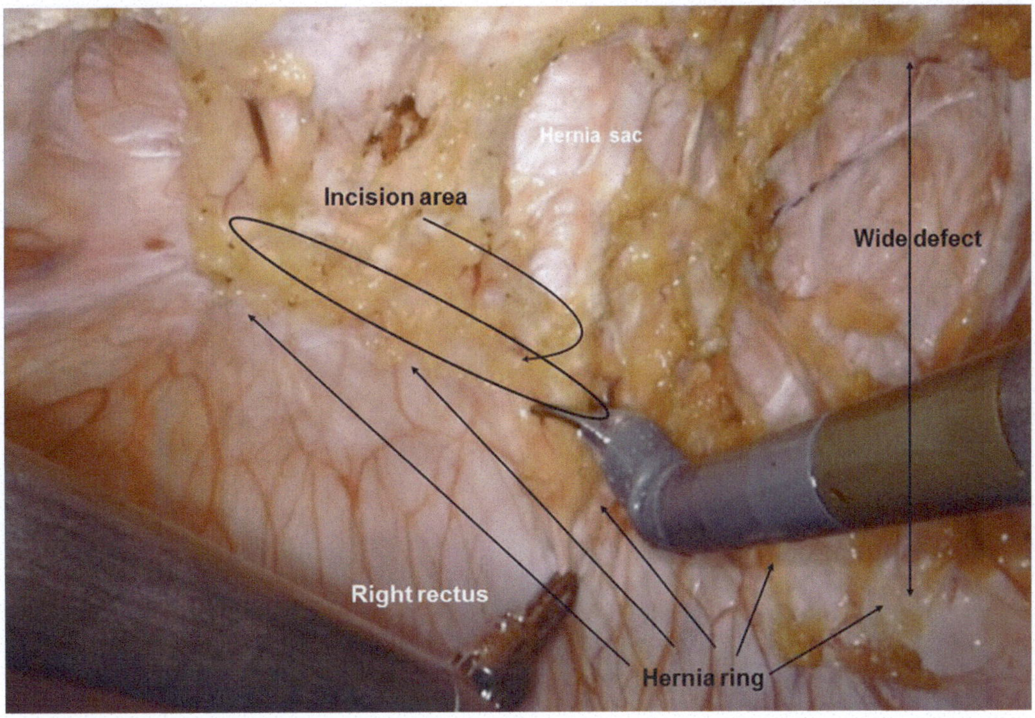


**Fig. 16.3** Incision area just at the hernia ring, on top of the fascial plane

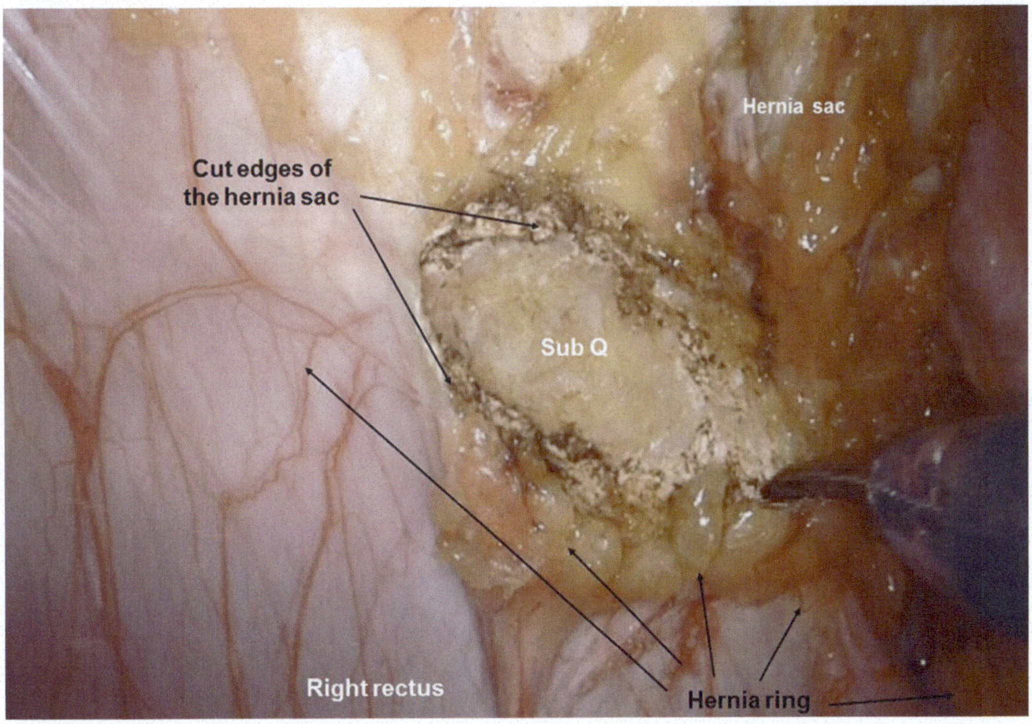


**Fig. 16.4** Initial incision on top of the hernia defect/edge. Transection of the hernia sac and exposure of the subcutaneous space

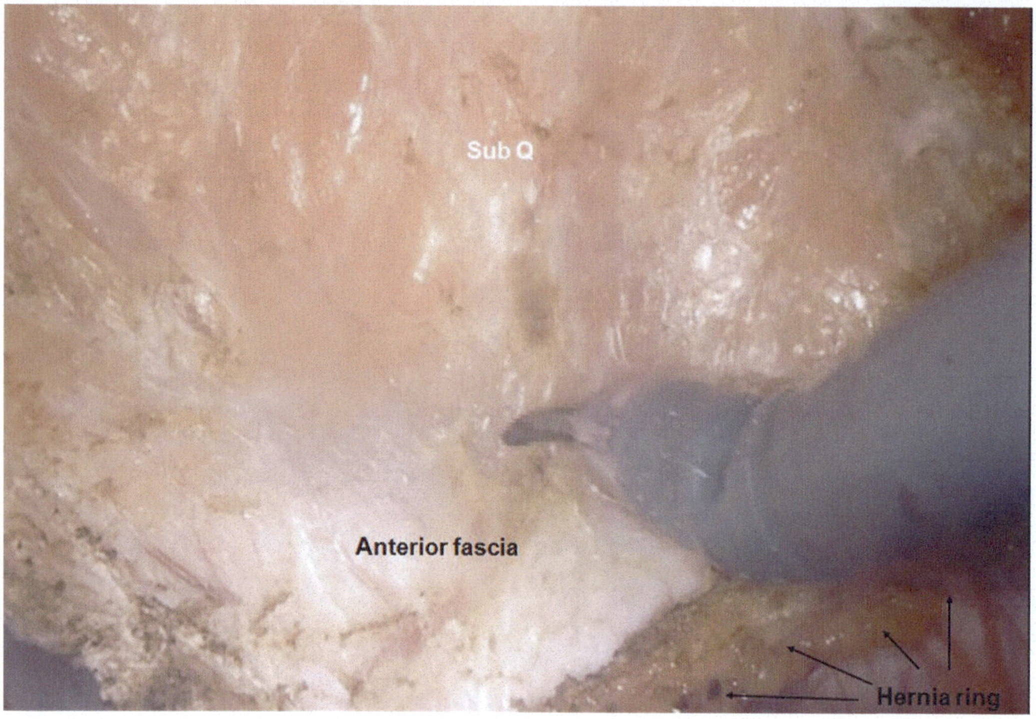


Fig. 16.5 Initial supra-aponeurotic dissection with anterior fascia below and subcutaneous plane (SubQ) on top

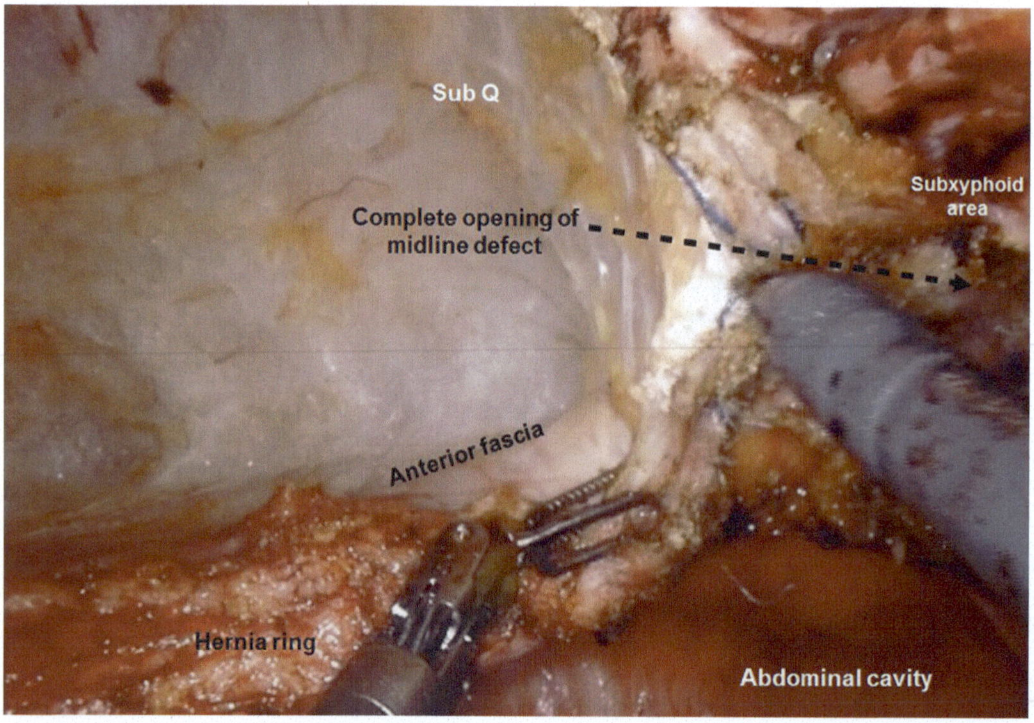


Fig. 16.6 Cephalad extension and opening of midline defect

At this point, it is important to reach the contralateral external oblique muscle, visualizing the entire anterior rectus sheath, and to be able to perform the anterior component separation (Figs. 16.8 and 16.9). A small incision is made 1–2 cm in the lateral direction of the border of the abdominal rectus (lateral to the semilunar line), in order to incise only the EOM fascia (Fig. 16.10). No fleshy muscular belly should be visualized at this time. After making

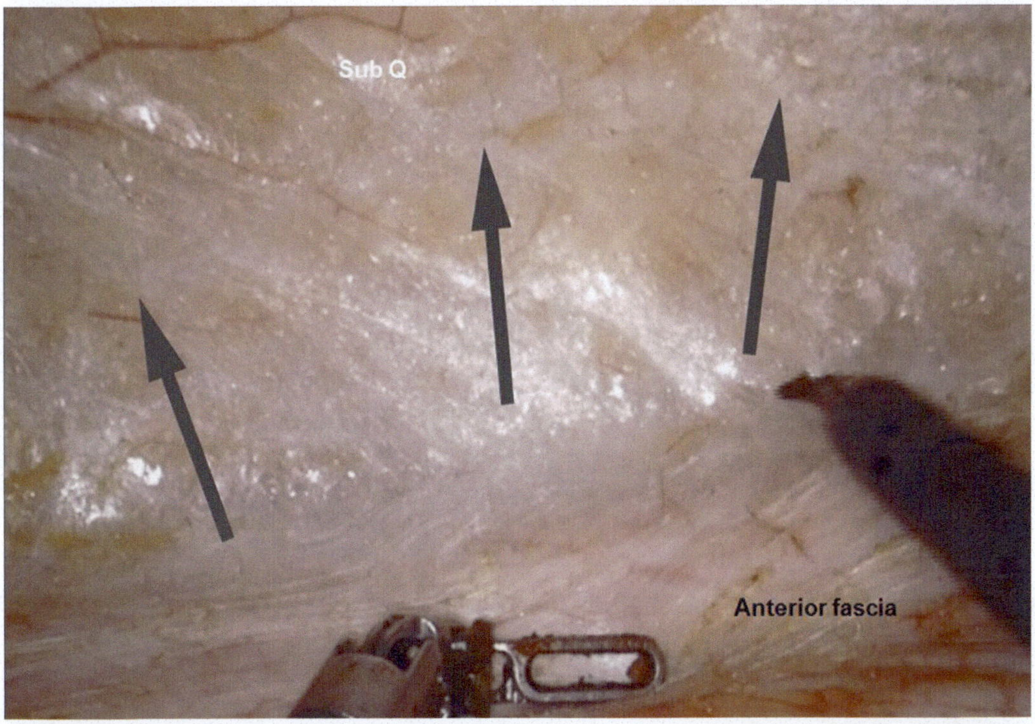


Fig. 16.7 Supra-aponeurotic dissection. Retraction from the pneumoperitoneum pressure (*bold arrows*) helps with exposure of the dissection plane

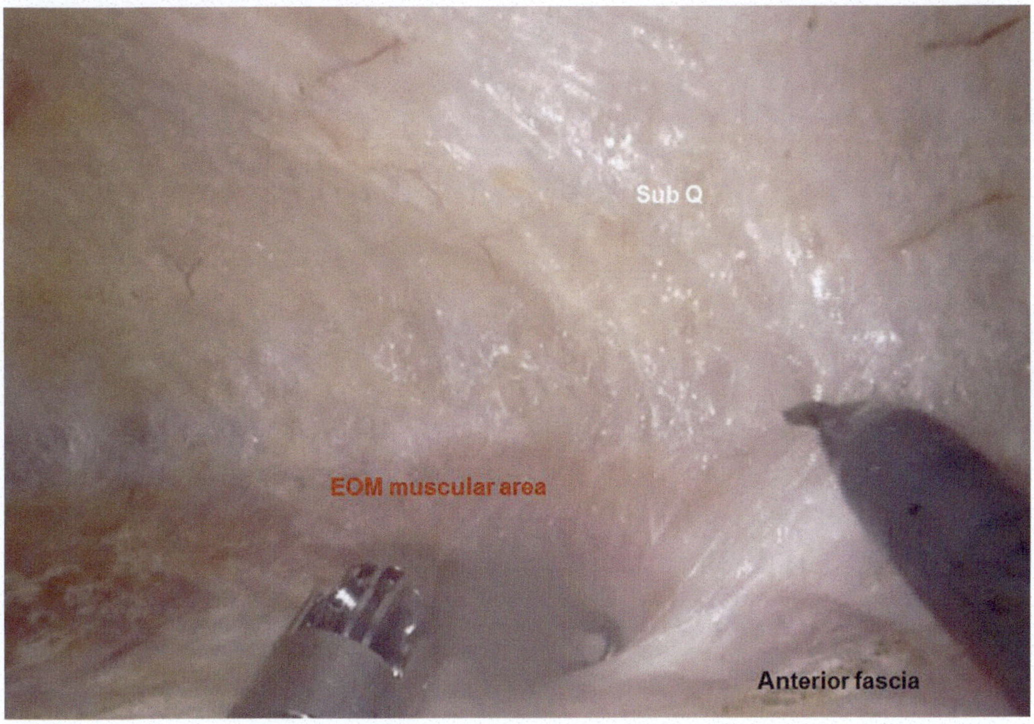


Fig. 16.8 As the dissection progresses laterally, muscular areas of the external oblique muscle (EOM) become evident

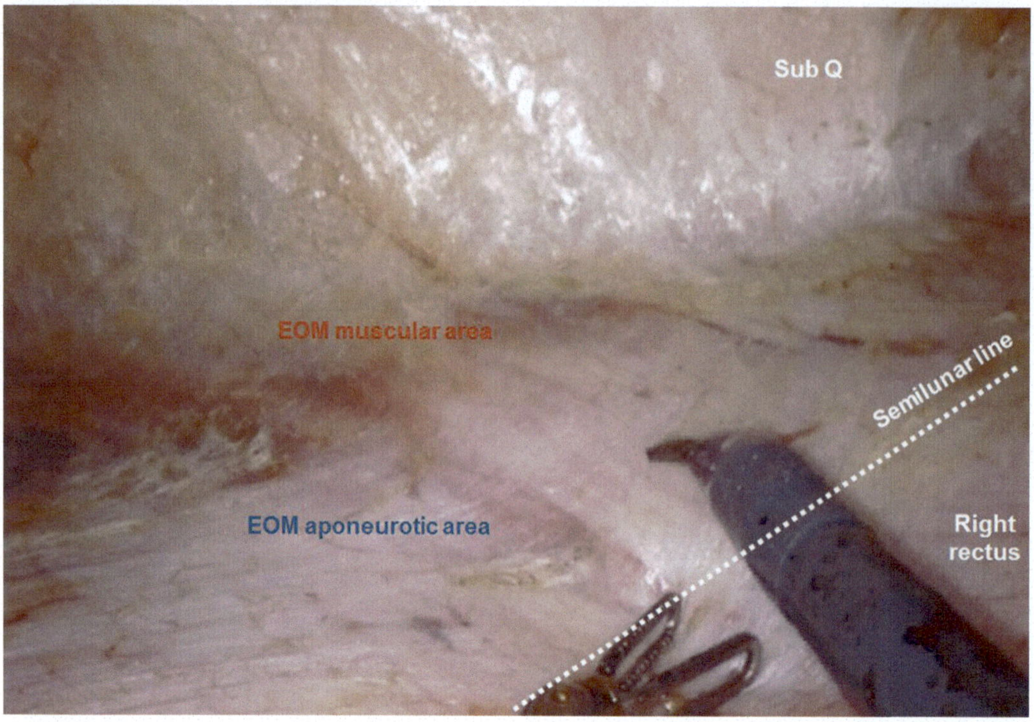


**Fig. 16.9** Once an adequate EOM muscular area is exposed, the rectus, semilunar line, and the aponeurotic extension of the EOM should be identified

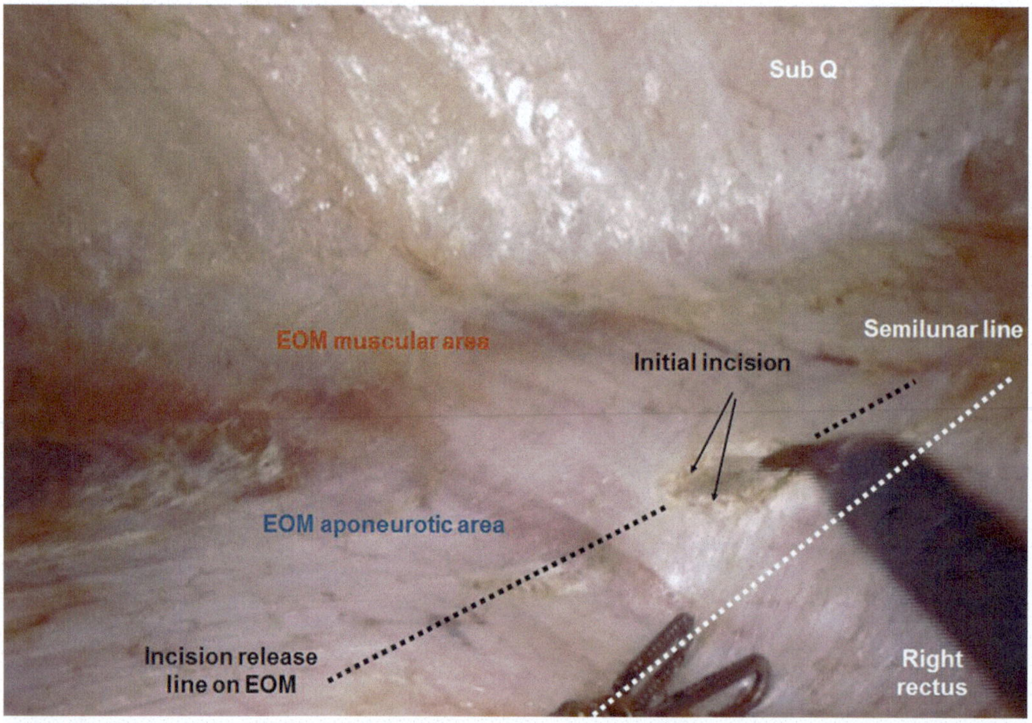


**Fig. 16.10** An initial incision of the aponeurosis of the EOM is done, lateral to the semilunar line. *Caution must be used to avoid injury to deeper planes involving the internal oblique muscle and transverse muscle*; the result could be a catastrophic injury to the full thickness of the semilunar line

sure that the internal oblique space is reached, the dissection is continued in the caudal direction to the inguinal ligament and cephalically to the costal border (Figs. 16.11 and 16.12).

Once this relaxation incision is created, the avascular interoblique plane should be freed by lateral blunt dissection in order to allow all possible sliding of the medial compartment (Figs. 16.13 and 16.14).

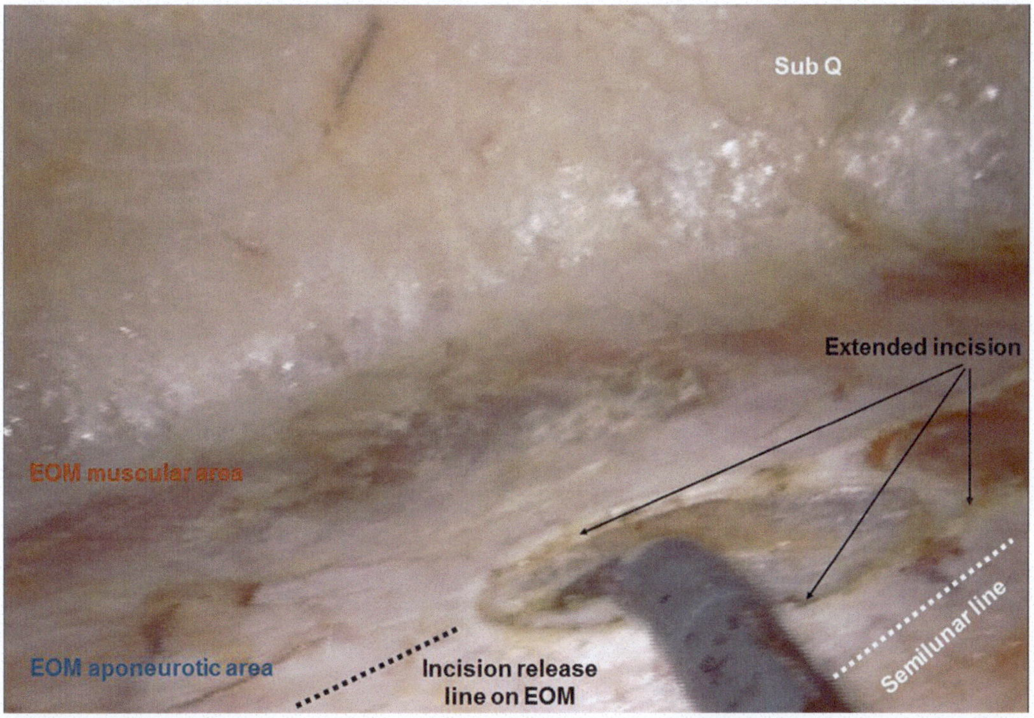


**Fig. 16.11** Caudal and cephalad progression of the incision of the aponeurosis of the EOM, parallel to the semilunar line

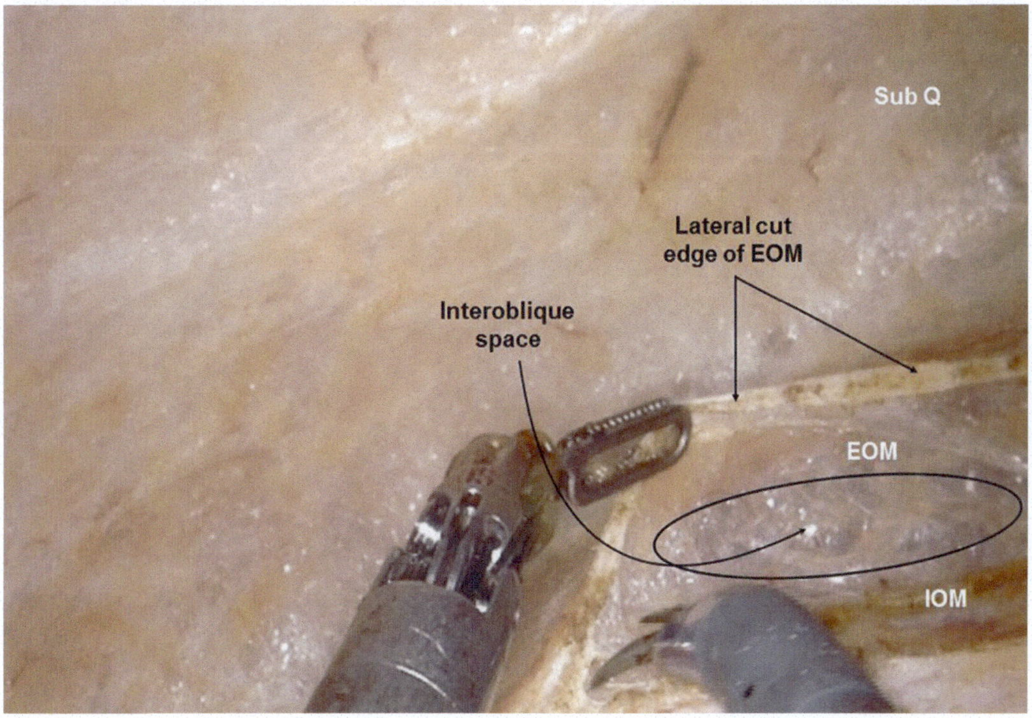


**Fig. 16.12** After the releasing incision is done, the interoblique plane MUST be opened and dissected to allow the proper component separation. IOM internal oblique muscle

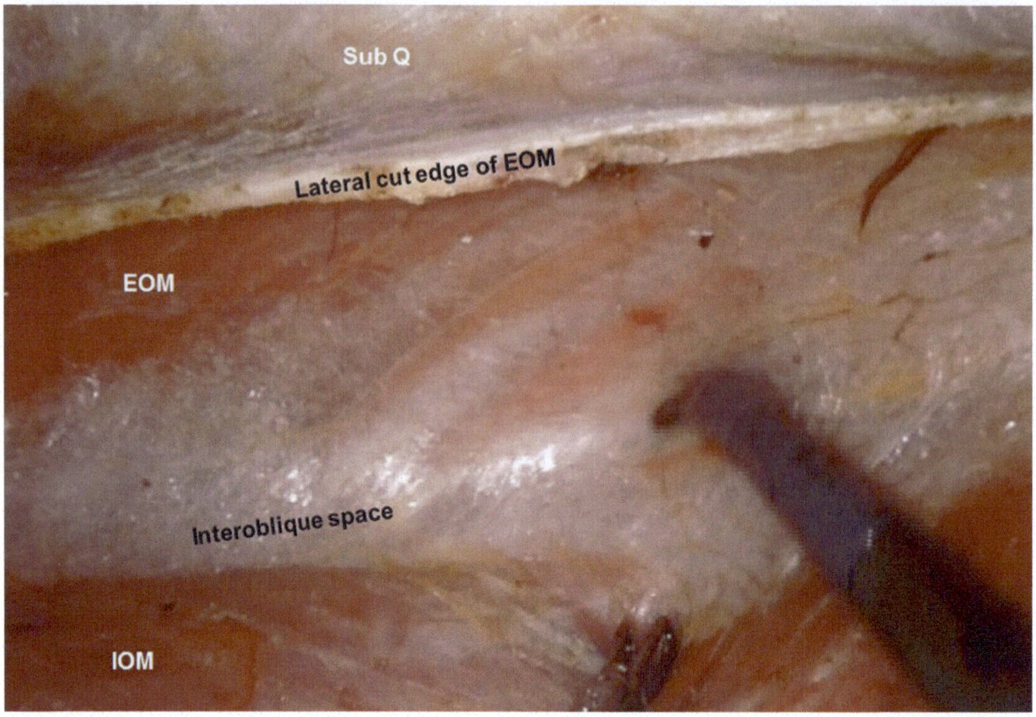


Fig. 16.13 The separation extends laterally as much as possible, to allow the medial mobilization of the midline. At this point, the different orientations of the muscle fibers of both oblique muscles can be appreciated

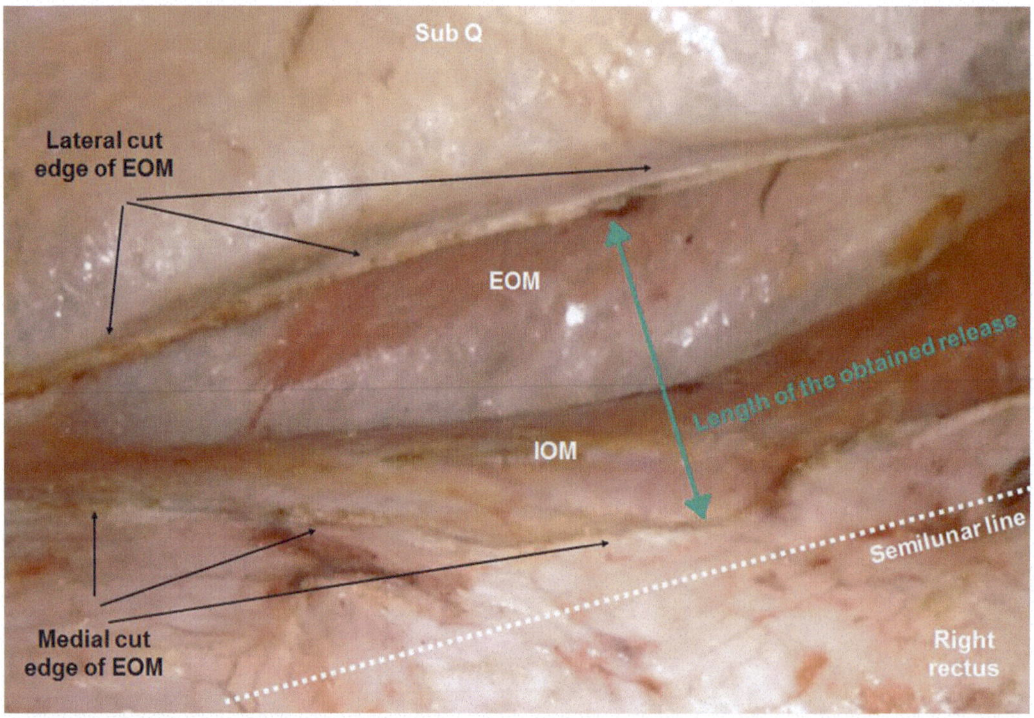


Fig. 16.14 Final aspect of the unilateral anterior component separation, with the separation of the cut edges of the EOM

Some clues that we learned from previous experience in Rives Double Docking Robotic Surgery are very important. At this point, we measure the size of the defect and the overlap that we are going to have after midline closure (Fig. 16.15).

Once this dissection is performed, lateral trocars are placed under direct vision in the contralateral side, in the subcutaneous space previously dissected (Figs. 16.16 and 16.17).

Then we insert and fixate the mesh, partially rolled, below the trocars positioned in the subcutaneous space (Fig. 16.18).

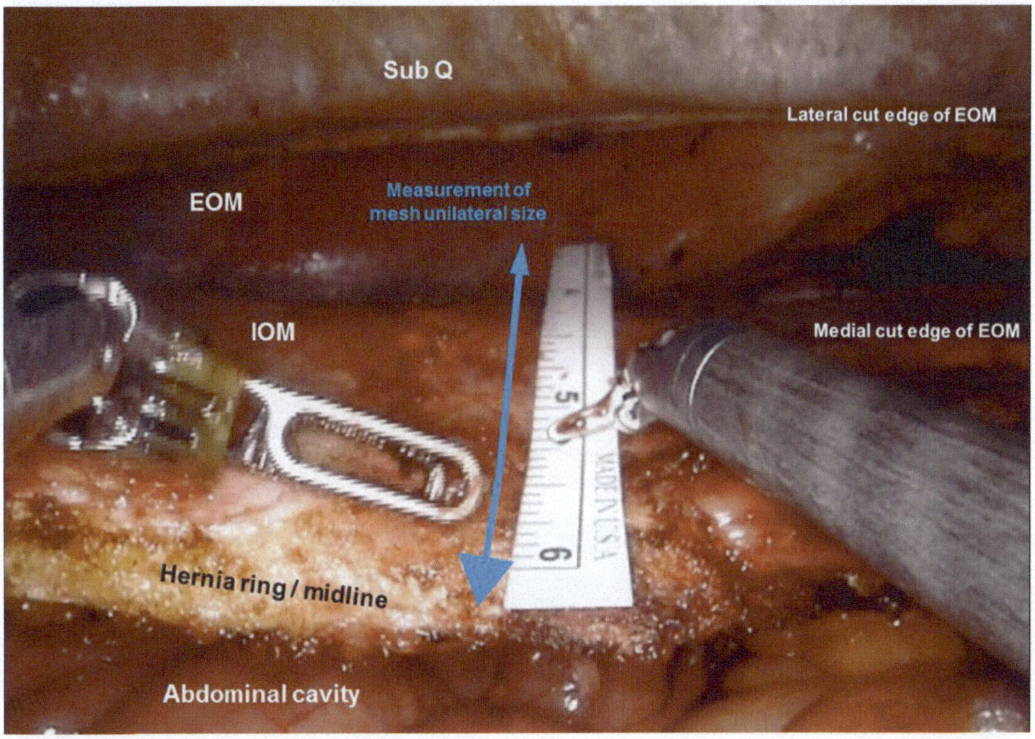


**Fig. 16.15** Measurement of the final unilateral onlay space for mesh trimming. In this case, 6 inches (15 cm) was reached, leading to a 30-cm-wide mesh trim

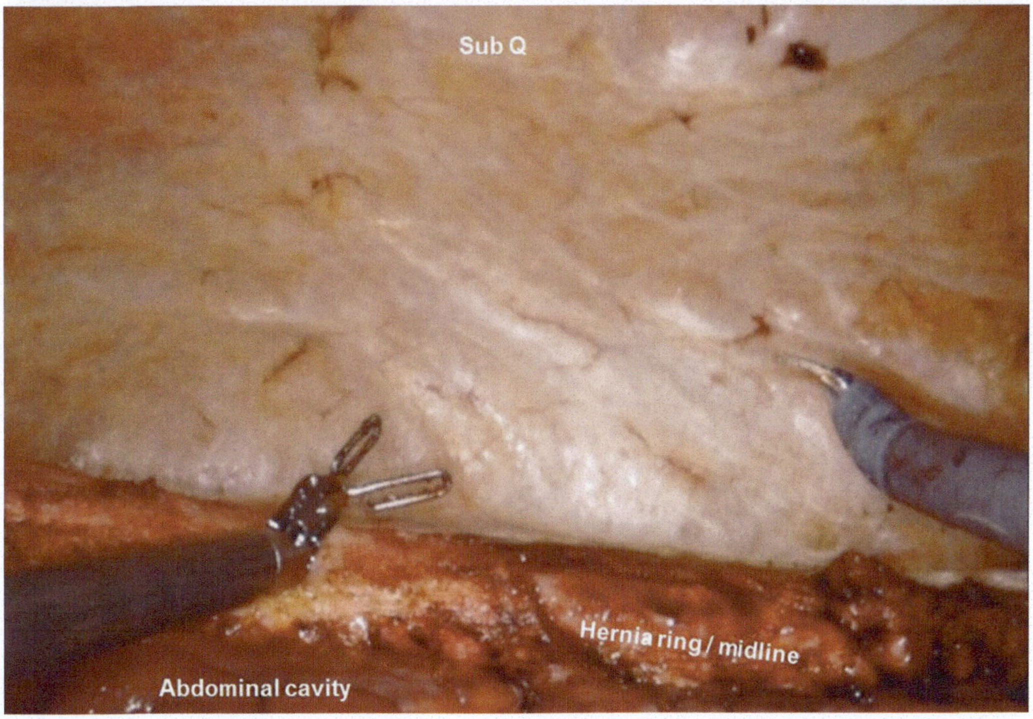


**Fig. 16.16** The camera is flipped 30° up, to allow a subcutaneous view

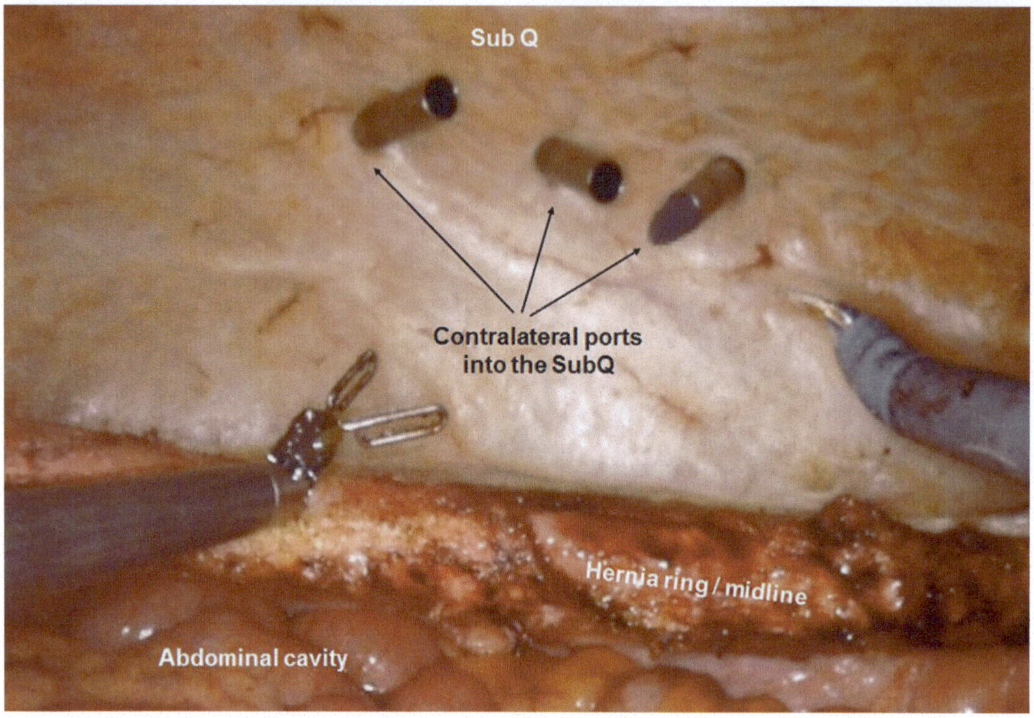


**Fig. 16.17** Insertion of three new robotics ports into the subcutaneous space at the right side

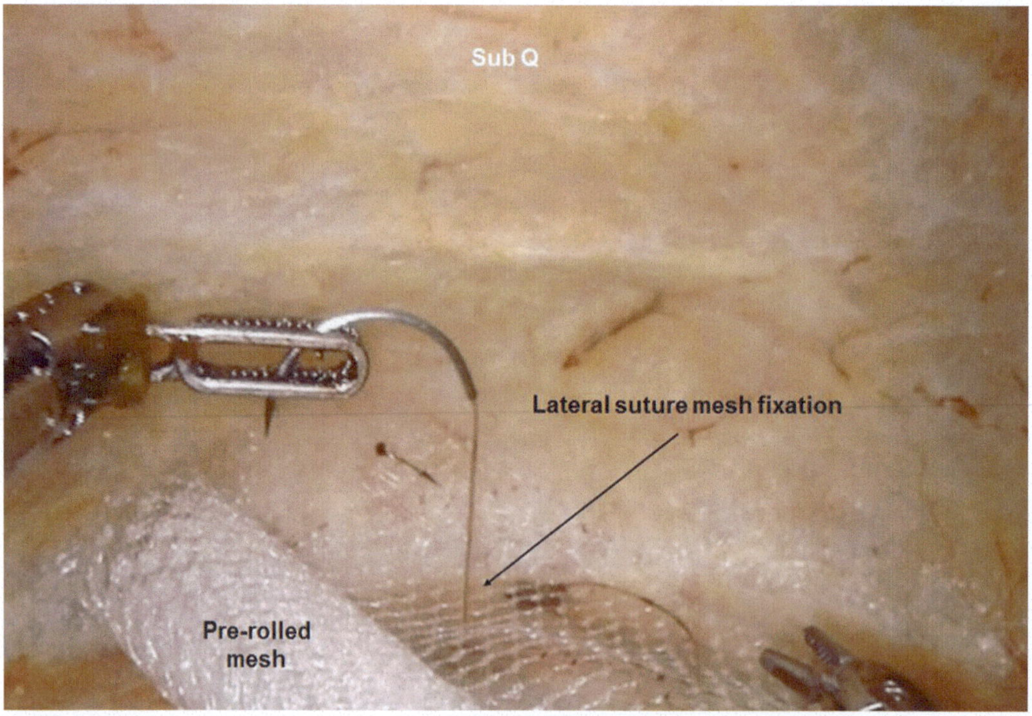


**Fig. 16.18** Mesh is rolled halfway widthwise and secured with a suture. It is inserted by a 12-mm port through the hernia defect, to be positioned and fixated over the released lateral edge of the EOM

This technique allows the mesh to be unrolled and fixated to complete the procedure (after dissection of the contralateral side) without the necessity of a third re-docking procedure [6, 11, 12].

The robot is re-docked in the opposite side (Fig. 16.19); now the dissection is carried out only in the subcutaneous space (in front of the rectus muscle) until adequate overlap is achieved (normally another 5 cm lateral to the medial rectus border), and the anterior component separation steps are repeated (Figs. 16.20, 16.21, and 16.22).

The initial trocar sites in the abdominal cavity are closed with 2-0 braided absorbable suture. Closure of the linea alba

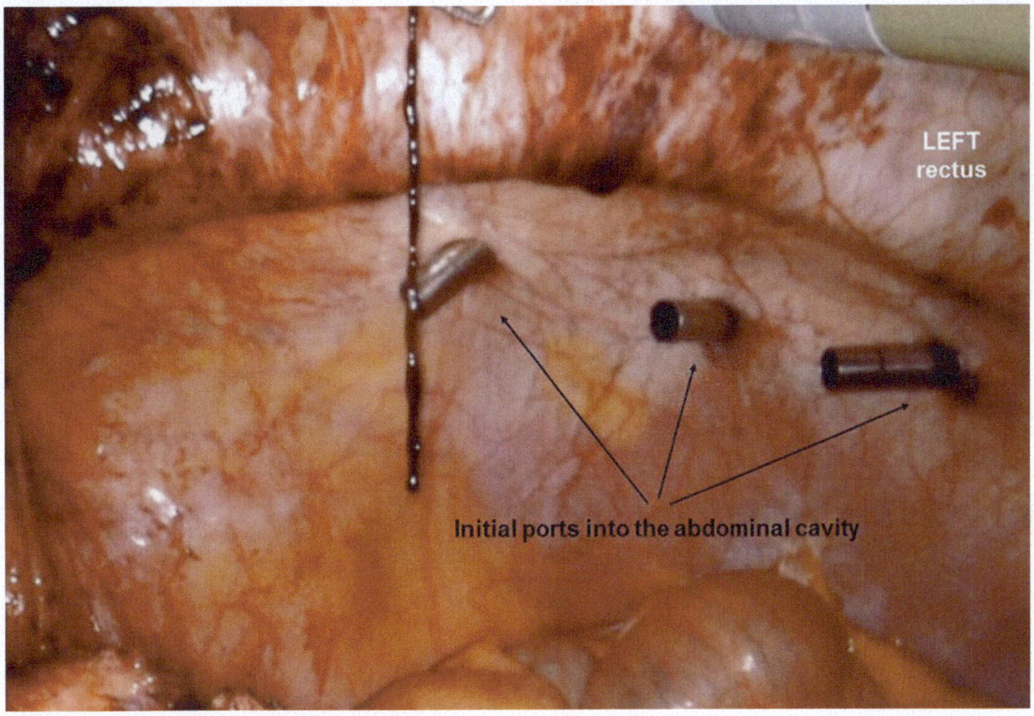


**Fig. 16.19** Initial aspect of re-docking from the patient's right side, with the view of the left side. The initial three intra-abdominal ports are visualized

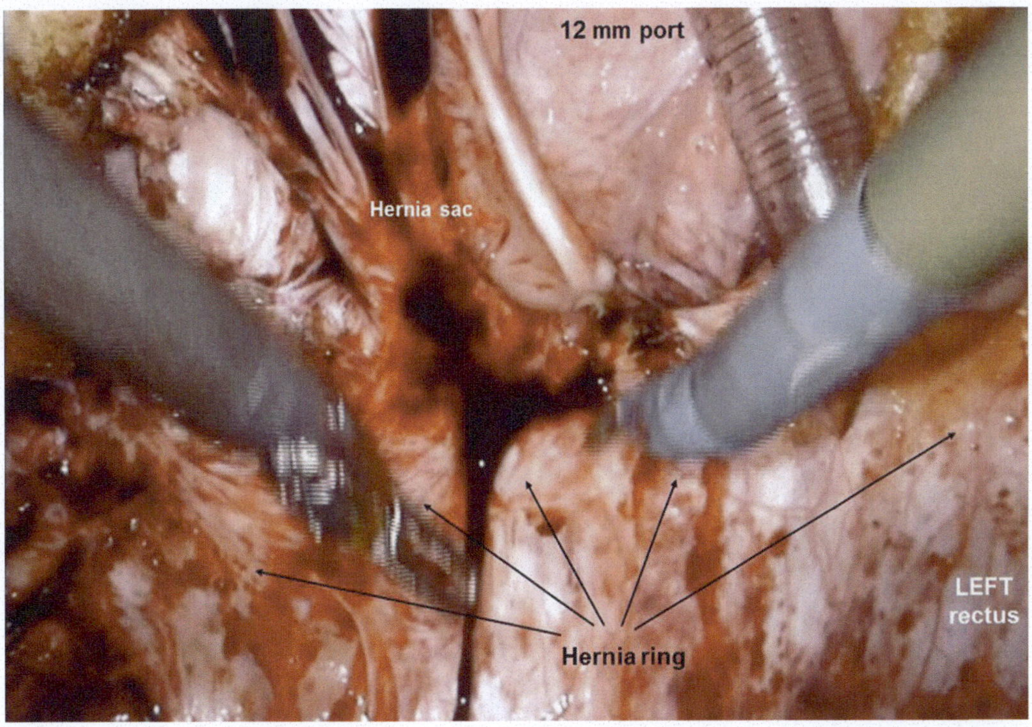


**Fig. 16.20** Identification of the left-side hernia defect edge. The 12-mm trocar can be seen coming from inside the hernia defect

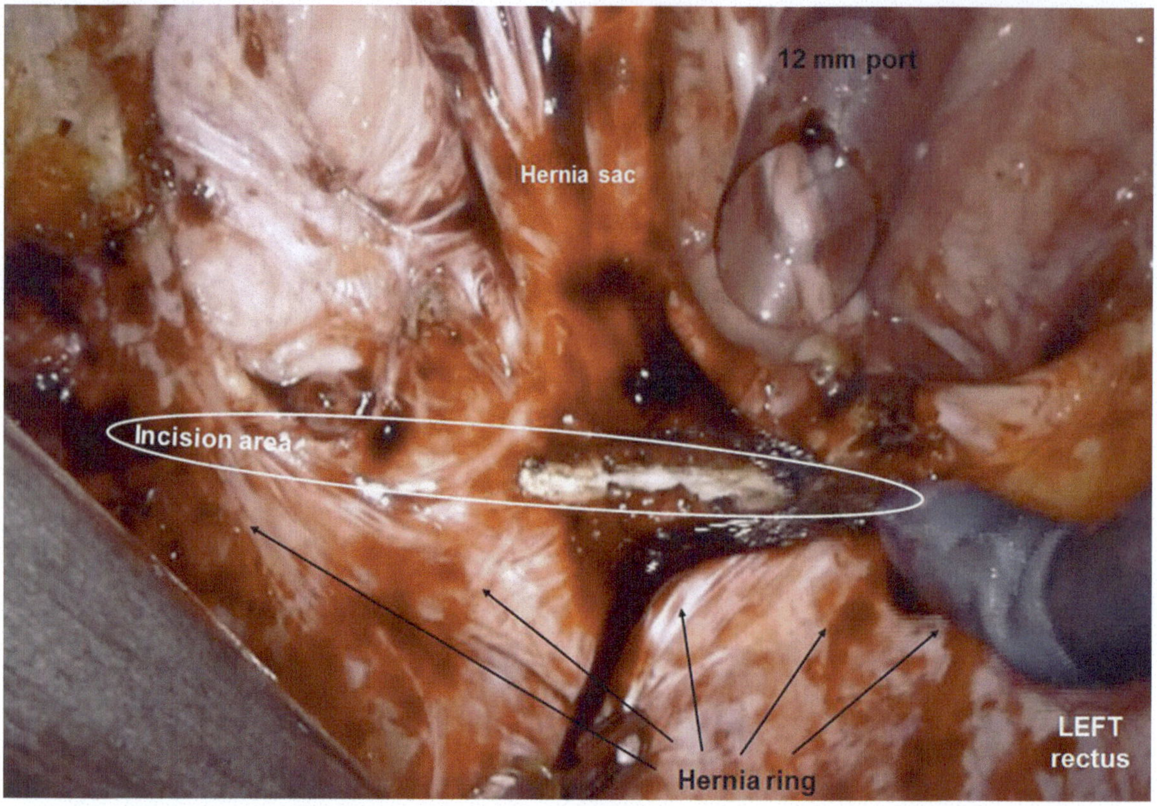


**Fig. 16.21** Initial incision on top of the hernia defect edge to access the subcutaneous space

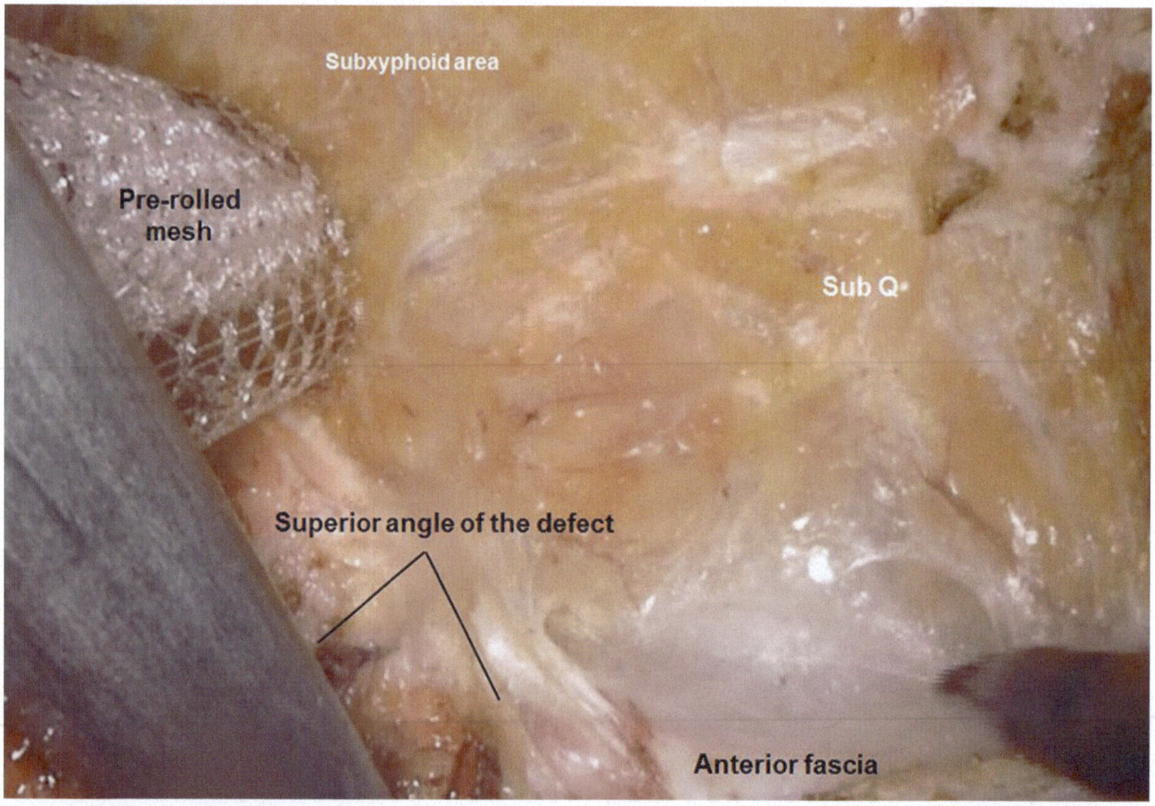


**Fig. 16.22** The same subcutaneous dissection is repeated on top of the anterior fascia. (Note the rolled edge of the mesh.) The superior and inferior angles of the midline defect are dissected to allow adequate overlap

is accomplished using a nonabsorbable #1 or #0 V-Loc™ suture in a running fashion (Figs. 16.23, 16.24, and 16.25). The mesh now can be unrolled from below the trocars and fixed on the contralateral side (Figs. 16.26, 16.27, 16.28, 16.29, and 16.30). Drains are placed under direct vision and retrieved in the lowest trocar position (Figs. 16.31 and 16.32). Skin incisions are closed with interrupted 4-0 monofilament absorbable suture.

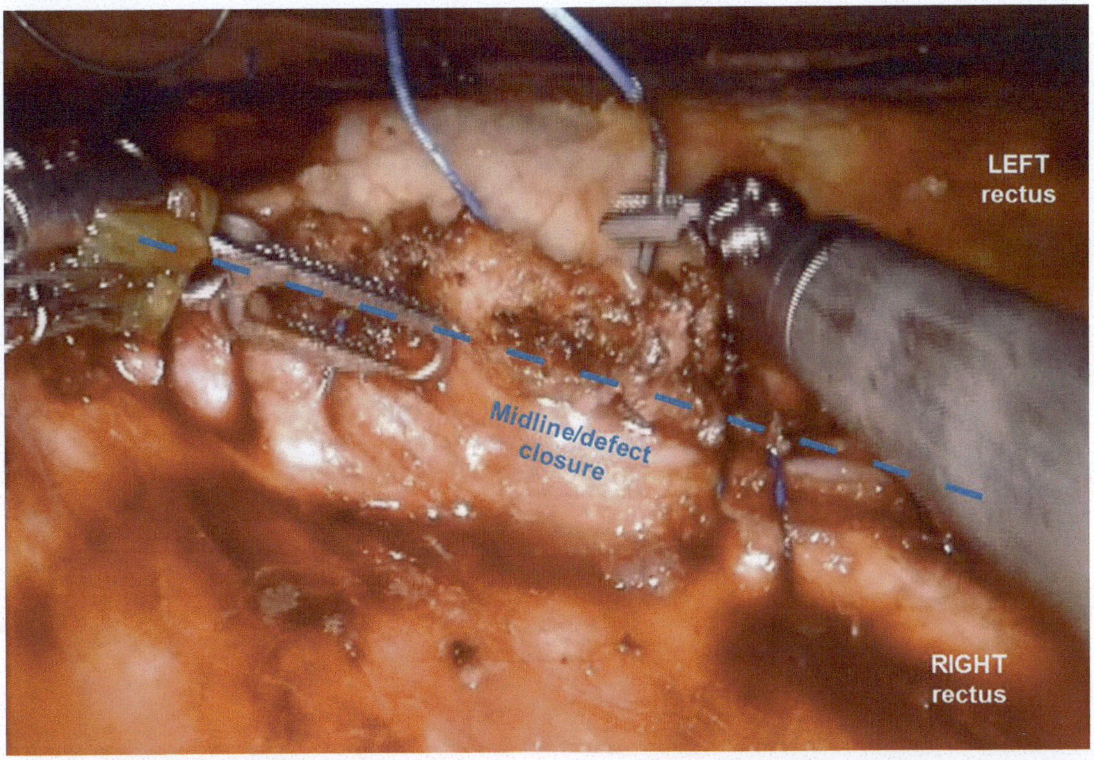


**Fig. 16.23** After the same steps of the anterior compartment separation (ACS) are repeated, the midline is closed with a running barbed suture. This suture is performed at the "floor" of the operative field, not in the "roof," as in preperitoneal and retromuscular approaches

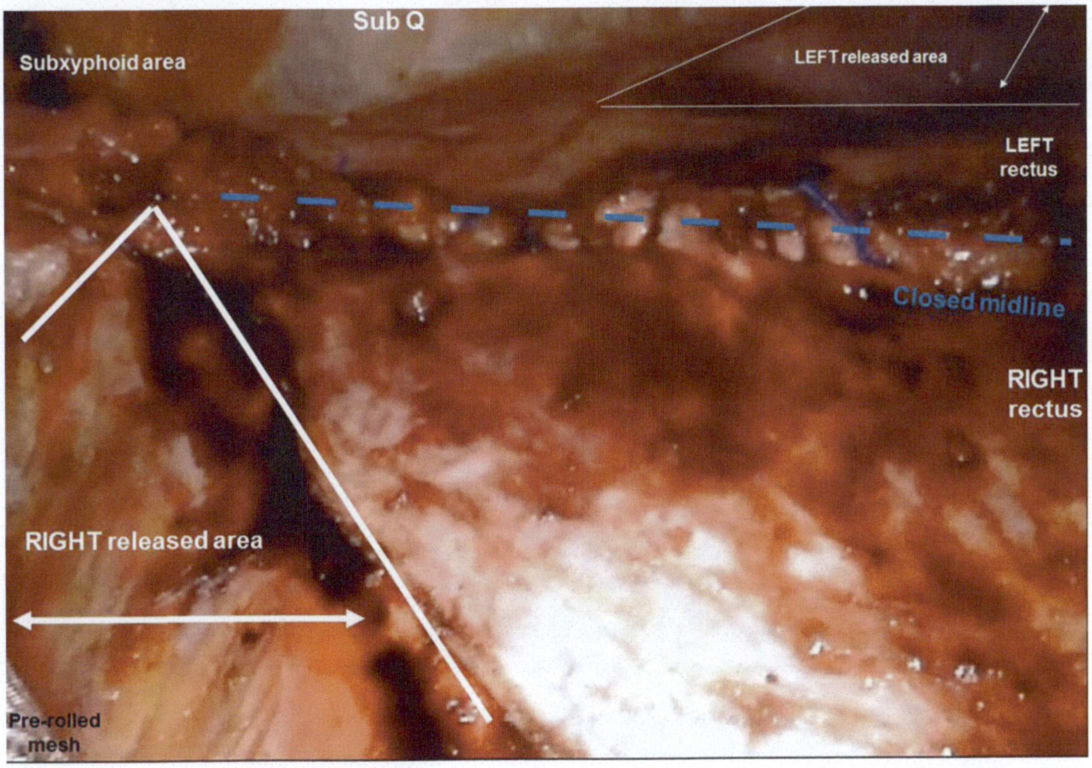


**Fig. 16.24** Final aspect of the closed midline. Both sides of the ACS can be appreciated

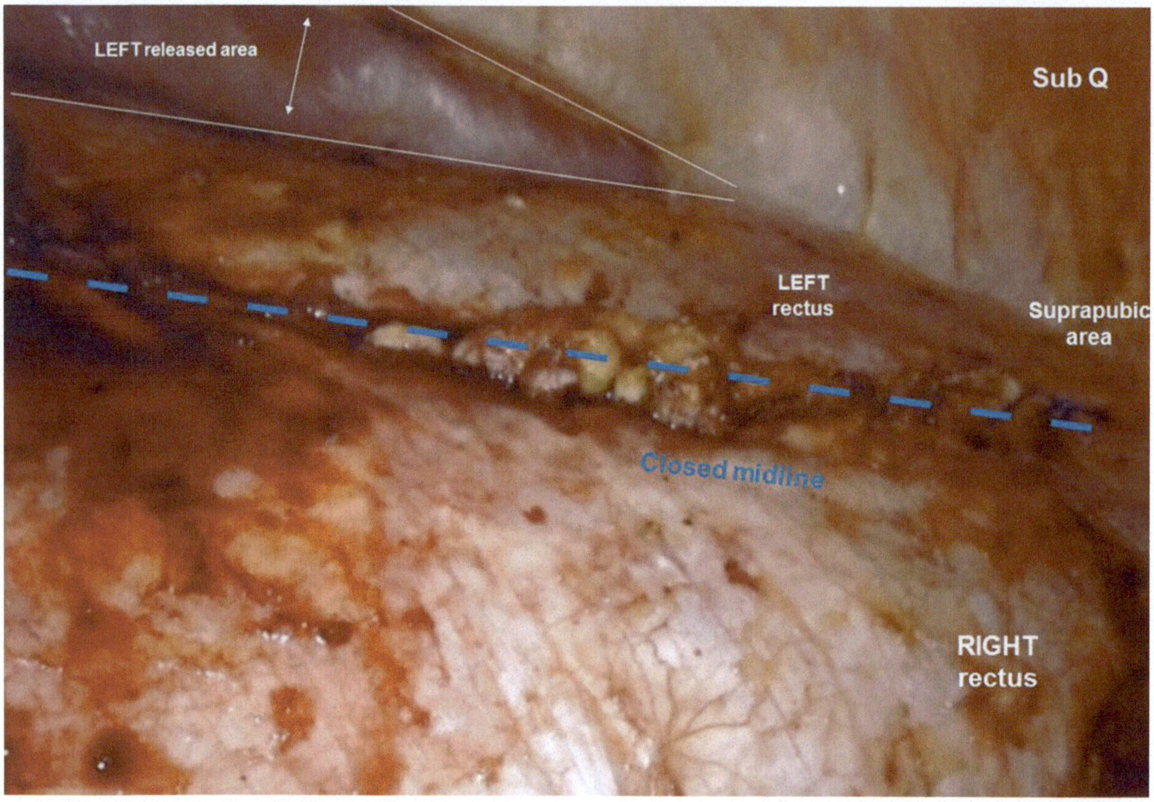


**Fig. 16.25** Caudal view of the closed midline

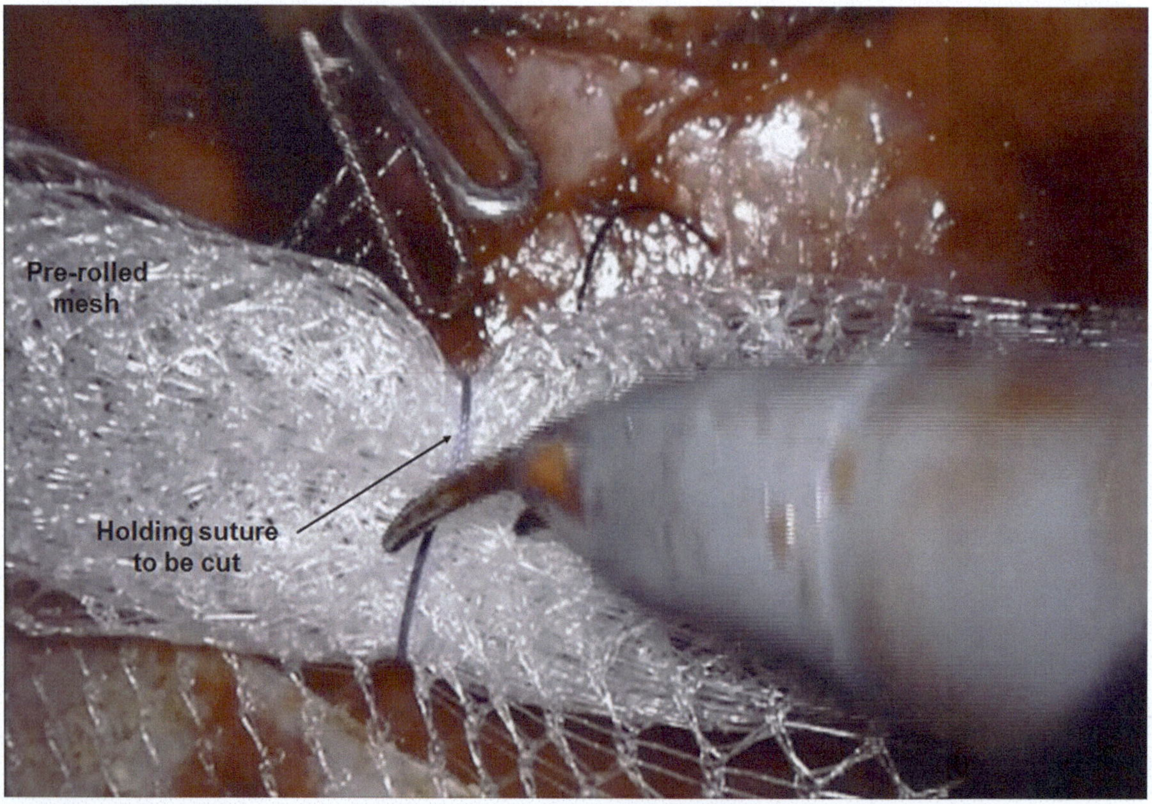


**Fig. 16.26** The suture that held the mesh rolled is cut to allow its opening

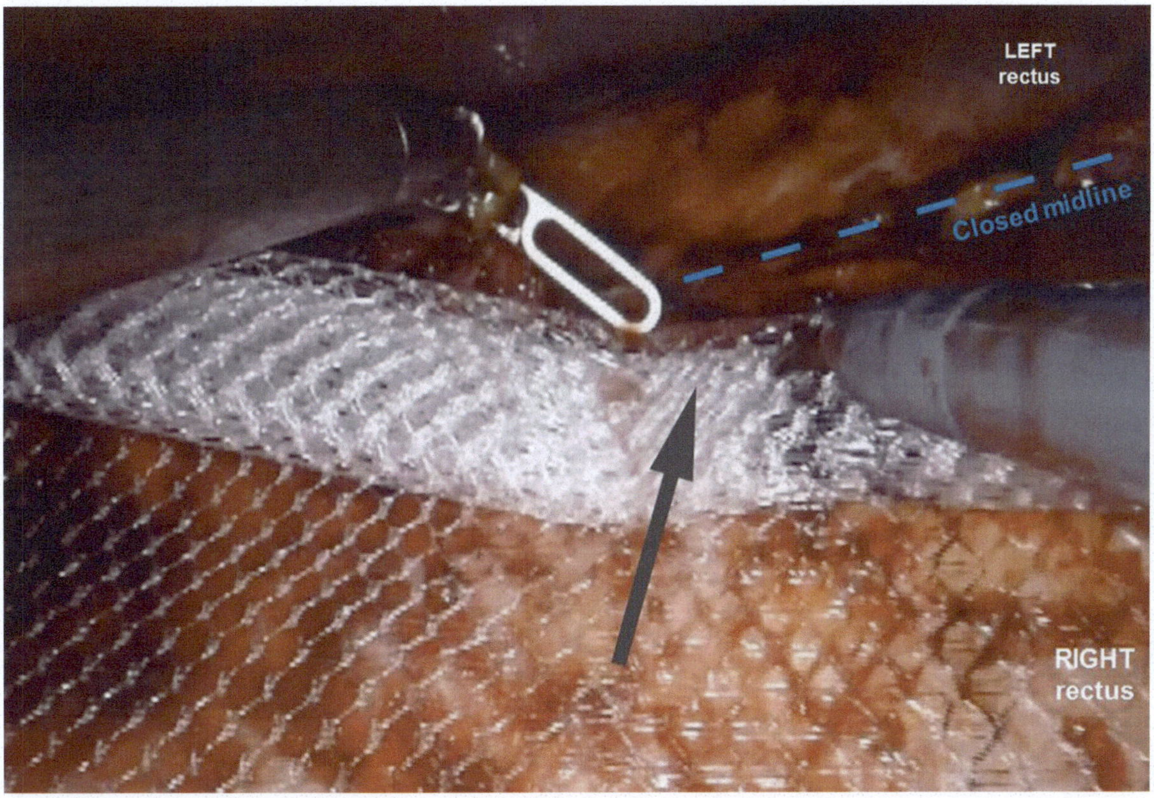


**Fig. 16.27** The mesh is unrolled in a lateral direction (*arrow*) to cover the entire supra-aponeurotic space

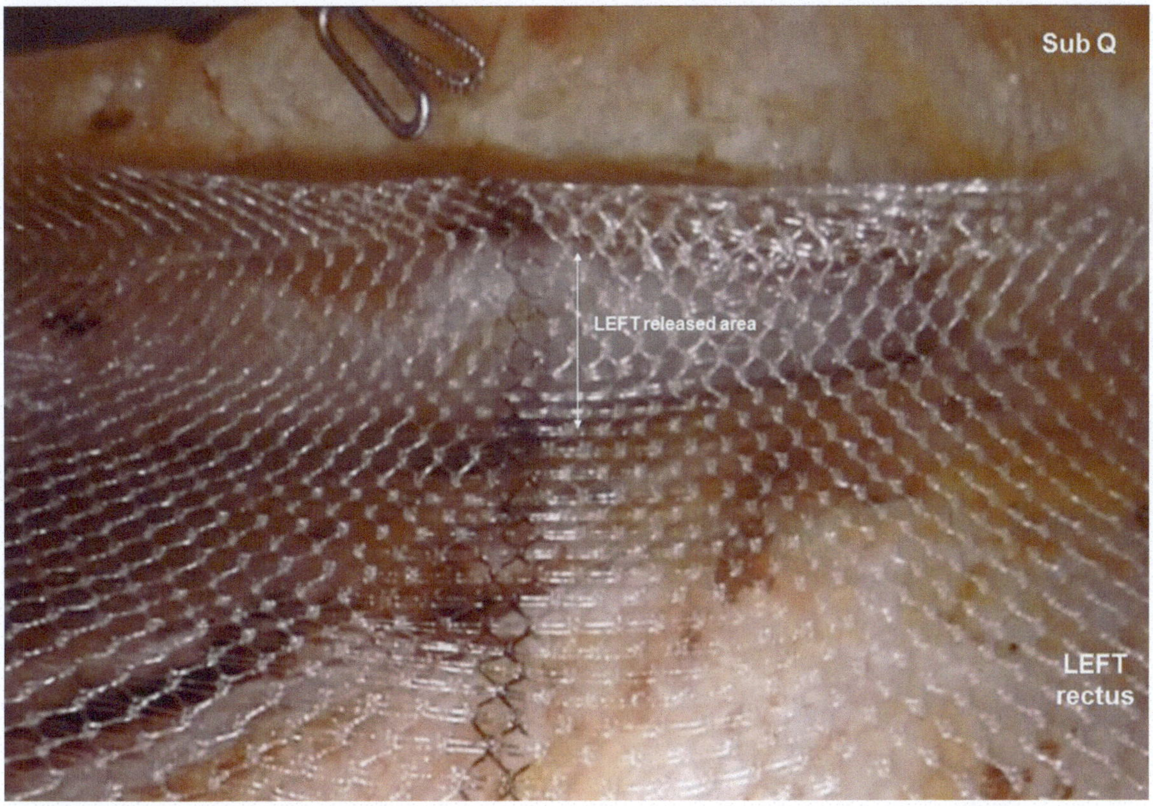


**Fig. 16.28** Once completely opened, the mesh should cover the midline and both released areas to prevent bulges

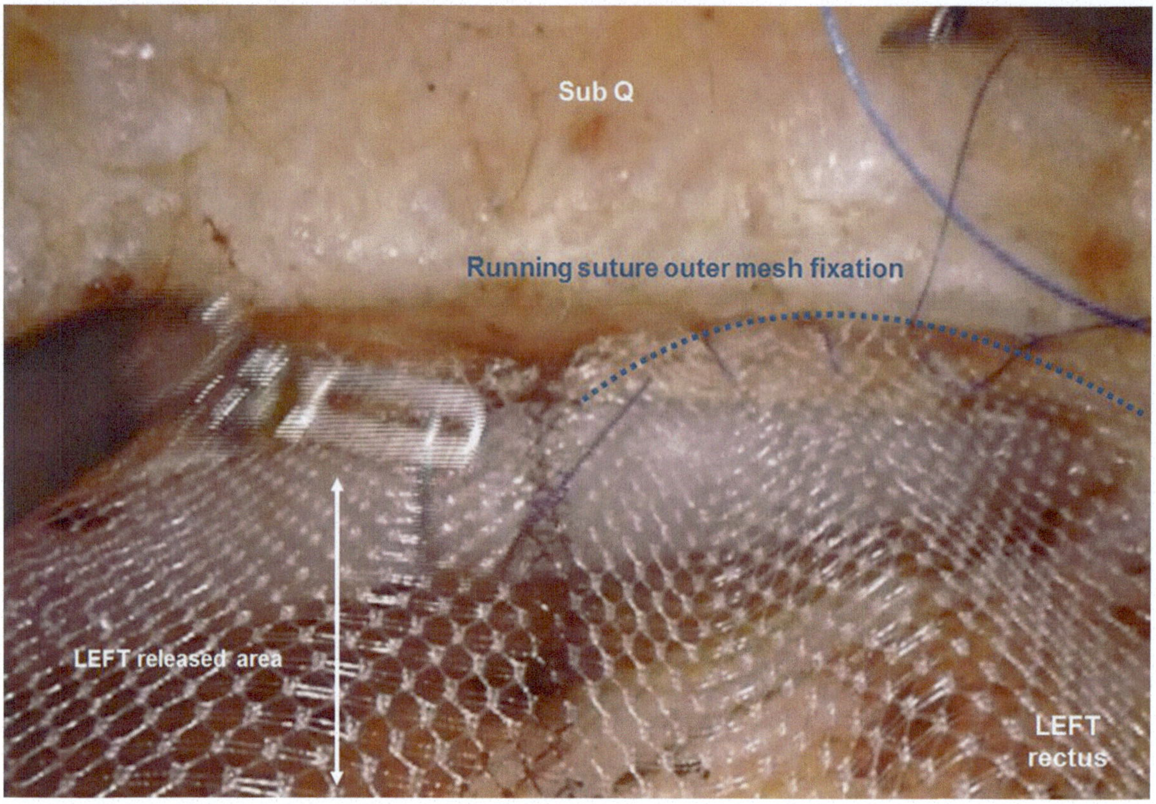


**Fig. 16.29** The mesh is fixed on its outer perimeter with interrupted or running sutures

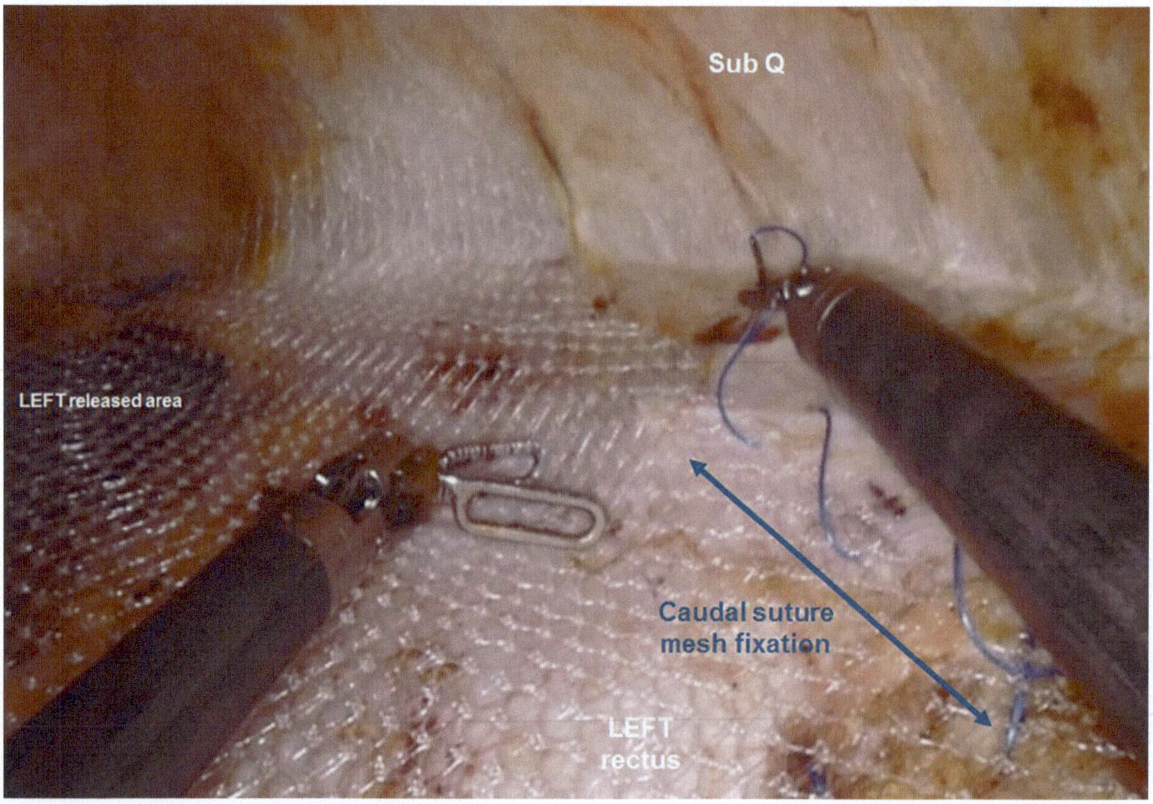


**Fig. 16.30** Suture fixation is performed all around the mesh edges

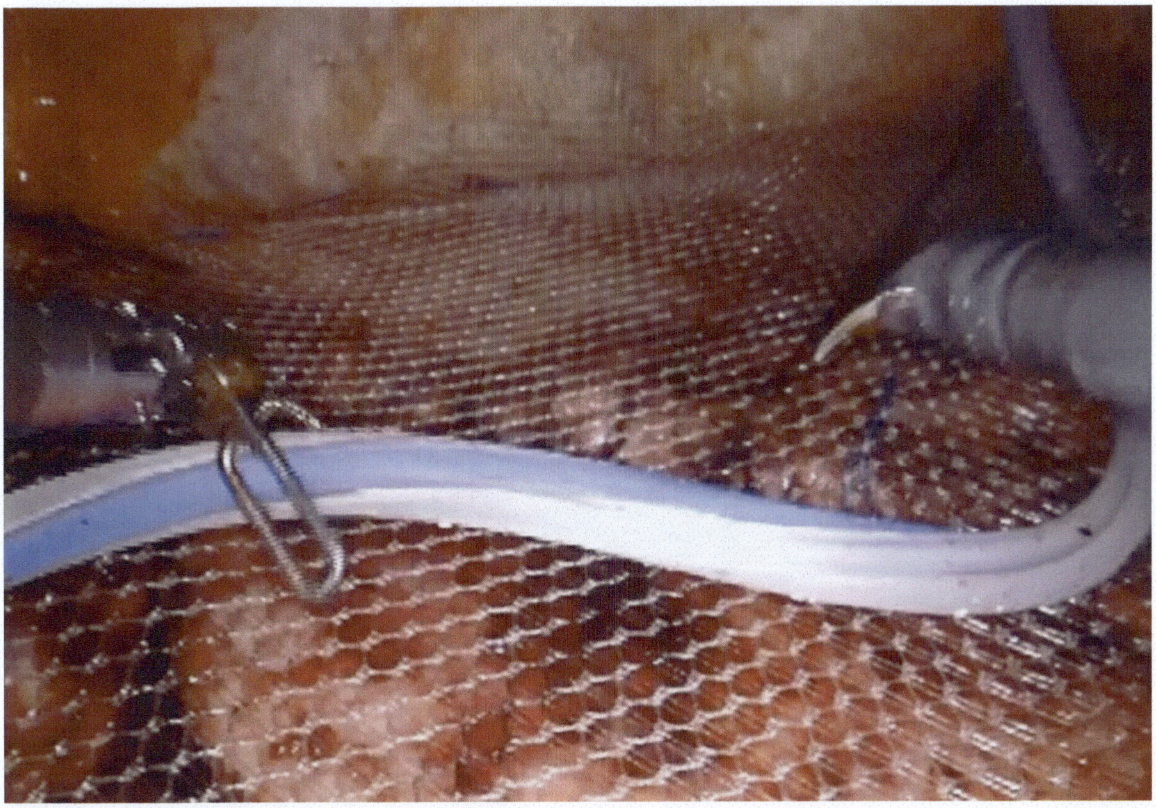

**Fig. 16.31** Suction-closed drains are positioned to avoid seroma formation after creation of the subcutaneous flaps

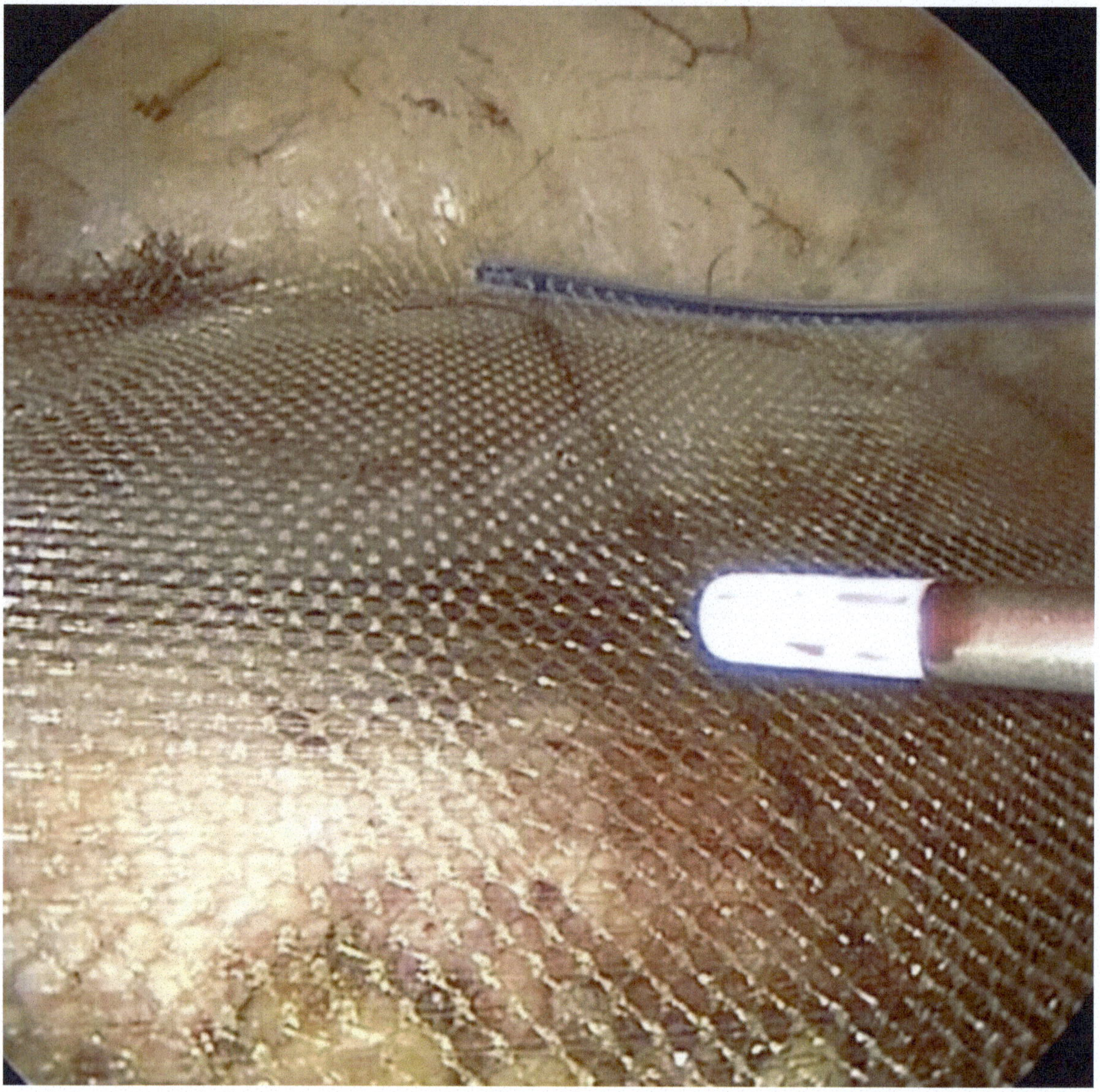

**Fig. 16.32** Laparoscopic view of additional fixation with application of fibrin glue to allow early integration of the mesh

## Conclusion

Robotic Anterior Component Separation is a novel concept derived from a mixed approach that includes open hernia repair characteristics and a robotic-assisted platform [6]. The idea is that this technique will allow the "regular surgeon" who is not a hernia specialist to be able to offer minimally invasive abdominal wall surgery, in a space that is already familiar, without any changes in the regular procedure other than the use of the robot [13, 14]. It will also allow the closure of the hernia defect and restoration of the linea alba, which is very challenging by traditional laparoscopy, and will prevent the mesh from being in contact with the abdominal viscera. This new approach may change the idea that minimally invasive abdominal wall surgery requires specific and tedious training. It should help to standardize ventral hernia repair by robotic surgery and facilitate training, allowing more surgeons to perform minimally invasive abdominal wall surgery. Clinical studies are needed to measure the impact and long-term results of the implementation of robotic onlay approaches in minimally invasive ventral hernia repair.

## References


1. Haskins IN, Voeller GR, Stoikes NF, Webb DL, Chandler RG, Phillips S, et al. Onlay with adhesive use compared with sublay mesh placement in ventral hernia repair: was Chevrel right? An Americas hernia society quality collaborative analysis. J Am Coll Surg. 2017;224:962–70. https://doi.org/10.1016/j.jamcollsurg.2017.01.048.
2. Muysoms FE, Miserez M, Berrevoet F, Campanelli G, Champault GG, Chelala E, Kingsnorth A. Classification of primary and incisional abdominal wall hernias. Hernia. 2009;13:407–14. https://doi.org/10.1007/s10029-009-0518-x.
3. Demetrashvili Z, Pipia I, Loladze D, Metreveli T, Ekaladze E, Kenchadze G, Khutsishvili K. Open retromuscular mesh repair versus onlay technique of incisional hernia: a randomized controlled trial. Int J Surg. 2017;37:65–70. https://doi.org/10.1016/j.ijsu.2016.12.008.
4. Holihan JL, Hannon C, Goodenough C, Flores-Gonzalez JR, Itani KM, Olavarria O, et al. Ventral hernia repair: a meta-analysis of randomized controlled trials. Surg Infect (Larchmt). 2017;18:647–58. https://doi.org/10.1089/sur.2017.029.
5. Liang MK, Holihan JL, Itani K, Alawadi ZM, Gonzalez JR, Askenasy EP, et al. Ventral hernia management: expert consensus guided by systematic review. Ann Surg. 2017;265:80–9. https://doi.org/10.1097/SLA.0000000000001701.
6. de Oliveira FM, Cavazzola LT, Weltz AS, Belyansky I. Ventral abdominal hernia repair: MIS extraperitoneal repair techniques: eTEP rives, MILOS/EMILOS, and onlay MIS repair. In: Davis Jr S, Dakin G, Bates A, editors. The SAGES manual of hernia surgery. Cham: Springer; 2019. p. 271–90. https://doi.org/10.1007/978-3-319-78411-3_20.
7. Carter SA, Hicks SC, Brahmbhatt R, Liang MK. Recurrence and pseudorecurrence after laparoscopic ventral hernia repair: predictors and patient-focused outcomes. Am Surg. 2014;80:138–48.
8. Nguyen DH, Nguyen MT, Askenasy EP, Kao LS, Liang MK. Primary fascial closure with laparoscopic ventral hernia repair: systematic review. World J Surg. 2014;38:3097–104. https://doi.org/10.1007/s00268-014-2722-9.
9. Malcher F, Cavazzola LT. Component separation of abdominal wall muscles. In: LeBlanc K, Kingsnorth A, Sanders D, editors. Management of abdominal hernias. Cham: Springer; 2018. p. 381–6. https://doi.org/10.1007/978-3-319-63251-3_26.
10. Switzer NJ, Dykstra MA, Gill RS, Lim S, Lester E, de Gara C, et al. Endoscopic versus open component separation: systematic review and meta-analysis. Surg Endosc. 2015;29:787–95.
11. Ballecer C, Parra-Davila E. Robotic ventral hernia repair. In: Novitsky YW, editor. Hernia surgery—current principles. Cham: Springer; 2016. p. 273–86.
12. Martin-Del-Campo LA, Weltz AS, Belyansky I, Novitsky YW. Comparative analysis of perioperative outcomes of robotic versus open transversus abdominis release. Surg Endosc. 2018;32:840–5. https://doi.org/10.1007/s00464-017-5752-1.
13. Carbonell AM, Warren JA, Prabhu AS, Ballecer CD, Janczyk RJ, Herrera J, et al. Reducing length of stay using a robotic-assisted approach for retromuscular ventral hernia repair: a comparative analysis from the Americas Hernia Society Quality Collaborative. Ann Surg. 2018;267:210–7. https://doi.org/10.1097/SLA.0000000000002244.
14. Gonzalez A, Escobar E, Romero R, Walker G, Mejias J, Gallas M, et al. Robotic-assisted ventral hernia repair: a multicenter evaluation of clinical outcomes. Surg Endosc. 2017;31:1342–9. https://doi.org/10.1007/s00464-016-5118-0.

# Index




O. Y. Kudsi (ed.), *Robotic Hernia Surgery*, https://doi.org/10.1007/978-3-030-46667-1

**U**



**V**

The manufacturer's authorised representative in the EU is Springer
Nature Customer Service Centre GmbH, Europaplatz 3, 69115 Heidelberg,
Germany. If you have any concerns regarding our products, please
contact ProductSafety@springernature.com

Printed and bound by CPI Group (UK) Ltd, Croydon, CR0 4YY
09/04/2026
02086936-0006